SALEM HEALTH
WOMEN'S HEALTH

SALEM HEALTH

WOMEN'S HEALTH

Volume 2

Human immunodeficiency virus (HIV) – Yoga

Edited by

Michael A. Buratovich, PhD

SALEM PRESS
A Division of EBSCO Information Services, Inc.
Ipswich, Massachusetts

GREY HOUSE PUBLISHING

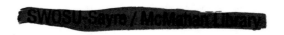

Publisher's Cataloging-In-Publication Data
(Prepared by The Donohue Group, Inc.)

Names: Buratovich, Michael A., editor.
Title: Women's health / editor, Michael A. Buratovich.
Other Titles: Salem health (Pasadena, Calif.)
Description: [First edition]. | Ipswich, Massachusetts : Salem Press, a division of EBSCO Information Services, Inc.; Amenia, NY : Grey House Publishing, [2019] | Includes bibliographical references and index.
  | Contents: Volume 1. Abdomen - Hormones – Volume 2. HIV - Yoga.
Identifiers: ISBN 9781642650464 (set) | ISBN 9781642653571 (v. 1) | ISBN 9781642653588 (v. 2)
Subjects: LCSH: Women–Health and hygiene–Encyclopedias. | Women–Diseases–Prevention–Encyclopedias.
Classification: LCC RA564.85 .W66 2019 | DDC 613/.04244–dc23

First Printing
PRINTED IN THE UNITED STATES OF AMERICA

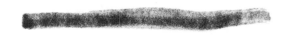

Contents

Volume 2

Complete List of Contents

Volume 1

Volume 2

H

Human immunodeficiency virus (HIV)

CATEGORY: Disease/Disorder

KEY TERMS:

antiretroviral treatment: treatment with drugs that inhibit the ability of the human immunodeficiency virus or other types of retroviruses to multiply in the body

CD4 lymphocytes (T cells): help coordinate the immune response by stimulating other immune cells, such as macrophages, B lymphocytes (B cells), and CD8 T lymphocytes (CD8 cells), to fight infection; HIV weakens the immune system by destroying CD4 cells

CDC: Centers for Disease Control and Prevention; serves as the national focus for developing and applying disease prevention and control, environmental health, and health promotion and health education activities designed to improve the health of the people of the United States

CAUSES AND SYMPTOMS

HIV infection in the USA peaks between the ages of 20–30 (35 people out of 100,000) whereas AIDS peak incidence happens at the approximate age of 45 (14 people out of 100,000). The overall prevalence in the USA is about 1.2 million, worldwide, the prevalence is at 37 million (approximately 0.5% of the population). According to the Centers for Disease Control and Prevention (CDC), women made up 19% of new HIV diagnoses in 2016, and 8% of those were from heterosexual contact. Incidence of new diagnoses were significantly higher in African American women (61%) than in other population groups.

Untreated, HIV has a mortality rate of >90% (8–10 years). Average life expectancy if treatment is received is 15–20 years lower. Prognosis depends on antiretroviral treatment, viral set point, CD4 count, and exposure to opportunistic pathogens, HIV type, and other conditions.

The virus infects CD4 lymphocytes (T cells). Three stages include acute infection, clinical latency and AIDS. In stage of acute infection, the virus reproduces quickly leading to acute (flu-like) symptoms within 2 – 4 weeks. During latency, many people remain asymptomatic. AIDS is defined by CD4 count <200. HIV can be detected via antigen / antibody-based tests. Monitoring the disease includes keeping track of CD4 count and viral load. There are 2 types of HIV: 1 (more common in industrialized countries), 2 (more common in poor countries and progresses more slowly).

There are mainly three routes of transmission:

Sexual: Responsible for about 80% of infections worldwide. Sexual act risk depends on the kind of behavior and practices one is employing. Risk for men who have sex with men (MSM) is 0.5% for receptive partner whereas risk for male to female sex is 0.1% for female partner and 0.05% for male partner. There are factors like the viral load, circumcision, or genital mucosal damage which may influence the likelihood of becoming infected.

Parenteral: Needle sharing accounts for 0.67% per exposure through needle – sharing contact. Needle stick injures account for 0.36% of risk per injury.

Vertical: During childbirth, the risk ranges from 5 – 15% whereas breastfeeding can lead to a risk between 5 – 20% of exposure.

It is important to note that the risk of transmission can be lowered significantly if HIV infection is

---

Information on Human Immunodeficiency Virus (HIV)

Causes: Transmission through exchange of body fluids (semen, vaginal fluid, blood, human milk)

Symptoms: Flulike or mononucleosis-like symptoms upon initial transmission; later, various opportunistic infections

Duration: Chronic, eventually fatal

Treatments: Highly active antiretroviral therapy (HAART) with nucleoside or nucleotide analogues, reverse transcriptase inhibitors, protease inhibitors, inhibitors of cellular entry

treated consistently and viral load is below the limit of detection.

HIV is symptomatic in early infection and the incubation period lasts 2–4 weeks. Acute infection includes symptoms of fever, fatigue, headache, lymphadenopathy, rash, myalgia, GI symptoms, oropharyngeal (sore throat, painful swallowing). Latency may be asymptomatic or may have symptoms like chronic sub febrile temperatures, lymphadenopathy, opportunistic infections (oral candidiasis, vaginal infections, oral hairy leukoplakia, diarrhea).

RISK FACTORS

Most women in the United States contract HIV from having sex with a man. During vaginal and anal sex, women are more likely to contract the virus than men. Compared to the penis, the vagina has much more surface area to which infected semen can be exposed. Semen can stay in a woman's system for days after sex, meaning that they are exposed to potentially infected semen for much longer than men. Infections, diseases and disorders that are more commonly found in women, such as yeast infections, bacterial vaginosis and sexually transmitted infections (STI).

Women in younger age groups tend to not use condoms or other protective measures when they have sex, meaning they are more likely to contract an STI. They are also at a higher risk than older women because their reproductive system is still developing.

DIAGNOSTICS AND SCREENING

The general indications are to test all patients with clinical features of acute or chronic HIV infection, all individuals with possible past exposure, especially high-risk individuals and one time testing is recommended early in every pregnancy. The diagnostic process is as follows;

Screening tests: Combination antigen / antibody tests which detect both HIV antigen and anti – HIV antibodies, a negative result essentially rules out HIV infection. An ELISA is a standard method for detecting antibodies within approximately 1 – 3 hours; requires laboratory. There are also rapid tests which can deliver results in about 20 minutes and do not require laboratory, which make them suitable as an alternative to more complex tests.

Confirmatory tests: HIV – 1 / HIV – 2 antibody differentiation immunoassay can detect both HIV – 1 and HIV – 2 in about 20 minutes and distinguish between the two types.

In the News: Experimental HIV Vaccine

Despite more than twenty-five years of intensive research— and a global expenditure of more than $6 billion— a vaccine that prevents HIV infection has remained elusive. One notorious trial was halted early when vaccinated subjects actually suffered an increased risk of infection. There are a number of complex reasons that candidate vaccines have proven ineffective. One reason is that the molecules on the surface of the virus to which the immune system's antibodies can bind are much more variable than in typical pathogens. The HIV genome, composed of ribonucleic acid (RNA), can accumulate mutations at frequencies up to 100 times higher than genomes composed of deoxyribonucleic acid (DNA) like the human genome. Thus, selection pressure due to an immune response against one set of HIV surface molecules will rapidly lead to the evolution of resistant strains displaying distinct sets of surface molecules. Indeed, multiple highly divergent strains are found in patients in different regions of the globe.

Finally, in September 2009, a U.S.-Thai team of investigators announced the first demonstration of reduced risk of HIV infection after immunization. The study employed a combination of two vaccines that had individually failed to be effective in previous experiments. Low-to-moderate- risk HIV-negative volunteers aged eighteen to thirty were given injections of vaccine or placebo and subsequently tested for infection every six months for three years. In the control group, 74 of 8,198 subjects were infected by the end of the study; in the vaccinated group, only 51 of 8,197 subjects became infected. Those figures reflect a statistically significant 31.2 percent reduction of probability of infection after vaccination.

Although the observed effect was encouraging, the results include a number of caveats. The vaccine combination targets the HIV strain encountered most frequently in Thailand and therefore would not be expected to provide immunity to the strains responsible for most infections in Africa, Europe, North America, and elsewhere. Vaccination had no apparent effect on the severity of infection in subjects who contracted HIV during the study. Lastly, the vaccine's efficacy is far below the 80 percent threshold required for approval for public distribution.

—*Carina Endres Howell, Ph.D.*

Detection of viral RNA: It can detect HIV infection earlier than antibody / antigen-based tests but FDA approved tests are limited to HIV – 1.

Post–treatment monitoring: Viral RNA load is an indicator of ART response, decrease in viral loads indicates effective treatment

TREATMENT AND THERAPY

The general approach to treat HIV infected people regardless of their CD4 count should be to begin combined antiretroviral therapy as soon as possible. Antiretroviral (ART) don't cure HIV but HIV medicines help people with HIV live longer, healthier lives. ART also reduces the risk of HIV transmission. The main goal of ART is to reduce a person's viral load to an undetectable level. The medication does this by preventing HIV from multiplying which reduces the amount of HIV in the body. Having less HIV in the body gives the immune system a chance to recover.

An undetectable level indicates that the viral load in the blood is too low to be detected by a viral load test. If the viral load is undetectable, this will prevent HIV transmission to a negative partner through sex. Medications side effects are varied, and it is recommended that patients talk to their health care provider about possible side effects of HIV medicine before starting the treatment. Overall, the benefits of taking the medication outweigh the side effects.

Includes HIV post – exposure prophylaxis should be initiated ASAP (one to two hours). A three-drug regimen is recommended (Tenofovir – emtricitabine + dolutegravir; tenofovir – emtricitabine + raltegravir). If needle stick then let the wound bleed, rinse / flush with water, soap or antiseptic, seek medical attention. Efficacy of vaccinations in HIV infected individuals is decreased. Live vaccines shouldn't be given if CD4 count < 200.

—Ralph R. Meyer, Ph.D.;
Updated by Richard Adler, Ph.D.
and David Hernandez

FOR FURTHER INFORMATION

Centers for Disease Control and Prevention. HIV Surveillance Report. url: https: //www.cdc.gov/hiv/pdf/library/reports/surveillance/cdc-hiv-surveillance-report-us.

Kasper DL, Fauci AS, Hauser SL, Longo DL, Lameson JL, Loscalzo J. Harrison's Principles of Internal Medicine. New York, NY: McGraw – Hill Education; 2015.

Agabegi SS, Agabegi ED. Step – Up To Medicine. Baltimore, MD, USA: Wolters Kluwer Health; 2015.

Hewitt RG. Abacavir Hypersensitivity Reaction. Clin Infect Dis. 2002; 34 (8); pp. 1137 – 1142. Doi: 10.1086 / 339751

Fan, Hung, Ross F. Conner, and Luis P. Villarreal. *The Biology of AIDS.* 4th ed. Sudbury, Mass.: Jones and Bartlett, 2000.

Farnan, Rose, and Maithe Enriquez. *What Nurses Know: HIV/AIDS.* New York: Demos Health, 2012.

"HIV among Women." Centers for Disease Control and Prevention, Centers for Disease Control and Prevention, 5 July 2018, www.cdc.gov/hiv/group/gender/women/index.html.

Matthews, Dawn D., ed. *AIDS Sourcebook.* 3d ed. Detroit, Mich.: Omnigraphics, 2003.

Sande Merle A., et al. *Sande's HIV/AIDS Medicine: Medical Management of AIDS, 2013.* Philadelphia: Elsevier Saunders, 2012.

Stine, Gerald J. *AIDS Update 2013.* New York: McGraw-Hill Higher Education, 2013.

Strauss, James, and Ellen Strauss. *Viruses and Human Disease.* 2d ed. Boston: Academic Press/Elsevier, 2008.

"Women and HIV." Womenshealth.gov, Office on Women's Health, 21 Nov. 2018, www.womenshealth.gov/hiv-and-aids/women-and-hiv.

Human papillomavirus (HPV)

CATEGORY: Disease/Disorder
Also known as: Papovaviruses

KEY TERMS:

cervical cancer: cancer of the cervix, the lower end of the uterus that projects into the vagina

genital warts: warts occurring in the genital and anal areas acquired by sexual contact and caused by HPV infection

Pap testing: a screening test to detect precancerous and cancerous cells of the cervix

CAUSES AND SYMPTOMS

Papillomaviruses are deoxyribonucleic acid (DNA) viruses that infect the skin and mucous membranes. Human papillomaviruses belong to a group of papillomaviruses that consists of nearly 120 strains. Most strains are relatively harmless, causing nothing more than benign skin warts (papillomas), while others cause genital warts (condyloma acuminate) and may cause some cancers.

Sexual contact is the primary mechanism by which the virus is acquired. About forty HPV strains are sexually transmitted and can infect the external genitalia, urethra, anus, rectum, and sometimes the mouth and throat. Some strains cause genital warts, while the more virulent, high-risk strains cause abnormal Papanicolaou (Pap) tests and can in some instances cause cancer of the cervix, vagina, vulva, penis, scrotum, anus, and/or the mouth and pharynx and possibly esophagus. An estimated 99% of cases of cervical cancer and 70% of vaginal and vulvar cancers are the result of persistent HPV infection.

HPV is the most common sexually transmitted infection. In 2017, the U. S. Centers for Disease Control and Prevention (CDC) estimated that 79 million Americans are infected with HPV. About 14 million new infections occur each year. About 46% of men and 40% of women are infected in the United States. Nearly 26% of men and 21% of women are infected by a high-risk HPV strain. About 80% of Americans will become infected by HPV at some time during their lives, but most people remain asymptomatic. In most cases, viral infection is cleared by the immune system within a few months without serious consequences. In some cases, however, the active infection becomes dormant and can later cause a reinfection. Babies of infected women may contract potentially life-threatening HPV infections during delivery.

Women are more susceptible to developing genital warts than men. However, not all HPV viruses cause genital warts. Often, infected women are asymptomatic, and HPV infection is only indicated by an abnormal Pap test. In the U. S., about 12,000 women are diagnosed with cervical cancer and about 4000 die from cervical cancer each year. Worldwide, the rates of HPV-associated cancers are much higher, especially in women who often receive limited routine gynecological care. Frequent Pap screenings are the best way to diagnose HPV infections in asymptomatic women.

TREATMENT AND THERAPY

As of 2017, the Food and Drug Administration (FDA) had approved three vaccines against HPV infections. The vaccines are effective only when

---

Information on Human Papillomavirus (HPV)

Causes: Viral infection spread through skin (usually sexual) contact

Symptoms: Warts or cancer in genital and anal areas

Duration: Acute in initial infection, then chronic and often recurrent

Treatments: For warts, topical ointments, creams, resins, or gels and electrocautery, cryosurgery, or laser surgery; for cancer, chemotherapy, radiation, surgery; prevention possible with vaccine. Persistent HPV infection is a hallmark of developing cervical cancer, and since the cancer usually develops slowly over five to ten years, early diagnosis and treatment can be effective in preventing cervical cancer.

---

given before HPV infection occurs. Thus, the vaccines are recommended for boys and girls at ages 11-12 just before they enter puberty. The vaccine is usually administered in two doses starting at ages 11-12 years with the two doses administered about 6 to 12 months apart. A third dose may be recommended if this protocol is not followed. Young women can get the vaccine until age 27.

HPV4 (Gardasil), licensed in 2006, immunizes against four strains of HPV, two of which cause about 70% of cervical cancers and two that cause about 90% of genital warts. The vaccine is approved for use in males and females ages 9 to 26 years. HPV2 (Cervarix) was licensed in 2009. It provides immunity against the two HPV strains that cause 70% of cervical cancers and is approved only for women and only between ages 10 to 25 years. Cervarix is no longer available in the U. S. In 2014, the FDA licensed HPV9 (Gardasil-9). It provides immunity against nine strains of HPV and is approved for both males and females ages 9 to 26. It can provide protection of up to 90% of genital cancers caused by HPV. All three HPV vaccines are 99% effective in creating immunity. Side effects are generally transient and mild.

Routine Pap screening for women is still recommended in both vaccinated and unvaccinated individuals, because the vaccines do not protect against all strains of HPV, and cervical cancer detected early can often be successfully treated. Risk reduction for HPV infection can be achieved by reducing the number of sexual partners. Condom use may partially reduce the risk of HPV infection in women. Since condoms do not cover all infected areas, however, their use does not eliminate the risk of infection.

As of 2017, HPV vaccination was controversial among some parents because it is recommended for children for a sexually active disease before they become sexually active. The medical reason for this recommendation is that the vaccine is ineffective once an infection has already been acquired. Some states that have required HPV vaccination for entry into junior high or high school have rolled back these requirements because the HPV infection, unlike, for example, measles, cannot be transmitted simply by sitting next to an infected individual in a classroom.

Since there is no cure for an HPV infection, the primary treatments are for warts and pre-cancerous cells. Some treatments for warts involve the use of topical ointments, creams, resins, and gels such as imiquimod (Aldara), podophyllin and podofilox (Condylox), and 5- fluorouracil, as well as trichloro-acetic acid. Alternatively, warts and precancerous tissue may be removed by electrocautery, cryosurgery, laser, loop electrosurgical excision or conventional surgery, but may recur.

PERSPECTIVE AND PROSPECTS

HPV was first described as a cause of skin warts in 1907. Not until the 1980s was HPV linked to cervical cancer. This relationship was noted when it was discovered that women who have had multiple sexual partners or who started to have sexual relations at a younger age are at greater risk of developing cervical cancer than women who have had few or no sexual partners.

The mechanism by which HPV causes cancer has recently been determined. Two proteins encoded by HPV DNA attach to and inactivate cellular proteins that control cell division. With these cellular proteins inactivated, the cell multiplies uncontrollably. Since sisters of women with cervical cancer have a higher risk of developing cervical cancer, it is thought that genetics may be involved in the progression of the disease.

—*Charles L. Vigue, Ph.D.*
Updated by Tish Davidson, A.M.;
and Charles L. Vigue, Ph.D

FOR FURTHER INFORMATION

Gearhart, Peter A. "Human papillomavirus." Medscape January 5, 2017. http://emedicine.medscape.com/article/219110-overview

Ghadishah, Delaram. "Genital Warts." Medscape November 17, 2016. http://emedicine.medscape.com/article/763014-overview

"HPV Infection". Mayo Clinic. https://www.mayoclinic.org/diseases-conditions/hpv-infection/symptoms-causes/syc-20351596

"Human Papillomavirus (HPV)". In: Davidson, Tish. *Vaccines: History, Issues, and Science.* Santa Barbara, CA: Greenwood, 2017; 94-6.

"———". U.S. Centers for Disease Control and Prevention (January 25, 2017). https://www.cdc.gov/hpv/index.html

U.S. National Library of Medicine. "HPV" MedlinePlus June 6, 2017. https://medlineplus.gov/hpv.html

Hypersexual disorder

CATEGORY: Disease/Disorder

KEY TERMS:

emotional dysregulation: the inability of a person to control or regulate their emotional responses to provocative stimuli

paraphilias: the experience of intense sexual arousal to atypical objects, situations, fantasies, behaviors, or individuals

DESCRIPTION AND DIAGNOSIS

Hypersexual disorder (HD) is interchangeably referred to as *sexually compulsive behavior, sexual dependency, problematic hypersexuality,* and *sex addiction.* Individuals with HD will excessively pursue solo or relational sexual activities; they may have difficulty controlling sexual thoughts, urges, and behavior; and the consequences adversely affect their interpersonal, social, or occupational areas of functioning. HD may result in unemployment, family breakdown, and divorce. Individuals with HD may take risks that put their own and their partners' health at risk, or risk criminal proceedings from participation in prostitution. HD adversely affects the overall emotional well-being and disrupts an individual's ecosystem.

Individuals with HD report high levels of shame and guilt about their urges and behavior.

Social workers variously conceptualize the condition as an impulsive disorder, an obsessive-compulsive disorder, or an addiction. HD is not in the fifth edition of the *Diagnostic and Statistical Manual of Mental Disorders (DSM-5)*, which is used to diagnose mental health disorders, because of insufficient research and concern that it may be misused in forensic court settings. The decision not to include HD in *DSM-5* is a controversial decision among social workers, many of whom treat the condition. The *ICD-10 Classification of Mental and Behavioral Disorders (ICD-10)*, which offers diagnostic definitions by the World Health Organization (WHO), includes the diagnosis of *excessive sexual drive* under the section of sexual dysfunction.

Research on HD in women is at an early stage and there is a lack of knowledge about its origins, features, and development. There may be differences in the form that HD takes in women as compared to men. Women tend to be more relationally concerned, though a 2010 study found that HD often presents in women as sexual activity with consenting adults. While men develop HD due to decreased sexual satisfaction and physical health, women develop it due to more psychological and social stressors. In the same 2010 study, it was found that women were concerned about unwanted pregnancies and sexually transmitted diseases as consequences of HD, while men were more concerned with legal and work-related consequences.

There is no one agreed-upon set of diagnostic criteria for HD. General consensus is that diagnosis requires persistent symptoms for at least 6 consecutive months. These symptoms may typically include excessive time spent on sexual fantasies or urges and/or planning for and executing these behaviors; repetitively engaging in these behaviors as a response to anxiety, depression, irritability, boredom, and so on; repetitively engaging in these behaviors as a response to life events that are stressful; unsuccessful but repeated attempts to reduce or control these fantasies, urges, or behaviors; repetitively engaging in these behaviors even when there is a risk of physical or emotional harm to self or others. The individual must also be experiencing significant distress or impairments in occupational, social, or other important areas of functioning.

In some cases, HD may be the result of a physical condition, such as a neurological disorder or substance use. Generally, however, the causes of HD are not known. Research into HD is in its infancy, which is the reason it has not been included in the *DSM-5*. The lack of studies that include diagnostic criteria in a large study population has hampered attempts to define HD as a distinct clinical disorder. Studies have correlated HD with a history of depression, substance use, and childhood abuse, and therefore the condition can be complex and difficult to evaluate. Emotional dysregulation and insecure attachment styles with partners are common. HD can also be comorbid and exist with paraphilias (conditions characterized by abnormal sexual desires). HD is often understood as a way for an individual to escape or relieve emotional pain. Social workers can assist patients in determining their own boundaries and what constitutes healthy sexuality. Social workers are advised to thoroughly assess underlying personal and interpersonal issues with patients seeking help. Additionally, Social workers should be aware of their own personal sexual issues and beliefs; understand the broad range of human sexual expression; and maintain strong professional boundaries. A number of self-reporting questionnaires have been developed to assess for HD.

Adults with histories of childhood maltreatment, including sexual, emotional, and physical abuse, are at risk for developing HD. Patients with depression or anxiety may be at risk.

SIGNS AND SYMPTOMS

HD can follow a cyclical pattern, similar to other addiction disorders. Possible symptoms may be physical, behavioral, or psychological.

Possible physical signs and symptoms of HD include possible exposure to HIV through sexual practices, and withdrawal symptoms that include sweating, increased heart rate, shortness of breath, fatigue, and nausea

Possible behavioral signs and symptoms of HD may include seeking new sexual partners frequently, frequent sexual encounters, compulsive masturbation, frequent use of pornography, engaging in risky sexual activities, paying for sexual services, using sexual activity to suppress unpleasant feelings, secrecy in regard to sexual behaviors, indifference towards regular sexual partner, a preference for sex that is anonymous or transactional, an intimacy disconnect, absence of control, and compulsive use of the Internet for sexual purposes.

Psychological signs and symptoms that may occur with a diagnosis of HD include obsessive thoughts about sex, feelings of guilt, loneliness, boredom, low self-esteem, or rationalizations related to the sexual behaviors and sexual choices, self-hatred, and feelings of shame.

Individuals with HD excessively pursue solo or relational sexual activities and are unable to control sexual behavior. They may be depressed and anxious. Individuals with HD frequently feel shame and guilt about their urges and behavior.

ASSESSMENT

Woman suspected of having HD should have a thorough biological, psychological, social, and spiritual assessment to determine treatment and diagnosis needs. Such an assessment should clarify the dysfunctional emotions and behaviors HD is causing in the patient's life, explore the possibility of other sexual dysfunctions, such as erectile or orgasmic difficulties, determine whether there are any biological factors, such as medical conditions, injury, or substance abuse that may be causing the sexual behaviors, understand the patient's early sexual and family experiences, including attitudes about sexuality, sex education, sexual or physical abuse, masturbation, and body image, explore any relationship problems in current and past relationships, and evaluate the presence of mental health problems.

ASSESSMENT AND SCREENING TOOLS

The assessment process may require the use of standardized assessment and screening tools. There are several screening and assessment tools that may be used when assessing the needs of patient with HD. Possible assessments that may be appropriate to use include the Kalichman Sexual Compulsivity Scale (SCS), which has 10 items on compulsive sexual behavior, excessive sexual activity, and sexual thoughts that are compulsive and has been widely used in assessment; the Sexual Addiction Screening Test (SAST), which has 52 items and is available online; the Sexual Addiction Screening Test – Women (WSAST), which has been studied with women; and the Hypersexual Behavior Inventory (HBI), which has 19 items and those listed symptoms and behaviors served as the outline for proposed criterion when HD

was being considered for inclusion in the *DSM-5* (but was subsequently excluded) and it does provide a clinical cutoff score.

Additional screening and assessment tools include the Experience in Close Relationship Scale (ECR), which is a 36-item questionnaire that explores avoidance of intimacy and attachment as well as anxious attachment related to abandonment and separation anxiety issues; the Internet Sex Screening Test (ISST), which is a 25-item tool that measures online sexual compulsivity; online sexual behavior, both social and isolated; online sexual spending; and interest in online sexual behavior; the Beck Depression Inventory (BDI) for adults, which has 12 multiple-choice questions and is widely used; The State-Trait Anxiety Inventory (STAI), which has 40 questions evaluating anxiety levels; and the Simple Screening Instrument for Alcohol and Other Drugs (SSI-AOD), which has 16 questions that require a yes or no response. Patients with HD may be referred for laboratory testing for sexually transmitted infections, if appropriate.

TREATMENT

Treatment often depends on how HD is conceptualized or manifested in the individual. For example, treatment for HD as an impulsive disorder may involve cognitive behavioral therapy (CBT), whereas when HD is viewed as an addiction, harm reduction and psychotherapy might be the primary techniques. There has been limited empirical support for any of the commonly used treatment approaches. CBT focuses on the individual's problematic urges and behavior, harm reduction advocates reducing problematic behavior rather than demanding abstinence, and psychotherapy addresses the underlying causes. Interventions combining CBT and psychotherapy are recommended. Couples therapy can help heal wounds, restore trust, and encourage forgiveness. Since research links depression and anxiety with HD, some social workers suggest pharmacotherapy (the use of medications), such as antidepressants. There are reports of success with 12-step programs; several organizations facilitate this self-help approach.

Mindfulness interventions as part of a treatment program are used by some social workers when treating HD. Mindfulness is a process in which patients are taught to bring awareness and acceptance to the thoughts, emotions, and physical sensations in their moment-to-moment experiences. The most common treatment approach for HD seems to be a combination of CBT, group therapy, and a 12-step program. There are no registered psychotropic medications for the treatment of HD, though there have been some trials completed with the use of antidepressants.

INTERVENTION

Women who experience unrelenting urges for, and the pursuit of, sexual activity accompanied by negative emotions (shame, guilt), should seek interventions to help reduce/ eliminate their urges. A social worker or therapist can explore her history, clarify areas of dysfunction, and evaluate her for the signs and symptoms of HD. If HD is suspected, she should have the social worker or therapist evaluate her for symptoms of depression, anxiety, and alcohol and other drug use. Psychotherapy, CBT, and pharmacology are all intervention options she may consider and if needed, she should ask for the appropriate referrals. Also, mental health professionals should assess her for any suicidal ideation or plans for self-harm

If the patient with HD experiences relationship distress and relationship breakdown due to hypersexual behaviors, a social worker or therapist can provide interventions to help repair trust in the relationship and strengthen the couple's connection. Alternatively, they may provide a referral, if needed.

RED FLAGS

HD can be complex to evaluate because of its potential comorbidity with mental health conditions such as depression and anxiety. HD may be a comorbid condition or cooccurring with paraphilias. Often it can be a struggle to have patients with HD acknowledge the disorder and take responsibility for their actions. Frequently, patients coming for counseling may not be coming as their own personal choice but instead are feeling forced into treatment after being caught and are coming to treatment to try to salvage a relationship. The social worker needs to recognize his or her role in helping patients come around to the position of wanting to genuinely make changes for themselves, regardless of what effect that may have on the relationship.

Individuals with HD may have trauma histories. Recovery from HD may have a negative impact on marital or partner relationships as the recovery process can result in new demands or requirements in the relationship. Caution should be utilized by social workers in diagnosing HD and note that not all individuals engaging in multiple affairs, being promiscuous, or exercising unusual expressions of sexuality are sex addicted.

—Jan Wagstaff, MA, MSW,
and Jessica Therivel, LMSW-IPR

FOR FURTHER INFORMATION

American Psychiatric Association. *Diagnostic and Statistical Manual of Mental Disorders, 5th Edition*, 2010.

Garcia, F. D., and F. Thibaut. "Sexual Addictions." *The American Journal of Drug and Alcohol Abuse*, vol. 36, no. 5, 2010, pp. 254–260.

Gilliland, Randy, et al. "The Roles of Shame and Guilt in Hypersexual Behavior." *Sexual Addiction & Compulsivity*, vol. 18, no. 1, 8 Mar. 2011, pp. 12–29.

Katehakis, Alexandra. "Affective Neuroscience and the Treatment of Sexual Addiction." Sexual Addiction & Compulsivity, vol. 16, no. 1, 21 Feb. 2009, pp. 1–31.

Kingston, Drew A., and Philip Firestone. "Problematic Hypersexuality: A Review of Conceptualization and Diagnosis." Sexual Addiction & Compulsivity, vol. 15, no. 4, 19 Nov. 2008, pp. 284–310.

Marshall, Liam E., and W. L. Marshall. "The Factorial Structure Of The Sexual Addiction Screening Testin Sexual Offenders and Socio-Economically Matched Community Non-Offenders." Sexual Addiction & Compulsivity, vol. 17, no. 3, July 2010, pp. 210–218.

Öberg, Katarina Görts, et al. "Hypersexual Disorder According to the Hypersexual Disorder Screening Inventory in Help-Seeking Swedish Men and Women With Self-Identified Hypersexual Behavior." *Sexual Medicine*, vol. 5, no. 4, 2017, pp. 229–236.

Opitz, Dawn M., et al. "Women's Sexual Addiction and Family Dynamics, Depression and Substance Abuse." *Sexual Addiction & Compulsivity*, vol. 16, no. 4, 30 Nov. 2009, pp. 324–340.

Samenow, Charles P. "A Biopsychosocial Model of Hypersexual Disorder/Sexual Addiction." *Sexual Addiction & Compulsivity*, vol. 17, no. 2, 26 May 2010, pp. 69–81.

———. "What You Should Know about Hypersexual Disorder." *Sexual Addiction & Compulsivity*, vol. 18, no. 3, 31 Aug. 2011, pp. 107–113.

Turner, Martha. "Uncovering and Treating Sex Addiction in Couples Therapy." *Journal of Family Psychotherapy*, vol. 20, no. 2-3, 22 July 2009, pp. 283–302.

Hyperthyroidism and hypothyroidism

CATEGORY: Disease/Disorder

KEY TERMS

goiter: an enlarged thyroid gland that appears as a swollen area in the front of the neck

Graves' disease: Autoimmune disease in which antibodies produced by the immune system stimulate the thyroid to overproduce thyroid hormone.

Hashimoto's disease: the autoimmune system produces antibodies that attack the thyroid gland leading to underproduction of thyroid hormone.

hyperthyroidism: the thyroid gland produces too much hormone

hypothyroidism: the thyroid gland produces too little hormone

thyroiditis: Inflammation of the thyroid gland.

CAUSES AND SYMPTOMS

More than 20 million people have some form of thyroid disease and almost 2/3 of that number is unaware of their affliction. More women than men develop thyroid disease, with the disease affecting one in eight (1 in 8) women. Thyroid disease often occurs immediately after pregnancy or menopause. The most common thyroid diseases affecting women are hypothyroidism, hyperthyroidism, postpartum thyroiditis, goiter, thyroid nodules and cancer. Women may notice feeling tired or restless, gaining or losing weight with no change in diet, changes in menstrual periods including irregular periods with changes in flow and even no period known as amenorrhea, hair loss and fast or irregular heart rate. A physician or other healthcare professional generally diagnose thyroid disease with examination and blood tests. Prompt treatment is indicated to address causes and symptoms.

Thyroid disease may also cause difficulty getting pregnant by interfering with hormones related to ovulation. An increase in prolactin hormone, the hormone related to breast milk production, may be caused by hypothyroidism and may prevent ovulation. Once a woman is pregnant, appropriate levels of thyroid hormone are necessary for brain development in the fetus. Hyperthyroidism left untreated during pregnancy may result in premature birth, preeclampsia causing high blood pressure and kidney issues, low birth weight and miscarriage. Hypothyroidism left untreated may lead to problems with the baby's growth and development, preeclampsia, miscarriage and stillbirth. Before trying to get pregnant, a woman should consider having her thyroid level checked.

The major functions of the human body are controlled by the endocrine system, which is a system of glands that make, store, and release hormones. Hormones are substances that help regulate the body's systems. The thyroid is a butterfly-shaped gland about two inches long that weighs less than an ounce and is located at the base of the throat. It produces two hormones: thyroxine, also known as T-4, and triiodothyronine, also known as T-3. The thyroid gland has influence over breathing, central and peripheral nervous system functions, muscle strength, body temperature, menstrual cycles, and body weight. These hormones play a key role in controlling heart rate and function as well as the body's temperature. Together, they regulate how food is metabolized to provide energy. They do this by controlling how the body uses carbohydrates and fats, how much protein the body produces, and how much calcium is released into the bloodstream. Thus, these two hormones influence every part of the body.

The main glands of the endocrine system, the hypothalamus and the pituitary gland, control the amount of T-3 and T-4 made and released by the thyroid. When the body needs these hormones, the hypothalamus signals the pituitary gland to release thyroid stimulating hormone, or TSH. TSH then tells the thyroid to release the appropriate hormones. Sometimes the process goes wrong, and the thyroid produces and releases the incorrect amounts of hormones. Infection, injury, or the ingestion of too much synthetic thyroid hormone can also interfere with the process. When a person has too much thyroxine in his or her system for any of these reasons, it results in a condition known as hyperthyroidism. When there is insufficient thyroxine produced by the thyroid, TSH is unable to stimulate the gland to produce sufficient hormones to manage body functions.

Thyroxine helps to regulate several of the body's systems, so both hyperthyroidism and hypothyroidism are often revealed by disruptions to these systems. With hyperthyroidism, a person might experience tachycardia, or a heart rate of more than one hundred beats per minute. The heart rate may also be irregular, a condition known as arrhythmia, or it may feel like the heart is pounding, which doctors refer to as palpitations. With hypothyroidism, a person may experience bradycardia, or slow heartbeat, overwhelming fatigue, weight gain and dry skin. Because of the wide range of symptoms, blood is drawn to determine the level of TSH and/or thyroxine circulating in the body. A high level of TSH and a low level of thyroid hormone indicates an underactive thyroid.

Hyperthyroidism is a medical condition in which the thyroid gland produces too much thyroid hormone. The presence of high thyroid hormone levels in the blood, regardless of source, is known as thyrotoxicosis, and may include high thyroxine levels as a result of an infection or ingesting too much synthetic thyroxine in tablet form. The most common cause of hyperthyroidism is Graves' disease, which is caused by the development of antibodies in the blood that activate the thyroid and increase production of thyroid hormone. Hyperthyroidism is also caused by tumors in the thyroid called adenomas that produce too much thyroid hormone (e.g., toxic adenoma, toxic multinodular goiter, Plummer disease), or, sometimes, inflammation of the thyroid (thyroiditis).

A person with hyperthyroidism will experience several symptoms, including nervousness, hand tremors, weight loss unrelated to diet, cardiovascular issues, and problems with food metabolism. Hyperthyroidism can be treated with medication or, in some cases, surgery.

Too much thyroxine can cause sudden weight loss despite the increased appetite that also is a sign of hyperthyroidism. In addition, the hormone's effect on temperature regulation might cause a person with hyperthyroidism to be more sensitive to heat and to experience an increase in sweat production. Other symptoms of hyperthyroidism include anxiety and nervousness, difficulty sleeping, fatigue, muscle weakness, a change in bowel habits, trembling hands, brittle hair, thinning skin, and the development of a goiter, or swelling, at the base of the neck. However, some older adults may not experience many of these symptoms or may experience them to a lesser degree. Some medications, most notably beta-blockers used for blood pressure control, may mask the symptoms and make them harder to detect.

The causes of hyperthyroidism and hypothyroidism vary. About 70 percent of hyperthyroidism cases are the result of a condition known as Graves' disease. In this condition, antibodies in the blood attack the entire thyroid, causing it to grow larger than normal and release too much thyroxine. While the cause of Graves' disease is not known, it does tend to run in families and is more likely to affect younger women. A benign tumor may also cause the release of too much thyroxine.

Some patients with hyperthyroidism experience a condition called Graves' ophthalmopathy. In these cases, the muscles behind the eye swell to the extent that the eyeball is pushed outside of the normal eye socket. This can cause the eye to become very dry and lead to redness, swelling, tearing, and irritation of the eye. This condition is more common in smokers.

Sometimes nodules, or small lumps of tissue, grow in and around the thyroid. These nodules can cause the thyroid to release more thyroxine than normal. This condition is known as a toxic nodule, or multinodular goiter.

In some cases, people can develop temporary hyperthyroidism due to an infection that interferes with the thyroid's function for a short period (thyroiditis). Additionally, sometimes people who have been prescribed a synthetic or artificial form of thyroxine as treatment for low thyroid function (hypothyroidism) might inadvertently take too high a dose. This also results in a temporary form of hyperthyroidism. High thyroxine levels from unintentional ingestion of too much thyroxine are also known as thyrotoxicosis. This differentiates this type of hyperthyroidism from the type caused by a malfunction of the thyroid gland.

If hyperthyroidism is suspected, a medical professional will check the patient's heart rate and look for telltale signs of the condition, such as moist and smooth skin, eye abnormalities, tremors, or an enlargement of the thyroid gland. Simple blood tests can assess the levels of thyroid hormone and TSH in the patient's system. When tests reveal low levels of TSH but high levels of thyroxine, or T-4, hyperthyroidism is likely present. This can be confirmed with an imaging procedure known as a thyroid scan. A thyroid uptake test, which checks how the thyroid processes iodine, may also be ordered to check the gland's functions.

In patients with hypothyroidism, the thyroid gland is unable to make enough thyroid hormone to support normal body functions and processes start to slow down. This may be caused by an autoimmune disease, Hashimoto's thyroiditis, radiation treatments, or surgical removal of the gland. Symptoms may include fatigue or easy tiring with normal activity, feeling colder, constipation, dry skin, weight gain, forgetfulness, and depression. There are more than three million cases of hypothyroidism diagnosed every year in the U.S.

TREATMENT AND THERAPY

Once hyperthyroidism is diagnosed, there are several ways to treat it. Some patients will be given antithyroid agents such as methimazole or propylthiouracil (PTU). These drugs stop the thyroid from making more thyroxine. In other cases, the patient will be given a single dose of radioactive iodine in capsule form. This will be absorbed by the overactive cells in the thyroid and will destroy them over the course of several weeks or months. The goal is to allow the thyroid to return to normal size and function. Antithyroid drugs and beta-blockers may be used during this time and even after to control any resulting symptoms of hyperthyroidism.

However, in some cases it is necessary to prevent any future recurrences of the condition. In these cases, a second dose of radioactive iodine may be given to destroy the thyroid, or the thyroid may be surgically removed or reduced in size. This will result in hypothyroidism, but this is easily treated with daily administration of synthetic thyroxine.

Risk factors for hypothyroidism include age, autoimmune diseases such as lupus (a chronic inflammatory condition) or rheumatoid arthritis, a family history of thyroid disease, and pregnancy or birth within six months before symptoms develop. Women over 60 are more likely to develop hypothyroidism, though symptoms may develop slowly over time, making it harder to diagnose. Hypothyroidism result from autoimmune diseases or an insufficient intake of

iodine. An autoimmune disease occurs when antibodies are produced that attack the body, and can be caused by genetic factors, a virus, or bacterium. More than likely, autoimmune diseases are a result of a combination of these factors. Patients with hyperthyroidism are often treated with radioactive iodine or anti-thyroid medications to decrease the overproduction of thyroxine. Treatments may decrease the thyroxine levels too drastically, leading to hypothyroidism which may be permanent. Thyroid surgery to remove part or all of the thyroid gland results in insufficient tissue left to produce thyroxine. Radiation treatments for head and neck cancers often cannot spare the thyroid gland, causing an inability to produce thyroid hormone. Replacement therapy will be necessary for life. Medicines taken for other conditions may also contribute to hypothyroidism. Lithium, a drug used to treat psychiatric conditions, is the most common example.

Less common causes of hypothyroidism may include congenital disease, a benign tumor of the pituitary gland that leaves it unable to produce thyroid-stimulating hormone (TSH), pregnancy, and iodine deficiency. Infants may be born without a thyroid gland or may have a defective gland due to an inherited disorder. Most states require newborn testing for thyroid disease. Hypothyroidism may be present during fetus development, before birth, or during childhood, leading to reduced physical growth and mental delays.

Pregnant women with hyperthyroidism or hypothyroidism should be monitored carefully during pregnancy. Iodine is an essential mineral for the production of thyroid hormones that can be obtained from seafood, plants grown in iodine rich soil, and iodized salt. Iodized salt has limited this causative factor in the U.S., but other parts of the world may routinely see iodine deficiency leading to hypothyroidism. It is important to read labels when purchasing salt as both iodized and non-iodized are available.

Too little thyroxine may cause a person to feel colder, experience fatigue, become forgetful and depressed, gain weight, develop elevated cholesterol levels, or experience thinning hair, a puffy face, muscle aches, joint swelling, or dry skin. Low levels of thyroid hormone may contribute to infertility, peripheral neuropathy (damage to nerves of the arms and legs) leading to pain, numbness and tingling, and an increased risk of heart disease resulting from an enlarged heart and heart failure. Myxedema, an advanced form of hypothyroidism, may be life threatening due to lowered blood pressure, slowed breathing, or a coma.

Treatment for hypothyroidism requires the patient to take a daily dose of a synthetic thyroid hormone such as levothyroxine (*Levothroid, Synthroid* and others) to restore normal levels of thyroxine thus reversing the symptoms of the disease. Dosage must be adjusted based on blood tests conducted every two to three months until levels are within acceptable range of normal. Once the appropriate dosage is determined, annual check-ups are used to monitor the disease. If the patient has existing heart disease, initial doses may start very low and gradually increase to allow the heart to get used to the increased metabolism. There are virtually no side effects related to levothyroxine, and treatment is almost always life-long. A patient should not stop taking thyroid replacement hormones unless told by the doctor, as symptoms will gradually return if a patient ceases taking medication. The patient should take the hormone first thing in the morning with water and then wait an hour before consuming coffee or food. Multivitamins with iron, some antacids, calcium, and other drugs may interfere with thyroid hormone, so a patent should confer with as doctor about when to take other substances in relation to the dose of hormone.

PERSPECTIVES AND PROSPECTS

Natural extracts that contain thyroid hormone derived from the thyroid glands of pigs are sometimes taken by patients with hypothyroidism. Such extracts are only available by prescription and should not be confused with the glandular concentrates sold in natural food store. These extracts are not approved by the U.S. Food and Drug Administration. The safety, potency and purity of these products is not guaranteed.

In the future, stem cell treatments for hypothyroidism may become a reality. In 2015, scientists from the Boston University School of Medicine and the Beth Israel Deaconess Medical Center reported the production of functional thyroid tissue from stem cells. This work solved a long-standing problem that prevented stem cell scientists from inducing the differentiation of pluripotent stem cells into mature thyroid tissue. With this new success, animal trials have begun, and human trials might be realized one day.

—*Janine Ungvarsky*
Updated by Patricia Stanfill Edens, PhD, RN, LFACHE

FOR FURTHER INFORMATION

Brady, Bridget. *Thyroid Gland: Overview.* EndocrineWeb, 6 July 2018, www.endocrineweb.com/conditions/thyroid-nodules/thyroid-gland-controls-bodys-metabolism-how-it-works-symptoms-hyperthyroi.

"Hashimoto Thyroiditis." *Genetics Home Reference,* U.S. National Library of Medicine, Feb. 2018, ghr.nlm.nih.gov/condition/hashimoto-thyroiditis.

"Hyperthyroidism." *MedlinePlus,* 24 July 2016, medlineplus.gov/ency/article/000356.htm.

"Hyperthyroidism." *National Institute of Diabetes and Kidney and Digestive Issues,* www.niddk.nih.gov/health-information/health-topics/endocrine/hyperthyroidism/Pages/fact-sheet.aspx.

"Hyperthyroidism." *University of Maryland Medical Center,* 27 Apr. 2016, umm.edu/health/medical/altmed/condition/hyperthyroidism.

"Hyperthyroidism (Overactive)." *American Thyroid Association,* www.thyroid.org/hyperthyroidism/

"Hypothyroidism (Underactive)" *American Thyroid Association,* www.thyroid.org/hypothyroidism/.

Kurmann, Anita A., et al. "Regeneration of Thyroid Function by Transplantation of Differentiated Pluripotent Stem Cells." *Cell Stem Cell,* vol. 17, no. 5, 5 Nov. 2015, pp. 527–542.

Lee, Stephanie L., et al. "Hyperthyroidism." *MedScape,* 13 July 2016, emedicine.medscape.com/article/121865-overview.

"Thyroid Disease." *Womenshealth.gov,* Office on Women's Health, 13 Nov. 2018, www.womenshealth.gov/a-z-topics/thyroid-disease.

"Thyroid Tests." *National Institute of Diabetes and Digestive and Kidney Diseases,* U.S. Department of Health and Human Services, May 2017, www.niddk.nih.gov/health-information/diagnostic-tests/thyroid.

Hypogonadism

CATEGORY: Disease/Disorder

KEY TERMS:

estrogen: a group of steroid hormones synthesized from cholesterol that promote the development and maintenance of female characteristics

follicle-stimulating hormone: a peptide hormone secreted by the anterior lobe of the pituitary gland, also called follitropin, that stimulates the growth of the ovum-containing follicles in the ovaries

gonadotropin releasing hormone: a peptide hormone synthesized in and secreted by the hypothalamus that stimulates the anterior lobe of the pituitary gland to secrete gonadotropins, which include follicle-stimulating hormone and luteinizing hormone

luteinizing hormone: a peptide hormone secreted by the anterior lobe of the pituitary gland that stimulates: ovulation of ova from Graafian follicles and the development of the corpora lutea after ovulation in the

testosterone: a sex steroid hormone synthesized from cholesterol that is the main male sex hormone, though is also present in women

CAUSES AND SYMPTOMS

Hypogonadism is a condition in which there is a decrease in one or both major functions of the gonads: the production of gametes and the production of sex hormones. Hypogonadism can arise at different times during human development, and the timing of its appearance determines the signs and symptoms it elicits. For example, when the body does not produce enough sex hormones during fetal development, the result might be that the external sex organs might fail to grow to the anticipated size. When hypogonadism occurs before puberty, a girl will not begin menstruating, and breast development and height might be limited. When hypogonadism occurs after puberty, women can experience symptoms such as hot flashes, loss of body hair, irregular menstruation, and low libido. The ovaries become suppressed, resulting in infertility, decreased libido, breast atrophy, and osteoporosis.

The ovaries work in concert with two parts of the brain: the hypothalamic region and the pituitary gland. The gonads (sex hormones), hypothalamus, and the pituitary gland function together to help the body reach and maintain puberty. The hypothalamus releases a hormone called gonadotropin-releasing hormone (GnRH). GnRH stimulates the pituitary gland to secrete two other hormones, follicle-stimulating hormone (FSH) and luteinizing hormone (LH). The FSH and LH stimulate the and ovary to function and produce sex steroids: predominantly estrogen. In turn, the increased blood levels of these sex steroids cause the pituitary gland

to reduce the amount of FSH and LH it produces. If this system is perturbed at any level, hypogonadism may arise.

Primary hypogonadism results from a disease of the ovaries, while secondary hypogonadism is caused by disease of the hypothalamus or pituitary gland. Hypogonadism can also be congenital, if due to conditions present at birth, or acquired, if a disease that affects the hypothalamus-pituitary axis is acquired after birth.

Some causes of primary congenital hypogonadism include chromosomal abnormalities such as Turner syndrome (X) in females; mutations in genes that encode receptors for gonadotropins (FSH receptor and LH receptor) or enzymes for sex steroid synthesis (e.g., 3β-hydroxysteroid dehydrogenase, 17α-hydroxylase), and mutations that cause premature ovarian failure in women (e.g., Fragile X syndrome, *BMP-15*).

Acquired primary hypogonadism may result from infection, autoimmune disorders, liver disease, certain drugs (alkylating and antineoplastic agents, ketoconazole, the anti-parasitic drug suramin, glucocorticoids), environmental toxins (e.g., dibromochloropropane), trauma to the ovaries, kidney disease, surgery, or radiation.

Congenital secondary hypogonadism can result from inherited mutations in GnRH, genes that encode gonadotropins (LH and FSH), leptin or the leptin receptor, or transcription factors required for pituitary development (*LHX3 & 4, HESX1, PROP1*). Additionally, congenital syndromes that affect the development of the hypothalamus, such as Prader-Willi syndrome, and Kallmann Syndrome, a disorder that also causes a reduced sense of smell, can also cause congenital secondary hypogonadism.

Acquired secondary hypogonadism typically occurs because of diseases of the hypothalamus or the pituitary gland. Therefore, trauma, excess iron, surgery, bleeding in the pituitary gland, tumors, strokes, or radiation that injures the hypothalamus and/or pituitary gland can cause acquired secondary hypogonadism. Additionally, prolonged use of GnRH analogs (e.g., triptorelin, goserelin, leuprolide, gonadorelin, histrelin), steroids, and opiates can suppress sex hormone production and cause hypogonadism, as can critical and chronic systemic illness, anorexia nervosa, nutritional deficiencies, rapid weight loss, obesity, sleep apnea, and diabetes mellitus.

Though not fatal, hypogonadism can cause additional health problems such as anemia, osteoporosis, and infertility in both men and women. To diagnose hypogonadism, medical professionals are likely to test hormone levels. In females, they will test for estrogen, and in males, for testosterone. Additionally, they will test levels of the hormones LH and FSH. Other commonly administered tests measure thyroid hormones and prolactin, which is a hormone released by the pituitary gland that stimulates breast development and milk production and decreases gonadotropin production. Some doctors might also test for anemia and possible genetic disorders. Women who are suspected to have hypogonadism might be sent for a sonogram of their ovaries. If doctors suspect pituitary disease, they might send her for an MRI or CT scan for a better examination of the pituitary gland.

TREATMENT AND THERAPY

Hormone replacement therapy can effectively treat hypogonadism in women who have not yet reached menopause. Estrogen and progesterone, either in pill or skin patch formulations, can be effectively prescribed to girls and women. Women who have a low sex drive might be prescribed a low dose of testosterone.

Restoring fertility to people with central hypogonadism can be difficult. For some women, hormones in the form of injections or pills can stimulate ovulation, which means the patient will produce eggs that can be fertilized to cause pregnancy. Successful pregnancies have been reported in women who were impregnated with embryos made from their own eggs and sperm from men with primary hypogonadism, such as Klinefelter syndrome. In these cases, sperm was surgically extracted from the testes and used to fertilize the eggs through in vitro fertilization by intracytoplasmic sperm injection.

– Gilan Gertz MSW
Updated by Michael A. Buratovich PhD

FOR FURTHER INFORMATION

Stamou M. I., and Georgopoulos, N. A. "Kallmann syndrome: phenotype and genotype of hypogonadotropic hypogonadism." *Metabolism*, vol. 86, 2018, 124-134. doi: 10.1016/j.metabol.2017.10.012.
Topaloglu, A. K., and Kotan, L. D. "Genetics of Hypogonadotropic Hypogonadism." *Endocr Dev*, vol. 29, 2016, 36-49. doi: 10.1159/000438841.
Trotman, G. E., "Delayed puberty in the female patient." *Current Opinion in Obstetrics and Gynecology*, vol. 28, no. 5, 2016, 366-372.
Vogiatzi, M. G. "Hypogonadism Treatment & Management." *Medscape*, 11 February, 2018, https://emedicine.medscape.com/article/922038-treatment.

Hysterectomy

CATEGORY: Procedure

KEY TERMS:

adenomyosis: a noncancerous disorder in which cells resembling the lining of the uterus are found within the muscle layer of the uterus, leading to abnormal vaginal bleeding and pain

estrogen: the female sex hormone produced by the ovaries and the adrenal gland that is responsible for the development of female secondary sex characteristics; the three types naturally produced by the body are estradiol, estrone, and estriol

Fallopian tubes: the structures located between the uterus and ovaries that are responsible for the transport of the egg; also called the oviducts

fibroid: a noncancerous tumor of the uterus, also known as leiomyoma; when large, these tumors can cause heavy menstrual bleeding leading to anemia or cause pressure symptoms in the pelvis

laparoscopy: a minimally invasive surgical procedure in which an instrument equipped with a small camera, called a laparoscope, is inserted through a small incision in the abdomen to visualize the pelvis or abdomen; surgical manipulation may be carried out during this procedure

menorrhagia: unusually heavy menstrual bleeding; when severe, it can lead to anemia

progesterone/progestin: a hormone produced in the ovaries that sustains pregnancy; birth control pills are composed primarily of progesterone, which works by suppressing ovulation

INDICATIONS AND PROCEDURES

The term "hysterectomy" comes from the Greek *hystera,* meaning "uterus," and *ektome,* meaning "to cut out." While hysterectomy refers to the removal of the uterus and, most commonly, the attached Fallopian tubes, there are several types of hysterectomies. Total hysterectomy, contrary to popular belief, does not mean that the ovaries are removed with the uterus. Rather, the term indicates the removal of the uterus and cervix. Subtotal, or partial, hysterectomy is the excision of the uterus above the cervix; the cervix is left in place. Either one or both ovaries may be removed with the uterus (unilateral oophorectomy or bilateral oophorectomy). Salpingo-oophorectomy refers to the removal of one of the Fallopian tubes along with the accompanying ovary, while bilateral salpingo-oophorectomy refers to the removal of both Fallopian tubes and ovaries.

Indications for hysterectomy can be divided into noncancerous and cancerous conditions. Within the noncancerous category, the most common indication for hysterectomy is symptomatic fibroids. Many women have fibroids, and the majority of fibroids do not cause symptoms and can be left alone. Symptomatic fibroids are those which are large enough to cause pressure symptoms in the pelvis, compress the bladder or rectum, or cause pain or discomfort during intercourse. Another type of symptomatic fibroids are those which cause excessively heavy menstrual bleeding and, when severe, anemia.

A hysterectomy is indicated in these situations if the patient fails to respond to less conservative therapy for symptomatic fibroids. Examples of conservative therapy for heavy bleeding include high-dose estrogen or birth control pills. A hysterectomy is usually performed only when childbearing is no longer desired, since removal of the uterus precludes pregnancy. Prior to hysterectomy, large fibroids may be shrunk with a course of a hormone called gonadotropin-releasing hormone. Unfortunately, this treatment results in menopausal symptoms, including hot flushes and bone density depletion, and therefore cannot be used for prolonged periods of time. More recently, treatments such as uterine artery embolization, in which the arteries feeding the uterus are blocked off using foreign particles such as gel foam, have been tried as an alternative to hysterectomy, in an attempt to preserve the uterus and avoid major surgery.

Another indication for hysterectomy is in patients who have had recurrent fibroids after myomectomy. A myomectomy is the surgical removal of isolated fibroids, rather than removal of the uterus itself. The benefit is that the uterus can be preserved, although the downside is that fibroids may regrow. Hysterectomy is the definitive treatment for uterine fibroids.

Another noncancerous indication for hysterectomy is adenomyosis, a painful condition whereby the cells of the uterine lining are abnormally embedded in the uterine muscle. No good treatments exist for this condition besides hysterectomy. Another indication for hysterectomy occurs in cases of abnormal uterine bleeding in which the bleeding is refractory to management with nonsurgical treatments, such as birth control pills or procedures that ablate the uterine lining.

Other less common indications for hysterectomy are uterine prolapse (in which the uterus descends into the vaginal canal, causing discomfort or urinary incontinence), chronic pelvic pain (refractory to more conservative management), and large infections of the uterus and pelvis that are unresponsive to antibiotics. Hysterectomy may also be performed as part of a cesarean section if the surgeon encounters uncontrollable bleeding after delivery of the infant.

Uterine cancer is a clear indication for hysterectomy. Often, the cancer causes abnormal uterine bleeding. Prior to hysterectomy, the cancer has usually been confirmed on biopsy of the uterine lining. If

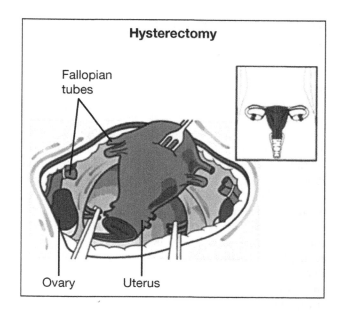

The uterus, and sometimes such accompanying organs as the ovaries and Fallopian tubes, may be removed to treat disease conditions or as a contraceptive measure; the inset shows the location of the uterus. © EBSCO

the cancer is small and localized to a small area of the uterus, then removal of the uterus alone may be curative. More often, however, uterine cancer may have spread more deeply into the uterine wall or even grown beyond the uterus. In these cases, hysterectomy may be accompanied by more extensive surgery that includes removing lymph nodes or other pelvic structures.

Most frequently, hysterectomy is accomplished through a 6- to 8-inch midline incision running either down from the navel or across the lower abdomen near or below the hairline (known as a "bikini incision"). This procedure is referred to as an abdominal hysterectomy. Vaginal hysterectomy is the removal of the uterus through the vaginal canal, rather than through a surgical opening in the abdomen. This procedure is most often performed to resolve prolapse (because the uterus has already descended into the vaginal canal) or when the uterus is not massively enlarged and can be pulled down and out through the vagina. If the hysterectomy is performed because of large fibroid tumors, then the abdominal approach is usually used. On rare occasions, a vaginal hysterectomy may be facilitated using laparoscopy. In these cases, laparoscopy enables visualization and manipulation of the uterus via small incisions in the abdomen to assist in removal of the uterus through the vaginal canal.

During the hysterectomy, the patient is almost always under general anesthesia. The patient lies on her back for abdominal hysterectomies. In vaginal hysterectomies, the patient's legs are placed in stirrups and the knees are spread apart to enable the gynecologist to gain access to the vaginal canal. The actual removal of the uterus involves clamping, transecting, and suture ligating the blood vessels that feed the uterus and the tissues that anchor the uterus in the pelvic cavity. Care is taken by the surgeon to avoid the ureters, the tubes carrying urine from the kidney to the bladder. The ureters are very close to the lower part of the uterus and can be damaged easily. If the entire uterus is removed, then the top end of the vagina, called the cuff, is sutured closed. If the cervix is left in place, then the top of the cervix is sutured closed.

After the surgery, the patient receives narcotic pain medication and antibiotics to prevent infection and is monitored carefully to confirm that vital signs are stable, and recovery is appropriate. Laboratory tests may be performed to ensure that the patient is not unusually anemic and that important organs such as the kidneys are functioning properly. Until a patient is able to walk, a catheter (a rubber tube attached to a collecting bag) will be used to pass urine. Patients may initially take liquids by mouth. When they can tolerate liquids, indicating no apparent injury to the bowels, patients may begin to take solid food. A patient may be hospitalized for two to four days after the hysterectomy, although hospital stays in general have been shortening in length. On the whole, patients who receive vaginal hysterectomies have shorter hospital stays than patients receiving abdominal hysterectomies, assuming that no complications arise. Patients can usually resume normal sexual functioning six weeks after the surgery.

USES AND COMPLICATIONS

Hysterectomy can be used to provide relief from pressure, pain, and bleeding from the uterus. It may also be curative in the early stages of uterine cancer and can increase survival in later stages. For women who are finished with childbearing and whose lifestyles or responsibilities do not allow them to try more conservative treatments, many of which require several months to take effect, hysterectomy can provide definitive relief from symptoms within the defined time period needed to undergo scheduled surgery. In cases of life-threatening uterine hemorrhage, hysterectomy can save a woman's life.

The common complications of hysterectomy are those which are common to many major surgeries. One complication is excessive blood loss. The average blood loss during a hysterectomy is estimated at between 400 and 500 cubic centimeters (about a pint). When removal of the uterus is difficult, for instance because of the position of large fibroids, increased blood loss is likely to occur. When excessive blood loss is of concern, the patient's blood levels may be checked during the procedure. A patient who is significantly anemic may receive blood transfusions to avoid poor oxygenation of the major organs and to increase blood volume, and hence avoid shock. The number of transfusions depends on the amount of blood estimated to be lost. If a blood vessel continues to bleed after the patient leaves the operating room, then the patient may need to return to the operating room to have the bleeding vessel identified and sutured.

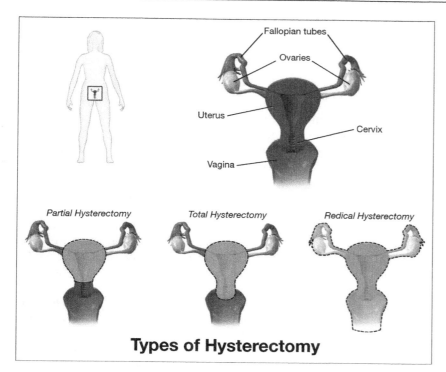

Types of Hysterectomy

(BruceBlaus via Wikimedia Commons)

Another common complication of hysterectomy is infection. Even when aseptic techniques are followed, an infection may develop several days after the surgery. This is particularly true in vaginal hysterectomies, where the surgeon works through the vaginal canal, considered a clean but contaminated field. For this reason, patients are given antibiotics immediately prior to surgery in order to prevent infection. A patient who shows signs of infection after the surgery may be placed on an extended course of antibiotics. The source of these infections can range from the vaginal cuff site to the peritoneum (the lining of the pelvic and abdominal cavity) and the urinary tract.

The third major complication that can occur with hysterectomy is inadvertent damage to internal organs. The urinary tract and the bowels are particularly at risk during hysterectomy because of their proximity to the uterus. The ureters can be occluded inadvertently by the misplacement of a suture. If discovered early, this damage can be repaired. If the problem is not recognized, however, then a damaged ureter can result in kidney malfunction. For this reason, kidney function is carefully followed after the hysterectomy through blood tests. Since the bladder sits on the bottom half of the uterus, it is a common organ that can be damaged during a hysterectomy. If the bladder is accidentally entered using the scalpel during surgery, then it can usually be repaired during the procedure. Postsurgery, the patient may need prolonged catheterization of the bladder to enhance bladder recovery.

The large and small intestines are another common site of surgical injury. They can be accidentally cut or sutured. Sometimes, this problem is not detected until after the patient has left the operating room, and the problem becomes apparent when normal bowel function does not return in a timely fashion postoperatively. The patient may experience nausea, vomiting, and abdominal distension and discomfort and may not be able to pass gas from the rectum.

Another complication that can occur after surgery is the formation of blood clots, particularly in the leg veins, as a result of the patient's immobility during and after surgery. These clots can be dangerous when they break off from their source and move into the lungs, a condition called pulmonary embolism. Large pulmonary emboli can be life-threatening. Pulmonary emboli can be prevented using warm compression stockings during and after surgery to promote blood flow. Early ambulation (walking) after surgery can also decrease the chances of developing leg vein clots and pulmonary emboli.

Long-term complications of hysterectomy also include scar formation in the pelvis, called adhesions, which can interfere with bowel function or cause pelvic pain. Some patients may experience the prolapse of the remaining pelvic organs (such as the bowels and bladder) into the space formerly occupied by the uterus. Procedures may be employed during the hysterectomy to anchor the vaginal cuff and close any spaces where prolapse might occur.

In rare cases, removal of the uterus can inadvertently decrease blood supply to any remaining ovaries, leading to ischemia and loss of ovarian function.

In these cases, the patient may experience the symptoms of estrogen deficiency, also known as menopausal symptoms. They include hot flashes, vaginal dryness, and, when estrogen deficiency is prolonged, bone density loss. In women whose hysterectomies included removal of the ovaries, the hot flashes may become apparent a few days after surgery. In these cases, estrogen therapy or other medications may be of benefit.

The impact of a hysterectomy on a woman's psychological state varies from woman to woman. In women who have been suffering a great deal from their symptoms, be it pressure and pain or abnormal bleeding, a hysterectomy can be a relief and enable them to return to their activities of daily living. Hysterectomy can improve sexual function in many cases. In other women, a hysterectomy can trigger a sense of loss and represent the end of the woman's fertility, which is often associated with youth and vitality.

PERSPECTIVE AND PROSPECTS

In ancient times, the complaints of women and the illnesses of the female organs were viewed as coming from an "unhappy uterus." It was believed that the uterus had the primary purpose of childbearing and that, when the uterus was not occupied with this function, it might show its wrath by abnormal bleeding and pain. These beliefs prevailed for centuries; early medical history indicates that women's gynecologic complaints were largely ignored. Moreover, no safe surgical procedures had been developed.

A noteworthy event in early American medical history was the operation attempted and documented by a frontier physician and surgeon, Ephraim McDowell. In 1809 in Danville, Kentucky, this daring young doctor carried out experimental surgery on a middle-aged woman to remove a huge ovarian tumor. Without the benefit of anesthesia and a sterile technique, he performed successful abdominal surgery on four out of five other patients.

Myomectomy, or removal of a fibroid tumor of the uterus, was the next procedure to be performed—first in France and later (about 1850) in Massachusetts by Washington Atlee. The first hysterectomy was successfully performed by Walter Burnham in the same decade, but he lost twelve of his next fifteen hysterectomy patients. In the text *Operative Gynecology* (1898), Howard A. Kelly of Baltimore describes one hundred hysterectomies that he performed in the late nineteenth century, all done because of pelvic infection. He lost only four patients, though convalescence for some survivors was prolonged.

Remarkable medical progress occurred in the nineteenth century in abdominal and vaginal surgical techniques. In the 1850s, Marion Sims of South Carolina was the first to perform vaginal surgery in the United States. He successfully repaired a vesicovaginal fistula, an abnormal opening between the bladder and the vagina through which urine escapes into the vagina. In the late nineteenth century, the "Manchester" operation for uterine prolapse was performed by A. Donald in Manchester, England. Prior to this procedure, uterine prolapse was treated with a pessary, a device inserted into the vagina to hold the uterus in place.

In the 1930s, N. Sproat Heaney of Chicago devised the present-day technique of vaginal hysterectomy. Vaginal (as opposed to abdominal) hysterectomy, it was believed, resulted in a less complicated procedure with shorter convalescence and more cosmetically pleasing results for most patients. For some time, vaginal hysterectomy was viewed as superior to abdominal hysterectomy. In the 1970s, between 25 and 40 percent of all hysterectomies were accomplished vaginally, depending on the age of the woman at the time of surgery. In 1981, however, a landmark study published by the US Congress, weighing the costs, risks, and benefits of hysterectomy, stated that women undergoing vaginal hysterectomy are more likely to have postoperative fever and to receive antibiotic treatment. Moreover, vaginal hysterectomy patients may undergo further surgery at a rate as high as 5 to 10 percent.

By the late 1980s and early 1990s, the trend among many gynecologists had shifted away from hysterectomy to more conservative treatments, when possible. Physicians began to question whether hysterectomies were, in some or even in most cases, medically necessary. As more information became available to women regarding alternatives to hysterectomy (a major revenue-producing surgical procedure in the United States), many women became more apt to question their physicians when told that hysterectomy was the only possible solution to their gynecological problems.

—*Genevieve Slomski, Ph.D.;*
Updated by Anne Lynn S. Chang, M.D.

FOR FURTHER INFORMATION

Clark, Jan. *Hysterectomy and the Alternatives: How to Ask the Right Questions and Explore Other Options.* Rev. ed. London: Vermilion, 2000.

Doherty, Gerard M., and Lawrence W. Way, eds. *Current Surgical Diagnosis and Treatment.* 12th ed. New York: Lange Medical Books/McGraw-Hill, 2006.

"Hysterectomy - Endometriosis - Fibroids." *Medline-Plus*, U.S. National Library of Medicine, 17 June 2016, medlineplus.gov/hysterectomy.html.

"Hysterectomy." *Womenshealth.gov*, Office on Women's Health, 15 Oct. 2018, www.womenshealth.gov/a-z-topics/hysterectomy.

"Hysterectomy—Laparoscopic Surgery." *Health Library*, March 15, 2013.

"Hysterectomy—Open Surgery." *Health Library*, September 27, 2012.

Ikram, M., et al. "Hysterectomy Comparison of Laparoscopic Assisted Vaginal Versus Total Abdominal Hysterectomy." *Professional Medical Journal* vol. 19, no. 2, March/April, 2012: 214–220.

Moore, Michele C., and Caroline M. de Costa. *Do You Really Need Surgery? A Sensible Guide to Hysterectomy and Other Procedures for Women.* New Brunswick, N.J.: Rutgers University Press, 2004.

Stenchever, Morton A., et al. *Comprehensive Gynecology.* 5th ed. St. Louis, Mo.: Mosby/Elsevier, 2007.

I

Immunodeficiency disorders

CATEGORY: Disease/Disorder

KEY TERMS:

antibody: protein immunoglobulin secreted by B lymphocytes; the production of antibodies is induced by specific foreign invaders, and they combine with and destroy only those invaders

B lymphocytes: also referred to as B cells; white cells of the immune system that produce antibodies; produced within the bone marrow

phagocytes: white cells of the immune system that destroy invading foreign bodies by engulfing and digesting them in a nonspecific immune response; include macrophages and neutrophils

stem cells: multipotential precursor cells within the bone marrow that develop into white cell populations, including lymphocytes and phagocytic cells

T lymphocyte: a type of immune cell that kills host cells infected by bacteria or viruses and secretes chemicals (interleukins) that regulate the immune response

CAUSES AND SYMPTOMS

The defense of the body against foreign invaders is provided by the immune system. In nonspecific immunity, phagocytic cells engulf and destroy invading particles. Specific immunity consists of very specialized cell types that are synthesized in response to a particular type of foreign invader. Self-replicating stem cells within the bone marrow give rise to lymphocytes, which mediate specific immunity. Lymphocytes establish self-replacing colonies within the thymus, spleen, and lymph nodes. The various categories of T lymphocytes are derived from the thymus colonies, while B lymphocytes develop and mature within the bone marrow. B lymphocytes secrete highly specific antibodies that attack bacteria and some viruses.

T lymphocytes do not secrete antibodies. Cytotoxic T cells directly attack body cells that have been infected with a bacterium or virus, while helper T cells regulate the immune response, either by directly interacting with other lymphocytes or by secreting chemicals, called interleukins, that regulate those cells. In immunodeficiency disorders, some or all of these defenses are compromised, which can have life-threatening consequences. Immunodeficiency diseases are generally the result of germinal cell lines or genetic abnormalities, are present from birth and can be passed to offspring; others may be somatically acquired through infection or exposure to damaging drug or radiation treatments and are not passed along to the next generation by sexual means. Depending upon the specific defect, the result may range from limited defects involving a class of cells to an entire shutdown of the immune system; prognosis depends on the severity of the defect.

The most severe immunodeficiency disorder is attributable to the absence of stem cells, which results in a total lack of both B and T lymphocytes. This rare genetic condition is referred to as severe combined immunodeficiency syndrome (SCID). Affected infants show a failure to thrive from birth and can easily die from common bacterial or viral infections. The term SCID encompasses a variety of genetic deficiencies. Certain forms are sex-linked, while other types may be autosomal (non-sex-linked). The most common autosomal form is a deficiency in the enzyme adenosine deaminase, resulting in disruption of deoxyribonucleic acid (DNA) synthesis in the stem cells.

Major syndromes that involve defects specific to the T lymphocyte population are characterized by recurrent viral and fungal infections. DiGeorge syndrome results from improper development of the thymus, which in turn results in insufficient production of T lymphocytes, often accompanied by other structural abnormalities in the infant. In severe cases, death results in early childhood from overwhelming viral infections.

The most common disorders affecting B lymphocytes are forms of hypogammaglobulinemia. This condition is characterized by insufficient levels of antibody. The cause is generally associated with increased rates of antibody breakdown or loss in the urine secondary to kidney malfunction. Bruton's agammaglobulinemia is a rare, sex-linked form of the condition, in which B cells fail to mature properly. Severe bacterial infections are the most common symptom. When the disorder is left untreated, infants generally die of severe pneumonia prior to six months of age.

Several immunodeficiency disorders may be the result of partial defects in the production and/or function of B and T lymphocytes. Wiskott-Aldrich syndrome is a genetically inherited disease manifested by recurrent infections and an itchy, scaly inflammation of the skin. Certain classes of antibodies are absent or scarce. Chronic mucocutaneous candidiasis is characterized by chronic fungal infection of the skin and mucous membranes; reduced levels of T cells are responsible for this disfiguring disorder.

Immunodeficiency disorders may also be the result of defects in phagocytic cells; the underlying cause of most of these disorders is ill-defined but often involves deficiencies in hydrolytic enzymes. In chronic granulomatosis, an inherited enzyme deficiency prevents the immune system from destroying bacteria that have been phagocytized. Infants affected by this disorder develop severe infections and chronic inflammations of internal organs and bones. The bacteria responsible for these infections are generally common flora that are not considered pathogens in healthy individuals. Immune disorders may involve defects in antibody production.

However, certain forms of inherited disorders involve another group of proteins called complement. Complement actually represents a group of serum proteins that interact with each other in a series. The pathway may be activated either specifically from antibody-target interactions or nonspecifically by surface components of certain bacteria. Intermediates in the complement pathway attract or stimulate phagocytosis (opsonins), induce inflammation, and play roles in cell destruction. Some of the intermediates are enzymes that regulate the activation of complement components. The most important intermediate in the pathway is the C3 component. C3 is a protein that acts as an opsonin and at the same time is involved in activating later steps in the sequence. Defects in C3 result in increased susceptibility to infection. Similar immune problems may result from defects in other complement intermediates.

DISEASES AND DISORDERS

Most of the disorders that affect the immune system are not inherited but develop sometime during the person's life. They are either the result of an infection or a consequence of another disease or its treatment. The use of corticosteroids to treat inflammations, or the illicit use of them in muscle-building, can interfere with the proper production and function of T lymphocytes. Other immunosuppressive drugs used to diminish the possibilities of graft or transplant rejection, or in the treatment of autoimmune diseases, can severely depress antibody production. Chemotherapeutic agents used in the treatment of cancer can affect DNA replication and severely compromise the entire immune system. Whole-body radiation can damage or destroy bone marrow stem cells.

The presence or absence of a Y chromosome influences the risk for autoimmune disease. For most autoimmune diseases, women are generally more affected than men. In multiple sclerosis (MS), the gap is modest, but in primary biliary cholangitis (PBC), that gap gets wider. MS is the most common neurological autoimmune disease, affects the brain and central nervous system; the immune system attacks the protective sheath that surrounds nerve fibers and disrupts the communication between the brain and other parts of the body. Women are around three times as likely to develop MS. PBC eventually results in the destruction of the bile ducts in the liver, possibly resulting in scarring of the tissue (cirrhosis). Data has suggested that women are ten times as likely to develop PBC.

The gender gap seen in cases of systemic lupus erythematosus (SLE) is very wide, with an estimated 9:1 ration of women to men developing the disease. SLE causes the immune system to attack healthy tissue found anywhere in the body, most commonly affecting the joints. The reason SLE affects more women is not officially determined, but many have suggested that sex hormones play an integral part. The age range during which most women develop SLE is the reproductive age, after puberty and before menopause, suggesting that high levels of estrogen and low levels of progesterone play a part.

Acquired immunodeficiency syndrome (AIDS) is caused by the human immunodeficiency virus (HIV). HIV is transmitted primarily through unprotected sexual contact, sharing of needles for intravenous drug use, transfusion with contaminated blood products, or contact with contaminated body fluids. HIV specifically infects one type of regulatory T lymphocyte, the helper T cell, resulting in severe immune depression. The virus may be harbored in an inapparent form for years. A much higher proportion of gay and bisexual men have HIV compared to any other group in the United States. Most gay and bisexual men get HIV from having anal sex without using condoms or taking medicines to prevent or treat HIV. Homophobia, stigma, and discrimination are potential drivers for increased prevalence of HIV in this population.

Initial symptoms of HIV may be quite mild, but they generally progress so that the affected individual becomes susceptible to a host of opportunistic bacterial and fungal infections. A rare form of cancer called Kaposi's sarcoma is associated with infection by a particular human herpesvirus, HHV8, in persons with AIDS. AIDS also produces neurological damage in about one-third of infected individuals.

TREATMENT AND THERAPY

Most treatment of immunodeficient individuals is palliative. Infections are treated with antibiotics whenever possible. Individuals are counseled to avoid situations in which they may be exposed to contagious agents.

Treatment of immunodeficiency disorders may also target the source of the deficiency. For example, in DiGeorge syndrome, characterized by the congenital absence of the thymus, fetal thymus transplants may correct the problem, with improvement in lymphocyte levels seen within hours after the transplants. The use of thymus extracts has also been beneficial. Syndromes such as hypogammaglobulinemia can be managed by injection with mixtures of antibodies. Drug therapy to substitute for some immune components absent in Wiskott-Aldrich syndrome has been shown to have variable effects. The most effective treatment for chronic mucocutaneous candidiasis is aggressive antifungal medication to eradicate the causative organism; treatment must continue for several months because fungal infections are slow to respond to therapy and frequently recur. Chronic granulomatosis is notoriously difficult to treat, and the most effective therapy has been antibiotic and antifungal agents used aggressively during an overt infection.

Because of the magnitude of the defects, many inherited immunodeficiency disorders are difficult to treat successfully and are commonly fatal early in life.

Chronic granulomatosis is usually fatal within the first few years of life, and only about 20 percent of patients reach the age of twenty. SCID is a serious disorder in which affected infants can die before a proper diagnosis is made. For individuals with these and other serious immunodeficiency disorders, maintenance in an environment free of bacteria, viruses, and fungi, such as a sterile "bubble," has been the best means to prevent life-threatening infections. Such an approach, however, precludes the possibility of a normal life. The most effective treatment for individuals with severely compromised immune systems is bone marrow transplantation. In this procedure, bone marrow from a compatible individual is introduced into the bone marrow of the patient. If the procedure works—and the success rate is high—in approximately one to six months the transplant recipient's immune system will be reconstituted and functional; full recovery may take up to one year. Bone marrow transplantation is a permanent cure for these disorders, since the transplanted marrow will contain stem cells that produce all the cell types of the immune system. The difficulties in transplantation include finding a compatible donor and preventing infections during the period after the transplant.

Prevention of HIV including using condoms is efficacious. Moreover, use of medications such as pre-exposure prophylaxis, a daily pill, lowers a patient's chance of acquiring HIV by over 90 percent. Candidates for pre-exposure prophylaxis include those who are not HIV positive and are at a higher risk of HIV infection such as gay and bisexual men, sex workers, and intravenous drug users.

Drug therapy for AIDS utilizes treatments that interfere with replication of the virus. The first drug to be approved for use was zidovudine (formerly AZT), a DNA analogue, but its success was somewhat limited, as it was associated with severe side effects and the creation of resistant virus. More recent treatments utilize drug "cocktails," combinations of drugs that act at different stages of viral replication. Vaccines and antibiotic therapy are used to prevent or treat the opportunistic illnesses that accompany AIDS. Various drugs may also help to ease symptoms of AIDS such as appetite disturbances, nausea, pain, insomnia, anxiety, depression, fever, and diarrhea. A combination of therapies has been shown to increase life expectancy in AIDS patients. Many patients choose to participate in clinical trials of experimental drugs not approved for general use in the hope that the new drug will be more effective at alleviating the disease. Others seek out alternative or nontraditional medical treatments that have a long history of use in Western cultures. These treatments include acupuncture, herbology, meditation, and homeopathy. An holistic aspect of therapy for HIV infected and AIDS patients is maintaining mental health through support groups and supportive caregivers.

Illicit use of corticosteroids can seriously compromise the immune system and may lead to permanent damage. The best therapy for this type of acquired immunodeficiency is prevention— that is, to not misuse the drugs. In their supervised use to control inflammation or other disease symptoms, normal immune function will return after treatment has been completed. A huge risk to cancer patients who are being treated with chemotherapy and/or radiation therapy is the depression of the immune system, which can lead to a host of infections being contracted and not easily fought off by the body's compromised immune system. These individuals should avoid exposure to infectious agents when possible and be attentive to lifestyle modifications that can strengthen the immune system and encourage its speedy recovery, including a nutritious diet, plenty of rest, and avoidance of stress. Appropriate dissemination of patient education about infection, and close monitoring for any signs of infection facilitates rapid antibiotic therapy, which can prevent serious complications.

PERSPECTIVE AND PROSPECTS

Prior to the gains in scientific knowledge about the mechanics of the immune system, individuals with genetic immunodeficiency disorders would die of serious infections during their first few years of life. Even when it was finally realized that these individuals suffered from defects of the immune system, little could be done for most of the disorders, except to treat infections as they developed and to avoid contact with potential disease-causing organisms—a near impossibility if one is to lead a normal life. Housing persons with SCID in sterile bubbles was uncommon because of the expense and impracticality. During the 1970s, bone marrow transplants were first developed; by the 1990s they had progressed to a greater than 80 percent success rate. As a result of improved transplant-rejection drugs, transplants from donors with less than- perfect tissue

---

Information on Immunodeficiency Disorders

Causes: Genetic disorders, infections, damage from drug or radiation treatments, environmental factors

Symptoms: Vary; can include recurrent infections, scaly inflammation of skin, chronic inflammations of internal organs and bones, fever, fatigue

Duration: Often chronic

Treatments: Prevention strategies for infections. Medicinal strategies typically target at source of deficiency; can include antibody injections, antifungal medications, bone marrow transplantation, drug cocktails, alternative medicine (acupuncture, herbal medicine, meditation, homeopathy)

---

matches are now possible. Bone marrow transplantation has been a source of cure for many individuals with immune disorders.

Bone marrow transplantation is not suitable or possible in every case of immunodeficiency disorder, and scientists have long sought a means to cure the genetic defects themselves. In 1992, French Anderson of the National Institutes of Health conducted the first gene therapy trial on a young girl suffering from SCID. Some of the girl's bone marrow cells were removed from her body and exposed to an inactivated virus containing a normal gene for ADA, the defective enzyme. Some of the stem cells in the marrow incorporated the healthy gene, and the engineered cells were returned to her body. The cells lodged in her bone marrow, where they produced healthy immune cells. The procedure was repeated successfully in three other children shortly afterward.

Among the exciting applications of research into the molecular biology of immunodeficiencies has been the identification of specific genetic defects. Bone marrow stem cells can now be isolated and identified. In the future, such cells may be engineered such that the defective gene associated with the deficiency may be replaced by a normal copy. Since the cells are those from the same individual, transplantation problems can be avoided. However, bone marrow or cord blood transplants remain the only cure for SCID.

—*Karen E. Kalumuck, Ph.D.;*
Updated by Christa Varnadoe Roe, BS, RN, OCN

FOR FURTHER INFORMATION

Abbas, Abul K., and Andrew H. Lichtman. *Basic Immunology: Functions and Disorders of the Immune System.* 4th ed. Philadelphia: Saunders/Elsevier, 2012.

Canellos George P., and Nancy Berliner. *Immunodeficiency, Infection, and Stem Cell.* Philadelphia: Saunders, 2011.

Centers for Disease Control and Prevention. *HIV and Gay and Bisexual Men.* 2018, https://www.cdc.gov/hiv/group/msm/index.html

Geha Raif S., and Luigi Notarangelo. *Case Studies in Immunology: A Clinical Companion.* 6th ed. New York: Garland Science, 2012.

Immune Web. http://immuneweb.org.

Mayo Clinic Staff. "Multiple Sclerosis." *Mayo Clinic,* Mayo Foundation for Medical Education and Research, 12 Mar. 2019, www.mayoclinic.org/diseases-conditions/multiple-sclerosis/symptoms-causes/syc-20350269.

———. "Primary Biliary Cholangitis." *Mayo Clinic,* Mayo Foundation for Medical Education and Research, 9 Mar. 2018, www.mayoclinic.org/diseases-conditions/primary-biliary-cholangitis-pbc/symptoms-causes/syc-20376874.

Ngo, S. T., et al. "Gender Differences in Autoimmune Disease." *Frontiers in Neuroendocrinology,* vol. 35, no. 3, Aug. 2014, pp. 347–369., doi:10.1016/j.yfrne.2014.04.004.

Soliman M, et al. "Mechanisms of HIV-1 Control." *Curr HIV/AIDS Rep,* vol. 14, no. 3, 2017, 101-109.

Stine, Gerald J. *AIDS Update 2013.* NewYork: McGraw-Hill, 2013.

Vickers, Peter S. *Severe Combined Immune Deficiency: Early Hospitalization and Isolation.* Hoboken, N.J.: John Wiley & Sons, 2009.

In vitro fertilization

CATEGORY: Procedure

KEY TERMS:

chromosome: a structure found in the cell nucleus that is composed of deoxyribonucleic acid (DNA) and associated proteins; chromosomes are responsible for carrying genetic information and can be observed under a microscope

clomiphene: a synthetic estrogenic substance used to induce ovulation in women who do not ovulate regularly; it is taken orally as a medication

endometriosis: a condition whereby cells of the uterine lining are found in abnormal locations, such as the pelvic cavity or ovary; endometriosis can lead to pelvic pain and the development of scars that can block the Fallopian tubes

Fallopian tube: one of two structures that conduct the egg, as it is released from the ovary, into the uterus

follicle: a spherical mass of cells and fluid within the ovary, from which the mature egg is produced

implantation: the process in which an embryo attaches and burrows into the lining of the uterus

in vitro: a Latin term used to indicate a process that has taken place outside an organism, such as in a laboratory test tube or petri dish

ovulation: the process whereby the egg is released from the ovary and can be fertilized by sperm; this event occurs approximately at the middle portion of a woman's menstrual cycle

semen analysis: analysis of a recently ejaculated semen specimen, which includes a sperm count and an estimate of the percentage of motile sperm

zygote: the single cell formed after fertilization that is the result of the fusion of egg and sperm; it can develop into a new individual organism

INDICATIONS AND PROCEDURES

The purpose of fertilization is to create a new organism or individual that has the same number of chromosomes as the parent individuals but that has a unique mixing of genetic traits from both the mother and the father. In animals, this is accomplished by the fusion of egg and sperm cells. Both egg and sperm contain half the number of chromosomes needed to produce a healthy individual. The fusion of egg and sperm results in a zygote, or fertilized egg, which can develop into an individual organism.

Eggs and sperm are both gametes, cells that are specialized to carry out reproductive functions. The sperm cells are produced in the testicles of the male. Sperm production is continuous in the male, and millions of sperm are made within the testicles each day. Sperm cells contain genetic material within their head and are equipped with a flagellum, or whip-like tail, to enable them to swim within a liquid medium.

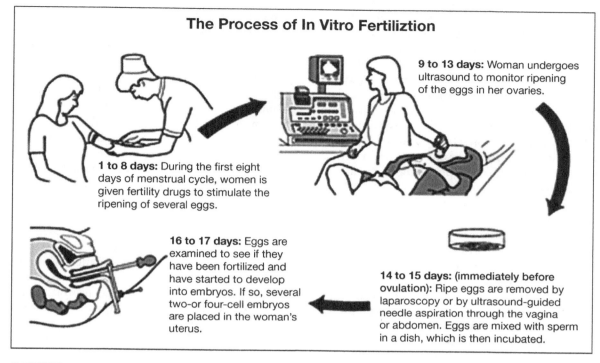

The Process of In Vitro Fertiliztion

1 to 8 days: During the first eight days of menstrual cycle, women is given fertility drugs to stimulate the ripening of several eggs.

9 to 13 days: Woman undergoes ultrasound to monitor ripening of the eggs in her ovaries.

14 to 15 days: (immediately before ovulation): Ripe eggs are removed by laparoscopy or by ultrasound-guided needle aspiration through the vagina or abdomen. Eggs are mixed with sperm in a dish, which is then incubated.

16 to 17 days: Eggs are examined to see if they have been fortilized and have started to develop into embryos. If so, several two-or four-cell embryos are placed in the woman's uterus.

© EBSCO

The egg, or ovum, is about .01 millimeter in size and hundreds of times larger than the sperm. It is produced in the ovaries of females and contains cytoplasm, the cellular substance and specialized cell structures that are needed for the zygote to form and grow. In women, a single mature egg is usually made with each menstrual cycle and is released from the follicle contained in one of the ovaries. As women age, their ovaries become depleted of follicles, and eventually, at the menopause, ovulation no longer occurs. Therefore, a woman's age can contribute significantly to her ability to conceive. Other causes of ovarian failure that may lead to infertility include the use of chemotherapeutic agents and premature ovarian failure syndrome.

In natural, or in vivo, fertilization, sperm from the male are deposited in the vaginal canal of the female during sexual intercourse. The sperm are contained in nutritive fluid, called semen. The sperm are able to swim up the cervical canal (the lower part of the uterus) only during and around the time of female ovulation, as the cervical mucus becomes permeable to sperm at this time. Once within the uterine cavity, the sperm make their way up into the Fallopian tubes, where they can meet the egg and proceed with fertilization.

Several steps lead to fertilization. The egg is surrounded by a layer of cells called the corona radiata. This layer is loose and easily penetrated by sperm. The next layer is the zona pellucida, which is a critical barrier in fertilization. One of the sugarcoated proteins in the zona pellucida, ZP2, captures a sperm cell by binding to its head. This causes a structure on the head of the sperm, called an acrosome, to release enzymes. This process is called the acrosomal reaction. These enzymes then digest the coat on the head of the sperm cell and digest a path for the sperm through the zona pellucida. After this, the sperm reaches the membrane of the egg, and the sperm and egg cells fuse. The chromosomes of the sperm and egg join, thus completing the process of fertilization. Subsequently, the fertilized egg travels back into the uterus and implants into the lining of the uterus, where it continues to develop as an embryo and then as a fetus.

When the natural anatomy or physiology of the reproductive system is abnormal, infertility can result. For instance, endometriosis in women can cause severe scarring of the pelvic cavity, leading to occluded Fallopian tubes or ovaries that are completely encased in scar tissue. In these cases, the egg may have difficulty reaching the Fallopian tube canal and hence is unable to meet sperm to achieve fertilization. Another cause of pelvic scarring is pelvic inflammatory disease (PID), which can be caused by sexually transmitted diseases (STDs) or ruptures in the gastrointestinal tract. In vitro fertilization (IVF) may be indicated when a couple experiences infertility. Infertility is defined as the lack of conception after one to two years of unprotected intercourse.

There are many causes of infertility, which may be attributable to either the male or the female partner. Usually when an infertile couple seeks medical attention, they are asked to give a detailed history and receive physical examinations by the physician. Depending on the findings, the couple will be asked to undergo testing to better identify the cause of the infertility. Men will be asked to give a semen sample. The sample will be analyzed in the laboratory to ensure that adequate numbers of sperm are present and that they are able to move appropriately, a procedure called semen analysis. Women may be assessed for anatomic defects, such as whether the Fallopian tubes are blocked or large fibroid tumors in the uterus may prevent sperm from entering the Fallopian tubes. This assessment may be accomplished using a technique called a hysterosalpingogram, in which dye is introduced into the uterine cavity and an X-ray picture is taken. If a woman's Fallopian tubes are blocked, then no dye will spill into the pelvic cavity. If a woman's tubes are open, then dye will be seen spilling into the pelvic cavity. In addition, women may also undergo assessments regarding their ovarian function and ability to produce eggs. Blood tests may be drawn to assess for appropriate hormone levels.

If the cause of infertility is found to be blocked Fallopian tubes, then IVF may be indicated. Sometimes, women with irregular menstrual cycles who do not ovulate at predictable intervals may be treated with a medication called clomiphene, in order to induce ovulation. If a woman fails to achieve spontaneous conception after several months of clomiphene therapy, then the physician may proceed with in vitro fertilization as the next step in the attempt to achieve conception.

Another example of when IVF may be indicated is in cases where the sperm are defective. For instance, some men may have sperm that have difficulty swimming appropriately or penetrating the egg. In such cases, the sperm may need to be injected artificially into the egg to achieve fertilization, a procedure called intracytoplasmic sperm injection (ICSI). To perform this procedure, eggs must be harvested from the woman. The eggs are then placed in a petri dish, where they are injected with the sperm. Because fertilization is occurring outside the body in this situation, this procedure is also a type of in vitro fertilization. After the eggs have matured for a few days in the laboratory, the healthiest-looking zygotes are placed into the woman's uterus, a procedure called embryo transfer.

Another example in which intracytoplasmic sperm injection might be used is when the couple's infertility is caused by the man's inability to ejaculate sperm. This might occur, for instance, with a lack or occlusion of the vas deferens, the tubes that carry sperm from the testicles to the urethra where the sperm can exit the body. To obtain sperm for IVF in these cases, the male partner may undergo testicular sperm extraction, in which sperm are removed from the testicles. The sperm are then injected into the ova to achieve fertilization in vitro.

The procedures for IVF involve the induction of ovulation in the woman using hormones that stimulate the ovaries. These are usually hormones that are similar to endogenous follicle-stimulating hormone (FSH), which is responsible for follicle growth within the ovary. These exogenous hormones lead to the development of multiple follicles within both ovaries.

The size and number of these follicles are observed by ultrasound, and when the appropriate number and size are achieved, the ovum harvest is performed. This procedure involves taking the woman to the operating room, where she is given anesthesia and placed on her back with her legs in stirrups and knees apart. A needle attached to a vacuum device is carefully introduced into the vaginal canal with ultrasound guidance. With the ultrasound helping to locate the ovaries and follicles precisely, the needle is inserted into the follicle through the posterior vagina. The fluid within the follicle is aspirated, and the egg usually is suctioned out of the follicle along with the follicular fluid and placed into a test tube. The same procedure is repeated until a sufficient number of eggs have been harvested or the follicles have been depleted. The eggs are then taken to the laboratory, where they are examined under a microscope.

A sperm sample is then collected from the male partner, and the sample is washed and analyzed to ensure that the sperm appear healthy and able to fertilize the eggs. The sperm are then introduced to the eggs within a petri dish containing tissue culture fluid. If intracytoplasmic sperm injection is to be performed, then single sperm are taken up into a glass needle and injected into individual eggs at this time. The petri dish is placed in an incubator for a few days. Once the embryos have developed sufficiently, a few healthy ones are chosen to be introduced into the woman's uterus through embryo transfer. This involves picking up the embryos into a semiflexible tube. The tube is then inserted carefully through the cervical canal into the uterine cavity, where the embryos are released. Embryos that are not transferred into the woman's uterus can be frozen using cryopreservation for future use.

Uses and Complications

IVF enables couples who suffer from infertility to conceive and bear children. Specifically, IVF is most helpful for couples whose infertility is caused by blocked Fallopian tubes or the inability of sperm to reach and penetrate the egg. In couples where the woman is unable to produce her own eggs, donor eggs from another woman may be used in IVF. If a man is unable to produce his own sperm, then sperm donors may be used in IVF.

Recent technology has enabled early prenatal diagnosis for inheritable conditions using cells taken from the early embryo during the six-to-eight-cell stage, called blastomere biopsy. Inheritable diseases caused by single gene defects, such as cystic fibrosis, Duchenne muscular dystrophy, sickle cell disease, hemophilia, and Tay-Sachs disease, have been detected using preimplantation diagnosis. This type of prenatal diagnosis is possible only through the IVF process, as the early embryo would not be accessible to the physician in cases of spontaneous conception. Procedures such as blastomere biopsy are far from common, however, given the technical difficulty and economic costs of such procedures.

The complications associated with the IVF process include a condition called ovarian hyperstimulation syndrome. This situation can occur when a woman receives hormones to stimulate ovulation. In these cases, the follicles within the ovary become excessively stimulated and grossly enlarge the ovary. When this condition is severe, the woman can suffer abdominal pain, fluid imbalances, electrolyte imbalances, abnormal kidney function, and an accumulation of fluid in the abdominal cavity or lungs. Her blood may have an abnormal tendency to form clots, and her blood pressure may become dangerously low. These patients are monitored carefully and require hospitalization, as severe ovarian hyperstimulation syndrome can be fatal.

Other complications of the IVF process can occur during the ovum harvest procedure. These include the risks of anesthesia and infection (because the needle is a foreign body introduced through the vagina, a nonsterile field). Another risk involves bleeding. Although the needle for harvesting the eggs is under ultrasound guidance, the risk of the needle inadvertently puncturing neighboring blood vessels still exists. In addition, the ovaries themselves may bleed when punctured, as they are highly vascular organs. Bleeding that is severe and life-threatening may require abdominal or pelvic surgery to identify the location of the bleeding and to stop the bleeding with sutures. If the patient becomes significantly anemic from the bleeding, she may require a blood transfusion.

Other risks of IVF are incurred during the embryo culture process. During this process, the petri dishes containing the embryos may become contaminated with microorganisms. In addition, problems with the tissue culture medium or with the incubation process may lead to poor embryo development and the lack of any viable embryos to transfer into the woman. Another risk is that embryos transferred into the uterus may not implant themselves in the lining.

The rate of achieving pregnancy after IVF is directly related to the number of embryos transferred into the uterus. When multiple embryos are transferred back into the uterus, however, the woman is at risk for a multiple gestation pregnancy. Multiple gestation pregnancies lead to an increased risk of spontaneous abortion (miscarriage) and preterm birth, as well as other pregnancy complications such as low birth weight, growth restriction in utero, increased risk of congenital anomalies, placental abnormalities, preeclampsia (a hypertensive disease of pregnancy), umbilical cord accidents, and malpresentations (when the fetus is not lying in the uterus with the head down, making vaginal birth difficult). More long-term risks of in vitro fertilization are the increased risk for complications during pregnancy.

For instance, women whose pregnancies were a result of assisted reproductive technologies such as IVF are at increased risk for preterm birth, when compared to age-matched women whose pregnancies were a result of spontaneous conception.

In addition, the long-term outcomes of children conceived using IVF is unknown, as the first children born as a result of this technique are beginning to enter middle age. Whether they will live normal life spans is unknown. Whether they will have normal reproductive outcomes themselves remains unclear. Whether they are more prone to diseases such as cancer later in life is also unknown.

PERSPECTIVE AND PROSPECTS

The first baby conceived through in vitro fertilization was Louise Brown, who was born in 1978. The English team responsible for this important breakthrough consisted of Patrick Steptoe, a surgeon from Oldham Hospital, and Robert Edwards, a reproductive physiologist from Cambridge University. In the 1960s, animal breeding programs had successfully utilized in vitro fertilization. In 1965, Edwards reported that he had successfully induced maturation of a human egg in vitro. Edwards teamed up with Steptoe and another colleague, Jean Purdy. In 1970, they reported that they had achieved in vitro fertilization and cleavage (cell division) in human eggs. The first successful birth of an IVF baby in the United States occurred in 1981 in Norfolk, Virginia. The first successful use of a previously frozen human embryo occurred in Australia in 1984; two years later, a similar procedure was employed successfully in the United States.

A couple can undergo multiple cycles of IVF. A 1996 study reported data from large centers in three countries that showed that the cumulative pregnancy rate after six cycles of IVF is approximately 60 percent. However, if a couple fails to achieve pregnancy after six cycles, then the chances of achieving pregnancy through IVF fall significantly. At that time, the infertile couple may be counseled to seek alternative means of becoming parents, such as adoption.

In vitro fertilization and its related procedures have provided opportunities to conceive for couples who would otherwise be childless. These opportunities have led to many ethical controversies as well. What should be done with frozen embryos that are not used? What are the rights of egg or sperm donors once the child is born? What are the rights of the child to know his or her parentage and family history of medical problems? What are the rights of surrogate mothers? How many embryos should be transferred back into the woman, given that multiple gestations are at increased risk for poor outcomes such as premature delivery? Is there a certain age at which women should not attempt pregnancy?

Some countries such as Australia, Norway, Spain, and the United Kingdom have responded to some of these questions by passing legislation regulating IVF. Other countries have been slower to respond, leaving decisions related to IVF to physicians, the patients themselves, and the court system. As more couples delay childbearing, the prevalence of infertility and the desire for IVF and other assisted reproductive technologies is likely to increase. Human reproduction is not an efficient process, and the older the female partner becomes, the less likely it is that natural conception will occur.

For instance, a 1986 survey in the United States reported that the proportion of married women who were infertile between the ages of twenty and twenty-four was only 7 percent. By the ages of forty to forty-four, this proportion became 28 percent. This statistic is partly attributable to the fact that the total length of time during which conception is possible is less in older women, as older women ovulate less frequently than do younger women.

—*Anne Lynn S. Chang, M.D.*

FOR FURTHER INFORMATION

Chisholm, Andrea, and Brian Randall. "In Vitro Fertilization." *Health Library*, May 22, 2013.

"FAQ – Treating Infertility." *ACOG*, American College of Obstetricians and Gynecologists, Oct. 2017, www.acog.org/Patients/FAQs/Treating-Infertility?IsMobileSet=false.

Gardner, David K., ed. *In Vitro Fertilization: A Practical Approach.* New York: Informa Healthcare, 2007.

"Infertility." *MedlinePlus*, U.S. National Library of Medicine, 3 Jan. 2017, https://medlineplus.gov/infertility.html

Lentz, Gretchen M., et al. *Comprehensive Gynecology.* 6th ed. Philadelphia: Mosby/Elsevier, 2013.

Sher, Geoffrey, Virginia Marriage Davis, and Jean Stoess. *In Vitro Fertilization: The A.R.T. of Making Babies.* 3d ed. New York: Facts On File, 2005.

Speroff, Leon, and Marc A. Fritz. *Clinical Gynecologic Endocrinology and Infertility.* 8th ed. Philadelphia: Lippincott Williams & Wilkins, 2011.

Wisot, Arthur L., and David R. Meldrum. *Conceptions and Misconceptions: The Informed Consumer's Guide Through the Maze of In Vitro Fertilization and Other Assisted Reproduction Techniques.* 2d ed. Point Roberts, Wash.: Hartley & Marks, 2004.

Infertility

CATEGORY: Disease/Disorder

KEY TERMS:

cervix: the bottom portion of the uterus, protruding into the vagina; the cervical canal, an opening in the cervix, allows sperm to pass from the vagina into the uterus

endometriosis: a disease in which patches of the uterine lining, the endometrium, implant on or in other organs

follicles: spherical structures in the ovary that contain the maturing ova (eggs)

hormone: a chemical signal that serves to coordinate the functions of different body parts; the hormones important in female reproduction are produced by the brain, the pituitary, and the ovaries

implantation: the process in which the early embryo attaches to the uterine lining; a critical event in pregnancy

ovaries: the pair of structures in the female that produce ova (eggs) and hormones

oviducts: the pair of tubes leading from the top of the uterus upward toward the ovaries; also called the Fallopian tubes

ovulation: the process in which an ovum is released from its follicle in the ovary; ovulation must occur for conception to be possible

pelvic inflammatory disease: a general term that refers to a state of inflammation and infection in the pelvic organs; may be caused by a sexually transmitted disease

uterus: the organ in which the embryo implants and grows

vagina: the tube-shaped organ that serves as the site for sperm deposition during intercourse

CAUSES AND SYMPTOMS

Infertility is defined as the failure of a woman to conceive despite regular sexual activity over the course of at least one year. Studies have estimated that in the United States, 10 to 15 percent of couples are infertile. In about half of these couples, it is the woman who is affected.

Female infertility may be caused by hormonal problems, or it may originate in the reproductive organs: the ovaries, oviducts, uterus, cervix, and vagina. The frequency of specific problems among infertile women is as follows: ovarian problems, 20 percent to 30 percent; damage to the Fallopian tubes, 30 percent to 50 percent; uterine problems, 5 percent to 10 percent; and cervical or vaginal abnormalities, 5 percent to 10 percent. Another 10 percent of women have unexplained infertility. Behavioral factors, such as diet and exercise and the use of tobacco, alcohol, or drugs, also play a role in infertility.

The ovaries have two important roles in conception: the production of ova (egg cells), culminating in ovulation, and the production of hormones. Ovulation usually occurs halfway through a woman's four-week menstrual cycle. In the two weeks preceding ovulation, follicle-stimulating hormone (FSH) from the pituitary gland causes follicles in the ovaries to grow and the ova within them to mature. As the follicles grow, they produce increasing amounts of estrogen. Near the middle of the cycle, the estrogen causes the pituitary gland to release a surge of luteinizing hormone (LH), which causes ovulation of the largest follicle in the ovary.

Anovulation (lack of ovulation) can result either directly, from an inability to produce LH, FSH, or estrogen, or indirectly, because of the presence of other hormones that interfere with the signaling systems between the pituitary and ovaries. For example, the woman may have an excess production of androgen (testosterone-like) hormones, either in her ovaries or in her adrenal glands, or her pituitary may produce too much prolactin, a hormone that is normally secreted in large amounts only after the birth of a child.

Besides ovulation, the ovaries have another critical role in conception, since they produce hormones that act on the uterus to allow it to support an embryo. In the first two weeks of the menstrual cycle, the uterine lining is prepared for a possible pregnancy by estrogen from the ovaries. Following ovulation, the uterus is maintained in a state that can support an embryo by progesterone, which is produced in the ovary by the follicle that just ovulated, now called a corpus luteum. Because of the effects of hormones from the corpus luteum on the uterus, the corpus luteum is essential to the survival of the embryo. If conception does not occur, the corpus luteum disintegrates and stops producing progesterone. As progesterone levels decline, the uterine lining can no longer be maintained and is shed as the menstrual flow.

Failure of the pregnancy can result from improper function of the corpus luteum, such as an inability to produce enough progesterone to sustain the uterine lining. The corpus luteum may also produce progesterone initially but then disintegrate too early. These problems in corpus luteum function, referred to as luteal phase insufficiency, may be caused by the same types of hormonal abnormalities that cause lack of ovulation. Some cases of infertility may be associated with an abnormally shaped uterus or vagina. Such malformations of the reproductive organs are common in women whose mothers took diethylstilbestrol (DES) during pregnancy. DES was prescribed to many pregnant women from 1941 to about 1970 as a protection against miscarriage; infertility and other problems have occurred in the offspring of these women.

Conception depends on normal function of the oviducts (or Fallopian tubes), thin tubes with an inner diameter of only a few millimeters; they are attached to the top of the uterus and curve upward toward the ovaries. The inner end of each tube, located near one of the ovaries, waves back and forth at the time of ovulation, drawing the mature ovum into the opening of the oviduct. Once in the oviduct, the ovum is propelled along by movements of the oviduct wall. Meanwhile, if intercourse has occurred recently, the man's sperm will be moving upward in the female system, swimming through the uterus and the oviducts. Fertilization, the union of the sperm and ovum, will occur in the oviduct, and then the fertilized ovum will pass down the oviduct and reach the uterus about three days after ovulation.

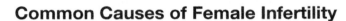

Common Causes of Female Infertility

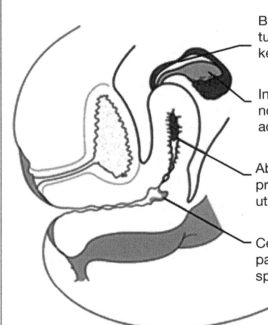

Blockage in Fallopian tubes, such as tubal kinking from adhesions, may keep sperm from reaching egg.

In ovaries, eggs may not mature or may not be released, as a result of tubo-ovarian adhesions or endometriosis.

Abnormality of uterus, such as fibroids, may prevent fertilized egg from being implanted in uterine wall.

Cervical mucus or cervicitis may prevent passage of sperm or damage or destroy sperm.

© EBSCO

Infertility can result from scar tissue formation inside the oviduct, resulting in physical blockage and inability to transport the ovum, sperm, or both. The most common cause of scar tissue formation in the reproductive organs is pelvic inflammatory disease (PID), a condition characterized by inflammation that spreads throughout the female reproductive tract. PID may be initiated by a sexually transmitted disease such as gonorrhea or chlamydia. Physicians in the United States have documented an increase in infertility attributable to tubal damage caused by sexually transmitted diseases. Damage to the outside of the oviduct can also cause infertility, because such damage can interfere with the mobility of the oviduct, which is necessary to the capture of the ovum at the time of ovulation. External damage to the oviduct may occur as an aftermath of abdominal surgery, when adhesions induced by surgical cutting are likely to form. An adhesion is an abnormal scar tissue connection between adjacent structures. Another possible cause of damage to the oviduct that can result in infertility is the presence of endometriosis.

Endometriosis refers to a condition in which patches of the uterine lining implant outside the uterus, in or on the surface of other organs. These patches are thought to arise during menstruation, when the uterine lining (endometrium) is normally shed from the body through the cervix and vagina; in a woman with endometriosis, for unknown reasons, the endometrium is carried to the interior of the pelvic cavity by passing up the oviducts. The endometrial patches can lodge in the oviduct itself, causing blockage, or can adhere to the outer surface of the oviducts, interfering with mobility.

Endometriosis can cause infertility by interfering with organs other than the oviducts. Endometrial patches on the outside of the uterus can cause distortions in the shape or placement of the uterus, interfering with embryonic implantation. Ovulation may be prevented by the presence of the endometrial tissues on the surface of the ovary. The presence of endometriosis, however, is not always associated with infertility: Thirty percent to forty percent of women with endometriosis cannot conceive, but the remainder appear to be fertile.

Another critical site in conception is the cervix. The cervix, the entryway to the uterus from the vagina, represents the first barrier through which sperm must pass on their way to the ovum. The cervix consists of a ring of strong, elastic tissue with a narrow canal. Glands in the cervix produce the mucus that fills the cervical canal and through which sperm swim en route to the ovum. The amount and quality of the cervical mucus change throughout the menstrual cycle, under the influence of hormones from the ovary. At ovulation, the mucus is in a state that is most easily penetrated by sperm; after ovulation, the mucus becomes almost impenetrable. Cervical problems that can lead to infertility include production of a mucus that does not allow sperm passage at the time of ovulation (hostile mucus syndrome) and interference with sperm transport caused by narrowing of the cervical canal. Such narrowing may be the result of a developmental abnormality or the presence of an infection, possibly a sexually transmitted disease.

TREATMENT AND THERAPY

The diagnosis of the exact cause of a woman's infertility is crucial to successful treatment. A complete medical history should reveal any obvious problems of previous infection or menstrual cycle irregularity. Adequacy of ovulation and luteal phase function can be determined from records of menstrual cycle length and changes in body temperature (body temperature is higher after ovulation). Hormone levels can be measured with tests of blood or urine samples. If damage to the oviducts or uterus is suspected, a hysterosalpingography will be performed. In this procedure, the injection of a special fluid into the uterus is followed by x-ray analysis of the fluid movement to reveal the shape of the uterine cavity and the oviducts. Cervical functioning can be assessed with the postcoital test, in which the physician attempts to recover sperm from the woman's uterus some hours after she has had intercourse with her partner. If a uterine problem is suspected, the woman may have an endometrial biopsy, in which a small sample of the uterine lining is removed and examined for abnormalities. Sometimes, exploratory surgery is performed to pinpoint the location of scar tissue or the location of endometrial patches.

Surgery may be used for treatment as well as diagnosis. Damage to the oviducts can sometimes be repaired surgically, and surgical removal of endometrial patches is a standard treatment for endometriosis. Often, however, surgery is a last resort because of the likelihood of the development of postsurgical adhesions, which can further complicate the infertility.

Newer forms of surgery using lasers and freezing offer better success because of a reduced risk of adhesions. Some women with hormonal difficulties can be treated successfully with so-called fertility drugs, which are intended to stimulate ovulation. There are several different drugs and hormones that fall under this heading: Clomiphene citrate (*Clomid*), human menopausal gonadotropin (hMG), gonadotropin- releasing hormone (GnRH), and bromocriptine mesylate (Parlodel) are among the medications commonly used, with the exact choice depending on the woman's particular problem. One problem with some of the drugs is the risk of multiple pregnancy (more than one fetus in the uterus). Other possible problems include nausea, dizziness, headache, and general malaise.

Aside from fertility drugs, there are a variety of methods in use to try to achieve pregnancy with external assistance, known collectively as assisted reproductive technology (ART). One example of this, artificial insemination, also known as intrauterine insemination (IUI), is an old technique that is still useful in various types of infertility. A previously collected sperm sample is placed in the woman's vagina or uterus using a special tube. Artificial insemination is always performed at the time of ovulation, in order to maximize the chance of conception. The ovulation date can be determined with body temperature records or by hormone measurements. In some cases, this procedure is combined with fertility drug treatment. Since the sperm can be placed directly in the uterus, it is useful in treating hostile mucus syndrome and certain types of male infertility. The sperm sample can be provided either by the woman's partner or by a donor. The pregnancy rate after artificial insemination is highly variable (anywhere from 10 to 70 percent), depending on the particular infertility problem in the couple.

Another assisted reproductive technology is gamete intrafallopian transfer (GIFT), the surgical placement of ova and sperm directly into the woman's oviducts. To be a candidate for this procedure, the woman must have at least one partially undamaged oviduct and a functional uterus. Ova are collected surgically from the ovaries after stimulation with a fertility drug, and a semen sample is collected from the male. The ova and the sperm are introduced into the oviducts through the same abdominal incision used to collect the ova. This procedure is useful in certain types of male infertility, if the woman produces an impenetrable cervical mucus, or if the ovarian ends of the oviducts are damaged. The range of infertility problems that may be resolved with GIFT can be extended by using donated ova or sperm. The pregnancy rate is about 33 percent overall, but the rate varies with the type of infertility present.

The most common assisted reproductive technology is in vitro fertilization (IVF), or the fertilization of the sperm and egg outside the woman's body, followed by implantation of the fertilized egg in the woman's uterus. In this procedure, ova are collected surgically after stimulation with fertility drugs and then placed in a laboratory dish and combined with sperm from the man. The actual fertilization, when a sperm penetrates the ovum, will occur in the dish. The resulting embryo is allowed to remain in the dish for two days, during which time it will have grown to two to four cells. Then, the embryo is placed in the woman's uterine cavity using a flexible tube. In vitro fertilization can be used in women who are infertile because of endometriosis, damaged oviducts, impenetrable cervical mucus, or ovarian failure. As with GIFT, in vitro fertilization may utilize donated ova or donated sperm, or extra embryos that have been produced by one couple may be implanted in a second woman. Embryos created through IVF can either be used immediately or frozen for later implantation. Success rates for in vitro fertilization have improved greatly over time, and in the United States in 2010, the proportion of IVF procedures that resulted in live births was about 56 percent for fresh embryos and 35 percent for frozen embryos, according to the Centers for Disease Control and Prevention.

Some women may benefit from nonsurgical embryo transfer. In this procedure, a fertile woman is artificially inseminated at the time of her ovulation; five days later, her uterus is flushed with a sterile solution, washing out the resulting embryo before it implants in the uterus. The retrieved embryo is then transferred to the uterus of another woman, who will carry it to term. Typically, the sperm provider and the woman who receives the embryo are the infertile couple who wish to rear the child, but the technique can be used in other circumstances as well. Embryo transfer can be used if the woman has damaged oviducts or is unable to ovulate, or if she has a genetic disease that could be passed to her offspring, because in this case the baby is not genetically related to the woman who carries it.

Information on Infertility

Causes: Endometriosis, cervical problems, anovulation, hormonal imbalance, abnormally shaped uterus or vagina, pelvic inflammatory disease

Symptoms: Often asymptomatic; can include lack of menstrual periods, blocked Fallopian tubes, abdominal pain with endometriosis

Duration: Short-term to chronic

Treatments: Fertility drugs, surgery, fertility procedures (e.g., in vitro fertilization)

Some infertile women who are unable to achieve a pregnancy themselves turn to the use of a surrogate, a woman who will agree to bear a child and then turn it over to the infertile woman to rear as her own. In the typical situation, the surrogate is artificially inseminated with the sperm of the infertile woman's husband. The surrogate then proceeds with pregnancy and delivery as normal but relinquishes the child to the infertile couple after its birth.

PERSPECTIVE AND PROSPECTS

One of the biggest problems that infertile couples face is the emotional upheaval that comes with the diagnosis of infertility, as bearing and rearing children is an experience that most people treasure. In addition to the emotional difficulty that may come with the recognition of infertility, more stress may be in store as the couple proceeds through treatment. The various treatments can cause embarrassment and sometimes physical pain, and fertility drugs themselves are known to cause emotional swings. For these reasons, a couple with an infertility problem is often advised to seek help from a private counselor or a support group.

Along with the emotional and physical challenges of infertility treatment, there is a considerable financial burden. Infertility treatments, in general, are expensive, especially for more sophisticated procedures such as in vitro fertilization and GIFT. Since the chances of a single procedure resulting in a pregnancy are often low, the couple may be faced with submitting to multiple procedures repeated many times. The cost over several years of treatment—a realistic possibility—can be very high. Many health insurance companies in the United States refuse to cover the costs of such treatment and are required to do so in only a few states.

Some of the treatments are accompanied by unresolved legal questions. In the case of nonsurgical embryo transfer, is the legal mother of the child the ovum donor or the woman who gives birth to the child? The same question of legal parentage arises in cases of surrogacy. Does a child born using donated ovum or sperm have a legal right to any information about the donor, such as medical history? How extensive should governmental regulation of infertility clinics be? For example, should there be standards for ensuring that donated sperm or ova are free from genetic defects? In the United States, some states have begun to address these issues, but no uniform policies have been set at the federal level.

The legal questions are largely unresolved because American society is still involved in religious and philosophical debates over the propriety of various infertility treatments. Some religions hold that any interference in conception is unacceptable. To these denominations, even artificial insemination is wrong. Other groups approve of treatments confined to a husband and wife but disapprove of a third party being involved as a donor or surrogate. Many people disapprove of any infertility treatment to help an individual who is not married. Almost all these issues stem from the fact that these reproductive technologies challenge the traditional definitions of parenthood.

—*Marcia Watson-Whitmyre, Ph.D.*

FOR FURTHER INFORMATION

American Society for Reproductive Medicine. http://www.asrm.org/.

"Assisted Reproductive Technology (ART) Report." *Centers for Disease Control and Prevention,* January 6, 2012.

"Female Infertility." *Mayo Clinic,* September 9, 2011.

Gordon, John David, et el. *Obstetrics, Gynecology and Infertility.* 7th ed., Arlington, VA: Scrub Hill Press, Scrub Hill Press; 2016.

Harkness, Carla. *The Infertility Book: A Comprehensive Medical and Emotional Guide.* Rev. ed. Berkeley, Calif.: Celestial Arts, 1996.

International Council on Infertility Information Dissemination. http://www.inciid.org. Phillips, Robert H., and Glenda Motta. *Coping with Endometriosis.* New York: Avery, 2000.

Quilligan, Edward J., and Frederick P. Zuspan, eds. *Current Therapy in Obstetrics and Gynecology.* 5th ed. Philadelphia: W. B. Saunders, 2000.

Riley, Julie. "Infertility in Women." *Health Library*, October 31, 2012.

Speroff, Leon, and Marc A. Fritz. *Clinical Gynecologic Endocrinology and Infertility*. 8th ed. Philadelphia: Lippincott Williams & Wilkins, 2011.

Turkington, Carol, and Michael M. Alper. *Encyclopedia of Fertility and Infertility*. New York: Facts On File, 2001.

Weschler, Toni. *Taking Charge of Your Fertility*. Rev. ed. New York: Collins, 2006.

Wisot, Arthur L., and David R. Meldrum. *Conceptions and Misconceptions: The Informed Consumer's Guide Through the Maze of In Vitro Fertilization and Other Assisted Reproduction Techniques*. 2d ed. Point Roberts, Wash.: Hartley & Marks, 2004.

Zouves, Christo. *Expecting Miracles: On the Path of Hope from Infertility to Parenthood*. New York: Berkley, 2003.

Intersex

CATEGORY: Disease/Disorder

KEY TERMS:

gonadal intersex: an individual with both ovarian and testicular tissue; this may be in the same gonad (an ovotestis), or the person might have one ovary and one testis; the individual may have XX chromosomes, XY chromosomes, or both; the external genitals may be ambiguous or may appear to be female or male

urogenital development: early development of the urinary system and genitals

fused labia: a condition where the two flaps of skin on either side of the opening to the vagina (the labia minora) are joined together

labioscrotal: relating to or being a swelling or ridge on each side of the embryonic rudiment of the penis or clitoris which develops into one of the scrotal sacs in the male and one of the labia majora in the female

hypospadias: a congenital condition in males in which the opening of the urethra is on the underside of the penis

CAUSES AND SYMPTOMS

Ambiguous genitalia is usually caused by a variation in the number of sex chromosomes or in prenatal exposure to key hormones. Males normally possess one X and one Y chromosome, while females normally have two X chromosomes. When an embryo has a different number or configuration of these chromosomes, normal urogenital development is disrupted and, in some cases, the resulting internal and external sex organs do not match. Inappropriate levels of male and female hormones during fetal development are also responsible for ambiguous genitalia. The main categories of ambiguous genitalia conditions are true gonadal intersex (formerly called "hermaphroditism"), 46, XY intersex ("male pseudohermaphroditism"), and 46, XX intersex ("female pseudohermaphroditism").

True gonadal intersex is a condition in which testicular and ovarian tissues are found in the same person and their urogenital development is ambiguous. A baby with an enlarged clitoris resembling a penis (clithoromegaly) and fused labioscrotal folds may be assigned to the male sex at birth, whereas a baby with a normal clitoris and open labial-scrotal folds might be considered a female at birth. Hypospadias, a condition in which urethra opens somewhere around or along the clitoris, penis, or vaginal canal, often occurs and lends further ambiguity to the appearance of the external genitalia. Similarly, testicles may be or believed to be undescended. The exact cause of this condition is generally unknown.

Persons with 46, XY intersex may develop internal testes, but their external genitals at birth appear female, incompletely male, or indeterminate. The undervirilization responsible for 46, XY intersex results from a lack of testosterone during fetal development. Among the causes are testicular malfunction; inadequate testosterone production; 5-alphareductase enzyme deficiency (sometimes called "guevedoces syndrome"), in which testosterone cannot be converted to 5-alpha-dihydrotestosterone (DHT), the inducer needed for the early development of male tissues; or malfunction in testosterone receptors, known as androgen insensitivity syndrome (AIS) or testicular feminization syndrome (TFS).

Individuals with AIS may lack ovaries, Fallopian tubes, and a uterus, but have a "blind" (dead-end) vagina and breasts; testes may or may not be present. As they enter puberty, they begin to grow genital hair and breasts and have the appearance of normal girls because they are unable to respond to testosterone.

Information on Intersex

Causes: Genetic defect of sex organs
Symptoms: Abnormal appearance of primary sexual characteristics
Duration: Chronic unless corrected
Treatments: Hormone therapy, surgery

Menstruation will not occur, however. When individuals with 5-alpha-reductase enzyme deficiency begin puberty, the clitoris enlarges into a penis-like structure without a urethra. The urethral opening is at the base of the enlarged clitoris. One or both of the internal testes descend into scrotal sacs, and the teenager begins to develop masculine body and facial hair, but there is no breast development. In some cases, the voice deepens, and muscle mass and body shape become more masculine. At puberty, the testes produce very large amounts of testosterone, which is able to make up for the lack of DHT and to stimulate some tissues to develop further.

Persons with 46, XX intersex often have clithoromegaly and fused labia, while the female internal organs develop normally. Female hormones produced at puberty lead to the development of female secondary sex characteristics, unless testosterone is administered. The virilization that causes 46, XX intersex may result from congenital adrenal hyperplasia, a kidney disorder that produces excess androgen in the fetus; ovarian tumors in the mother; aromatase enzyme deficiency, in which male hormones cannot be converted to female hormones; or other sources of prenatal testosterone exposure.

TREATMENT AND THERAPY

The most common forms of treatment are hormone therapy and surgery. Hormone therapy might be of value in helping to establish the gender roles affected individuals desire in their culture. Surgery may be required at birth to correct hypospadias or other conditions that impair proper urinary function. Concerned parents should consult with their physicians about the child's specific condition, the possible underlying causes, and the risks and benefits of various treatment options. Psychological counseling is recommended for parents and individuals with ambiguous genitalia, particularly with respective to making treatment decisions.

PERSPECTIVE AND PROSPECTS

In the past, parents and physicians were quick to assign a sex to an infant with ambiguous genitalia and pursue surgery to make the genitalia more recognizably male or female. Immediate surgery is now recommended only to improve or restore function, and families are encouraged to involve the intersex person in making decisions about gender and sexual identity and treatments that support those decisions.

In general, persons with ambiguous genitalia are content with their sexual assignments and are no more likely to seek sex reassignment or to change gender later in life than are persons born with normal genitalia; however, gender-atypical behavior may be associated with some intersex conditions. Intersex individuals also appear just as likely to be heterosexual as the general population. Normal puberty may be absent in affected individuals, and fertility can be an issue in adulthood.

—Jaime S. Colomé, Ph.D.

FOR FURTHER INFORMATION

"46, XXXTesticular Disorder of Sex Development." *Genetics Home Reference*, May 20, 2013.

"Ambiguous Genitalia." *MedlinePlus*, May 7, 2012.

"Ambiguous Genitalia." *Mayo Foundation for Medical Education and Research*, March 16, 2012.

"Androgen Insensitivity Syndrome." *MedlinePlus*, July 19, 2012.

"Answers to Your Questions about Individuals with Intersex Conditions." *American Psychological Association*, 2013.

Dreger, Alice Domurat. *Hermaphrodites and the Medical Invention of Sex*. Cambridge, Mass.: Harvard University Press, 2003.

Hida. "What is Intersex?" *Intersex Campaign for Equality*, 13 Nov. 2017, www.intersexequality.com/intersex/.

Kaneshiro, Neil, et al. "Intersex." *MedlinePlus*, U.S. National Library of Medicine, 5 Sept. 2017, medlineplus.gov/ency/article/001669.htm.

Karkazis, Katrina Alicia. *Fixing Sex: Intersex, Medical Authority, and Lived Experience*. Durham, N.C.: Duke University Press, 2008.

Moore, Keith L., and T. V. N. Persaud. *The Developing Human*. 8th ed. Philadelphia: Saunders/Elsevier, 2008.

Morland, Iain, ed. *Intersex and After*. Durham, N.C.: Duke University Press, 2009.

Intimate partner violence

CATEGORY: Disease/Disorder

KEY TERMS:

danger assessment tool: An instrument that helps determine the level of danger an abused woman has of being killed by her intimate partner.

mandatory reporting requirements: laws designating groups of professionals that are required to report specific types of violence, abuse, and neglect. In the U.S. these laws vary by state.

posttraumatic stress disorder: A maladaptive condition resulting from exposure to events beyond the realm of normal human experience and characterized by persistent difficulties involving emotional numbing, intense fear, helplessness, horror, reexperiencing of trauma, avoidance, and arousal.

The U.S. Center for Disease Control (CDC) has developed standardized definitions for the four subcategories of interpartner violence:

1. Physical is the use of physical force, possibly causing disability, injury, or death.
2. Sexual includes the use of physical aggression to force a person to engage in a sex act, when a sex act is attempted or completed with a person who is unable to understand or communicate their unwillingness to be complicit in the act, and abusive sexual contact.
3. Threats of physical or sexual violence are when words, gestures, or weapons are used to threaten bodily harm.
4. Psychological/emotional abuse describes harm caused by acts, threats of acts, or coercive tactics, and are acts largely defined based on the victim's perception of an act being abusive.

EPIDEMIOLOGY

Interpartner violence affects women at a higher rate than men. It is likely that incidents are underreported, so prevalence data are estimates. In the United States, 35.6 percent of women and 28.5 percent of men report physical violence, stalking, or rape during their lifetimes. Women are more often victims of sexual violence, with 9.4 percent of women in the United States experiencing rape in their lifetimes. Nearly 17 percent of women and 8 percent of men report being victims of sexual violence other than

rape during their lifetimes. On the other hand, rates of psychological abuse by an intimate partner are almost equal among genders, with 48.4 percent of men and 48.8 percent of women reporting psychological abuse in their lifetimes.

Worldwide, rates of interpartner sexual and physical violence against women were measured in a World Health Organization (WHO) multicountry study. Among 15 study sites, rates of women reporting they had experienced either sexual or physical violence in their lifetimes ranged from 15 to 71 percent. The rate of participants who reported that they experienced either form of violence in the past year ranged among sites from 4 to 53 percent.

HEALTH EFFECTS OF INTERPARTNER VIOLENCE

Interpartner violence may lead to direct physical harm. It has also been associated with higher rates of other physical symptoms and comorbid conditions that may persist long after the violent episode has ended. These conditions include headaches, back, musculoskeletal, or chest pain, gynecological disorders, gastrointestinal disorders, sexually transmitted infections, and respiratory infections.

Studies have found a correlation between incidence of interpartner violence and pregnancy. The effects of violence for the year prior to pregnancy have been observed to be far reaching and include poor physical outcomes for the mother and fetus, as well as increased risk for postpartum depression in the mother.

Victims of interpartner violence also exhibit increased levels of psychological conditions, especially posttraumatic stress disorder and major depressive disorder. Victims are also more likely to engage in negative health behaviors, such as substance abuse and high-risk sexual behaviors. These comorbidities can equate to long-term health consequences and disability across the lifespan for those who suffer from interpartner violence.

PREVENTION

The approach to preventing interpartner violence is multifaceted. Prevention efforts must begin by encouraging healthy relationships and emotionally supportive environments. Services must be readily available for victims, including healthcare, legal assistance, and mental health counseling to enable intervention and prevent reoccurrence. Healthcare providers should be trained to intervene when a victim of interpartner violence is identified. WHO and the Family Violence Prevention Fund have both outlined approaches to addressing patients who are victims of interpartner violence.

First and foremost, the patient's immediate risk for danger should be assessed, followed by support and possible referral for counseling. The Danger Assessment Tool is one instrument that can be used to assess how at-risk a female patient is for being murdered by her intimate partner. Some states require clinicians to report acts of violence communicated by patients. Clinicians should be familiar with the mandatory reporting requirements in their state of practice.

—Beth Williams

FOR FURTHER INFORMATION

Bonomi, A.E., et al. "Medical and Psychosocial Diagnoses in Women with a History of Intimate Partner Violence Diagnoses in Women Abused by Intimate Partners." *Archives of Internal Medicine*, vol. 169, no. 18, 2009, 1692-1697.

Campbell, J.Q. "Danger Risk Assessment Tool." Johns Hopkins University, School of Nursing, 2004.

Devries, K.M., et al. "Intimate Partner Violence and Incident Depressive Symptoms and Suicide Attempts: A Systematic Review of Longitudinal Studies." *PLoS Medicine*, vol. 10, no. 5, 2013, e1001439.

Garcia-Moreno, C., et al. "Prevalence of Intimate Partner Violence: Findings from the WHO Multi-Country Study on Women's Health and Domestic Violence." *The Lancet*, vol. 368, no. 9543, 2006, 1260-1269.

Gazmararian, J.A., et al. "Prevalence of Violence against Pregnant Women." *JAMA: The Journal of the American Medical Association*, vol. 275, no. 24, 1996, 1915-1920.

Ludermir, A. et al. "Violence against Women by Their Intimate Partner during Pregnancy and Postnatal Depression: A Prospective Cohort Study." *The Lancet*, vol. 376, no. 9744, 2010, 903-910.

Roberts, T. A., et al. "Longitudinal Effect of Intimate Partner Abuse on High-risk Behavior among Adolescents." *Archives of Pediatrics & Adolescent Medicine*, vol. 157, no. 9, 2003, 875.

Saltzman, L.E., et al. *Intimate Partner Violence Surveillance: Uniform Definitions and Recommended Data Elements: Version 1.0.* Atlanta, GA: Centers for Disease Control and Prevention, National Center for Injury Prevention and Control, 2002.

Intimate partner violence and pregnancy

CATEGORY: Social issue

DESCRIPTION

Intimate partner violence (IPV) is any physical, sexual, psychological, or emotional harm inflicted by one person on another within an intimate, romantic, and/or spousal relationship that is ongoing or that has ended. Such violence may also be referred to as spousal abuse or domestic violence, which is a broader term that can include child abuse and elder abuse.

Intimate partner violence is described as a severe and escalating form of violence characterized by multiple forms of abuse, terrorization, and controlling behavior on the part of the abuser. It rarely consists of a single episode, but usually instead occurs in a recurring pattern of intimidation and abuse. Relationships of this kind can be very difficult to leave, although abused women often make many attempts to leave perpetrators of IPV. Pregnant women can feel especially trapped in such relationships. Child abuse occurs in 30 to 60 percent of cases of IPV.

Intimate partner violence may begin or increase during pregnancy or the postpartum period. The biophysical effects of IPV on pregnant women include physical injury, gastrointestinal disorders, chronic pain syndromes, depression, and suicidal behavior. Victims of physical violence are more than twice as likely as nonvictims to experience postpartum depression (PPD). The frequency of abuse can increase in the postpartum period, and especially during the first 3 months following birth.

Up to half of reported cases of IPV include sexual violence, which can deter a female partner from wanting to become pregnant. Women are sometimes forced to have sex and sometimes also forced to bear children as a form of abuse, a risk that is greater for younger women and adolescent girls than for other women. Women who are victims of IPV have an increased risk of abortion, miscarriage, stillbirth, preterm delivery, and low birthweight. IPV can also result in gynecological disorders and sexually transmitted diseases (STDs), including human immunodeficiency virus (HIV) infection and acquired immune deficiency syndrome (AIDS).

FACTS AND FIGURES

Research indicates that perpetrators of IPV are more likely to be younger men with low self-esteem, emotional dependency, and limited income. Anger, hostility, sexist beliefs and values, and personality disorders are common aspects of a perpetrator's profile. A history of poverty in childhood, with low academic achievement and delinquency, is also described as a strong predictor of abusive behavior. Another indicator is having witnessed or experienced violence as a child. Alcohol use is frequently present in cases of reported abuse.

In the United States, IPV has reached epidemic proportions, with 50 million women experiencing some form of such abuse during their lives, and women being much more likely than men to be injured by IPV. In the United States, women are much more likely than men to be injured by IPV. Intimate partner violence accounts for half of all murders of women, with IPV related to the victim's pregnancy considered a significant factor in many these deaths. In 2010 in the United States, 1,295 deaths involved IPV, accounting for approximately 10 percent of homicides in that year. IPV is considered an antecedent in 25 percent of female suicides.

Internationally, the number of pregnant women being abused may be as high as 1 in 5, and IPV accounts for a substantial proportion of maternal deaths.

Psychosocial effects of living under a constant threat of physical harm include anxiety, degradation, humiliation, and ridicule. Victims of IPV often become isolated and dependent upon their abusive partners. Female victims of IPV are more likely than male victims to use violence in self-defense and are more likely to use weapons. Perpetrators of IPV often prevent their victims from maintaining functional relationships with family members and friends. Victims may also be prevented from taking employment, or may find it difficult to maintain a job and may become economically dependent on their abusers.

Particular attention should be given to the impact of IPV on children, because abuse of both women and children often occurs in family systems. Childhood exposure to IPV is linked to low self-esteem, social withdrawal, depression, and anxiety. Children exposed to IPV are more likely to exhibit cognitive, behavioral, and emotional problems, and some will exhibit symptoms of trauma. These problems can lead to difficulties in education and future employment and result in early school dropout, criminal behavior, and early pregnancy in children exposed to IPV. Separation from the abuser can significantly reduce the maltreatment of children.

RISK FACTORS

The high rates of IPV against female victims suggest that all women are potentially at risk for it. However, females ages 16 to 24 years and women with physical or mental disabilities are at the greatest risk for IPV, with women who have histories of child abuse, women with mental disorders, and women who abuse substances also at risk. The risk of IPV is also increased for women living in communities characterized by poverty, crowding, and low social capital. Reporting IPV or involving others can increase the likelihood of violence immediately after a victim reaches out for help, and experiencing physical violence during pregnancy more than doubles the risk of postpartum depression. Intimate partner violence is also an antecedent in suicide attempts by women, and increases the risk for further violence and murder. Despite this, many victims do not report IPV to family, friends, coworkers, service providers, or police, and healthcare workers such as doctors and nurses often underreport IPV.

Also creating a high risk of IPV are tolerance of sexism and traditional beliefs that endorse gender norms in which women stay at home to care for children while men make household and economic decisions. Educational disparities between partners may increase the risk of IPV for women.

Family pets are sometimes beaten and abused by perpetrators of IPV to gain emotional and psychological control over their victims.

SIGNS AND SYMPTOMS

Many pregnant victims of IPV are frequent users of healthcare services, with enduring and chronic pains. Signs of IPV include marks caused by strangulation, slapping, biting, and burns, with injuries of the head, face, and neck described as significant red flags for IPV. Victims of IPV often attribute these physical signs of abuse to household falls and accidents. Mental signs of IPV may include depression, anxiety, panic attacks, phobias, post-traumatic stress disorder, and suicidal ideation. Signs of coerced or forced sex and sexual acts may also indicate IPV.

Treatment

Pregnant victims of IPV need legal, financial, emotional, and psychological support services; health services; and assistance with housing, employment, and childcare. The social worker of a woman who experiences IPV during pregnancy must work in collaboration with her and suggest possible resources for advice and help. This includes inquiring about the victim's intimate relationship and the support networks available to her during her pregnancy and postpartum period. The social worker should ask about the frequency of her visits to a physician, note the number of her emergency room visits, and observe her for head, face, and neck injuries that may indicate IPV. The social worker should also record health complaints, including gastrointestinal disorders, chronic pain syndromes, depression, and suicidal behavior. Testing the victim for HIV/AIDS and STD may be indicated.

Intervention

Planning for the safety of pregnant victims of IPV and for their escape from their harmful milieu is important, and local shelters for victims of IPV can provide information about the services available in the area in which they live. If the victim has specific questions, the social worker can call the shelter on her behalf.

Social workers should be aware of their own cultural values, beliefs, and biases and develop specialized knowledge about the histories, traditions, and values of the women they serve. They should adopt treatment methodologies that reflect their knowledge of the cultural diversity of the communities in which they practice.

Safety measures that may help a pregnant victim of abuse include:

- Identifying a safe refuge from abuse.
- Referral to a local refuge or shelter.
- Having a telephone accessible at all times, and knowing the appropriate telephone numbers (such as the police) to call for help.
- Telling trusted friends and neighbors about the abusive situation and developing a plan and visual signal for help when it is needed.
- Teaching children how to get help.
- Planning safety measures with children and identifying a safe place for them, such as a room with a locking door or a friend's house where they can go for help.

- Setting money aside or asking friends or family members to hold money for instances in which it may be needed.
- Having an extra set of car keys.
- Obtaining a restraining order or order of protection and keeping a certified copy of it where it can be immediately available at all times.
- Changing locks and telephone numbers.
- Interventions focusing on school-aged children that teach respect in relationships and appropriate behavior have proven successful in reducing some forms of intimate violence.

Applicable Laws and Regulations

In the United States, laws and regulation that require healthcare and social workers to report IPV vary from state to state, with some states having no requirement at all for IPV to others requiring the reporting of any injury caused by a weapon. Detailed information about state reporting requirements can be found at the Health Cares About IPV website.

—*Jan Wagstaff, MA, MSW*

For Further Information

Bell, H., Busch-Armendariz, N. B., Sanchez, E., & Tekippe, A. (2008). Pregnant and parenting battered women speak out about their relationships and challenges. *Journal of Aggression, Maltreatment & Trauma, 17*(3), 318-335.

Bianchi, A., McFarlane, J., Nava, A., Gilroy, H., Maddoux, J., & Cesario, S. (2014). Rapid assessment to identify and quantify the risk of intimate partner violence during pregnancy. *Birth: Issues in Perinatal Care, 41*(1), 88-92. doi:10.1111/birt.12091

Hellmuth, J., Gordon, K., Stuart, G., & Moore, T. (2013). Intimate partner violence perpetration during pregnancy and postpartum. *Maternal & Child Health Journal, 17*(8), 1405-1413. doi:10.1007/s10995-012-1141-5

Hughes, M. J., & Rasmussen, L. A. (2010). The utility of motivational interviewing in domestic violence shelters: A qualitative exploration. *Journal of Aggression, Maltreatment & Trauma, 19*(3), 300-322.

"Intimate Partner Violence." Centers for Disease Control and Prevention. October 23, 2018. http://www.cdc.gov/ViolencePrevention/intimatepartnerviolence/index. html. Accessed March 8, 2019.

Kulkarni, S. (2007). Romance narrative, feminine ideals, and developmental detours for young mothers. *Journal of Women & Social Work, 22*(1), 23-38.

Sadusky, J. M., Martinson, R., Lizdas, K., & McGee, C. (2010). The Praxis Safety and Accountability Audit: Practicing a "sociology for people". *Violence Against Women, 16*(9), 1031-1044.

Shneyderman, Y., & Kiely, M. (2013). Intimate partner violence during pregnancy: Victim or perpetrator? Does it make a difference?. *BJOG: An International Journal of Obstetrics and Gynaecology, 120*(11), 1375-1385. doi:10.1111/1471-0528.12357

Spivak, H. R., Jenkins, L., Van Audenhove, K., Lee, D., Kelly, M., & Iskander, J. (2014). CDC Grand Rounds: A public health approach to prevention of intimate partner violence. *MMWR. Morbidity and Mortality Weekly Report, 63*(2), 38-41.

Intimate partner violence in same-sex relationships

CATEGORY: Social issue

CAUSES AND SYMPTOMS

Intimate partner violence (IPV) is any physical, sexual, psychological, or emotional abuse inflicted by one person on another within an intimate, romantic, or spousal relationship. The relationship may be ongoing or it may have ended but the violence has continued. IPV is also referred to as domestic violence, interpersonal violence, and family violence, which are broader terms that include child abuse and elder abuse. IPV is characterized as an escalating form of violence involving multiple forms of abuse, terrorization, and controlling behavior on the part of an abuser. There are similarities and differences between opposite-sex and same-sex IPV. The social, cultural, and legal complexities of the abuse can differ dramatically, but the relational dynamics are the same: individual power is used to control, exploit, and abuse the victim.

The victims of IPV live under constant threats of physical harm, degradation, humiliation, and ridicule. The relationships with children and friends of victims of IPV are undermined. As a way of gaining control over the victim of IPV, some perpetrators of IPV in same-sex relationships may threaten victims with exposing their sexual orientation to family and friends. In an effort to minimize the abuse, perpetrators may attempt to convince victims that they are "mutual batterers." This false perception of "common couple violence" can hide the perpetrator and the pattern of abuse and often prevents victims from reporting IPV and seeking help. Lesbians report difficulties in acknowledging that what they are experiencing is abuse. Unique legal complexities surrounding the custody of children and property can occur. In many states, victims of IPV in same-sex relationships do not have the same legal rights and options for recourse as victims of IPV in opposite-sex relationships. IPV can have a dramatic impact upon a victim's physical health and in extreme cases can be fatal. Research indicates that sexual risk-taking can co-occur with IPV, increasing the risk of acquiring sexually transmitted infections (STIs). There is a lack of specialized services for gay and lesbian victims of IPV in many parts of the United States.

Signs of physical IPV may be visible or hidden. Visible signs may include red marks around the neck from strangulation, bruising, and bite and burn marks. Physical signs of coerced or forced sex may also indicate IPV. Head, face, and neck injuries are described as significant red flags for IPV. These physical signs are commonly attributed by victims of IPV to be primarily due to household falls and accidents: social workers need to be alert to any disparities in the victim's accounts of the attribution of the injuries. Mental health symptoms that may be present when IPV occurs include symptoms of depression, anxiety, panic attacks, phobias, posttraumatic stress disorder (PTSD), and suicidal ideation.

FACTS AND FIGURES

Researchers have found that male victims of same-sex IPV are 50 to 60 percent more likely to be HIV-positive than males in non-abusive same-sex relationships. In a study on sexual violence perpetration by adolescents, males were two times more likely to perpetrate sexual violence against male peers than females were against other females. According to a 2012 report by the National Coalition of Anti-Violence Programs on IPV in the lesbian, gay, bisexual, transgender, and queer/questioning (LGBTQ) and HIV-affected community, 41.7 percent of those reporting IPV in 2012 identified as gay and 24.5 percent as lesbian; 40.3

percent were between 19 and 29 years old and 1.6 percent were over age 60; and transgender persons reporting IPV were 4.4 times more likely to encounter violence perpetrated by the police while they were reporting IPV than persons who did not identify as transgender.

In one recent study, almost 75 percent of lesbian women reported that they were victims of psychological IPV. Emotional and psychological abuse is more likely in lesbian couples than gay couples. Compared to heterosexual couples, lesbian and gay couples experienced higher life-time prevalence of IPV: 44 percent of lesbian women and 26 percent of gay men. Bisexual people seem to experience the most IPV, especially bisexual women. The stereotype of lesbian relationships being peaceful and ideal due to the absence of masculine aggression and violence can result in lesbian and bisexual women not recognizing abusive behavior.

RISK FACTORS

There are common risk factors for IPV victimization between same-sex relationships and opposite-sex relationships including substance abuse, personality disorders, relationship dependency, violence in family of origin, rigid adherence to socially and culturally constructed norms of masculinity (such as suppressing emotional vulnerability, avoiding dependency, aggressiveness, striving to succeed at work at the cost of relationships). The risk factors unique to same-sex relationships are the possible presence of identity concealment (being in the closet), internalized homonegativity (self-loathing due to sexual orientation, also conceived of as internalized homophobia), and the stress placed on both the individuals and the relationship by societal homophobia. Economic disparity between same-sex partners may also present a risk to IPV victimization, as may a low income, unemployment, and depression. In addition, research suggests that Latino gay men are particularly vulnerable to IPV. Adolescent males studied in an urban community in the United States were at higher risk for both IPV perpetration and victimization if they had personal histories of heavy episodic drinking and/or drug use, childhood sexual abuse, and exposure to violence in the community. The experience of adverse events in youth such as parental substance abuse, parental IPV, and physical and sexual abuse may increase the likelihood that gay men in the United

States will engage in alcohol/drug abuse, IPV, and risky sexual behaviors.

ASSESSMENT AND SCREENING

A complete biological, psychological, social, and spiritual assessment, including the risk for suicide and harming others should be completed and the victim should be assessed for immediate safety.

Gender-neutral questions should be used to elicit more information from persons in same-sex relationships. The disclosure of less violent forms of IPV is considered a first step in articulating abuse for victims in same-sex relationships. Assessment tools include the following.

The Partner Violence Screen (PVS) has three yes-or-no questions: if the victim has been physically hurt, whether she or he feels safe in the present relationship, and whether she or he fears a previous one.

The Hurt, Insulted, Threatened with Harm, or Screamed at (HITS) instrument has four questions that ask whether the victim's partner has hurt, insulted, threatened, or screamed at him or her.

The Intimate Partner Violence among Gay and Bisexual Men (IPV-GBM) contains 23 items, including previously ignored domains such as controlling behavior, monitoring behaviors, emotional violence, and HIV-related violence. Healthcare settings may utilize a revised and shortened scale of the IPV-BGM.

TREATMENT AND INTERVENTION

The IPV services for victims in same-sex relationships are limited. Services for victims of IPV are especially scarce for gay men. Lesbians who seek assistance from shelters may experience homophobia from shelters that are designed to serve heterosexual women and children fleeing violence from male partners. As with all victims of IPV, safety is the first consideration, and it is important that victims of IPV are assisted with making a safety plan. A strengths-based approach is recommended in which the social worker explores with the victim any positive actions he or she can take in the present situation. Therapeutic group work is also suggested to help explore and name experiences of abuse. Skill development to learn how to access resources, garner social support, and communicate with one's intimate partner may also be beneficial.

Victims receiving care or treatment for the victimization of IPV may need assistance with obtaining immediate shelter. A social worker or other helping professional assisting the victim may call the local shelter and LBGTQ center for advice and suggestions on safe and temporary accommodations for the victim.

When a victim of IPV is ready to leave an abusive relationship, a social worker or other helping professional should assist in developing a safety plan and plan of action for leaving the relationship.

Steps should be taken to help the victim find legal advice; find safe accommodations, including new schools if needed; identifying available support networks; and find work, training, or financial assistance. The social worker should assist in developing the safety plan while the victim is still in the relationship and preparing to leave.

Victims of IPV may need support including counseling and therapeutic services. The social worker or other helping professional should call the local shelter and/or LGBTQ center to find available therapists that provide individual and group services.

RED FLAGS

The fear of being outed to family, friends, employers, law enforcement, and the community at large is one of the biggest barriers to same-sex victims and perpetrators seeking help. The legal issues surrounding same-sex couples are more complex than are the legal issues for opposite-sex couples and may require specialized legal knowledge. Male victims of IPV are less likely to report IPV because of the belief that police either will not believe them or will be ineffective. Same-sex IPV often goes unrecognized by professionals at primary care facilities.

—*Jan Wagstaff, MA, MSW*

FURTHER READING

Brown, Carrie. "Gender-Role Implications on Same-Sex Intimate Partner Abuse." *Journal of Family Violence*, vol. 23, no. 6, 25 Mar. 2008, pp. 457–462., doi:10.1007/s10896-008-9172-9.

Eaton, Lisa, et al. "Examining Factors Co-Existing with Interpersonal Violence in Lesbian Relationships." *Journal of Family Violence*, vol. 23, no. 8, 26 July 2008, pp. 697–705., doi:10.1007/s10896-008-9194-3.

Hassouneh, Dena, and Nancy Glass. "The Influence of Gender Role Stereotyping on Women's Experiences of Female Same-Sex Intimate Partner Violence." *Violence Against Women*, vol. 14, no. 3, 1 Mar. 2008, pp. 310–325., doi:10.1177/1077801207313734.

Irwin, Jude. "(Dis)Counted Stories." *Qualitative Social Work: Research and Practice*, vol. 7, no. 2, 1 June 2008, pp. 199–215., doi:10.1177/1473325008089630.

Lindley, Lisa L., et al. "Becoming Visible: Assessing the Availability of Online Sexual Health Information for Lesbians." *Health Promotion Practice*, vol. 13, no. 4, 15 June 2011, pp. 472–480., doi:10.1177/1524839910390314.

Waters, Emily, et al. "Lesbian, Gay, Bisexual, Transgender, Queer, and HIV-affected Intimate Partner Violence in 2015." *National Coalition of Anti-Violence Programs*. New York City Gay and Lesbian Anti-Violence Project, 2016.

Oswald, Ramona F., et al. "Lesbian Mothers' Counseling Experiences in the Context of Intimate Partner Violence." *Psychology of Women Quarterly*, vol. 34, no. 3, 2 Aug. 2010, pp. 286–296., doi:10.1111/j.1471-6402.2010.01575.x.

Patzel, Brenda. "What Blocked Heterosexual Women and Lesbians in Leaving Their Abusive Relationships." *Journal of the American Psychiatric Nurses Association*, vol. 12, no. 4, 1 Aug. 2006, pp. 208–215., doi:10.1177/1078390306294897.

Rollè, Luca, et al. "When Intimate Partner Violence Meets Same Sex Couples: A Review of Same Sex Intimate Partner Violence." *Frontiers in Psychology*, vol. 9, 21 Aug. 2018, doi:10.3389/fpsyg.2018.01506.

Intimate partner violence: Women as perpetrators

CATEGORY: Social issue

DESCRIPTION

Intimate partner violence (IPV) is any physical, sexual, psychological, or emotional abuse inflicted by one person on another within an intimate, romantic, and/or spousal relationship that is ongoing or that has ended. IPV is also referred to as domestic violence, interpersonal violence, and family violence. Little is understood about the individual experiences of men who are abused by an intimate partner. One helpline reported that men experience intimidation, isolation, threats, and emotional abuse similar to that experienced by women. Men can also be blamed for the abuse or it may be minimized by the female perpetrator. Although women experience higher rates of physical and mental health problems as a result of victimization of IPV, male victims of IPV also experience negative physical and mental effects, including frequent headaches, chronic pain, difficulty sleeping, depression, anxiety, and symptoms of posttraumatic stress disorder (PTSD).

In addition to physical assaults, men have reported being victimized through sexual violence and stalking. Abused men have high rates of depression, although it is hard to determine whether the depression is a result from the IPV or was already present and increasing the vulnerability for IPV. Unemployment and alcohol abuse are also likely to be features of abusive relationships for either or both partners, male or female. Males who are physically assaulted by their female partners may also be perpetrators of violence. Social workers should provide services to both victims and abusers of IPV.

Men who experience IPV are unlikely to report the IPV to law enforcement or to healthcare professionals and social workers. Men who do seek help for IPV encounter difficulties because most IPV shelters, help centers, and medical facilities provide services for female victims only. Many victims of IPV including men, have reported shame, fear, social stigmatization, and negative self-image as a result of IPV. In addition, norms of masculinity (toughness, stoicism, not showing emotions) may act as significant barriers for men seeking help. When men disclose IPV, they are sometimes judged to be weak and may experience ridicule.

The motives of female perpetrators of IPV are similar to the motives of male perpetrators. These common motives for IPV include self-defense, control, jealousy, fear, retribution, defense of children, and to maintain a tough guise. Mental health issues, including traits of personality disorders such as narcissistic and antisocial personality disorder, are common in the typical IPV perpetrator profile. The symptoms of depression, emotional regulation problems, anxiety, substance abuse, and PTSD are also predominant in perpetrators of IPV. Women who use violence in their relationships have personal histories that typically include high levels of childhood trauma and abuse.

FACTS AND FIGURES

In the United States 28.5 percent of men experience rape, physical violence, or stalking by an intimate partner. In cases of IPV against men, the majority of the perpetrators are female. IPV and child abuse often cooccur in families. Emotional abuse has a higher correlation with depressive symptoms for male victims of IPV than physical abuse or sexual assault and men who experience IPV are nearly three times more likely to report symptoms of depression than men who do not experience IPV. Of men surveyed in a rural community and those surveyed in a national sample, 30.1 percent and 18.1 percent, respectively, reported emotional victimization in the past year by a female intimate partner. The National Intimate Partner and Sexual Violence Survey revealed that 4.7 percent of male respondents reported physical IPV victimization in 2010. Arrests of women for IPV were reported to make up 8 to 20 percent of all arrests for IPV as of 2007, which is an increase of 25 to 35 percent since the 1980s.

RISK FACTORS

The risk factors for IPV for both female perpetrators and male victims may include alcohol and other substance abuse, low income or financial stress, unemployment, and mental health problems, such as depression, anxiety, and PTSD symptoms. Men have an increased risk for IPV perpetration and victimization if they witnessed family violence as children.

SIGNS AND SYMPTOMS

Signs of IPV may be visible or hidden. Female perpetrators are more likely to use physical forms of IPV such as slapping, biting, kicking, punching, or hitting their partner with an object; physical injuries consistent with these actions may suggest that abuse has occurred. Other physical symptoms of IPV victimization may include frequent headaches, chronic pain, and difficulty sleeping. Male victims of IPV may see mental health professionals for the treatment of depressive symptoms.

ASSESSMENT

A thorough biological, psychological, social, and spiritual assessment of the victim or perpetrator of IPV should be completed by social workers and other mental health professionals. The assessment should be sensitive, particularly during disclosure, to the male culture and ethnic background of the victim. An accurate screening of male victims of IPV is critical. The history of witnessing family violence may contribute to the minimization by men of IPV victimization. It is also important that social workers completing an assessment keep in mind that women who are violent may also be victims of IPV.

ASSESSMENT AND SCREENING TOOLS

Screening tools that may be used by social workers, clinical psychologists, or other mental health professionals to gather information for an assessment of IPV may include the following.

A. The Partner Violence Screen (PVS) questionnaire consists of three yes-or-no questions: if the victim has been physically hurt, whether he or she feels safe in the present relationship, or whether he or she fears a previous relationship.

B. The physically Hurt, Insulted, Threatened with Harm, Screamed at (HITS) instrument has four questions: whether the victim's partner has hurt, insulted, threatened, or screamed at him or her.

INTERVENTION

The safety of the individual is paramount. Although services for male victims of intimate partner violence are scarce, social workers can help clarify their immediate and long-term needs, as well as assist in finding appropriate services. Women who are violent towards their male partners may also be victims of IPV, and therefore services may be offered to the female partners of male victims of IPV. Service providers are advised to assess couples for all forms of abuse, not only physical abuse.

Men and women who have experienced IPV may experience emotional distress as a result of the IPV. If appropriate, the social worker should provide counseling and support or assist in finding a therapist to help the victim feel supported, safe, and reduce distress. The National Domestic Violence Hotline has a database that can help men find support services.

The social worker or helping professional working with a victim of IPV who is ready to leave an abusive relationship should assist the victim with developing a safety plan to leave the relationship. The victim should be guided through figuring out what is needed for the move, including finding legal advice, sourcing accommodations and new schools, identifying support networks, and finding work, training, or financial assistance. The National Domestic Violence Hotline has a database that can help men find shelters and other services.

APPLICABLE LAWS AND REGULATIONS

In the United States, only three states (Alabama, New Mexico, and Wyoming) do not require mandatory reporting of domestic violence. For the states that do require reporting, this reporting falls into three categories: reporting of injuries caused by weapons, reporting of injuries caused by violation of criminal laws, and reporting of injuries that are specific to domestic violence. Additional IPV statutes may be found on the U.S. Department of Health and Human Services website.

FOOD FOR THOUGHT

Unlike male-perpetrated intimate partner violence, female-perpetrated intimate partner violence is not a predictor of relationship breakups. Similar rates of IPV victimization have been reported in male populations in Sweden, the Netherlands, Ecuador, and Spain. The reasons male victims report they stay in an abusive relationship are financial security and continued contact with their children.

RED FLAGS

Male victims who are physically attacked may also be perpetrators of IPV and not solely victims of IPV.

IPV and child abuse can co-occur in families. Some male victims may remain in the abusive relationship in order to protect their children. Many children that are exposed to IPV experience symptoms of low self-esteem, social withdrawal, depression, and anxiety and they are more likely to exhibit cognitive and behavioral problems.

NEXT STEPS

It is important that social workers and mental health professionals work in collaboration with the victim of IPV. Men and women experiencing IPV should be provided contact details for the National Domestic Violence Hotline and/or the local IPV help center where information and services can be sought. If the victim intends to leave the relationship, he/she should talk with the social worker about having a plan to do this. In cases where the victim is not ready to leave the relationship, a safety plan should be created with the victim.

—Jan Wagstaff, MA, MSW,
and Jennifer Mary Dorrell, ASW

FOR FURTHER INFORMATION

Barber, C. F. (2008). Domestic violence against men. *Nursing Standard, 22*(51), 35-39.

Drijber, B. C., et al. "Male victims of domestic violence." *Journal of Family Violence*, 28, no.2, 2013, 173-178. doi: 10.1007/ s10896-012-9482-9

"Intimate Partner Violence." Centers for Disease Control and Prevention. October 23, 2018. http://www.cdc.gov/ViolencePrevention/intimatepartnerviolence/index. html.

Pornari, C. D., Dixon, L., & Humphreys, G. W. (2013). Systematically identifying implicit theories in male and female intimate partner violence perpetrators. *Aggression & Violent Behavior, 18*(5), 496-505. doi: 10.1016/j.avb.2013.07.005

Winstok, Z., & Strauss, M. A. (2014). Gender differences in the link between intimate partner physical violence and depression. *Aggression & Violent Behavior, 19*(2), 91-101. doi: 10.1016/j.avb.2014.01.003

Tsui, V. (2014). Male victims of intimate partner abuse: Use and helpfulness of services. *Social Work, 59*(2), 121-130.

Intimate partner violence: Women as victims

CATEGORY: Social issue

DESCRIPTION

Intimate partner violence (IPV) is any physical, sexual, psychological, or emotional abuse inflicted by one person on another within an intimate, romantic, and/ or spousal relationship that is ongoing or has ended. It is also referred to as domestic violence and/ or family violence, which includes child and elder abuse. Studies have included stalking and control of a partner's reproductive or sexual health as aspects of IPV. Globally, up to half of reported cases of IPV include sexual violence, which is used by the perpetrator to maintain power and control. The physical effects of IPV can be fatal. Of the 2,032 females murdered in the United States in 2010, 39.2 percent were killed by an intimate partner, and on a worldwide scale, IPV is considered a preexisting event in 25 percent of female suicides. Internationally, IPV is described as a human rights issue that is reaching epidemic proportions. It is overwhelmingly a crime perpetrated by men against women, but affects both women and men regardless of age, race, economic status, ethnicity, sexual orientation, and education level.

IPV is characterized by multiple forms of abuse, terrorization, and controlling behavior on the part of the abuser. Its effects on victims include living in fear as a result of constant threats of physical harm, degradation, humiliation, and ridicule. Such violence rarely consists of a single incident but is instead a pattern of abuse that is often prolonged and may continue for years, disrupting an individual's entire pattern of living. It often involves behavior that limits the victim's access to the outside world in order to increase the victim's dependency on the abuser. This is often accomplished through psychological threats and intimidation as well as physical violence. The goal of the abuser is to establish and maintain power over the abuser's partner. Abusers will often prevent their partner-victims from maintaining functional relationships with family members and friends. They may also prevent the partner from working or may make it difficult for the partner to maintain a job, which as a consequence may make the partner economically dependent on the abuser. Relationships involving IPV can be very difficult for women to leave, and they may make multiple attempts to do so.

FACTS AND FIGURES

On a worldwide scale, about one in three women has experienced IPV. According to the 2011 National Intimate Partner and Sexual Violence Survey, 8.8 percent of women in the United States had been raped by an intimate partner in the past 12 months, 15.5 percent had experienced another form of sexual violence by an intimate partner, and 9.2 percent had been stalked by an intimate partner.

RISK FACTORS

Intimate partner violence may create long-term health problems for its victims. These include physical injury, gastrointestinal disorders, chronic pain, depression, and suicidal behavior. It can also result in gynecological disorders, unwanted pregnancy, premature labor and birth, and sexually transmitted infections, including HIV/AIDS. Women who are highly committed to maintaining the relationship with an abusive partner will often minimize and excuse the abuse and are more likely to blame themselves for their circumstances.

Child maltreatment occurs together with IPV, and children often suffer from witnessing abuse. In either case, affected children may exhibit symptoms of trauma and can develop low self-esteem, social withdrawal, depression, and anxiety. Children who witness IPV are more likely to exhibit cognitive, behavioral, and emotional problems than other children. In some cases, family pets are beaten or otherwise abused to gain emotional and psychological control over victims of IPV.

Immigrants who remain enculturated in the traditions of their country of origin are at higher risk of IPV.

Studies done by the U.S. Centers for Disease Control and Prevention (CDC) of perpetrators of IPV have found that they are more likely to be younger men with low self-esteem, emotional dependency, and low income. Anger, hostility, beliefs, and values learned from a perpetrator's father, and personality disorders are often found in the psychological profiles of perpetrators of IPV. A history of poverty, low academic achievement, and delinquency is also a strong predictor of abusive behavior, as is having witnessed or experienced violence as a child. Alcohol use is another feature of reported abuse.

Women between the ages of 18 and 24 and those with a physical or mental disability have an increased risk of IPV, as do women with a history of child abuse and/or women exposed to violence between their parents. Pregnancy and low education levels, and living in rural communities, can also increase a woman's risk of IPV, as can a disparity in education between the partners in a relationship. Families living in communities characterized by poverty, crowding, and low social capital can be at risk. Cultural and traditional beliefs that support and reinforce patriarchy can encourage IPV, and an increased risk of IPV exists in families in which women stay at home to care for children while men make household and economic decisions.

Reporting IPV or involving others can increase the likelihood of violence immediately after a victim reaches out for help.

SIGNS AND SYMPTOMS

Psychological signs in a victim of IPV include fearfulness, emotional distress, depression, anxiety, thoughts of suicide, panic attacks, difficulty in sleeping, and low self-esteem. Physical signs include cuts, scratches, bruises, bite marks, burns, broken bones, welts, internal bleeding, head injuries, frequent headaches, chronic pain, and poor physical health. Behavioral effects of IPV can include drug and alcohol use, denial or minimization of violence, and self-blame for a partner's violence. Social effects can include isolation from friends and family, difficulty in trusting others, and being in relationships. Sexual consequences of IPV include unwanted pregnancy, STIs, frequent vaginal or urinary tract infections, and pelvic pain.

TREATMENT

A complete assessment of the victim of IPV is essential for understanding the nature and extent of its impact on the victim and for successful intervention. The assessment should include a complete medical, psychological, social, and spiritual evaluation, including specific questions about the victim's safety and any thoughts about suicide. Questions should include the frequency of the victim's physician visits and number of emergency room visits. Indications of IPV may be head, face, and neck injuries; gastrointestinal disorders; chronic pain; depression; and suicidal behavior. The victim may attribute physical injuries from IPV to unwitnessed household accidents.

A childhood history of witnessed IPV or child maltreatment may indicate a potential for being abused as an adult.

INTERVENTION

Intervention should include education about the psychological and other risk factors that lead to violent relationships. Group therapy, along with individual therapy, can be beneficial to individuals who suffer from a traumatic experience. A range of interventions considered to be promising and/or evidence-based are available to address the mental health needs of women who have endured IPV.

CBT is often used to address posttraumatic stress disorder (PTSD) and related mental health issues for women who have suffered trauma resulting from IPV. CBT focuses on examining the relationships between thoughts, feelings, and behaviors, with the goal of assisting victims of IPV to modify their patterns of thinking and improve their coping ability. Techniques of CBT such as thought-stopping, recording of thoughts, and role playing can be used to increase skills and provide the victim with insight into beliefs about herself, dysfunctional thinking, and maladaptive strategies for coping.

Trauma-focused CBT integrates cognitive and behavioral interventions with trauma-specific interventions such as education of the victim about the psychological effects of trauma and common reactions to it, coping skills to manage emotional and behavioral reactions, and individualized stress-management techniques. A key component is the trauma narrative, in which the victim describes in detail the most important parts of the trauma she has experienced.

The social worker assisting a victim of IPV must work in collaboration with the victim and suggest possible resources for help and advice, including both formal and informal sources of support. Victims often need multiple types of services. The local IPV shelter is able to provide the latest information on the legal, financial, and counseling services available in the victim's area. If the victim has specific questions (for instance, about financial assistance), the social worker can call the shelter on her behalf.

Social workers assisting victims of IPV should be aware of their own cultural values, beliefs, and biases and develop specialized knowledge about the histories, traditions, and values of their clients. Social workers should adopt treatment methodologies that reflect their knowledge of the cultural diversity of the communities in which they practice. It is also important to know that doctors, nurses, and other healthcare workers may underreport IPV.

Safety measures that may help a victim of abuse include:

1. Identifying a safe refuge from abuse.
2. Referral to a local refuge or shelter.
3. Having a telephone accessible at all times and knowing the appropriate telephone numbers (such as the police) to call for help.
4. Telling trusted friends and neighbors about the abusive situation and developing a plan and visual signal for help when it is needed.
5. Teaching children how to get help.
6. Planning safety measures with children and identifying a safe place for them, such as a room with a locking door or a friend's house where they can go for help.
7. Setting money aside or asking friends or family members to hold money for instances in which it may be needed.
8. Having an extra set of car keys.

9. Obtaining a restraining order or order of protection and keeping a certified copy of it where it can be immediately available at all times.
10. Changing locks and telephone numbers.

APPLICABLE LAWS AND REGULATIONS

In the United States, laws or regulations that require healthcare and social workers to report IPV and child abuse vary from state to state, with some states having no requirement at all for reporting IPV to others requiring the reporting of any injury caused by a weapon. Detailed state-by-state reporting requirements can be found at the Health Cares About IPV website.

The Violence Against Women Act of 1994 (VAWA) provides for the investigation and prosecution of violent crimes against women and to male victims of domestic violence, dating violence, sexual assault, and stalking. The Violence Against Women Reauthorization Act of 2013 extended protections to Native American women, immigrants, and LGBT persons. The U.S. Victims of Trafficking and Violence Protection Act, including the Battered Immigrant Women's Protection Act, of 2000, created the nonimmigrant visa, which enables immigrant women in abusive marriages and family situations to leave their spouses without fear of change in their immigration status.

—Jan Wagstaff, MA, MSW,
and Jennifer Mary Dorrell, ASW

FOR FURTHER INFORMATION

Anderson, K. M., Renner, L. M., & Bloom, T. S. (2014). Rural women's strategic responses to intimate partner violence. *Health Care for Women International*, 35(4), 423-441. doi:10.1080/07399332.2013.815757

Breiding, M. J., Smith, S. G., Basile, K. C., Walters, M. L., Chen, J., & Merrick, M. T. (2014). Prevalence and characteristics of sexual violence, stalking, and intimate partner violence victimization – National Intimate Partner Sexual Violence Survey, United States, 2011. *MMWR, SS63*(8), 1-18.

"Intimate Partner Violence." Centers for Disease Control and Prevention. October 23, 2018. http://www.cdc.gov/ViolencePrevention/intimate-partnerviolence/index. html. Accessed March 8, 2019.

Macy, R. J., Rizo, C. F., Guo, S., & Ermentrout, D. M. (2013). Changes in intimate partner violence among women mandated to community services. *Research on Social Work Practice, 23*(6), 624-638.

Okano, M., Langille, J., & Walsh, Z. (2016). Psychopathy, alcohol use, and intimate partner violence: Evidence from two samples. *Law and Human Behavior,* 1-7. Advance online publication.

Wahab, S., Trimble, J., Mejia, A., Mitchell, S. R., Thomas, M. J., Timmons, V. W., & Nicolaidis, C. (2014). Motivational interviewing at the intersections of depression and intimate partner violence among African American women. *Journal of Evidence-Based Social Work, 11*(3), 291-303. doi:10.1080/15433714.2013.791502

Iron

CATEGORY: Biology

KEY TERMS:

ferritin: the primary intracellular storage form of iron
total iron-binding capacity (TIBC): a measure of the iron-binding capacity in blood (via transferrin)
transferrin: the primary transport form of iron; transferrin exhibits an inverse relationship to ferritin

STRUCTURE AND FUNCTIONS

Iron (Fe) is an essential trace mineral that was first recognized as an essential nutrient in the 1860s. The average adult human body contains 3–4 g of iron, nearly 70% of which is found in RBCs as part of the heme portion of the hemoglobin molecule that transports oxygen to cells. In the body, iron is stored as ferritin and hemosiderin; these stored forms of iron account for about 25% of total body iron. The remainder exists in myoglobin (i.e., the oxygen-carrying molecular found in cardiac and skeletal muscles); as a key component of numerous enzymatic pathways; as transferrin, a blood plasma protein that is the transport form of iron; and as the labile iron pool, a rapidly recycling form of iron that is directly involved in cell iron production.

About 90% of iron is recycled and reused by the body. Iron is essential for oxygen and carbon dioxide transport. It is necessary for aerobic energy production due to its role as a component of enzymes, and as an electron transporter in the metabolic pathway (called the Krebs cycle) that converts carbohydrate, protein, and fat into usable energy.

Key functions of iron arise from its role in oxidation and reduction (called redox) reactions, which is the ability to donate and accept electrons. This electron transport activity is critical to hemoglobin- and myoglobin-mediated transport of oxygen and carbon dioxide.

Iron is present in enzymes that drive the conversion of energy from food, in the form of calories, into cellular energy, which is supplied by adenosine triphosphate (ATP).

The cytochrome P-450 system, which breaks down compounds that are foreign to the body (called xenobiotics) requires iron to convert water-insoluble medications into water-soluble compounds for excretion.

Iron is chemically reactive and must be protein-bound in the body to prevent damage to cell membranes and DNA. The tissue damage associated with iron overload syndromes (e.g., hemochromatosis) is due to iron's highly reactive nature.

The many important roles of iron in the body are evident in the wide range of signs and symptoms present in persons with iron deficiency, including lethargy, breathlessness, headaches, irritability, dizziness, weight loss, deficits in learning and concentration, difficulty maintaining body temperature, and reduced immunity.

SOURCES OF IRON

Dietary iron is present in heme and non-heme forms. Heme iron is bound in the hemoglobin molecule. Because hemoglobin is present only in organisms with blood, heme iron comes exclusively from foods of animal origin, including meat, fish, and poultry. Plants and iron-fortified foods provide non-heme iron, which is not part of the hemoglobin molecule, to the diet. Heme iron is more absorbable than non-heme iron (15–45% compared with 1–15%), but non-heme iron accounts for more total iron in the diet. Good sources of heme iron include beef, chicken, and fish, oysters, crab, shrimp, and other shellfish, and organ meats, such as liver and kidneys. Good sources of non-heme iron include fortified cereals, bread, pasta, rice, beans, lentils, chickpeas, green leafy vegetables (especially spinach), tofu and other soy products, canned tomato products, molasses, and raisins. Dietary supplements can be used to increase iron intake and correct deficient serum levels of iron-containing compounds in individuals with inadequate dietary intake or impaired iron absorption.

The preferred route of iron administration is oral. 325 mg of ferrous sulfate 3 times daily is recommended for individuals with iron deficiency. Current recommendations for pregnant women include iron supplementation both during surgery and after delivery, often in combination with the B-vitamin, folate.

Iron supplementation can cause gastrointestinal (GI) effects, including nausea, constipation, and diarrhea. Reduction of the dose of iron supplementation, followed by a gradual increase in dose over several days, may improve tolerance.

Increasing fiber intake may help alleviate constipation associated with iron supplementation.

Patients prescribed oral iron supplements should be advised that iron will darken stools. In liquid iron preparations, a straw or spoon should be used to place the liquid iron at the back of the mouth to avoid staining the teeth.

Ferrous sulfate is best absorbed on an empty stomach. Vitamin C–rich foods, such as citrus fruit, can increase non-heme iron absorption. Other iron formulations, such as ferrous gluconate and ferrous fumarate, typically cause fewer GI adverse effects; these forms of iron are less readily absorbed and should be prescribed only for patients who do not tolerate ferrous sulfate.

Iron supplementation should continue for several months after resolution of iron-deficiency anemia to allow for rebuilding of iron stores.

RECOMMENDED INTAKE OF IRON

Recommended dietary intake of iron (mg/day) has been established for various age groups and are shown in the table below.

DISORDERS AND DISEASES

The World Health Organization (WHO) cites iron deficiency as the number one nutritional disorder in the world. It is reported that up to 80% of people worldwide are iron deficient, and 30% exhibit clinically evident iron-deficiency anemia. Iron-deficiency anemia is the most common form of anemia worldwide, and can arise from low dietary intake of iron, or inadequate absorption of iron.

Excessive blood loss is another major underlying cause, especially in women who experience heavy or prolonged menstrual bleeding. Additionally, increased requirements for iron during pregnancy can predispose women to gestational iron deficiency. In sum, iron deficiency anemia affects up to 47% of preschool children, 30% of women of childbearing age, and 42% of pregnant women worldwide.

Specific populations are at risk for iron deficiency. Such at-risk populations include:

1. preterm and low birth weight infants
2. breastfed infants who do not receive iron supplementation
3. infants and young children who consume large quantities of milk and insufficient iron-containing foods; milk contains minimal iron and calcium inhibits iron absorption from the diet as well
4. pregnant women, especially those with a history of 2 or more previous pregnancies or who have had several pregnancies in a short period of time
5. women of childbearing age and women with heavy menstrual blood loss
6. women with certain gynecological/uterine conditions, including fibroids
7. female athletes or women on low-calorie diets (e.g., < 1,500 calories/ day); for smaller individuals, a low-calorie intake may be adequate to maintain weight but lacks sufficient dietary iron
8. persons with protein-energy malnutrition (e.g., persons failing to consume adequate calories and protein to sustain health and/or promote growth in children)
9. persons with kidney failure, especially those treated with dialysis
10. patients who have had a partial or complete gastrectomy (i.e., removal of parts of the stomach)
11. persons with achlorhydria (i.e., low or absent gastric acid production)
12. patients receiving medical treatments that decrease the number of red blood cells and/or platelets (e.g., chemotherapy)
13. patients who have experienced significant blood loss due to injury or surgery
14. persons with vitamin A deficiency
15. persons with conditions involving inflammation of the small intestine (e.g., Crohn's disease)

Of note, body stores of iron vary from person to person; however, women and children often have little ferritin and hemosiderin (e.g., stored forms of iron) compared to men. Coupled with generally increased iron demands, women are made particularly susceptible to developing iron deficiency. In iron-deficient postmenopausal women, determining the source of iron loss is critical; gastrointestinal blood loss represents the most common cause of iron deficiency in this population.

Signs, symptoms and health consequences of more pronounced iron deficiency include fatigue; lethargy; weakness; breathlessness; headaches; irritability; dizziness; weight loss; deficits in learning and concentration; difficulty maintaining body temperature; impaired immunity, exercise intolerance; constipation, menstrual irregularity; muscle twitching; tingling and numbness in the extremities; tinnitus; heart palpitations; growth retardation, reduced school achievement, and impaired motor and cognitive development in children, pallor, fingernail "spooning;" blue-tinged sclera (i.e., whites of the eyes have blue tint); pica (i.e., craving for non-nutritional items such as ice, chalk, or clay); esophageal stricture (e.g., as occurs in Plummer-Vinson syndrome); glossitis; and angular stomatitis (i.e., irritation and cracking at the corners of the mouth).

Excluding blood loss, the body does not readily secrete iron. As such, chronic iron toxicity, which may result from long-term, excessive iron intake (e.g., high dose supplementation in a non-deficient person), or from medical conditions leading to excessive iron absorption (e.g., hemochromatosis), is a serious concern.

Iron poisoning, which refers to acute iron overload typically resulting from a one-time iron overdose, is the most common cause of fatal poisoning in children under the age of 5 years. Signs and symptoms of acute iron poisoning in adults begin to appear after a one-time ingestion of >20 mg of iron per kg of body weight. More severe acute iron poisoning, in which some of the toxic effects may not be reversible, occurs in adults when one-time iron intake exceeds 40 mg of iron per kg of body weight. A one-time iron dose exceeding 60 mg of iron per kg of body weight can result in severe toxicity and can be lethal in persons of all ages.

Signs and symptoms of acute iron poisoning occur in 5 somewhat overlapping stages, and are defined as gastrointestinal (stage 1), latent (stage 2), metabolic/cardiovascular (stage 3), hepatic (stage 4), and delayed (stage 5)

Acute iron poisoning is a medical emergency; treatment includes stomach and whole bowel irrigation to remove unabsorbed iron from the GI tract and administration of iron binders (e.g., deferoxamine) by injection or intravenously; serum iron levels roughly correlate with clinical severity of acute iron poisoning as follows: a) normal serum iron: 65–165 µg/dL; b) mild acute iron poisoning: 165–300 µg/dL; c) moderate acute iron poisoning: 300–500 µg/ dL; and d) severe acute iron poisoning: >500 µg/dL.

Iron overload is caused most often by excessive iron absorption in the GI tract from hemochromatosis, ineffective erythropoiesis (i.e., decreased RBC production), or repeated transfusions; chronic high-dose iron supplementation in the absence of iron deficiency may also lead to iron overload.

Untreated iron overload leads to iron deposition in soft tissues, resulting in liver dysfunction, diabetes mellitus and other endocrine abnormalities, and/or cardiovascular complications. Iron overload is treated with regular phlebotomy (i.e., intentional blood removal, including for donation). In cases of iron overload in the presence of severe anemia, a medical condition in which hemoglobin values are low but levels of stored iron are excessively high, chelation therapy (e.g., administration of iron binders) may be initiated.

Depletion of ferritin and hemosiderin, the stored forms of iron, occurs prior to a drop in hemoglobin concentration, so low hemoglobin concentrations indicate long-standing anemia.

Indicators of iron deficiency that are more sensitive than serum hemoglobin are serum ferritin and transferrin, and total iron-binding capacity (TIBC). The normal values for ferritin levels are 12–150 ng/mL for females, and 12–300 ng/mL for males. The normal range for blood transferrin levels are 200–360 mg/dL. Finally, a normal TIBC is between 240 and 450 µg/dL.

Other laboratory tests relevant to evaluation of iron levels include hematocrit, red blood cell distribution width (RDW), mean corpuscular volume (MCV), mean corpuscular hemoglobin (MCH), and mean corpuscular hemoglobin concentration (MCHC); normal values are as follows: a) HCT: 36–44% for females, 40–50% for males; b) RDW: 11–15%; c)

MCV: 80–95 femtoliters; d) MCH: 27–31 pg/cell; and e) MCHC: 32–36 gm/dL.

Low values for ferritin, hemoglobin (<12 g/dL for females), MCV, MCH, and MCHC indicate iron-deficiency anemia; values for TIBC, transferrin, and RDW increase with iron deficiency

Supplemental iron can bind tightly with certain compounds to form iron-drug complexes, if iron is taken concurrently with certain medications. This greatly decreases medication effectiveness; medications with which iron can form iron-drug complexes include tetracycline (i.e. an antibiotic) and its derivatives (e.g., demeclocycline, doxycycline, methacycline, minocycline, oxytetracycline), penicillamine (i.e. a copper binder), methyldopa, levodopa, carbidopa (i.e. medications for Parkinson's disease), ciprofloxacin (i.e. and antibiotic), thyroxine (i.e. hypothyroidism medication), captopril (i.e. blood pressure lowering medication), and folic acid.

Iron supplements can also decrease the efficacy of other medications, including chloramphenicol (i.e. an antibiotic), cimetidine (i.e. heartburn and ulcer medication), nalidixic acid (i.e. an antibiotic), and ofloxacin (i.e. an antibiotic) and its derivatives (e.g., cinoxacin, enoxacin, levofloxacin, lomefloxacin, and norfloxacin).

To reduce the likelihood that iron will form iron-drug complexes with medications or decrease medication efficacy, it is typically recommended that iron supplements be taken 2 hours before or 2 hours after taking medication.

RESEARCH FINDINGS

Researchers examined the Childhood Autism Risks from Genetics and the Environment (CHARGE) study to determine if a relationship exists between maternal iron intake and autism spectrum disorder (ASD) risk in offspring. Resulting data indicates that low iron intake, in combination with advanced maternal age (i.e., >35 years) and metabolic conditions (e.g., DM2 and obesity), is associated with a 5-fold increase in risk of ASD in offspring.

Correction of anemia with IV iron in patients with heart failure (HF) may improve HF outcomes, but randomized trials are necessary to confirm that this approach is universally beneficial to persons with HF.

Observational studies suggest that higher iron intake may be associated with increased risk of Parkinson's disease, particularly in persons with low serum cholesterol levels and low intake of vitamin C.

The hypothesis that high iron intake and high levels of stored iron contribute to cardiovascular disease through promotion of oxidation is not supported by current literature.

A systematic review of 67 randomized controlled trials (representing a composite of 8506 women, the majority between 13 and 45 years old) demonstrated a significant improvement in hemoglobin concentrations and iron indices (e.g., ferritin) with daily iron supplementation, with or without vitamin C and folate. Most of the trials included in this review lasted one to three months. Low-dose (30 mg or less) supplementation effectively lowered rates of anemia and iron deficiency, while minimizing adverse gastrointestinal effects. The effect, as expected based on previous research, was potentiated by vitamin C co-supplementation. Accompanying meta-analyses suggested an improvement in exercise performance, as well as a decrease in fatigue.

Similar studies have been conducted on pregnant women, in the setting of prenatal care. The impact of long-term iron supplementation with respect to important clinical outcomes for the mother and child (such as preterm delivery or infant mortality) remains largely unclear. A systematic review of 11 trials demonstrated consistent improvement in iron and hematological indices, but not in said clinical outcomes.

Research surrounding management and treatment of postpartum iron deficiency anemia remains largely inconclusive. A recent systematic review of 22 studies (2858 postpartum women) tested various treatment permutations, including red blood cell transfusion, oral/IV iron, and erythropoietin (EPO). Superior functional outcomes (fatigue reduction) were generally observed with IV iron relative to oral iron, though in conjunction with worse cardiac, anaphylactic (allergic), and gastrointestinal outcomes overall. The effectiveness of EPO treatment in this population remains unclear, though EPO appeared to benefit participants by supporting higher breastfeeding rates.

Obesity has been linked to iron deficiency in previous studies. Researchers suggest that obesity increases the susceptibility to iron deficiency due to higher iron needs that are not easily met through diet. More specifically, maternal obesity among pregnant women appears to pose harm to future offspring. The results of a prospective, observational study conducted on 316 newborns with risk factors of infantile iron deficiency anemia indicate that maternal obesity and excessive weight gain during pregnancy are independent risk factors for iron deficiency in offspring.

SUMMARY

Consumers should become knowledgeable about the role and importance of iron. Iron is necessary for the production of red blood cells, DNA, and energy. A well-balanced diet includes good sources of iron such as beef, chicken, fish, green vegetables, and beans. Vitamin C rich foods are known to increase the body's absorption if iron. Iron-deficiency anemia is the most common form of anemia worldwide. Certain populations are particularly susceptible, including women of child-bearing age and pregnant women. Signs and symptoms of iron deficiency include fatigue, weakness, and dizziness. The body does not readily excrete iron so certain individuals should be aware of the potential for iron poisoning from excessive intake or supplementation. One should also recognize the potential for interactions between iron and certain medications. Research studies on the physiological impact of iron intake and supplementation suggest the following: maternal iron intake may decrease the risk of autism in children; higher iron intake may reduce the risk of developing Parkinson's disease; IV iron correction of anemia in heart failure patients may improve outcome; daily, long-term iron supplementation plays an important role during and after pregnancy; obesity may be linked to iron deficiency.

—Cherie Marcel, BS
and Suzanne Dixon, MPH, MS, RD
Updated by Ariel Choi, ScB

FOR FURTHER INFORMATION

Boyle, J. S., "Pediatric iron toxicity." *Medscape.* Feb 04, 2019, https://emedicine.medscape.com/article/1011689-overview.

Low, M.S., et al. "Daily iron supplementation for improving anaemia, iron status and health in menstruating women." *Cochrane Database of Systematic Reviews,* vol. 4, 2016, CD009747.

Markova, V., et al. Treatment for women with postpartum iron deficiency anaemia. *Cochrane Database of Systematic Reviews,* vol. 8, 2015, CD010861.

McDonagh, M., et al. *Routine Iron Supplementation and Screening for Iron Deficiency Anemia in Pregnant Women: A Systematic Review to Update the U.S. Preventive Services Task Force Recommendation.* Rockville, MD: Agency for Healthcare Research and Quality (US), 2015.

National Institutes of Health. Medline Plus. "Iron supplements." 28 January 2019, https://medlineplus.gov/druginfo/meds/a682778.html.

O'Malley, G. F., & O'Malley, R. "Iron poisoning." *Merck. Manual for Health Care Professionals.* January 2018, https://www.merckmanuals.com/en-pr/professional/injuries-poisoning/poisoning/iron-poisoning.

Schmidt, R. J., et al. "Maternal intake of supplemental iron and risk of autism spectrum disorder." *American Journal of Epidemiology,* vol. 180, no. 9, 2015, 890-900. doi:10.1093/aje/kwu208

Spanierman, C. S. "Iron toxicity" *Medscape.* 4 Feb, 2019, https://emedicine.medscape.com/article/815213-overview.

World Health Organization. *Guideline: Iron Supplementation in Postpartum Women.* Geneva: World Health Organization, 2016.

Irritable bowel syndrome (IBS)

CATEGORY: Disease/Disorder
Also known as: Irritable colon, mucous colitis, nervous colon, spastic colon or bowel

KEY TERMS:

biofeedback: the technique of making unconscious or involuntary bodily processes perceptible to the senses in order to manipulate them by conscious mental control

cognitive behavioral therapy: a type of psychotherapy that focuses on feelings and actions, specifically replacing negative thoughts with positive thoughts, thereby resulting in more desirable outcomes

colon: the large intestine

colonoscopy: the use of a small-diameter, flexible tube of optical fibers with an external light source to visually examine the interior of the body, specifically the colon

Crohn's disease: a disease characterized by inflammation of all layers (full thickness) of the intestines or any part of the digestive tract; early symptoms may resemble those of irritable bowel syndrome

gastroenterology: study of the function and diseases associated with the stomach, intestines, and other organs of the digestive tract such as the liver and pancreas

ileum: distal part of the small intestine, closest to the starting part of the colon; can be involved in ulcerative colitis.

ischemic colitis: inadequate blood supply to the colon

lactose: a sugar found in milk and milk products; some people cannot digest lactose, causing lactose intolerance, which can produce symptoms that resemble those of irritable bowel syndrome

organic: arising from an organ

peristalsis: a series of muscular contractions that move food through the intestines during the process of digestion

sigmoid: the distal part of the large colon, just before the rectum

sigmoidoscopy: similar to colonoscopy, with the tubular instrument with light instead inspecting only the anus, rectum, and sigmoid colon

ulcerative colitis: an inflammatory disease that causes superficial ulcers in the colon and rectum

CAUSES AND SYMPTOMS

Irritable bowel syndrome (IBS) is a gastrointestinal (GI) disorder characterized by abdominal pain or discomfort associated with diarrhea, constipation, or alternations between these two types of bowel motions. Other GI symptoms are related to this syndrome, including chronic abdominal pain, bloating, cramping, gas, heartburn, nausea, passage of mucus, an increased urge to defecate, and a feeling of incomplete defecation. Moreover, non-GI symptoms may accompany IBS, such as discomforts during menstruation, urination, and sexual activities. Although symptoms vary in intensity, they do not grow steadily worse over time but may wax and wane over the years.

IBS is sometimes referred to as a functional disorder, meaning that no anatomical issue or specific pathology can be identified through examination. Several causes of IBS have been suggested, but there is no single organic cause that can explain this condition. IBS is understood as a disease with a common set of symptoms that are evaluated based either on the Manning criteria (established in 1978) or the Rome III criteria (updated in 2006) for standardized diagnosis of IBS and for distinguishing organic causes for the syndrome. The Manning criteria include the following: pain relief with defecation, sensation of incomplete defecation, passage of mucus, and frequent and looser stools associated with the onset of pain. The more symptoms are present, the higher the probability of IBS diagnosis. The Rome III criteria include recurrent abdominal pain or discomfort associated with two or more of the following: relief after defecation, change in frequency of stools in association with pain, and change in form or appearance of stools associated with pain. The duration of these symptoms should at least be three days per month for the past three months or the onset of symptoms should at least be six months prior to diagnosis.

Three traditional physiological factors contribute to the symptoms of IBS: changes in GI motility, psychological aspects such as stress, and GI hypersensitivity. The GI motility responds to various stimuli such as food, stress, and gut distension; the resulting changes in activity of the major part of the large intestine or colon can lead to IBS symptoms. Following food digestion by the stomach and the small intestine, the undigested material is propelled toward the rectum by peristalsis. When peristalsis becomes disrupted by IBS, the flow becomes too slow, causing constipation, or too fast, causing diarrhea.

Some foods and drinks appear more likely to trigger IBS attacks by disrupting peristalsis. Fatty foods, fried foods, milk products, chocolate, drinks with caffeine, and alcohol.

The nervous system processing between the brain and the intestines suggest that stress may be the culprit in IBS. Many IBS sufferers report symptoms following a meal when they experience stress. Psychologic stress has been shown to exacerbate GI symptoms in IBS. Stress may also be involved in some people who develop IBS following infection or inflammation of the bowel. In addition, psychiatric diseases are common among IBS patients, especially in those who are hospitalized.

A hypersensitive gut is characterized by enhanced perception of normal motility throughout the digestive tract. Recent studies have shown that specific parts of the brain show greater activation in IBS patients; these activated brain regions are associated with attention and response selection. IBS is more commonly seen in women than in men, with up to 20 percent of

Information on Irritable Bowel Syndrome (IBS)

Causes: Unclear; possibly changes in activity of colon resulting from dietary factors, stress, female reproductive hormones

Symptoms: Abdominal pain and cramps, diarrhea or constipation, bloating, nausea

Duration: Chronic

Treatments: Dietary changes, antispasmodic drugs, psychological counseling, behavioral therapy (e.g., hypnosis and biofeedback, relaxation techniques) can alleviate the symptoms of IBS, as well as eliminating some fruits or vegetables, such as cabbage, broccoli, cauliflower, and Brussels sprouts. In some cases, however, no specific foods cause specific symptoms, as any food intake seems to worsen symptoms. Often, IBS-aggravating foods vary from person to person.

the American population affected. Although it can occur at any time, IBS generally appears in the patient's teens and twenties, and it frequently is found in members of the same family. Americans and Europeans have similar frequencies of IBS.

IBS IN WOMEN

Women in western countries, particularly young women, are more likely to be affected by IBS than men. It is most prevalent during the years a woman is menstruating and may cause the most distress during the second half of the menstrual cycle (after ovulation and before menses). While menstruation can exacerbate IBS symptoms, pregnancy has shown to improve these symptoms. It can be a common cause of lower abdominal pain, leading women to visit their gynecologist.

Endometriosis and hysterectomy have also been found to be more common amongst women with IBS. While hysterectomy has been found to coincide with IBS, neither hysterectomy nor tubal ligation relates to increased severity of IBS symptoms. On the other hand, endometriosis has only been shown to correlate to increased bloating and is not related with other IBS symptoms.

One explanation for the higher prevalence amongst women is that sexual abuse is a strong risk factor for the development of IBS. Sexual abuse also

correlated with severity of IBS symptoms often resulting in more IBS-related sick days, non-GI symptoms, increased psychological/physiological stress, increased pain, and increased lifetime surgeries. Another explanation to the increased prevalence amongst women is that women are more likely to seek medical care.

The impact of IBS in women can also affect sexual function and thereby impact intimate relationships. Sexual dysfunction ranges from decreasing sex drive to dyspareunia, or pain with sex. Due to the complexity of IBS, it is imperative that women seek out healthcare from a care team including specialists in pelvic physiology, gastroenterology, psychiatry, and gynecology to best treat their symptoms and other comorbid conditions.

TREATMENT AND THERAPY

Diagnosis of IBS is an involved process that is accomplished through a series of steps. A thorough history should be provided to the physician. Symptom-based criteria (Manning or Rome III) will be used to identify IBS. Moreover, alarming symptoms such as weight loss, unrelenting diarrhea, family history of colon cancer, and psychiatric aspects such as depression and suicidal thoughts will be ruled out. A physical examination will be performed on the first visit. Laboratory tests and a colonoscopy or sigmoidoscopy may be performed, and a stool sample may be obtained—all of which will rule out serious diseases such as colon cancer, infection, and inflammatory diseases. Traditionally, IBS has been a diagnosis of exclusion.

Treatment options will include dietary and lifestyle changes, medications targeted toward the predominant symptoms, and psychological modalities. Generally, a low-fat, high-fiber diet lessens symptoms, although the tolerance of fiber (as is true of all foods) varies from person to person. Dietary changes vary according to the severity of the patient's symptoms. In mild cases of IBS, known-aggravating foods should be identified and avoided. Many doctors recommend eliminating dairy products for a period of time as lactose-intolerance can aggravate IBS symptoms. Symptoms may also be eased by eating smaller meals. Since no diet has been found that controls all symptoms, a diary of symptoms and food intake is valuable in determining which foods are offensive. Establishment of

In the News:
A Novel Approach to Treating IBS Symptoms

A new target for treatment of the symptoms of irritable bowel syndrome (IBS) is presented by the serotonin (5-HT) receptors that are present in nerves of the gastrointestinal (GI) tract and other organs. Receptors are proteins involved in the response of organs to various signals. Blocking these receptors can modify responses of the nerves in the GI tract. There are several types of 5-HT receptors; they are designated by numbers such as 5-HT3 and 5-HT4.

Alosetron (*Lotronex*) targets the 5-HT3 receptors in the GI tract. The desired effects of the drug include pain relief, normalization of bowel frequency, and decreased urgency for bowel movements in female patients with diarrhea-predominant IBS. The restrictive guidelines for alosetron were established because of its serious side effects: severe constipation and ischemic colitis that can potentially be fatal. Alosetron was withdrawn from the market but eventually reapproved by the Food and Drug Administration (FDA) with restrictive guidelines for its prescription.

A similar drug called cilansetron also targets the 5-HT3 receptors in the GI tract, and studies have shown that its effects on individuals with IBS are the same as for alosetron. It is the first 5-HT3 blocker specific for both male and female IBS patients suffering from diarrhea. In April 2005, the FDA did not approve the product registration for cilansetron in the United States, even though the phase III registration trials were complete, and requested additional data from Solvay, the manufacturer. The FDA denial may be related to the challenges undergone by alosetron. By the end of 2005, Solvay suspended its product application in the United States, but it continues to discuss the introduction of cilansetron in the United Kingdom through the Medicines and Healthcare Products Regulatory Agency. The United Kingdom is the reference country for the introduction of cilansetron to the member countries of the European Union.

Tegaserod is a drug for treating constipation in IBS patients. It is marketed by Novartis as Zelnorm in the United States and Zelmac outside the United States. Tegaserod was approved by the FDA in 2002 for treatment of female patients suffering from constipation-predominant IBS. Tegaserod targets the 5-HT4 receptors in the GI tract. The desired effects of the drug include decreasing pain perception and reversing constipation through faster food transit in the GI tract. Tegaserod seems to be well tolerated by most patients, with most common side effects including headache, abdominal pain, and diarrhea.

Evidence showed a link between the drug and an increased risk of heart attack and stroke, however, and it was withdrawn from the U.S. market in March 2007.

More treatment options using the novel approach of targeting the serotonin (5-HT) receptors may be on the horizon as researchers learn more about the efficacy and safety of these new drugs in IBS patients.

—*Miriam E. Schwartz, M.D., M.A., Ph.D., and Colm A. Ó'Moráin, M.A., M.D., M.Sc., D.Sc. Updated by Ananya Anand, M.Sc. and Tatianna Pryce*

fixed times for meals and bathroom visits helps regulate bowel habits as well.

In addition to dietary changes, medications are given to alleviate predominant IBS symptoms. Abdominal pain is treated with antispasmodic drugs such as dicyclomine and hyoscyamine, especially if the pain is associated with meals; these drugs relax the smooth muscles of the intestines. An antidiarrheal agent such as loperamide is used to reduce loose stools and slow gastric motility to relieve abdominal pain. A medication called alosetron (*Lotronex*) is also used for diarrhea. Because alosetron has serious side effects, such as severe constipation and ischemic colitis, it was withdrawn from the market for a while; it is now available again, but with specific restrictions and only for severe IBS with diarrhea in women. Physicians must enroll in a special program with the manufacturer in order to prescribe alosetron. For constipation, bulk laxatives that supply increased dietary fiber such as psyllium (*Metamucil*, *Fiberall*, *Konsyl*, Colon Cleanse, and other similar products) are recommended. A medication for constipation called tegaserod (*Zelnorm*) was made available in 2002 but was withdrawn in 2007 when evidence suggested that it raised the risk of heart attack and stroke. Lubiprostone (*Amitiza*), which helps promote chloride channel secretions in the bowel and thus aids peristalsis, has been approved for use in women with constipation-predominant IBS and patients with chronic constipation. Linaclotide (*Linzess*), a guanylate cyclase-C agonist, increases the motility and blocks pain signals in the bowels. It is approved for adults eighteen and older who have IBS with constipation or chronic constipation, but further studies are required to assess its effectiveness. Antibiotic treatment has not been well studied, but rifaximin has been approved for treatment of IBS without constipation.

Psychological treatments are imperative for IBS patients whose quality of life is severely impaired. Patients who have concomitant psychiatric conditions such as depression, history of sexual abuse, or any major life stress should be treated for their psychiatric ailments so that they can cope better with IBS. Psychological counseling, cognitive behavioral therapy, hypnosis, biofeedback, and relaxation techniques are recommended to reduce anxiety and encourage learning to cope better with the pain of IBS. Severe pain from IBS can be treated with antidepressants such as tricyclics. Anxiolytic medications such as diazepam and lorazepam can be given to patients who have short-term anxiety that exacerbates their IBS symptoms, but these medications should be used with caution given their addictive potential. Moderate exercise has also been shown to be beneficial. In addition to dietary changes prescribed by doctors, alternative practitioners may advise herbal remedies to treat symptoms of IBS, such as Chinese herbal medicines, aloe vera, ginger, evening primrose, fennel, peppermint extract, chamomile, and rosemary. Aromatherapy, hydrotherapy, acupuncture, chiropractic, and osteopathy as alternative treatments may also be useful in some individuals.

PERSPECTIVE AND PROSPECTS

IBS was once believed to be a psychological disorder, but recent studies have shown that it is a true medical disorder with specific physiological characteristics and a significant impact on individuals who are afflicted with it. In addition, IBS has considerable effects on the society's health care burden. It has been reported that IBS is the second most common reason for seeing a physician and missing work (the first being the common cold) and accounts for 12 percent of visits to primary care and for the largest group seen by gastroenterologists. In terms of GI diseases, IBS is second only to gastroesophageal reflux disease (GERD) as most prevalent GI disorder in the United States, and it

is the most commonly diagnosed GI condition. IBS affects 15.4 million people, and the economic costs (both direct and indirect) are in the billions of dollars. These costs are derived from work absenteeism, doctor visits, medical tests, and procedures, as well as other related expenses. Although there is no cure for IBS, it is not a life-threatening condition. It has not been shown to cause intestinal bleeding or inflammation, as in Crohn's disease, ulcerative colitis, or cancer. Long-term management, though frustrating, involves commitment to therapy for six months or more to find the best combinations of medicine, diet, counseling, and support for control of IBS symptoms.

—Mary Hurd
Updated by Miriam E. Schwartz, M.D., M.A., Ph.D.,
and Colm A. Ó'Moráin, M.A., M.D., M.Sc., D.Sc.
and Tatianna Pryce

FOR FURTHER INFORMATION

"American Gastroenterological Association Technical Review on Irritable Bowel Syndrome." *Gastroenterology*, vol. 123, no. 6, 2002, 2108–2131.

Chey, William D., et al. "Bacterial Overgrowth and IBS: Bridging the Gap." *Gastroenterology and Hepatology* vol. 2, no. 8, supp., 2006, 5–13.

Darnley, Simon, and Barbara Millar. *Understanding Irritable Bowel Syndrome*. New York: Wiley, 2003.

Hadley, Susan K., and Stephen M. Gaarder. "Treatment of Irritable Bowel Syndrome." *American Family Physician* vol. 72, no. 12, 2005, 2501–2506.

International Foundation for Functional Gastrointestinal Disorders. "Targeted IBS Medications." *AboutIBS*, March 23, 2013.

Irritable Bowel Syndrome Self Help and Support Group. *IBS Group*, April 25, 2013. MedlinePlus. "Irritable Bowel Syndrome." *MedlinePlus*, May 20, 2013.

Mertz, Howard R. "Irritable Bowel Syndrome." *New England Journal of Medicine* vol. 349, no. 22, 2003, 2136–2145.

National Digestive Diseases Information Clearinghouse (NDDIC). "Irritable Bowel Syndrome." *National Digestive Diseases Information Clearing House (NDDIC)*, July 2, 2012.

Wood, Debra. "Irritable Bowel Syndrome." *Health Library*, September 30, 2012.

K

Ketogenic diet in adults

CATEGORY: Biology

KEY TERMS:
ketone: an organic compound containing a carbonyl group bonded to two hydrocarbon groups, made by oxidizing secondary alcohols; the simplest such compound is acetone

ketosis: a metabolic state characterized by raised levels of ketone bodies in the body tissues, which is typically pathological in conditions such as diabetes, or may be the consequence of a diet that is very low in carbohydrates

STRUCTURE AND FUNCTION
The ketogenic diet (KD) refers to a diet that is high in fat, low in carbohydrates, and moderate in protein. KD has historically been used to control seizure activity but more recently researched to address weight loss and other health concerns. Eating a KD replaces glucose-based energy sources with fat-based energy sources, resulting in a physiologic state of ketosis. Ketosis is evidenced by the build-up of ketone bodies, or ketones, in the blood and urine. Ketones are water-soluble compounds that are produced as byproducts when fat-based energy sources are utilized. Although the process is not entirely understood, the increase in ketones is correlated with improved control of seizures. The KD is structured and mathematically calculated and should be initiated only with close medical supervision. It is a challenging diet for patients with seizures to learn and follow and is not usually suggested by a clinician until at least 2 attempts of pharmacotherapy have failed.

Although the KD is predominantly prescribed as a therapy for children with epilepsy or other seizure disorders, it has been used with good results in treatment of adults to control seizure activity. Most individuals tolerate the KD better than pharmacotherapy, but potential adverse effects include elevated low-density lipoprotein (LDL) cholesterol levels, constipation, kidney stones, and acidosis.

The exact mechanism that causes the KD to be effective in reducing seizures is not fully understood. It is possible that ketones, namely acetone, acetoacetate, and beta-hydroxybutyrate, cross the blood/brain barrier (i.e., filtering system that carries blood to the brain) and affect the onset, propagation, and/or cessation of seizures. Ketones may also be indicators of the presence of certain other substances or metabolic changes that have not been identified.

The switch from glucose-burning to fat-burning that takes place on the KD may affect physiologic use and production of insulin in such a way that improves seizure control.

IMPLEMENTATION
Traditionally, the KD is initiated over a period of 3 days after a 48-hour fast, although the necessity of fasting has been questioned in results of recent research. The KD requires commitment, education from a physician and/or dietitian, and the ability to learn about calculating meal plans, weighing food, and initiating strategies for eating away from home. Completing these requirements takes time. Achieving and maintaining good adherence to the KD is a process that occurs over time. The carbohydrate content of all medications should be included in the meal plan calculations in order to maintain appropriate carbohydrate intake.

RESEARCH FINDINGS
Research results show that when adults adhere strictly to the KD, they achieve significant improvement in seizure control. However, establishing good adherence to the KD is challenging for adults. Research studies have also examined the use of the KD to address certain women's health concerns such as polycystic ovary syndrome (PCOS), endometriosis, and uterine fibroids. A study by Cohen et al published in the August 2018 *Journal of Nutrition* suggests the KD may be helpful to patients with ovarian or endometrial cancer. However, further research is needed in these areas. Also, women who are pregnant, breastfeeding,

or have other health issues should only try the KD under the care of their healthcare provider.

It can be very difficult to follow such a rigid diet after years of established dietary patterns and traditions. Another concern for recommending the KD to adults is the possibility of elevated LDL levels. Results of studies show the therapeutic potential of consuming a modified Atkins diet or a low glycemic index diet to achieve better long-term adherence and fewer adverse effects among adults.

Authors of a retrospective case review of 10 cases of critically ill adult patients with super refractory status

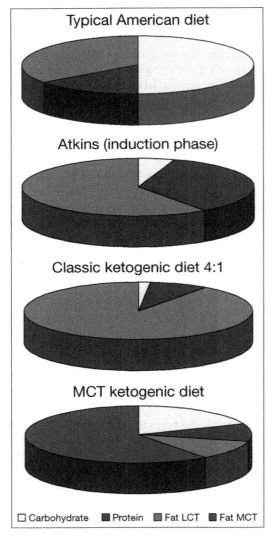

The ketogenic diet compared with other diets. (Wikimedia Commons)

epilepticus (SRSE) reported that treatment with the KD resulted in resolution of status epilepticus in 90% of the patients.

SUMMARY

Individuals should become knowledgeable about the physiologic effects of the ketogenic diet (KD). The KD, which is high in fat and low in carbohydrates, is prescribed to help control seizure disorders, lose weight, and address other health issues. Patients and their family members should follow strict adherence to the prescribed KD with continued medical surveillance to monitor health status. Research suggests the KD may result in elevated LDL levels and less strict carbohydrate-controlled diets may be a good alternative.

—*Cherie Marcel, BS*
Updated by Marylane Wade Koch, MSN, RN

FOR FURTHER INFORMATION

Cohen, W. C., et al. "Ketogenic Diet Reduces Central Obesity and Serum Insulin in Women with Ovarian or Endometrial Cancer." *The Journal of Nutrition*, Vol. 148, no. 8, 2018, 1253–1260, doi: 10.1093/jn/nxy119

Kossoff, E. H., & Freeman, J. M. "The ketogenic diet: An effective therapy for seizure control." *Nutrition in Clinical Care*, vol. 8, no. 4, 2005, 149-157.

Kossoff, E. H., Freeman, J. M., Turner, Z., & Rubenstein, J. E. "What is the ketogenic diet?" *Ketogenic diets*, 5th ed., New York, NY: Demos Medical Publishing, 2011, 15-75.

Kossoff, E. H., & Harman, A. L. "Ketogenic diets: New advances for metabolism-based therapies." *Current Opinion in Neurology*, vol. 25, no. 2, 2012, 173-178.

Masino, S. A., & Rho, J. M. "Mechanisms of ketogenic diet action." J. L. Noebels, M. Avoli, & M. A. Rogawski, editors. *Jasper's Basic Mechanisms of the Epilepsies*, 4th ed., Bethesda, MD: National Center for Biotechnology Information (US), 2012.

Schultz, R. J., & Hockenberry, M. J. "The child with cerebral dysfunction." M. J. Hockenberry & D. Wilson, editors. *Wong's nursing care of infants and children*, 9th ed., St. Louis, MO: Elsevier Mosby, 2011, p. 1553

Thakur, K.T., et al. "Ketogenic diet for adults in super-refractory status epilepticus." *Neurology*, vol. 82, no. 8, 2014, 665-670. doi:10.1212/WNL.0000000000000151

L

Laparoscopy

CATEGORY: Procedure

KEY TERMS:

abdomen: the area of the body between the diaphragm and the pelvis; it contains the visceral organs

cholecystectomy: the surgical removal of the gallbladder

ectopic pregnancy: the development of a fertilized egg in a Fallopian tube instead of the uterus; can be fatal to the mother unless it is corrected surgically

endometriosis: a female reproductive disease in which cells from the uterine lining (the endometrium) grow outside the uterus, causing severe pain and infertility and sometimes the need for hysterectomy

Fallopian tubes: the two tubes through which eggs pass on the way from the ovaries to the uterus

general anesthesia: anesthesia that induces unconsciousness

implant: a section of endometrial tissue found outside the uterus

local anesthesia: anesthesia that numbs the feeling in a body part, administered by injection or direct application to the skin

INDICATIONS AND PROCEDURES

Laparoscopy is a surgical technique for examining the abdominal organs and for treating surgically many diseases of these organs. The instrument used is called a laparoscope. It is a flexible tube that contains fiber optics for visualization purposes and a channel through which physicians can pass special surgical instruments into the abdominal cavity.

Upon insertion of a laparoscope into the abdomen through a small surgical incision (usually near the navel), physicians can observe the liver, kidneys, gallbladder, pancreas, spleen, and exterior aspects of the intestines in both sexes. Hence the technique is useful for detecting cirrhosis of the liver, the presence of stones and tumors, and many other diseases of the abdominal organs. The female reproductive organs can also be examined in this manner.

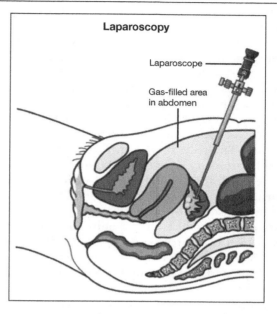

Many surgical procedures involving the abdomen, such as appendectomy or the removal of eggs from the ovaries for in vitro fertilization, can be performed using laparoscopy. Gas is pumped into the abdominal cavity, and a fiber-optic scope and instruments are inserted through a small hole in the skin. © EBSCO

Before laparoscopy can be carried out, the patient must fast for at least twelve hours. The patient is given a local or general anesthetic, depending on the purpose of the procedure. In exploratory abdominal examinations, the instrument is inserted into the abdomen through a small incision in the abdominal wall after local anesthesia has numbed it. Often, especially when extensive surgery is anticipated, the procedure begins after general anesthesia produces unconsciousness.

Upon the completion of exploration or surgery, the laparoscope is withdrawn, and the incision is closed. Laparoscopic abdominal examination is often used to detect endometriosis, the presence of endometrial cells outside the uterus. This procedure begins

551

with the administration of local anesthesia when only exploration or biopsy is planned. General anesthesia is used when the removal of implants (endometrial tissue) is anticipated. The entry incision is made near the navel, and the laparoscope is inserted. The fiberoptics system is used to search the abdominal organs for implants. Visibility of the abdominal organs is usually enhanced by pumping in a harmless gas, such as carbon dioxide, to distend the abdomen. After the confirmation of endometriosis, surgical implant removal is carried out immediately, unless the decision is made to institute drug therapy instead. Full recovery from this surgery requires only a day of postoperative bed rest and a week of curtailing activities.

Laparoscopy can also be employed for female sterilization. The patient is given a general anesthetic. After laparoscopic visualization of the Fallopian tubes in the gas-distended abdomen is achieved, surgical instruments for tube cauterization or cutting are introduced and the sterilization is carried out. The entire procedure often requires only thirty minutes, which is one reason for its popularity. In addition, patients can go home in a few hours and have fully recovered after a day or two of bed rest and seven to ten days of curtailing activities.

Laparoscopy is also useful for diagnosing adnexal disease in young women; adnexal masses are abnormal growths near the uterus, commonly located in the ovaries, fallopian tubes, or connective tissues. Most are benign, but they can occasionally be malignant. Adnexal disease in young women can mimic acute appendicitis. The use of diagnostic laparoscopy can decrease the number of laparotomies by a third. Further, ruptured ovarian cysts, ovarian torsion, PID (pelvic inflammatory disease), and tubal pregnancies—which again can present as appendicitis and can be diagnosed with laparoscopy.

USES AND COMPLICATIONS

Common laparoscopic surgeries are cholecystectomy (the removal of the gallbladder), the removal of gallstones and kidney stones, tumor resection, female sterilization by cutting or blocking the Fallopian tubes, the treatment of endometriosis through the removal of implants from abdominal organs, and the removal of biopsy samples from abdominal organs. Traditional uses of laparoscopy in female reproductive surgery are to identify and correct pelvic pain resulting from endometriosis, ectopic pregnancy, and pelvic tumors.

Laparoscopy has several advantages. There is rarely a need for patients on chronic drug therapy to discontinue medication before laparoscopy. In addition, the use of laparoscopy dramatically lowers surgical incision size, surgical trauma, length of hospital stay, and recovery time. Laparoscopy should be avoided, however, in cases of advanced abdominal wall cancer, severe respiratory or cardiovascular disease, or tuberculosis. Extreme obesity does not disqualify a patient from undergoing laparoscopy but makes the procedure much more difficult to perform.

As laparoscopic surgery has increased in scope, more procedures yield surgical tissues that are larger in size than the laparoscope channel (for example, the removal of gallbladders, gallstones, and ovaries). In many cases these organs and structures are cut into small pieces for removal. If potentially dangerous items are involved—such as malignancies that can spread on dissection—larger, more conventional incisions are often combined with laparoscopy.

PERSPECTIVE AND PROSPECTS

Since the 1970s, the uses of laparoscopy have constantly expanded. Once confined to the exploratory examination of the abdomen, the methodology has been applied to a large number of different types of surgery in addition to those already mentioned. Such versatility is attributable to the development of better laparoscopes, advanced instrumentation for diverse surgeries, and improved fiber-optic and video technologies. As a consequence of these advances, many surgeons predict that most future abdominal surgery will be laparoscopic.

The driving force for such innovation includes the public demand for quicker recovery times. In the United States, this desire is intensified by the requirements of insurance companies, employers, and the federal government for shorter hospital stays. Both changes are made possible by decreased severity of surgical trauma in laparoscopy when compared to traditional surgery, a result of the smaller incisions. The dramatic trend toward laparoscopy can be seen with cholecystectomies: Of those done in 1992, 70 percent were laparoscopic, compared to less than 1 percent in 1989; according to a 2010 report, about 75 percent of cholecystectomies are done with laparoscopic surgery.

—Sanford S. Singer, Ph.D.
Updated by Michael J. O'Neal

FOR FURTHER INFORMATION

Graber, John N., et al., eds. *Laparoscopic Abdominal Surgery*. New York: McGraw-Hill, 1993.

Henderson, Lorraine, and Ros Wood. *Explaining Endometriosis*. 2d ed. St. Leonards, N.S.W.: Allen and Unwin, 2000.

Kapadia, Cyrus R., James M. Crawford, and Caroline Taylor. *An Atlas of Gastroenterology: A Guide to Diagnosis and Differential Diagnosis*. Boca Raton, Fla.: Pantheon, 2003.

Ost, Michael C. *Robotic and Laparoscopic Reconstructive Surgery in Children and Adults*. New York: Humana Press, 2011.

Reddick, Eddie Joe, ed. *An Atlas of Laparoscopic Surgery*. New York: Raven Press, 1993.

Terzicİ_, Hana. *Laparoscopy: New Developments, Procedures, and Risks*. Hauppauge, N.Y.: Nova Science, 2012.

Zollinger, Robert M., Jr., and Robert M. Zollinger, Sr. *Zollinger's Atlas of Surgical Operations*. 9th ed. New York: McGraw-Hill, 2011.

Zucker, Karl A., ed. *Surgical Laparoscopy*. 2d ed. Philadelphia: Lippincott Williams & Wilkins, 2001.

Leiomyoma

CATEGORY: Biology

KEY TERMS:

menarche: the first occurrence of menstruation

ultrasound: sound or other vibrations having an ultrasonic frequency, particularly as used in medical imaging; most commonly used to examine the fetus of a pregnant woman

uterine fibroids: benign smooth muscle tumors of the uterus

INTRODUCTION

Leiomyomas, commonly called uterine fibroids, are a common abnormal tumor growth that occurs in the uterus. The vast majority of leiomyomas are benign and tend to occur more frequently with increased age. Leiomyoma development is dependent on estrogen and progesterone, and most leiomyomas that develop during sexual maturity reduce in size after menopause. A small percentage of leiomyomas develop into uterine cancer, but they are not considered an independent risk factor for cancer development.

RISK FACTORS

Leiomyomas begin forming at menarche and increase in size and prevalence during the reproductive years, typically up to age 50. Early onset of menarche and a family history of uterine fibroids have been associated with an increased risk of fibroids. They are less likely in women who have been pregnant. There is ongoing research suggesting various dietary risk factors for fibroids, including increased consumption of red meat, sugar, alcohol, and caffeine. Leiomyoma is up to 2 or 3 times more prevalent in African American women when compared to other ethnic groups.

SYMPTOMS AND DIAGNOSIS

The most common symptoms of leiomyomas include heavier than usual menstrual periods, feelings of pelvic pressure or pain, abdominal distention, or infertility issues not attributable to other malnutrition or hormonal irregularity. In cases of large fibroids, some women may have constipation or urinary retention symptoms. Less common symptoms include painful sexual intercourse or pain associated with menses.

Leiomyomas are diagnosed based on a careful history and physical exam including imaging studies, such as a pelvic ultrasound. Ultrasounds are typically able to accurately differentiate between a leiomyoma or a cancerous growth (known as a uterine carcinoma or uterine cancer). If a tumor is visualized on ultrasound, it may be removed surgically or further evaluated using an MRI.

SYMPTOM MANAGEMENT

Although leiomyomas are common and typically not concerning for cancerous process, the symptoms experienced by the patient may affect quality of life and overall sense of health and wellness. Concerns about bowel and bladder continence, abdominal pain, painful intercourse and infertility should be handled with care. Management of leiomyoma symptoms may warrant referral to mental health, fertility counseling, or pain management.

NUTRITION THERAPY FOR THE PREVENTION OF LEIOMYOMAS

In general, the best recommendation for a diet focused on the prevention of leiomyomas is to eat a high-fiber diet, which includes a wide variety of fruits, vegetables, lean proteins, and unsaturated fats. In particular, women should eat a diet rich in cruciferous vegetables, such as broccoli, cabbage, cauliflower. These foods contain phytonutrients that assist in the metabolism of estrogen. Also, when choosing foods, try to pick whole-grain, high-fiber foods, since the consumption of a high-fiber diet is generally associated with a lower risk of mortality. Additionally, women should try to balance their caloric intake and physical activity to achieve or maintain a healthy body weight.

RESEARCH FINDINGS

Results of several studies have noted potential benefits from increased intake of fruits and vegetables for the prevention of leiomyomas. Researchers have reported that women who consume a primarily plant-based diet that is high in green vegetables, fruit, and fish have a lower likelihood of developing leiomyomas compared with women who eat a meat-based diet.

Black women develop leiomyomas at a rate that is 2–3 times that of White women. Researchers are not certain if the disparity is due to genetic differences or to cultural and dietary differences. Results of a large prospective study of the dietary intake of Black women in relation to leiomyoma incidence showed that the women who consumed higher amounts of dairy products were less likely to develop leiomyomas, suggesting that diet influences risk.

SUMMARY

Individuals should learn about how a healthy diet may help prevent leiomyomas. Patients diagnosed with leiomyoma should report any health-related changes to the treating clinician as soon as possible, follow the prescribed treatment regimen and continue medical surveillance to monitor health status. Research suggests that a primarily plant–based diet may help reduce the risk of developing leiomyomas.

—*Cherie Marcel, BS*
Updated by Patrick Richardson

FOR FURTHER INFORMATION

Chiaffarino, F., et al. "Diet and uterine myomas." *Obstetrics and Gynecology*, 94, no. 3, 1999, 395-398.
He, Y., et al. "Associations between uterine fibroids and lifestyles including diet, physical activity and stress: A case-control study in China." *Asia Pacific Journal of Clinical Nutrition*, vol. 22, no. 1, 2013, 109-117. doi:10.6133/ apjcn.2013.22.1.07
Nagata, C., et al. "Association of intakes of fat, dietary fibre, soya isoflavones and alcohol with uterine fibroids in Japanese women." *British Journal of Nutrition*, 101, no. 10, 2009, 1427-1431. doi:10.1002/uog.7319
Tempest, M. "Uterine fibroids and nutrition." *Today's Dietitian*, vol. 14, no. 5, 2012, 40-43.
Wise, L. A., et al. "Intake of fruit, vegetables, and carotenoids in relation to risk of uterine leiomyomata." *American Journal of Clinical Nutrition*, vol. 94, no. 6, 2011, 1620-1631.
Wise, L. A., et al. "A prospective study of dairy intake and risk of uterine leiomyomata." *American Journal of Epidemiology*, vol. 171, no. 2, 2010, 221-232.

Leptin

CATEGORY: Biology

KEY TERMS:

adipocytes: cells specialized for the storage of fat, found in connective tissue
hormone: a chemical substance produced in the body that controls and regulates the activity of certain cells or organs
insulin: a hormone produced in the pancreas by the islets of Langerhans, which regulates the amount of glucose in the blood
obesity: a condition characterized by the excessive accumulation and storage of fat in the body

STRUCTURE AND FUNCTIONS

Leptin (from the Greek *leptos*, meaning "thin") is a protein hormone with important effects in regulating body weight, metabolism, and reproductive function by working to promote sufficient caloric intake (i.e., sending "full" signals to the brain when an individual has consumed an adequate amount of calories) and regulate glycemic control in healthy individuals. It is the product of the obese (*ob*) gene occurring on chromosome 7 in the human. Leptin is produced primarily by adipocytes (white fat cells), but is also produced by cells of the epithelium of the stomach and in the placenta. It appears that as adipocytes increase in size because of accumulation of triglycerides (fat molecules), they synthesize more and more leptin. However, the mechanism by which leptin production is controlled is largely unknown. It is likely that a number of hormones modulate leptin output, including corticosteroids and insulin. Insulin and leptin work hand-in-hand to control energy homeostasis, with insulin providing fuel to cells and leptin regulating energy stores in the cells. It is hypothesized that as the leptin levels increase, it's efficacy at maintaining energy intake decreases. Therefore, as an individual continues to consume an energy-dense diet, leptin and insulin levels rise but fail to maintain homeostasis and provide proper signaling to the brain.

Disorders and Diseases

At first leptin was assumed to be simply a signaling molecule involved in limiting food intake and increasing energy expenditure. Studies published as early as 1994 showed a remarkable difference in weight gain in mice deficient in leptin (mice with a nonfunctional *ob* gene). Daily injections of leptin into these animals resulted in a reduction of food intake within a few days and a 50 percent decrease in body weight within a month.

More recent studies in the human have not been as promising. It appears that leptin's effects on body weight are mediated through effects on hypothalamic (brain) centers that control feeding behavior and hunger, body temperature, and energy expenditure. If leptin levels are low, appetite is stimulated and use of energy limited. If leptin levels are high, appetite is reduced, and energy use stimulated. The most likely target of leptin in the hypothalamus is inhibition of neuropeptide Y, a potent stimulator of food intake. However, this inhibition alone could not account for the effects seen, and studies looking at other hormones are under way.

Leptin also affects reproductive function in humans. It has long been known that very low body fat in human females is associated with cessation of menstrual cycles, and the onset of puberty is known to correlate with body composition (fat levels) as well as age. Several studies have suggested that leptin stimulates hypothalamic output of gonadotropin-releasing hormone, which in turn causes increases of luteinizing and follicle-stimulating hormones from the anterior pituitary gland. These hormones stimulate the onset of puberty. Prepubertal mice treated with leptin become thin and reach reproductive maturity earlier than control mice. One report has also indicated that humans with mutations in the *ob* gene that prevent them from producing leptin not only become obese but also fail to achieve puberty.

Leptin has been identified in placental tissues; newborn babies show higher levels than those found in their mothers. Leptin has also been found in human breast milk. Together, these findings suggest that leptin aids in intrauterine and neonatal growth and development, as well as in regulation of neonatal food intake.

Finally, leptin appears to have a role in immune system function. Studies have suggested a role for leptin in production of white blood cells and in the control of macrophage function. Mice that lack leptin have depressed immune systems, but the mechanisms for this remain unclear.

Perspective and Prospects

Although early reports claimed that leptin could be useful in treating human obesity, clinical reports to date have not looked promising. It appears that deficiencies in leptin production are a rare cause of human obesity. However, since most obese individuals have plenty of leptin available, additional leptin will have no effect. In those individuals with a genetic deficiency of leptin, clinical use would require either daily injections of leptin or gene therapy. At this point neither of these options looks particularly promising.

—*Kerry L. Cheesman, Ph.D.*
Updated by Emma Kleck, MSN, RN, FNP

For Further Information

Barinaga, Marcia. "Obesity: Leptin Receptor Weighs In." *Science* 271 (January 5, 1996): 29.

Castracane, V. Daniel, and Michael C. Henson, eds. *Leptin*. New York: Springer, 2011.

Goodman, H. Maurice. *Basic Medical Endocrinology*. 4th ed. Boston: Academic Press/Elsevier, 2009.

Hemling, Rose M., and Arthur t. Belkin. *Leptin: Hormonal Functions, Dysfunctions, and Clinical Uses*. New York: Nova Science, 2011.

Henry, Helen L., and Anthony W. Norman, eds. *Encyclopedia of Hormones*. 3 vols. San Diego, Calif.: Academic Press, 2003.

Holt, Richard I.G., and Neil A. Hanley. *Essential Endocrinology and Diabetes*. 6th ed. Chichester, West Sussex: Wiley-Blackwell, 2012.

Perez-Tilve, D. (2019). Et Tu, Leptin?. *Trends in Endocrinology & Metabolism*. pii: S1043-2760(19)30025-6. doi: 10.1016/j.tem.2019.02.001.

Rink, Timothy J. "In Search of a Satiety Factor." *Nature* 372 (December 1, 1994): 372–373.

Society for Neuroscience. "Food for Thought: Obesity and Addiction." *BrainFacts*, April 20, 2012.

Lesbian, Gay, Bisexual, Transgender, and Queer (LGBTQ)

CATEGORY: Development

KEY TERMS:

asexual: an individual who identifies on a spectrum of non-sexuality, not having sexual attraction and/or not having romantic attraction

bisexual: an individual who is sexually, and/or romantically, attracted to both men and women, or to more than one gender of people.

gay: may refer to same-sex attraction (i.e. male-male or female-female) generally. Self-identified men who are attracted to other men may consider themselves gay.

gender: generally classified by societal expectations of feminine or masculine roles in social, psychological, or emotional expression.

gender identity: self-identification as man, woman, both, or something else entirely.

gender-confirming surgery or gender-affirming surgery: also known as sex reassignment surgery; surgery aimed to alter a person's primary and/or secondary sex characteristics to resemble that of their expressed gender (e.g., vaginoplasty or phalloplasty).

lesbian: a self-identified woman who is sexually, or romantically, attracted to other women.

queer: sexual or gender identity that is categorized outside of established gender roles or sexuality. Usually a self-identification. May be considered offensive term by some in LGBT community but has been increasingly reclaimed by community members.

sex: typically assigned at birth, refers to biological, genetic, or physical characteristics associated with gender. *Also used to refer to sexual intercourse.*

sexuality: an individual's sexual preference or orientation, also refers to feelings about sexual intercourse, arousal, and one's relationship to sexual activity.

trans or transgender: an umbrella term often used to describe those who do not ascribe to a binary means of gender, as it relates to their gender assigned at birth or their cultural norms. Transgender is a self-identified term and some gender nonbinary (i.e. not identifying as "men" or "women") individuals do not use this term

HISTORY OF LGBTQ POPULATION

The history of sexuality demonstrated a fluid movement since Grecian times. From engaging in sexual activity with animals to man, Zeus defied the stereotypical Westernized man one might think of today. In one story of Greek mythology, it was suggested that Zeus was in love with Ganymede and abducted him from his father's home. Ganymede was made to be the cupbearer, as well as Zeus' lover. Historians provided reasons for this myth's importance as a justification, within religion, for gay sexuality; others indicated this story was a part of the culture in Greek history. Nonetheless, this myth was important in development of the idea that sexuality is fluid.

During the 18th century it was determined by various cultures (e.g., bourgeois society; capitalism; ruling class) that sexual activity not meant for procreation, was a sin. Sex was viewed as an activity that only occurred between a man and a woman. While this thought continued into the 20th Century, Freud began frank discussions on sexuality. Yet, the idea of sexuality was still limited to discussion and research within psychiatry. It was considered taboo to discuss sex, sexuality, and gender outside of a research context. From many religious standpoints, it was not acceptable to engage in any form of sex, whether it be masturbatory or with another, nor was it acceptable to be attracted sexually and/or romantically to the same-sex. These viewpoints were labeled a repressive state-of-mind, which in some respects, continues in the 21st century. The public continues to scrutinize others for the sex, sexuality, gender, or gender expression.

Ideas about sex and sexuality have made significant changes throughout time. In 1948, Alfred Kinsey's book on male sexuality was released. The book described that gay sexuality was more common than initially believed. It was then that gay and lesbian rights organizations began to form. In 1961, Illinois became the first state to decriminalize homosexuality between two consenting adults. In 1969, the Stonewall Riots occurred in New York City, which brought LGBTQ+ issues to the forefront, as protesters demanded equal rights and acceptance. More recently, in 2004, Massachusetts was the first state to allow same-sex marriage. This allowance then became widespread throughout the United States, with *Obergefell v. Hodges,* which ruled that bans on same-sex marriage are unconstitutional. In 2016 then-President Obama discussed legislation regarding allowance of transgender persons using bathrooms according to their self-identified gender. The Obama Administration provided federal guidelines for schools and workplaces regarding antidiscrimination policies. However, the guidelines have since been rescinded by the current administration.

As with sexuality, gender may also be viewed as a social construct, taught to children from the moment of birth. Other cultures view gender expression and sexual orientation as a more fluid process compared to the Western culture. For example, in Chile identifying as a transgender male or a lesbian is more acceptable, given that the Chilean culture is a "machista" or one that values masculinity. However, when a transgender female identifies as such, they may experience discrimination such as physical and verbal aggression. Another example is found within the Spanish culture. Sexual orientation, specifically identifying as lesbian, gay, or bisexual, is more accepted within Spain. Further, Spanish media, music, and arts have significantly increased incorporation of LGBTQ into their culture. The idea of gender and sexual fluidity differs from the traditional thoughts regarding gender as a binary – limited to male/man and female/woman -typically found within the United States.

TREATMENT AND THERAPY

LGBTQ individuals experience a variety of physical and mental health disparities. A 2016 report by the National LGBT Health Education Center indicated that LGBT populations experience higher rates of substance abuse, HIV and sexually transmitted infections, unhealthy weight, smoking, violence victimization, depression, anxiety and suicide. Researchers noted that these disparities can be understood within the context of minority stress theory. Ilian Meyer, a prominent researcher on minority stress in LGBTQ populations, suggests that minority stress results from external, objective stressful events and conditions, expectations of instances of discrimination and stigma, and internalizations of negative societal attitudes. The distress experienced by LGBTQ individuals is largely due to experiences of stigma, discrimination, and social marginalization. Medical and mental health providers should be prepared to address concerns related to various psychosocial factors.

Treatment options can include educating patients about positive health behaviors and providing medical treatment for smoking, weight gain, HIV and sexually transmitted infections. LGBTQ people may need access to birth control and/or PrEP (HIV "pre-exposure prophylaxis", pills that can prevent contracting HIV) depending on who they have sexual activity with. How someone identifies (i.e. gay, lesbian, transgender) does not dictate the kind of activity they engage in. Additional treatment factors to consider are providing information about local LGBTQ organizations or communities, and referrals for individuals or family members to legal supports and mental health providers. Furthermore, hormone replacement therapy and gender-affirming surgeries can be a helpful option for transgender individuals who desire to have their outward appearance better match their gender. Health providers should also critically examine their own attitudes and beliefs about LGBTQ individuals to ensure that they are not unintentionally adding to distress experienced by this population by furthering negative stereotypes or incorrect assumptions. Staff at service agencies should be trained in the specifics of being welcoming and accommodating to LGBTQ populations, and institutional policies should be evaluated for inclusivity of unique needs of LGBTQ people and families.

PERSPECTIVE AND PROSPECTS

While there are many theories on gender development, one in particular focuses on those individuals who identify as gender-nonconforming. In 2011, Diane Ehrensaft, a developmental psychologist, named this theory the Gender Journey. The core of the theory is that gender identity is an individual's

Information on LGBTQ

Causes: Psychological, biological, familial, and sociocultural factors.

Symptoms: There are no symptoms associated with lesbian, gay, or bisexual individuals, as these terms are not a disorder or medical diagnosis. For transgender individuals, they may report an incongruence between their expressed versus assigned gender; may want to wear clothing that is typical of the opposite gender; or report a dislike of their primary and/or secondary sex characteristics.

Duration: Childhood or adulthood; may be static or dynamic.

Treatments: Psychological and social interventions, or gender-affirming surgery.

sense of psychological self as a man, a woman, both, or neither. Another aspect of the theory is that gender is a combination of nature (e.g., sex chromosomes XX, XY, or a combination) and nurture, and that gender development continues throughout the lifespan. It is important to note that there is physical gender (primary and secondary sex characteristics) as well as brain gender (how the brain structures function with respect to gender). Gender also refers to how someone self-identifies and presents in the world.

Gender and sexuality were previously studied in order to determine if there was a biological underpinning to the individual's decision with how they identify their gender and/or sexuality. There appears to be some genetic contribution to gender identity, but experts do not agree on the mechanisms, other than to say genetic and psychosocial factors are at play. Pediatric endocrinologists, Daniel Klink and Martin Den Heijer, note sex differences within the functional and anatomical structures of the brain in males and females. Some examples of the differences are that females have a larger hippocampus (emotion processing, memory, and autonomic nervous system activation), Broca's area (speech production), and the right parietal lobe (integration of sensory information); where as males have a larger hypothalamus (coordinates autonomic nervous system with the pituitary gland), and amygdala (integrates emotions, emotional behavior, and motivation). It appears that sex steroids affect gender identity in that they impact brain and body differentiation, but no one gene has

been identified to yield gender dysphoria or, for that matter, gender or sexual identity.

With respect to sexuality, this perspective is developed from a bio-psycho-social model. Biological factors are more controversial, as researchers attempt to find a "gay gene." As for psychological factors, an individual's personality may play a role in one's attitude towards their sexual development. Further, social factors are included in development of sexuality. For example, parental acceptance, support, style, as well as peer relationships and cultural influences, are all encompassing with respect to sexual interests and attitudes. Results from these studies are inconclusive and continue to be a source of debate among the LGBTQ community and medical professionals alike.

—Lindsey L. Wilner, Psy.D. & Jacob S. Sawyer, Ph.D.
Updated by Geraldine F. Marrocco, EdD., APRN, CNS,
ANP-BC, FAANP
and Eli Stark, RN, MSN

FOR FURTHER INFORMATION

Ehrensaft, Diane, and Edgardo Menvielle. *Gender Born, Gender Made: Raising Healthy Gender-Nonconforming Children*. The Experiment, 2011.

Erickson-Schroth, Laura, editor. *Trans Bodies, Trans Selves: A Resource for the Transgender Community*. Oxford Univ. Press, 2014.

Foucault, Michel. *The History of Sexuality*. Vintage, 1976.

"Media Reference Guide." GLAAD. www.glaad.org/.

PFLAG. https://pflag.org

"LGBTTIQQ2SAA+ Definitions." *Revel Riot*, www.revelandriot.com/

"Standards of Care for the Health of Transsexual, Transgender, and Gender Nonconforming People." *World Professional Association for Transgender Health*, vol. 7, 2012.

"Trans Student Educational Resources." *Trans Student Educational Resources*, www.transstudent.org/gender.

Liposuction

CATEGORY: Procedure

KEY TERMS:
abdomen: the area of the body between the diaphragm and the pelvis; it contains the visceral organs
adipose tissue: the tissue that stores fat

cannula: a tube used to drain body fluids or to administer medications

general anesthesia: anesthesia that induces unconsciousness

local anesthesia: anesthesia that numbs the feeling in a body part; administered by injection or direct application to the skin

subcutaneous: under the skin

INDICATIONS AND PROCEDURES

The fat contained in adipose tissue makes up 15 to 20 percent of the body weights of most healthy individuals. Much adipose tissue is found inside the abdominal cavity, but significant amounts are located under the skin of the abdomen, arms, breasts, hips, knees, legs, and throat. The quantity of this subcutaneous fat at any such site is based on individual heredity, age, and eating habits. When excessive eating greatly elevates body fat, a patient becomes obese, a condition that can be life-threatening. Until recently, the sole means for decreasing fat content resulting from obesity was time-consuming dieting, which requires much patience and will power. In addition, the positive consequences of long diets can be easily obliterated if dieters begin to overeat again. Recurrent overeating is common and often followed by the rapid regaining of the fat.

Persons who have undesired, unattractive fat deposits as a result of age, heredity, or obesity may undergo cosmetic surgery, such as so-called tummy tucks, to remove them. Such major procedures, however, often remove muscle along with fat and cause considerable scarring. Liposuction is a relatively easy way to lose unattractive body fat; it also is seen as a fast way to reverse obesity and is touted as more permanent than dieting. A cannula connected to a suction pump is inserted under the skin in the desired area. Then a chosen amount of fat is sucked out, the cannula is withdrawn, and the incision is closed. The result is a recontouring of the body part. Hence, liposuction has become a very popular cosmetic surgery procedure for the abdomen, arms, breasts, hips, knees, legs, and throat; many pounds can be removed from large areas such as the abdomen.

Liposuction begins with the administration of antibiotics and the anesthesia of the area to be

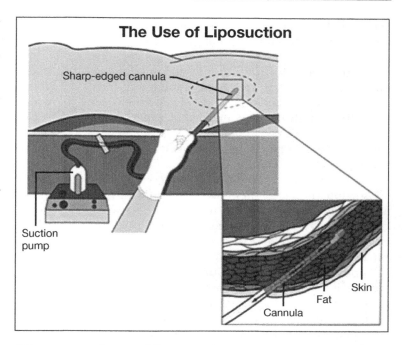

The Use of Liposuction

Sharp-edged cannula

Suction pump

Skin

Fat

Cannula

When unwanted areas of fat seem resistant to dieting and exercise, some patients turn to liposuction, the physical removal of fat deposits with a tube and a suction pump. The cosmetic results of this procedure may vary considerably. © EBSCO

recontoured. Local anesthesia is safer, but general anesthesia is used when necessary.

The process usually begins after a 1.3-centimeter (0.5-inch) incision is made in a fold of the treated body region, so that the scar will not be noticeable after healing. At this time, a sterile cannula is introduced under the skin of the treatment area. Next, the surgeon uses suction through the cannula to remove the fat deposits. Liposuction produces temporary tunnels in adipose tissue. Upon completion of the procedure, the incision is closed and the surgical area is wrapped with tight bandages or covered with support garments. This final stage of recontouring helps the tissue to collapse back into the desired shape during healing. In most patients, the skin around the area soon shrinks into the new contours. When this does not happen easily, because of old age or other factors, liposuction is accompanied by surgical skin removal.

USES AND COMPLICATIONS

Liposuction can be used for body recontouring only when undesired contours are attributable to fat deposits; those attributable to anatomical features such as bone structure cannot be treated in this manner.

A major principle on which liposuction is based is the supposition that the body contains a fixed number of fat cells and that, as people become fatter, the cells fill with droplets of fat and expand. The removal of fat cells by liposuction is deemed to decrease the future ability of the treated body part to become fat because fewer cells are available to be filled. Dieting and exercise are less successful than liposuction because they do not diminish the number of fat cells in adipose tissue, only decreasing fat cell size. Hence, when dieters return to eating excess food again or exercise stops, the fat cells expand again.

Another aspect of liposuction which is becoming popular is the ability to remove undesired fat from some body sites and insert it where the fat is wanted for recontouring. Most often, this transfer involves enlarging women's breasts or correcting cases in which the two breasts are of markedly different size. Liposuction also can be used to repair asymmetry in other body parts as a result of accidents.

Liposuction, as with any other surgery, has associated risks and complications. According to reputable practitioners, however, they are temporary and relatively minor, such as black-and-blue marks and the accumulation of blood and serum under the skin of treated areas. These complications are minimized by fluid removal during surgery and by the application of tight bandages or garments after the operation. Another related complication is that subcutaneous fat removal leads to fluid loss from the body. When large amounts of fat are removed, shock occurs if the fluid is not replaced quickly. Therefore, another component of successful liposuction is timely fluid replacement.

The more extensive and complex the liposuction procedure attempted, the more likely it is to cause complications. Particularly prone to problems are liposuction procedures in which major skin removal is required. Hence, surgeons who perform liposuction suggest that potential patients be realistic about the goals of the surgery. It is also recommended that patients choose reputable practitioners.

PERSPECTIVE AND PROSPECTS

Liposuction, currently viewed as relatively safe cosmetic surgery, originated in Europe in the late 1960s. In 1982, it reached the United States. Since that time, its use has burgeoned, and about a half million liposuction surgeries are carried out yearly. Although its first use was as a purely cosmetic procedure, liposuction is now done for noncosmetic reasons, including repairing injuries sustained in accidents. Women were once the sole liposuction patients, though that gap is closing. Men make up about 15 percent of treated individuals.

In the United States, liposuction is not presently accepted by insurance companies or considered tax deductible. This situation may change because several studies have found that obese people have a greater chance of developing cardiovascular disease and cancer. It must be noted, however, that liposuction offers only temporary relief from body fat. Although it does decrease fat deposition in a treated region, lack of proper calorie intake and exercise will deposit fat elsewhere in the body.

—*Sanford S. Singer, Ph.D.*

FOR FURTHER INFORMATION

Rubin, J. Peter, et al. *Body Contouring and Liposuction.* New York Elsevier Saunders, 2013.

Schafer, Jeffry B. *A Patient's Guide to Liposuction: How to Make an Informed Decision.* Denver, Colo.: Outskirts Press, 2011.

Shelton, Ron M., and Terry Malloy. *Liposuction.* New York: Berkley, 2004.

Shiffman, Melvin A., and Alberto Di Giuseppe, eds. *Liposuction: Principles and Practice.* New York: Springer, 2006.

Wilkinson, Tolbert S. *Atlas of Liposuction.* Philadelphia: Saunders/ Elsevier, 2005.

US Food and Drug Administration. "The Skinny on Liposuction." Author, April 12, 2013.

Zollinger, Robert M., Jr., and Robert M. Zollinger, Sr. *Zollinger's Atlas of Surgical Operations.* 8th ed. New York: McGraw-Hill, 2003.

M

Malignancy and metastasis

CATEGORY: Disease/Disorder

KEY TERMS:

benign tumors: tumors that grow relatively slowly, do not interfere with normal body functions, and do not metastasize

carcinogen: a natural or artificial substance inducing the transformation of cells toward the malignant state

chemotherapy: the use of chemicals to kill or inhibit the growth of cancer cells

multistep progression: the typical pathway of induction of cancer, beginning with an initial alteration to a gene and progressing to the fully malignant state

oncogene: a gene directly or indirectly inducing the transformation of cells from the normal to the malignant state; most oncogenes have normal counterparts in body cells

retrovirus: a virus infecting mammalian and other cells that sometimes carries and introduces oncogenes into host cells

transfection: a technique used to introduce genes into cells by exposing the cells to fragmented deoxyribonucleic acid (DNA) under conditions that promote the uptake and incorporation of DNA

tumor suppressor gene: a gene that, in its normal form, inhibits cell division

CAUSES AND SYMPTOMS

Cancer cells are characterized by two primary features: uncontrolled cell division and metastasis. Normal cells enter an unregulated, rapid growth phase by losing the controls that normally limit division rates to the amount required for normal growth and maintenance of body tissues. During metastasis, tumor cells lose the connections that normally hold them in place in body tissues, break loose, and spread from their original sites to lodge and grow in other body locations. Tumor cells with these characteristics are described as malignant.

The detrimental effects of malignant tumors are caused by the interference of rapidly growing masses of cancer cells with the activities of normal tissues and organs or by the loss of vital functions due to the conversion of cells with essential functions to nonfunctional forms. Some malignant tumors of glandular tissue upset bodily functions by producing and secreting excessive quantities of hormones.

As malignant tumors grow, they compress surrounding normal tissues, destroying normal structures by cutting off blood supplies and interrupting nerve function. They may also break through barriers that separate major body regions, such as internal membranes, the gut wall, or even the skin. Such breakthroughs cause internal or external bleeding and infection, and destroy the organization and separation of body regions necessary for normal function. Both compression and breakthroughs can cause pain that, in advanced cases, may be extreme.

Malignant tumors of blood tissues involve cell lines that normally divide to supply the body's requirements for red and white blood cells, contained within the bone marrow. Cancer in these cell lines crowds the bloodstream with immature, nonfunctional cells that are unable to accomplish required activities, such as the delivery of oxygen to tissues or the activation of the immune response. When the total mass of actively growing and dividing malignant cells becomes large, their demands for nutrients may deprive normal cells, tissues, and organs of needed supplies, leading to generally impaired functions, fatigue, weakness, and weight loss.

Not all unregulated tissue growths are malignant. Some tumors, such as common skin warts, are benign—they do not usually interfere with normal body functions. They grow relatively slowly and do not metastasize. Often, benign tumors are surrounded by a closed capsule of connective tissue that prevents or retards expansion and breakup. Some initially benign tumors may change to malignant forms, however, including even common skin warts.

Individual cells of a malignant tumor exhibit differences from normal cells in activity, biochemistry, physiology, and structure. First and foremost is the characteristic of uncontrolled division. Cancer cells typically move through the division cycle much more rapidly than normal cells. This rapid division is accompanied by biochemical changes characteristic of dividing cells, such as high metabolic rates; increases in the rate of transport of substances across the plasma membrane; increases in protein phosphorylation; raised cytoplasmic concentrations of sodium, potassium, and calcium ions; and an elevated pH. Often chromosomal abnormalities are present, including extra or missing chromosomes, exchanges of segments between chromosomes, and breakage.

Cancer cells also typically fail to develop all the characteristics and structures of fully mature cells of their type. They may lose mature characteristics if these were attained before conversion to the malignant state. Frequently, loss of mature characteristics involves disorganization or disappearance of the cytoskeleton. Alterations are also noted in the structure and density of surface carbohydrate groups. Cancer cells lose tight attachments to their neighbors or to supportive extracellular materials such as collagen; some cancer cells secrete enzymes that break cell connections and destroy elements of the extracellular matrix, aiding their movement into and through surrounding tissues. If removed from the body and placed in test-tube cultures, most cancer cells have the capacity to divide indefinitely. In contrast, most normal body cells placed in a culture medium eventually stop dividing.

The conversion of normal cells to malignant types usually involves multiple causes inducing a series of changes that occur in stages over a considerable length of time. This characteristic is known as the multistep progression of cancer. In most cases, the complete sequence of steps leading from an initiating alteration to full malignancy is unknown.

The initial event in a multistep progression usually involves the alteration of a gene from a normal to an aberrant form known as an oncogene. The gene involved is typically one that regulates cell growth and division or takes part in biochemical sequences with this effect. The alteration may involve the substitution or loss of DNA sequences, the movement of the gene to a new location in the chromosomes, or the movement of another gene or its controlling elements to

the vicinity of the gene. In some cases, the alteration involves a gene that in normal form suppresses cell division in cells in which it is active. Loss or alteration of function of such genes, known as tumor suppressor genes, can directly or indirectly increase growth and division rates.

An initiating genetic alteration may be induced by a long list of factors, including exposure to radiation or certain chemicals, the insertion of viral DNA into the chromosomes, or the generation of random mutations during the duplication of genetic material. In a few cancers, the initiating event involves the insertion of an oncogene into the DNA by an infecting virus that carries the oncogene as a part of its genetic makeup.

In some cases, an initiating oncogene or faulty tumor suppressor gene is inherited, producing a strong predisposition to the development of malignancy. Among these strongly predisposed cancers are familial retinoblastoma, familial adenomatous polyps of the colon, and multiple endocrine neoplasia, in which tumors develop in the thyroid, adrenal medulla, and parathyroid glands. In addition to the strongly predisposed cancers, some, including breast cancer, ovarian cancer, and colon cancers other than familial adenomatous polyps, show some degree of disposition in family lines, meaning that members of these families show a greater tendency to develop the cancer than individuals in other families.

Subsequent steps from the initiating change to the fully malignant state usually include the conversion of additional genes to oncogenic form or the loss of function of tumor suppressor genes. Also important during intermediate stages are further alterations to the initial and succeeding oncogenes that increase their activation. The initial conversion of a normal gene to oncogenic form by its movement to a new location in the chromosomes may be compounded at successive steps, for example, by sequence changes or the multiplication of the oncogene into extra copies. The subsequent steps in progression to the malignant state are driven by many of the sources of change responsible for the initiating step. Because genetic alterations often occur during the duplication and division of the genetic material, an increase in the cell division rate by the initiating change may increase the chance that further alterations leading to full malignancy will occur.

A change advancing the progression toward full malignancy may take place soon after a previous change or only after a long delay. Moreover, further changes may not occur, leaving the progression at an intermediate stage, without the development of full malignancy, for the lifetime of the individual. The avoidance of environmental factors that induce genetic alterations, including overexposure to radiation sources such as sunlight, x-rays, and radon gas and chemicals such as those in cigarette smoke, increases the chance that progression toward malignancy will remain incomplete. The last stage in progression to full malignancy is often metastasis. After the loss of normal adhesions to neighboring cells or to elements of the extracellular matrix, the separation and movement of cancer cells from a primary tumor to secondary locations may occur through the development of active motility or through breakage into elements of the circulatory system.

Relatively few of the cells that break loose from a tumor survive the rigors of passage through the body. Most are destroyed by various factors, including deformation by passage through narrow capillaries and destruction by blood turbulence around the heart valves and vessel junctions. Furthermore, tumor cells often develop changes in their surface groups that permit detection and elimination by the immune system as they move through the body. Unfortunately, the rigors of travel through the body may act as a sort of natural selection for the cells that are most malignant—that is, those most able to resist destruction—which can then grow uncontrollably and spread further by metastasis.

Many natural and artificial agents trigger the initial step in the progression to the malignant state or push cells through intermediate stages. Most of these agents, collectively called carcinogens, are chemicals or forms of radiation capable of inducing chemical changes in DNA. Some, however, may initiate or further this progression by modifying ribonucleic acids (RNAs) or proteins, or they may act by increasing the rate of DNA replication and cell division.

Treatment and Therapy

Cancer is treated most frequently by one or a combination of the following primary techniques: surgical removal of tumors, radiation therapy, and chemotherapy or immunotherapy. Surgical removal is most effective if the growth has remained localized so that the entire tumor can be detected and removed. Often, surgery is combined with radiation or chemotherapy in an attempt to eliminate malignant cells that have broken loose from a primary tumor and lodged in other parts of the body. Surgical removal followed by chemotherapy is presently the most effective treatment for most forms of cancer, especially if the tumor is detected and removed before extensive metastasis has taken place. Most responsive to surgical treatments have been non-melanoma or low grade melanoma skin cancers, many of which are easily detected and remain localized and accessible.

Radiation therapy may be directed toward the destruction of a tumor in a specific body location. Alternatively, it may be used in whole-body exposure to kill cancer cells that have metastasized and lodged in many body regions. In either case, the method takes advantage of the destructive effects of radiation on DNA, particularly during periods when the DNA is under duplication. Because cancer cells undergo replication at higher rates than most other body cells, the technique is more selective for tumors than for normal tissues. The selection is only partial, however, so that body cells that divide rapidly, such as those of the blood, hair follicles, and intestinal lining, are also affected. As a consequence, radiation therapy often has side effects ranging from unpleasant to serious, including hair loss, nausea and vomiting, anemia, and suppression of the immune system. Because radiation is mutagenic, radiation therapy carries the additional disadvantage of being carcinogenic; the treatment, while effective in the destruction or inhibition of a malignant growth, may also initiate new cancers or push cells through intermediate stages in progression toward malignancy. Immunotherapy involves modifying the patient's immune system to attack the cancer directly but may also result in autoimmune side effects such as rash, diarrhea, or even severe allergic reaction.

When possible, radiation is directed only toward the body regions containing a tumor in order to minimize the destruction of normal tissues. This may be accomplished by focusing a radiation source on the tumor or by shielding body regions outside the tumor with a radiation barrier such as a lead sheet. Chemotherapy involves the use of chemicals that retard cell division or kill tumor cells more readily than normal body cells. Most of the chemicals used in chemotherapy have been discovered by routine screening of

Information on Malignancy and Metastasis

Causes: Genetic factors, carcinogens, retroviruses

Symptoms: Vary; can include loss or impairment of normal bodily functions, interrupted nerve function, internal or external bleeding and infection, pain, swelling, fatigue, weakness, weight loss

Duration: Often chronic with recurrent episodes

Treatments: Surgery, radiation, chemotherapy

substances for their effects on cancer cells in cultures and test animals. Several hundred thousand chemicals were tested in the screening effort that produced the thirty or so chemotherapeutic agents available for cancer treatment.

Many of the chemicals most effective in cancer chemotherapy alter the chemical structure of DNA, produce breaks in DNA molecules, slow or stop DNA duplication, or interfere with the natural systems repairing chemical lesions in DNA. These effects inhibit cell division or interfere with cell functions sufficiently to kill the cancer cells. Because DNA is most susceptible to chemical alteration during duplication and cancer cells duplicate their DNA and divide more rapidly than most normal tissue cells, the effects of these chemicals are most pronounced in malignant types. Normal cells, however, are also affected to some extent, particularly those in tissues that divide more rapidly. As a result, chemotherapeutic chemicals can produce essentially the same detrimental side effects as radiation therapy. The side effects of chemotherapy are serious enough to be fatal in 2 to 5 percent of persons treated. Because they alter DNA, many chemotherapeutic agents are carcinogens and carry the additional risk, as with radiation, of inducing the formation of new cancers.

Not all chemicals used in chemotherapy alter DNA. Some act by interfering with cell division or other cell processes rather than directly modifying DNA. Two chemotherapeutic agents often used in cancer treatment, vinblastine and taxol, for example, slow or stop cell division through their ability to interfere with the spindle structure that divides chromosomes. The drugs can slow or stop tumor growth as well as the division of normal cells.

Tumors frequently develop resistance to some of the chemicals used in chemotherapy, so that the treatment gradually becomes less effective. Development of resistance is often associated with random duplication of DNA segments, commonly noted in tumor cells. In some, the random duplication happens to include genes that provide resistance to the chemicals employed in chemotherapy. The genes providing resistance usually encode enzymes that break down the applied chemical or its metabolic derivatives or transport proteins of the plasma membrane capable of rapidly excreting the chemical from the cell. One gene in particular, the multidrug resistance gene (MDR), is frequently found to be duplicated or highly activated in resistant cells. This gene, which is normally active in cells of the liver, kidney, adrenal glands, and parts of the digestive system, encodes a transport pump that can expel a large number of substances from cells, including many of those used in chemotherapy. Over activity of the MDR pump can effectively keep chemotherapy drugs below toxic levels in cancer cells. Cells developing resistance are more likely to survive chemotherapy and give rise to malignant cell lines with resistance. The chemotherapeutic agents involved may thus have the unfortunate effect of selecting cells with resistance, thereby ensuring that they will become the dominant types in the tumor.

Success rates with chemotherapy vary from negligible to about 80 percent, depending on the cancer type. For most, success rates do not range above 50 to 60 percent. Some cancer types, including lung, breast, ovarian, and colorectal tumors, respond poorly or not at all to chemotherapy. The overall cure rate for surgery, radiation, and chemotherapy combined, as judged by no recurrence of the cancer for a period of five years, is between 50 and 60 percent.

It is hoped that full success in the treatment of cancer will come from the continued study of the genes controlling cell division and the regulatory mechanisms that modify the activity of these genes in the cell cycle. An understanding of the molecular activities of these genes and their modifying controls may bring with it a molecular means to reach specifically into cancer cells and halt their growth and metastasis.

PERSPECTIVE AND PROSPECTS

Indications that malignancy and metastasis might have a basis in altered gene activity began to appear in the nineteenth century. In 1820, a British physician,

Sir William Norris, noted that melanoma, a cancer involving pigmented skin cells, was especially prevalent in one family under study. More than forty kinds of cancer, including common types such as breast cancer and colon cancer, have since been noticed to occur more frequently in some families than in others. Another indication that cancer has a basis in altered gene activity was the fact that the chromosomes of many tumor cells show abnormalities, such as extra chromosomes, broken chromosomes, or rearrangements of one kind or another. These abnormalities suggested that cancer might be induced by altered genes with activities related to cell division.

These indications were put on a firm basis by research with tumors caused by viruses infecting animal cells, most notably those caused by a group of viruses called retroviruses. Many retroviral infections cause little or no damage to their hosts, but some are associated with induction of cancer. (Another type of pathogenic retrovirus is responsible for acquired immunodeficiency syndrome, or AIDS.) The cancer-inducing types of retroviruses were found to carry genes capable of transforming normal cells into malignant ones. The transforming genes were at first thought to be purely viral in origin, but DNA sequencing and other molecular approaches revealed that the viral oncogenes had normal counterparts among the genes directly or indirectly regulating cell division in cells of the infected host. Among the most productive of the investigators using this approach were J. Michael Bishop and Harold E. Varmus, who received the 1989 Nobel Prize in Physiology or Medicine for their research establishing the relationship between retroviral oncogenes and their normal cellular counterparts.

The discovery of altered host genes in cancer-inducing retroviruses prompted a search for similar genes in non-viral cancers. Much of this work was accomplished by transfection experiments, in which the DNA of cancer cells is extracted and introduced into cultured mouse cells. Frequently, the mouse cells are transformed into types that grow much more rapidly than normal cells. The human oncogene responsible for the transformation is then identified in the altered cells. Many of the oncogenes identified by transfection turned out to be among those already carried by retroviruses, confirming by a different route that these genes are capable of contributing to the transformation of cells into a cancerous state.

The transfection experiments also identified some additional oncogenes not previously found in retroviruses. In spite of impressive advances in treatment, cancer remains among the most dreaded of human diseases. Recognized as a major threat to health since the earliest days of recorded history, cancer still counts as one of the most frequent causes of human fatality. In technically advanced countries, it accounts for about 15 to 20 percent of deaths each year. Smoking, the most frequent single cause of cancer, is estimated to be responsible for about one-third of these deaths.

—*Stephen L. Wolfe, Ph.D.*
Updated by Patrick Richardson

FOR FURTHER INFORMATION

Alberts, Bruce, et al. *Molecular Biology of the Cell.* 5th ed. New York: Garland, 2008.

"Cancer." *MedlinePlus,* May 2, 2013.

Eyre, Harmon J., Dianne Partie Lange, and Lois B. Morris. *Informed Decisions: The Complete Book of Cancer Diagnosis, Treatment, and Recovery.* 2d ed. Atlanta: American Cancer Society, 2002.

Ko, Andrew, Malin Dollinger, and Ernest H. Rosenbaum. *Everyone's Guide to Cancer Therapy.* 5th ed. Kansas City, Mo.: Andrews McMeel, 2008.

Lackie, J. M., ed. *The Dictionary of Cell and Molecular Biology.* 4th ed. Boston: Academic Press, 2007.

Lodish, Harvey, et al. *Molecular Cell Biology.* 7th ed. New York: W. H. Freeman, 2012.

"Metastatic Cancer Fact Sheet." *National Cancer Institute,* March 28, 2013.

Mammography

CATEGORY: Procedure

KEY TERMS:

architectural distortion: when a mammogram shows a region where the breasts normal appearance looks like an abnormal arrangement of tissue strands, but without any associated mass as the apparent cause of this distortion

contrast: a substance used to increase the contrast of structures or fluids within the body in medical imaging

microcalcifications: calcium deposits within breast tissue; they appear as white spots or flecks on a mammogram

signal-to-noise: a measure used in science and engineering that compares the level of a desired signal
to the level of background noise

INDICATIONS AND PROCEDURES

X-ray mammography is a complicated procedure.
The quality of the mammographic image is proportionately dependent upon the imaging equipment in
use and the way in which it is utilized.

Critical factors include compression and positioning of the breast, the use of the right image
receptor, and exposure of the x-ray tube. Improper
use of equipment and procedures contributes to an
image that is suboptimal. With proper care and thorough knowledge in the use of instruments designed
for mammography, however, excellent image quality
can be obtained.

In mammography, four physical constraints must
be considered when evaluating the performance of
the systems.

First, contrast is of utmost importance because
minute differences in soft tissue density are essential.
Second, resolution is important because of the need
to identify microcalcifications as small as 100 microm-
eters, which are often associated with abnormalities.
Third, an adequate x-ray dose is vital to obtain an
image with the proper signal-to-noise ratio. Too much
radiation, however, means added risk for the patient.
Fourth, a decrease in noise (background) is important to achieve an image with an adequate signal-
to-noise ratio for proper diagnosis.

The examination can be conducted with the
patient standing or sitting. To achieve the desired
radiographic projection, the x-ray tube is set at an
optimal angle. The mammography unit has a support
plate onto which the breast is positioned.
A plastic paddle assists in compressing the breast onto
this plate. The pressure applied to achieve proper
compression can be applied manually, but most mammography technicians prefer power-assisted compression, as this permits the radiographer to use both
hands to position the breast properly.

The shape, rigidity, and composition of the compression or support plate are crucial factors. The support plate is composed of a carbon-fiber composite
capable of a high x-ray transmission. The support is in
front of the tunnel, and the tunnel receives the image
receptor. The standard image receptor uses a high-
resolution mammographic screen-film combination.

With receptor technology advancing rapidly, however, digital receptors are fast becoming available.
The big advantage of digital receptors is that they
offer either a limited field of view for stereotactical
localization or a full field of view for standard mammographic imaging.

Since all mammography units are intended to
show the soft tissue of the breast while displaying differences in contrast and since proper compression is
vital, the natural mobility of the breast should be considered. The breast is easiest to compress from the
inferior and lateral aspects. The preliminary automatic compression between the paddle and the support plate should never go beyond forty-five pounds
of pressure, and the patient should not be in pain.
Nevertheless, the breast must be taut to the touch.

Improper compression can lead to erroneous
results. The outcome of proper compression is a reduction of x-ray radiation to the breast by reducing tissue
thickness; the bringing of lesions closer to the film,
thus facilitating an accurate reading; a reduction in
movement blurriness because the breast is held immo-
bile; increased contrast as a result of flattened breasts,
thereby decreasing thickness; elimination of confusion caused by superimposition shadows; and easier
visualization of the borders of circumscribed lesions.

It is helpful if magnification of the image is possible, particularly if small areas are being examined.
Magnification is of greater importance in areas of suspicious microcalcifications or at surgical sites. Unfortunately, the greater the magnification, the higher the
patient's radiation dose because the breast is placed
much closer to the source of radiation.

In addition to compression, image quality depends
on a number of factors: positioning, radiation exposure, contrast, sharpness, noise, artifacts, and labeling.
The craniocaudal position (compression of the breast
from top to bottom) and the mediolateral oblique
position (compression of the breast from side to side)
are the two standard positions employed in mammography. Each position provides specific views, and
proper positioning reveals as much of the tissue as
possible for diagnosis. Any area that is omitted will
create false results that may endanger the patient's
life. Adequate exposure to radiation is essential. If this
is not achieved, then it is difficult to identify the skin
and subcutaneous tissue. Usually, contrast is highest
for thinner breasts and lowest for thicker breasts; this
is primarily the result of more scattered radiation and

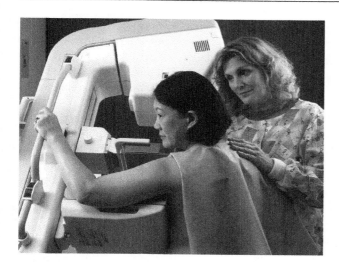

A woman receive a mammogram. (National Cancer Institute via Wikimedia Commons)

greater tissue absorption of low radiation in thicker breasts. Without contrast, particularly in thicker breast tissue, different tissue densities will have very similar appearances.

Sharpness, or the visualization of fine details in the image, is one of the central factors in achieving a correct diagnosis. If the desired sharpness is not obtained, then the image is referred to as "unsharp." Unsharpness may be the result of motion blur, poor screen-film contrast, or other technical factors. Noise and sharpness are closely linked. "Noise" is defined as increased background and a decreased ability to see tiny structures, such as calcifications. The major contributors of noise are scatter and quantum mottle, which is fluctuation in the number of x-ray photons needed to form the image. Examples of artifacts are scratches, fingerprints, dirt, lint, and dust. Standardized labeling in mammography to identify the left side from the right side, so that the films cannot be subject to misinterpretation, is vital, especially because mammograms can be legal documents.

A slightly different approach is used to screen women with breast implants. Two craniocaudal views are obtained, one with the implant in the field of view and one with the implant as much out of the field as possible. In a similar way, two mediolateral oblique views are imaged.

Digital mammography differs from regular mammography in that in the former, electronic detectors capture and facilitate the display of the x-ray signals on a computer or laser-printed film. In all other aspects, it is still the same procedure— proper positioning and compression of the breast are still critical for obtaining quality digital images. The goal of digital mammography also remains the same: to detect and localize breast abnormalities.

As exposure to radiation is a major concern with traditional mammography, the primary force to developing digital x-ray mammography is the idea that it has the potential to enhance image quality—and therefore lesion detection, especially for dense breasts—with a lower dose of radiation. The greatest advantage in digital mammography is its ability to separate image acquisition from image display, thus providing the ability to manipulate contrast, brightness, and magnification with one exposure.

Dynamic or real-time imaging, especially with biopsies, is possible with digital mammography, providing a better understanding of breast tumors with regard to localization and boundaries. This procedure can also facilitate the direct use of computers for detection and diagnosis. Such computer-aided detection (CAD) programs can identify areas of abnormal or suspicious tissue for the radiologist. In addition, with digital technology, it is possible to form three-dimensional (3-D) images by combining x-rays images from all angles along an arc around the breast. The ease of digital image archiving, retrieval, and transmission is another advantage. One disadvantage is that while digital mammograms require lower doses of radiation than traditional film mammograms, 3-D imaging is often conducted simultaneous to traditional 2-D mammography, thus elevating the total radiation administered.

USES AND COMPLICATIONS

There are two basic types of mammographic examinations: screening mammography and diagnostic mammography. "Screening mammography" refers to examinations of women with no obvious symptoms to detect breast cancers. A standard screening examination includes two views of each breast, sometimes referred to as the "standard views."

General agreement has been reached that screening mammography reduces mortality from breast cancer in women fifty years of age or older, but an ongoing debate exists over the effectiveness of screening mammography in women aged forty to forty-nine. Randomized clinical trials have confirmed the validity of screening mammography. Deaths attributable to breast cancer have been reduced. The American Cancer Society and most other well-known professional societies have continued to recommend screening mammography for women in the younger age group because of the results of several studies that advocate the benefits of screening in this age group. Likewise, the frequency of screening mammography remains a subject of debate. Since 2009, the US Preventative Services Task Force has recommended biennial screening for women over fifty, while most other major organizations continue to recommend annual screening. The National Cancer Institute also recommends that screening mammography begin earlier and be conducted more frequently in women who have a family history of breast cancer.

A negative result produced by screening mammography would not include straight lines, unless there is a history of surgery or trauma, and would not show bulging contours from tissue into fatty areas. Characteristics in a screening view that suggest the need for follow-up diagnostic screening are masses, microcalcifications, architectural distortion, and parenchymal asymmetry. Palpable abnormalities described by the patient, focal tenderness, and spontaneous nipple discharge also warrant diagnostic screening.

As with all preventive measures, screening mammography cannot eliminate all deaths from breast cancer, for several reasons. It does not detect all types of cancers, including some that are actually detected by physical examination. Also, some tumors may appear and develop too quickly to be detected and identified at an early, more curable stage. Mammograms are particularly difficult to interpret for women with dense breast tissue, which is especially common in young women. The dense tissue prevents the identification of abnormalities associated with tumors, thereby leading to a higher rate of false-positive and false-negative test results.

Diagnostic mammography, also referred to as "consultative mammography" or "problem-solving mammography," is the type of study preferred when there are clinical findings, such as a palpable lump or an abnormal screening mammogram requiring additional analysis. Additionally, each diagnostic mammography examination is performed to suit the individual patient who has symptoms or abnormal findings.

Diagnostic mammography may warrant additional views of the breast (such as spot compression and magnification), a correlative clinical examination, and ultrasonography. In almost all instances, barring a few exceptions, a radiologist is present during a diagnostic mammography study.

Diagnostic mammography should be carried out when a biopsy is being considered for a palpable lump in a woman over thirty years of age. The reason for doing a mammogram preceding a biopsy is to better define the nature of the clinical abnormality and to find other unexpected lesions. Mammographic characteristics of possible benign lesions are a cluster of small round or oval calcifications; nonpalpable, noncalcified, solid round or oval, and predominantly well-circumscribed masses; nonpalpable focal symmetry with concave margins and interspersed fat; asymptomatic single dilated duct (no nipple discharge); and multiple (three or more) similar findings, distributed randomly and often bilaterally. Mammographic characteristics of malignant lesions are a mass with no history of previous surgery, trauma, or mastitis that is ill defined and microtubulated; malignant microcalcifications; skin thickening and retraction; nipple retraction; and architectural distortion with no history of previous surgery or trauma.

The ruling concern in mammography is the amount of radiation to which the patient is exposed. Therefore, an automatic radiation exposure control device is necessary to avoid overexposure. The radiation detector is placed behind the image receptor so that its image does not appear on the mammogram. Exposure is terminated when the signal recorded by the monitor reaches a predefined level. Unfortunately, the x-ray photons reaching the detector fluctuate considerably depending on the size and composition of the breast. As a result, the signal recorded by the detector is only an approximate indication of the energy absorbed. Therefore, it is unlikely that an accurate reading will be available. In any therapeutic model that is considered a source of risk to the patient, it is essential to bear in mind the number of deaths caused by the technique as opposed to the number of deaths that it actually prevents. Fortunately, the benefits of mammography supersede the risk of radiation exposure. Furthermore, risk estimates have decreased following the adoption of a relative risk model and allowance for the variation of risk with age at exposure.

PERSPECTIVE AND PROSPECTS

Though much progress has been made in the field of cancer medicine, early detection remains the best approach in the war against breast cancer. Ample clinical data have shown that women diagnosed with breast cancers in the early stages are more likely to survive than those diagnosed with more advanced stages of the same disease. A systematic physical breast examination by a clinician once a year may help in identifying tumors that are fairly small and that may go unnoticed in the absence of such examinations. The relative benefits and risks of regular breast self-examination remain a subject of debate among medical experts.

Nearly all medical experts agree that in women over fifty, routine x-ray mammography, with or without clinical examination, has been valuable in detecting tumors and at earlier stages. This has been very effectively shown in randomized clinical trials to reduce disease-specific mortality. Consequently, routine mammographic screening, especially for women over fifty years of age, has been actively promoted in many countries and nongovernmental agencies.

Breast imaging technologies that are being developed are progressing with three distinct goals in mind: to identify the most minute tumor lesions; to localize abnormalities to aid further examination, analysis, or treatment; and to characterize the abnormalities and assist in the decision-making process following identification. Radiologists and patients alike dream of an ideal imaging modality that would achieve all three goals in a single use. In reality, most current technologies fail to do so; hence, many developers are intent on perfecting one goal at a time. In addition to these technical goals, developers hope to generate methods that are more practical, inexpensive, harmless, and appealing to the patient.

—*Giri Sulur, Ph.D.*

FOR FURTHER INFORMATION

Kopans, Daniel B. *Breast Imaging.* 3d ed. Baltimore: Lippincott Williams & Wilkins, 2007.

Love, Susan, and Karen Lindsey. *Dr. Susan Love's Breast Book.* 5th ed. Cambridge, Mass.: Da Capo Press, 2010.

"Mammography." *MedlinePlus*, U.S. National Library of Medicine, 22 Oct. 2018, medlineplus.gov/mammography.html.

National Cancer Institute. "Mammograms." *National Institutes of Health,* July 24, 2012.

RadiologyInfo.org. "Mammography." *Radiological Society of North America*, May 7, 2013.

Sutton, Amy L., editor. *Cancer Sourcebook for Women: Basic Consumer Health Information About Leading Causes of Cancer in Women.* 3d ed. Detroit, Mich.: Omnigraphics, 2006.

What Is a Mammogram? Centers for Disease Control and Prevention, 11 Sept. 2018, www.cdc.gov/cancer/breast/basic_info/mammograms.htm.

Mastectomy and lumpectomy

CATEGORY: Procedures

KEY TERMS:

BRCA1: an abbreviation for breast cancer 1; the mutant chromosomal factor, when found in chromosome 17, which indicates that a woman is vulnerable to developing breast cancer

estrogen: any of several hormones produced by the ovaries that regulate some female reproductive processes and maintain secondary sex characteristics in the female

fibrocystic breasts: the lumpy breasts that some women routinely develop, particularly in the seven or eight days before menstruation

mammography: an X-ray examination of the breasts, the purpose of which is to reveal tumors and other abnormalities

metastasis: the spreading of cancer cells from the original site to other parts of the body

palpation: a digital examination of affected parts of the body

quadrantectomy: a form of lumpectomy that removes more tissue than the usual lumpectomy, leaving little visible scarring but slightly diminishing the size of the affected breast

sonogram: an image of body organs produced through focusing sound waves on the part to be examined

ultrasound: a method of diagnostic imaging that focuses sound waves inaudible to humans on a given organ to produce detailed images of that organ

INDICATIONS AND PROCEDURES

The early indications of breast cancer are often quite subtle, although in this stage it may be revealed by routine mammograms. In some cases, no overt symptoms exist until the cancer is well advanced. Women between forty and fifty years of age without risk factors are advised to have a mammogram every two years. Women over fifty or in the high-risk category because of a family history of breast cancer should have a mammogram once every year. If palpation of the breast reveals a lump, then immediate mammography is indicated.

It is necessary to be constantly vigilant for any sign that an abnormality exists in the breast. Clear indications of possible breast cancer include lumps or thickening of the tissue in the breast or in the area under the arms. Symptoms such as discoloration of the breasts or dimpling, thickening, scaling, or puckering of one or both breasts may also arouse suspicion of breast cancer. A significant change in the shape of the breast or a swelling of it are also symptomatic. A bloody discharge from the nipple, scaly skin on the nipple or surrounding area, inversion of the nipple, or discoloration of the area surrounding the nipple may presage the presence of breast cancer. Monthly palpation of the breasts, preferably seven or eight days after menstruation, may reveal lumps that could be harmless growths but that might be cancerous. This procedure is referred to as breast self-examination (BSE). Because the female breast contains many glands, it is not uncommon in some women for lumps to appear regularly—often profusely— particularly in the week prior to menstruation.

Women with notably lumpy breasts are said to have fibrocystic breasts. Often, the lumps diminish in size in the week following menstruation. If they do not recede, however, then these lumps should be regarded with suspicion and the patient should be examined by a physician, preferably a surgeon, gynecologist, or oncologist.

Once a problem is detected, a number of procedures must be considered for dealing with it. The initial procedure in treating suspected breast cancer usually involves a mammogram to reveal irregularities in the breast. If the results of the mammogram are negative and the patient is still convinced that there is a lump in the breast, an ultrasound or sonographic examination may be indicated. In such tests, harmless sound waves are focused on the breast. These sound waves are reflected so that they create an image of formations within the breast. Although ultrasound cannot definitively indicate whether a lump is cancerous, it can at least verify whether a lump exists.

It can also show whether the lump is hollow and filled with fluid, in which case it is usually a benign cyst rather than a cancerous growth.

If a growth is detected, the next, least-invasive means of determining whether it is cancerous is through a needle biopsy. In this procedure, the patient, under local anesthetic, has a hollow needle inserted into the growth. Fluids and cells are then harvested from it. If the growth is a cyst, a clear or light-yellow fluid will be withdrawn, causing the cyst to collapse. This may be all the treatment required. In all cases, however, the substances withdrawn from the growth are examined by a pathologist for the presence of cancer cells.

Not all growths are so positioned that needle biopsies are possible. In such cases, a surgical biopsy is probably necessary. If the lump is small, then a lumpectomy, or the removal of the entire lump, may occur. Larger lumps often cannot be removed at this stage, so portions are excised for pathological examination. A pathologist carefully studies the tissue removed to determine whether it contains cancer cells.

In the past, biopsies often occurred while patients were anesthetized and, if the pathological report was positive for cancer, then a radical mastectomy was performed immediately while the patient was still under anesthetic. Since the late twentieth century, however, a two-step procedure has usually replaced this one-step method. If cancer is detected, then surgery is delayed, giving physicians the opportunity to consult with their patients about the treatments available to them. The major decision in such cases usually is whether a total mastectomy or a partial mastectomy, commonly referred to as a lumpectomy, should be performed. Total mastectomy involves the total removal of the breast and the surrounding lymph nodes.

A radical mastectomy, done under general anesthetic, involves making a large, elliptical incision on the breast, including the nipple and often the entire breast. The incision normally extends into the armpit. All the breast tissue is excised, including the skin and the fat down to the chest muscles. The incision extends into the armpit to remove as much of the breast tissue as possible, including the lymph nodes, which may be cancerous. Once the bleeding has been controlled, a drainage tube is inserted, and the incision is closed with sutures, clips, or adhesive substances. This drastic form of treatment can be traumatic both physically and psychologically to patients. Many women fear the disfigurement that follows it. Some women, especially those with a family history of breast cancer, may decide that the total removal of the breast is their safest option. In some cases, to prevent future threats of breast cancer, they demand the removal of both breasts.

A lumpectomy, usually performed under local anesthetic, involves the removal only of cancerous tissue. The incision is made under the breast, and the lump, with surrounding tissue, is removed. The appearance of the breast remains much the same as it was before the surgery. In some cases, physicians recommend a quadrantectomy, which involves the removal of the cancerous tissue as well as significant amounts of the surrounding tissue. Quite often, the lymph nodes are removed as well. When this treatment is used, the breast will appear slightly smaller than it previously was, but it can be enhanced through plastic surgery.

Subcutaneous mastectomy is frequently indicated in situations in which the tumor is small. In this procedure, the surgeon makes an incision under the breast. Most of the skin and the nipple remain intact, although the milk ducts that lead into the nipple are cut. Following the surgery, sometimes immediately, a breast implant can be inserted, restoring the breast to its normal appearance. Mastectomy and lumpectomy are routinely followed by a course of radiation and/or chemotherapy designed to kill any fugitive cancer cells that the surgery has missed. While the goal of mastectomy is to create as little scarring as possible, considerable scarring may occur, particularly with radical mastectomy, and the absence of one or both breasts usually requires significant psychological adjustments on the part of women who have undergone the procedure. The breast reconstruction performed by a plastic surgeon following a mastectomy is often accompanied by treatment from a psychologist or psychiatrist. Some women with family histories of breast cancer, particularly if the disease has occurred in first-level relatives (mother or sisters), may opt for a mastectomy rather than a lumpectomy to relieve themselves of the fear of contracting the disease, although most oncologists make such women fully aware of other, less drastic procedures available to them.

Certainly, a consideration in reaching a decision about whether to have a lumpectomy or the more drastic mastectomy must include many factors. High on the list of such factors is heredity. In many patients who suffer from this disease, *BRCA1* and *BRCA2*, mutated genes, are an early indication that breast cancer may eventually occur. The *BRCA* gene is frequently present in the female members of families with histories of breast cancer and ovarian cancer. About 85 percent of women with the *BRCA* gene will develop breast cancer if they live a normal life span. Women who have the *BRCA* gene may decide to have a prophylactic mastectomy before symptoms occur, although many women in this situation prefer treatment with tamoxifen, which appears to hold breast cancer at bay.

Advances in treating cancers of all kinds progressed rapidly during the last half of the twentieth century, and even greater impetus characterizes current advances. The four major treatments—often used in combination with each other— are surgery, radiation therapy, chemotherapy, and hormonal therapy. In the treatment of breast cancer, radiation may be used initially to shrink existing tumors that, once reduced in size, will be removed surgically. However, when surgeons remove cancerous tumors, they also remove large numbers of surrounding cells that might be affected; such a procedure is usually followed by additional radiation aimed at killing any lingering cancer cells the surgery has missed.

USES AND COMPLICATIONS

The salient use of surgery in cases of breast cancer is to remove its source, not only clearing away any tumors that may be found but also removing additional cancerous tissue as well as lymph nodes that might be affected.

Cancer cells can exist either in the breast's lobules, which contain the cells that produce milk, or in the ducts that carry the milk to the nipples. Cancer cells in either of these locations can be of two types, invasive or noninvasive (also called in situ). The major complication with invasive cancer is that it can and usually does metastasize, spreading often to the lymph nodes, into the lungs and to other parts of the body. In such cases, a radical mastectomy is indicated. It must be performed as quickly as possible and followed by a strenuous course that typically includes radiation or chemotherapy. Noninvasive cancer is less likely to metastasize, although it sometimes does. Lumpectomy or quadrantectomy is often used to treat such cancers, but these procedures must be followed by close monitoring over the rest of the patient's life and by radiation or chemotherapy following surgery.

Chemotherapy is used less often than radiation in the postsurgical treatment of breast cancer but is occasionally used along with it. Some physicians use anticancer drugs to reduce the possibility of recurrence. This treatment, as well as hormone treatment, is designed to kill any fugitive cancer cells that have strayed from the immediate site of the cancer that has been removed. Whereas surgery and radiation are local, affecting only the part of the body being focused upon, chemotherapy is systemic: the drugs used in chemotherapy travel through the bloodstream to all parts of the body. The disadvantage of chemotherapy is that it nearly always has significant side effects. In rare cases, complications are so extreme that they result in death. Usually, chemotherapy is indicated only for women who have not yet undergone the menopause and whose tumors are an inch or larger in size. It may also be employed in cases in which the patient's tumor shows signs of growing rapidly and aggressively invading and attacking other parts of the body.

Related to chemotherapy is hormonal therapy. Hormones are chemicals produced by the body for various purposes. For example, when one is under sudden, undue stress, the body produces adrenaline, which provides a rush of energy and causes the heartbeat to accelerate. In women, the body produces estrogen every month during the menstrual cycle. Estrogen causes the cells in the milk ducts and lobules to grow in preparation for pregnancy. This chemical stimulates the growth of normal cells but can also stimulate the growth of cancer cells. Hormonal therapy is systemic. It involves introducing into the bloodstream a synthetic chemical, usually tamoxifen, which makes it impossible for the body's natural estrogen to find its way to cancer cells that would be nourished by it. A complete biopsy report can determine whether hormonal therapy is appropriate in individual cases.

PERSPECTIVE AND PROSPECTS

Until the middle of the twentieth century, a diagnosis of cancer, particularly of breast cancer, was viewed as a death sentence. Diagnosis generally occurred after the cancer had metastasized. In the first half of the

century, general practitioners were much more prevalent than the specialists who, working as a team, are now generally mustered to provide cancer treatment once a diagnosis is made.

With the proliferation of sophisticated medical equipment, including the highly sensitive X-ray machines used in mammography and the various forms of ultrasound and sonography equipment that are part of nearly every hospital's arsenal of diagnostic equipment, an increasing number of cancers are discovered before they become symptomatic, so that they can be treated with considerable success.

Historically, mastectomies have been performed for centuries. President John Adams's daughter underwent this excruciating surgery early in the nineteenth century, enduring this procedure without the benefit of anesthesia. As was usually true in such cases, the surgery extended her life for only a little while because her cancer was discovered in an advanced stage and had metastasized.

By the late nineteenth and early twentieth centuries, accepted treatment for breast cancer was a radical mastectomy that involved the removal of the affected breast and of as many surrounding cancer cells and lymph nodes as possible. William Halsted, a pioneer in the field of breast cancer surgery and a professor of surgery at the highly respected Johns Hopkins University Medical School, championed the cause of the radical mastectomy, which he viewed as a procedure that could extend substantially the survival of his patients. Little was said about curing breast cancer patients of their cancers. The radical surgery that physicians across the country performed following Halsted's lead was viewed simply as a means of adding months or years to the life of the cancer patient. Until 1970, about 70 percent of women in the United States who had breast cancer were subjected to radical mastectomy.

Several factors brought about a major change in the treatment of breast cancer during the 1960s and 1970s, when social activism was very much in the forefront of American life. Feminists pointed out that most of the surgeons treating breast cancer were men. As an increasing number of women entered medical schools and eventually established medical practices, greater attention was paid to treating breast cancer in less disfiguring ways than had been common earlier. Along with this change came advances in medical technology that made early diagnosis and more focused treatment a reality. As the chemical treatment of all cancers came to be better understood and more widely employed, the focus was more on preventing and curing cancer than on merely prolonging the lives of those who suffered from it.

Laboratory tests for detecting a woman's predisposition for breast cancer have become increasingly sophisticated and accurate. Where the *BRCA1* or *BRCA2* gene is present, the possibility of developing breast cancer is greatly increased; women shown to possess this gene have been made more vigilant than ever before in monitoring their conditions and in seeking immediate medical intervention if even the slightest symptom appears.

Shortly after the end of World War II, some oncologists rejected Halsted's emphasis on radical mastectomy. Surgeon Jerome Urban garnered numerous followers in his call for extremely radical surgeries in cancer cases. His procedures involved the removal of ribs, various internal organs, and even limbs in order to find and destroy every cancer cell. Surgeon Bernard Fisher stood in opposition to Urban, championing the effectiveness of smaller surgeries, such as the simple mastectomy, which involved the removal of one breast but not of all the lymph nodes and, in some cases, the lumpectomy, involving the removal only of the tumor and its surrounding cells.

The lumpectomy has gained acceptance through the intervening years. It is less disfiguring than either the radical or the simple mastectomy, leaving only a small scar on the underside of the breast. In cases where lumpectomy is viewed as a viable option, survival rates and cure rates are comparable to those of patients who have undergone more radical surgery. Advances in medical science are accelerating substantially. Stem cell research offers great promise in the treatment and cure of diseases such as breast cancer. Researchers appear to be on the threshold of developing cells designed to destroy specific errant cells, such as those that cause cancer, while leaving healthy cells intact.

—*R. Baird Shuman, Ph.D.*

FOR FURTHER INFORMATION

Abouzied, Mohei. "Lumpectomy." *Health Library,* Nov. 26, 2012.
"Breast Cancer." *MedlinePlus,* June 12, 2013.
Chisholm, Andrea. "Mastectomy." *Health Library,* Oct. 31, 2012.
Friedewald, Vincent, and Aman U. Buzdar, with Michael Bokulich. *Ask the Doctor: Breast Cancer.* Kansas City, Mo.: Andrews McMeel, 1997.
Hirshaut, Yashar, and Peter I. Pressman. *Breast Cancer: The Complete Guide.* 5th ed. New York: Bantam Books, 2008.
Lange, Vladimir. *Be a Survivor: Your Guide to Breast Cancer Treatment.* 5th rev. ed. Los Angeles: Lange Productions, 2010.
Lerner, Barron H. *The Breast Cancer Wars: Hope, Fear, and the Pursuit of a Cure in Twentieth-Century America.* New York: Oxford University Press, 2001.
Link, John S. *The Breast Cancer Survival Manual: A Step-by-Step Guide.* 5th ed. New York: Henry Holt, 2012.
"Mastectomy." *MedlinePlus,* May 24, 2013.
Sproul, Amy, ed. *A Breast Cancer Journey: Your Personal Guidebook.* 2d ed. Atlanta: American Cancer Society, 2004. "Surgery for Breast Cancer." *American Cancer Society,* Feb. 26, 2013.
Sutton, Amy L., ed. *Breast Cancer Sourcebook: Basic Consumer Health Information About Breast Cancer.* 4th ed. Detroit: Omnigraphics, 2012.

Mastitis

CATEGORY: Disease/Disorder

KEY TERMS:
mastitis: inflammation of the glands in the breast
periareolar: around the areola (dark part of the breast just around the nipples)
periductal: around the duct (drainage system of the mammary glands)

CAUSES AND SYMPTOMS

Mastitis is defined as inflammation of the breast tissue that may or may not be caused by infection. Although mastitis most commonly occurs in lactating women (lactational mastitis), it is important to note that mastitis can also occur in the absence of lactation (nonlactational mastitis).

Lactational mastitis is usually caused by a staphylococcal infection of the breast. The bacteria may enter the breast through a sore or crack in the nipple, although some patients do not report having sore or cracked nipples. The onset of the infection is often associated with stress, reduced immunity, missed or increased intervals between breastfeeding a baby.

There are two forms of nonlactational mastitis. These types are known as periductal mastitis and idiopathic granulomatous mastitis. Periductal mastitis occurs when the subareolar ducts of the breast become inflamed. The cause of periductal mastitis is unknown, but one well-known risk factor is smoking. It most commonly affects young women and can also occur in men. Long-term reoccurring periductal mastitis has been associated with squamous metaplasia. Idiopathic granulomatous mastitis is known as breast tissue inflammation of unknown cause. It is a rare and benign disorder that has not been associated with breast cancer. It sometimes occurs in the presence of sarcoidosis tuberculosis, histoplasmosis, *Corynebacterium kroppenstedtii* infection as well as other illnesses.

Common symptoms of mastitis are swelling, redness, hotness, tenderness, an area of hardness, and pain in part or the entire infected breast. In some cases, there is a localized area of soreness in the breast, while in other cases; the entire breast may be inflamed. The victim typically has flu-like symptoms, such as tiredness, aches, chills, fever, and fatigue. These feelings often occur prior to breast soreness. If the cause is engorgement with breast milk or a plugged duct, then the patient will start feeling better instead of worse. Blocked ducts usually resolve themselves naturally within twenty-four to forty-eight hours, although a blocked duct may sometimes lead to mastitis. Patients with periductal mastitis may present with periareolar inflammation. Similarly, inflammation of various breast tissues may occur with idiopathic granulomatous mastitis with symptoms such as nipple retraction and sinus formation.

TREATMENT AND THERAPY

To manage mastitis patients can alternately apply hot and cold packs to the affected area of the breast. This will help reduce the pain caused by inflammation by providing comfort. Gently massaging the tender area increases circulation and helps loosen any plugged ducts. Fever can be treated with acetaminophen or ibuprofen without any harm to a breastfeeding baby. Patients should also drink plenty of fluids. For nursing mothers, unless the pain is too intense, breastfeeding should be continued during the

---

Information on Mastitis

Symptoms: Breast swelling, redness, hotness, tenderness, hard area, pain; typically begins with flu-like symptoms (tiredness, aches, chills, fever, fatigue)

Duration: Two to five days for bacterial infections; one to two days for blocked duct; up to a year for idiopathic granulomatous mastitis.

Treatments: Alternate hot and cold packs, gentle massage, acetaminophen or ibuprofen for fever; continued breastfeeding; antibiotics if necessary (cephalexin, cloxacillin, erythromycin, flucloxacillin)

---

treatment of mastitis. If breastfeeding is discontinued, then the breast should be drained regularly with a breast pump.

Once a diagnosis of mastitis is made and the cause is bacterial the proper antibiotics should be administered. The soreness usually begins to disappear within two to five days of appropriate antibiotic treatment. Redness may continue for up to a week or more. Bed rest helps relieve stress and builds up the immune system. If not treated properly and in a timely manner, mastitis can lead to a breast abscess that requires surgical draining. For patients with periductal mastitis needle aspiration or incision may and antibiotics may be needed for treatment. Idiopathic granulomatous mastitis often resolves without medical intervention but may take up to a year to heal. Patients with idiopathic granulomatous mastitis and pain can use nonsteroidal anti-inflammatory drugs to help relieve symptoms.

PERSPECTIVE AND PROSPECTS

It is important to note that there are different types of mastitis, which may be a result of different mechanisms. Lactational mastitis is the most common form of mastitis and occurs frequently among nursing mothers during the first three months postpartum. The most important preventive measure against mastitis for these women is regular breastfeeding. Recurrent mastitis is associated with irregular breastfeeding patterns, fatigue, and stress. Frequent breastfeeding and lifestyle changes that promote good health and a strengthened immune system are key ingredients for reducing the occurrence of mastitis.

—*Alvin K. Benson, Ph.D.*
Updated by Ashley Henry, MPH, RN

FOR FURTHER INFORMATION

Alan, Rick. "Mastitis." *Health Library*, May 11, 2013.

Colson, Jenni Lynn, ed. *Breastfeeding Sourcebook*. Detroit: Omnigraphics, 2002.

Berens, P. "Breast Pain: Engorgement, Nipple Pain, and Mastitis." *Clinical Obstetrics and Gynecology*, vol. 58, no. 4, 2015, 902-914. doi: 10.1097/grf.0000000000-000153

Hunt, K. M., et al. "Mastitis is Associated with Increased Free Fatty Acids, Somatic Cell Count, and Interleukin-8 Concentrations in Human Milk." *Breastfeeding Medicine*, vol. 8, no. 1, 2013, 105–110.

Dixon, J., & Pariser, K. (2019). "Nonlactational mastitis in adults." *UpToDate*, Nov 27, 2017, https://www-uptodate-com.arbor.idm.oclc.org/contents/nonlactational-mastitis-in-adults?search=mastitis&source=search_result&selectedTitle=2~70&usage_type=default&display_rank=2.

Icon HealtIcon Health. *Mastitis: A Medical Dictionary, Bibliography, and Annotated Research Guide to Internet References*. San Diego: ICON Health Publications, 2004.

Jahanfar, S., et al. "Antibiotics for Mastitis in Breastfeeding Women." *The Cochrane Database of Systematic Review*, vol. 2, 2013, CD0054582013.

Reddy, Pavani. "Postpartum Mastitis and Community-Acquired Methicillin-Resistant *Staphylococcus aureus* "*Emerging Infectious Diseases*, vol. 13, no. 2, 2007, 298.

Swenson, Deborah E. *Telephone Triage for the Obstetric Patient: A Nursing Guide*. Philadelphia: W. B. Saunders, 2001.

Masturbation

CATEGORY: Development

PHYSICAL AND PSYCHOLOGICAL FACTORS

Masturbation is the first sexual experience for a great majority of people. Some young people inadvertently stumble on sexual arousal and orgasm in the course of engaging in some other physical activity. Others purposely stimulate themselves, aroused by curiosity after reading erotic literature, watching sexually explicit films, or listening to the imaginary or real sexual adventures of their peers.

Most women practice masturbation to relieve sexual tension, achieve sexual pleasure, enjoy sexual stimulation in the absence of an available partner, and experience relaxation. Stimulation of the clitoral shaft and clitoral area, and/or the vagina, with a hand or an object is the method that women most commonly employ. Some women masturbate by using a vibrator. Mutual masturbation provides a satisfying and pleasurable form of sexual intimacy and release for many couples. It is also one of the most common techniques that gay and lesbian couples use during sexual intimacy.

DISORDERS AND EFFECTS

Under certain circumstances, masturbation may result in some undesirable consequences. If a child masturbates constantly, it may be an indication of excessive anxiety and tension. Compulsive and frenzied masturbation may reflect abuse or maltreatment in a child's home life. Frequent masturbation may be a child's way of relieving tension or unconsciously reenacting past or present traumatic sexual episodes.

Among adults, excessive masturbation may point toward a lack of self-esteem and the resultant fear and inability to develop healthy intimate relationships with others. Psychiatry, psychotherapy, and sex therapy have proven helpful in successfully alleviating these problems.

PERSPECTIVE AND PROSPECTS

Throughout history, attitudes toward the practice of masturbation have been riddled with misconceptions, guilt, and fear. Fear of masturbation and its supposed harmful effects, such as loss of memory and intelligence, was widespread through the nineteenth century. Medical authorities today do not find any evidence of physical damage from masturbation. In fact, many modern sex therapists encourage self-stimulation as part of healthy sexuality. In modern sex therapy, masturbation has become part of the therapeutics used in treating certain sexual dysfunctions. Patients with difficulties or inability to have orgasm are encouraged by their therapists to engage in masturbation. It is widely believed that orgasm once achieved through masturbation will eventually generalize and transfer to satisfactory sexual intercourse.

—*Tulsi B. Saral, Ph.D.*

FOR FURTHER INFORMATION

Bockting, Walter, and Eli Coleman, eds. *Masturbation as a Means of Achieving Sexual Health*. New York: Haworth Press, 2003.

Laqueur, ThomasWalter. *Solitary Sex: A Cultural History of Masturbation.* New York: Zone Books, 2003.

"Masturbation." *HealthyChildren.org,* May 11, 2013.

"Masturbation." *InteliHealth,* June 10, 2008.

Rowan, Edward L. *The Joy of Self-Pleasuring: Why Feel Guilty About Feeling Good?* Amherst, Mass.: Prometheus Books, 2000.

Sarnoff, Suzanne, and Irving Sarnoff. *Masturbation and Adult Sexuality.* Bridgewater, N.J.: Replica Books, 2001.

Melanoma

CATEGORY: Disease/Disorder

KEY TERMS:

dysplasia: the aberrant growth or development of cells

melanocytes: cells in the upper layer of skin which produce the pigment melanin

metastasis: the spread of cells from a primary site of cancer to areas throughout the body

nevus: a pigmented site on the skin which is composed of melanocytes

INTRODUCTION

Melanoma is an aggressive form of skin cancer that originates in melanocytes, the skin cells responsible for pigmentation. Most melanocyte growth (known as a nevus or mole) is benign, however excessive mutations can result in cancer development. Melanoma is most commonly associated with excessive exposure to ultraviolet radiation, such as blistering sunburns or use of tanning beds. But research has demonstrated that there is a strong genetic component to the development of the disease, and alterations in the immune system may leave patients more susceptible to cancer causing mutations. While the total number of patients diagnosed with melanoma every year is relatively small, nearly 80% of deaths from skin cancer are due to melanoma rather than the more common basal cell or squamous cell carcinomas. Women under 50 have a higher probability of developing melanoma than any other cancer, except breast or thyroid cancer. Rates of young women presenting with melanoma have been on the rise, possibly resulting from tanning both outside and at tanning salons. If caught in the very early stages, 5-year survival for melanoma is approximately 95%. However, this number drops dramatically if melanoma spreads to the lymph nodes (Stage III, survival rate is approximately 60%) or if the cancer becomes metastatic and spreads to other organs (Stage IV, approximately 25%).

RISK FACTORS

Risk factors for melanoma include fair skin, freckles, red hair, a large number of atypical moles (also known as dysplastic nevus), a childhood history of blistering sunburns, use of tanning beds, hobbies that involve increased sun exposure such as golf or hiking, inadequate sun protection, or a family history of skin cancers. While most melanomas occur in people over the age of 70, it affects patients younger than 30 at a much higher rate than most cancer types.

SYMPTOMS AND DIAGNOSIS

The common pneumonic device for the warning signs of a mole that is concerning for melanoma is "ABCDE: Asymmetry (one side is different than the other), Border (jagged rather than smooth), Color (dark or multicolored), Diameter (larger than the size of a pencil eraser) and Elevation (raised instead of flat)/ Evolution (mole has recently changed in appearance).

Women most often see melanomas develop on their legs or arms, while men usually present on the chest and back. As with many other cancers, women have better mortality rates for melanoma than men.

Diagnosis of melanoma must be made by a pathologist who will examine the mole under a microscope. Staging is based on the Breslow's Depth, or how far into the skin layers the melanoma has penetrated. Accurate staging of melanoma is essential, as it impacts treatment decisions. Stage 0 melanoma (in which the mole is entirely superficial) are considered curable by excision alone, while more invasive melanomas have a very high risk of spreading and are commonly treated with chemotherapy to prevent recurrence.

TREATMENT

Treatment of melanoma varies widely based on the stage of the disease at diagnosis, the goals of the patient, and the patient's ability to tolerate intensive treatment. Early detection and surgical removal

Information on Melanoma

Causes: Exposure to ultraviolet light and resulting mutations

Symptoms: Nevus (usually a mole) that changes in shape, size, or pigmentation; may spread to lymphatic system and other regions

Duration: Chronic, sometimes fatal

Treatments: Surgery, chemotherapy, radiation, biological therapy using protein extracts from the melanoma

FOR FURTHER INFORMATION

"About Melanoma." *Melanoma Research Foundation,* 2011.

Gore, Martin, and Julie Newton-Bishop. *Melanoma: Critical Debates.* Malden, Mass.: Blackwell, 2002.

LaRusso, Laurie, and Brian Randall. "Melanoma." *Health Library,* Apr. 9, 2013.

Melanoma. (National Cancer Institute)

Miller, Arlo, and Martin C. Mihm, Jr. "Melanoma." *New England Journal of Medicine,* vol. 355, no. 1, 2006, 51–65.

Poole, Catherine. *Melanoma: Prevention, Detection, and Treatment.* 2d ed. New Haven, Conn.: Yale University Press, 2005.

Sharfman, William. *Melanoma.* New York: Demos Medical, 2012.

"What You Need to Know about Melanoma and Other Skin Cancers." *National Cancer Institute,* June 2010.

Skin Cancer." *American Cancer Society,* May 2016.

remain the gold standard for treatment of melanoma. More aggressive melanomas can be treated with close observation or chemotherapy after excision. Melanomas that have spread to the lymph nodes are usually treated with a combination of radiation, chemotherapy, or immunotherapy. Metastatic melanoma is treated with combined immunotherapy or chemotherapy and is an active area of clinical research. Unfortunately, treatment goals for metastatic melanoma are generally to control the spread of the cancer and to prolong life, rather than to cure.

PREVENTION AND FUTURE RESEARCH

Primary prevention of melanoma in the form of good skin protection from ultraviolet radiation remains of critical importance. Fair-skinned individuals at high risk of increased sun exposure must take additional care to practice adequate sun protection and should be evaluated by a dermatologist trained in skin cancer detection on a yearly basis.

Additional research into genetic predisposition to melanoma and the role of the immune system in the development of the disease are areas of intense research. The most promising development in the treatment of aggressive melanoma has been the approval of immunotherapy, which modifies the patient's immune system to attack the cancer cells rather than attacking the cells directly like a conventional chemotherapy. The improved success of these treatments has provided hope for patients facing this deadly disease and has also provided insight into researchers looking to unlock the genetic or immune basis for the development of this cancer.

—*Richard Adler, PhD*
Updated by Patrick Richardson

Menopause

CATEGORY: Biology

KEY TERMS:

climacteric: that phase in the aging process of women marking the transition from the reproductive stage of life to the nonreproductive stage

estrogen: the female hormones estradiol and estrone, produced by the ovaries and responsible for the development of secondary sex characteristics

exogenous: originating outside an organ or part

osteoporosis: a condition characterized by a loss of bone density and an increased susceptibility to fractures

progesterone: a hormone, released by the corpus luteum and placenta, responsible for changes in the uterine endometrium

PROCESS AND EFFECTS

The word "menopause" comes from two Greek words meaning "month" and "cessation." It is used medically to mean a cessation of, not a "pause" in, menstrual periods. Technically, the menopause begins the moment a woman has had her final menstrual period; until then, her menstrual periods may have shown a wide variety of irregularities, including missed periods. Medical experts refer to the time when the body is noticeably preparing for the menopause as the perimenopause, which can begin anywhere from five to ten years before the menopause. While estrogen levels begin to decrease gradually, periods are normal, but memory may be less sharp and mood swings may occur. During that time, a woman still experiences menstrual periods, but they are erratic. Some women stop menstruating suddenly, without irregularities; however, they are in the minority. For some women, signs of the menopause, such as hot flashes, may begin during the perimenopause. For even more women, such signs begin, or at least increase in intensity, at the menopause.

The term "climacteric" covers a longer span and includes all the years of diminishing estrogen production, both before and after a woman's last menstrual period. Some experts believe that women may undergo declines in their levels of estrogen even when they are in their late twenties; almost all experts believe that estrogen levels drop at least by a woman's mid-thirties, and the process accelerates in the late forties. The average age at which the menopause occurs is fifty-one years, with the usual range between ages forty-five and fifty-five. For some it occurs much earlier, for others much later. Only 8 percent of women reach the menopause before age forty, and only 5 percent continue to menstruate after age fifty-three. Avery few have menstrual periods until they are sixty.

Even after the menopause, the climacteric continues. Declining hormonal levels bring more changes, until the situation stabilizes. A decade or more of noticeable changes can take place before the climacteric is completed. Unlike the climacteric, the menopause itself is usually considered completed after one full year without a period. After two years, a woman can be reasonably certain that her periods have ceased permanently. The signs and symptoms of the menopause, however, can linger for years longer.

Starting in her mid-forties, a woman's ovaries gradually lose their ability to respond to the follicle-stimulating hormone (FSH), which is released by the pituitary into the blood, triggering the release of estrogen from the ovaries. A few eggs do remain even after menstrual flows have ceased, and the production of estrogen does not stop completely after the menopause; in much smaller amounts, it continues to be released by the adrenal glands, in fatty tissue, and

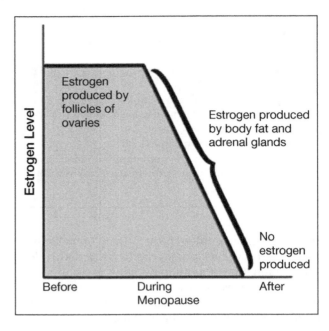

During menopause, which may last for several years, estrogen production diminishes; after the menopause, estrogen is no longer produced by the body. © EBSCO

in the brain. At the menopause, however, the blood levels of estrogen are drastically reduced—by about 75 percent.

About two to four years before the menopause, many women stop ovulating or ovulate irregularly or only occasionally. Although almost all the follicles enclosing the eggs are depleted by this time, the ovaries continue to produce estrogen. Estrogen continues to build up the endometrium (the lining of the uterus), but without ovulation no progesterone is produced to shed the extra lining. Therefore, instead of regular periods, a woman may bleed at unexpected times as the extra lining is shed sporadically.

During the perimenopause, menstrual periods may be late or early, longer than usual or shorter, and lighter than before or heavier. They may disappear for several months, then reappear for several more. It has been noted that in 15 to 20 percent of women the typical menopausal symptoms, sometimes accompanied by noticeable mood swings similar to premenstrual tension, begin during the perimenopausal period.

According to the National Institutes of Health (NIH), about 80 percent of women experience mild or no signs of the menopause. The rest have symptoms troublesome enough to seek medical attention. The two most important factors in determining how a woman will fare are probably the rate of decline of her female hormones and the final degree of hormone depletion. A woman's genes, general health, lifetime quality of diet, level of activity, and psychological acceptance of aging are also major influences. The most severe symptoms occur in women who lose their ovaries through surgery or radiation when they are perimenopausal.

When only the uterus is removed (hysterectomy) and the ovaries remain intact, menstrual periods stop but all other aspects of the menopause occur in the same way and at the same age. When only one ovary is removed, the menopause occurs normally. If both ovaries are removed, a complete menopause takes place abruptly, sometimes with intense effects. Women who have had a tubal ligation to prevent pregnancy will experience a normal menopause because tubal ligation does not affect ovaries, the uterus, or hormonal secretions.

Although experts disagree about the causes of a variety of symptoms that may appear at the menopause, there is no disagreement about the fact that the majority of women experience hot flashes, or flushes. For two out of three women, hot flashes can start well before the last menstruation. Generally, however, hot flashes increase dramatically at menopause and continue to occur, with intermittent breaks (sometimes lasting several months), for five years or so.

While hot flashes are not dangerous, they are uncomfortable. Many women have only three or four episodes a day— or even a week—and hardly notice them. Others have as many as fifty severe flashes a day. The intense waves of heat generally last several minutes, but some unusual flashes have been reported to last as long as an hour. Usually there is some perspiration; with a severe flash, there is heavy perspiration. Because the blood vessels dilate (expand) and then contract, the hot flash is often followed by chills, even intense shivering. Since the flashes are usually worse at night, they can cause insomnia.

Other vasomotor symptoms can also appear with the menopause. Experts believe that they are the result of disruptions of the same mechanisms—vasomotor instability—that are manifested as hot flashes. Palpitations, which are distinct and rapid heartbeats, may also occur. A woman may experience dizziness or may feel faint or nauseated at times. She may have peculiar sensations in her arms and hands, especially her fingers. Some feel these sensations as tingling, or pins and needles, while others say that their fingers occasionally feel numb. One of the oddest, most frightening sensations associated with the menopause is formication, a feeling of insects crawling over the skin.

Headaches, depression, mood swings, insomnia, and weight gain often affect women at the menopause and may be related to the body's hormonal readjustments. Insomnia is second only to hot flashes as the symptom that causes women to seek out their doctors' help at the menopause. The hypothalamus controls sleep as well as temperature and hormone production; insomnia is caused by changes in sleep patterns and brain waves from the same hypothalamic disturbances that result in the hot flashes and an overstimulated central nervous system.

COMPLICATIONS AND DISORDERS

During the menopause, the walls of the vagina become smooth and dry and produce less lubrication, producing a condition called atrophic vaginitis. It has been assumed that this condition is attributable to a lack of estrogen. Despite doubts concerning the relationship between circulating estrogen and objective measures of vaginal atrophy, estrogen (often topical) is frequently prescribed and effectively used in the alleviation or elimination of symptoms.

One of the problems that women encounter with the menopause is calcium deficiency. Many experts believe that before the menopause a woman requires a minimum of 1,000 milligrams of calcium a day in food or supplements. At the menopause, however, a woman who is not taking estrogen needs 1,500 milligrams of calcium a day. Since it is very difficult to obtain these daily allotments from food without consuming considerable amounts of milk or milk products, calcium supplements are often recommended for menopausal and postmenopausal women.

If the calcium deficiency is allowed to persist, osteoporosis, a loss of bone density that can lead to dangerous fractures, can result. Osteoporosis is known to have less of a damaging effect on women who are somewhat overweight because estrogen continues to be produced in fatty tissues after the menopause. Cigarettes, alcohol, and caffeine increase bone loss because they interfere with the body's ability to absorb calcium. A well-balanced diet, calcium supplements, and regular exercise—especially weight-bearing exercise—are effective ways of controlling osteoporosis. Hormone therapy is another means of coping with osteoporosis brought on by the menopause. Since nearly half of all women do not develop osteoporosis, however, many physicians do not believe that administering estrogen therapy to combat this disease is worth the risks, except in women at high risk for osteoporosis.

Although estrogen was isolated as a substance in the 1920s, the modern study of hormones—how they work, where they are produced, and what their benefits are—began in the 1940s. Originally, estrogen was administered cautiously to women who had lost their ovaries through surgery and to those with severe distress after the menopause. It was not until the 1960s that estrogen replacement therapy became widespread, however, when books such as Robert A. Wilson's *Feminine Forever* (1966) promoted its use as the newfound "fountain of youth" for women. The replacement of estrogen was suddenly fashionable, with the hormone being viewed as a miracle drug that could keep women looking and feeling youthful well into their later years. Physicians began prescribing it for women well before the menopause, and it was recommended for use throughout life. Often, large doses were prescribed.

By the mid-1970s, millions of women were taking estrogen. A decade later, however, the numbers had fallen. Beginning in 1975, research studies began documenting dramatic increases—sometimes as high as 500 percent—in cases of cancer of the lining of the endometrium among women taking estrogen, compared with those not taking it. Other studies at that time found higher rates of breast cancer as well as other problems, such as gallbladder conditions, among women taking estrogen.

Some studies found the overall risk of contracting uterine cancer increased 350 percent for women who took estrogen for a year or more. Some women who were on the therapy for long periods were judged to be as much as 100 percent more likely to contract uterine cancer. Furthermore, contrary to expectations, some studies claimed that the risk persisted even ten years after the estrogen use was discontinued. Other studies also found that the risk of cancer persisted, though for a shorter period.

These studies were based on replacement therapy using estrogen only. Estrogen stimulates the growth of cells in the endometrium, which is one of the aspects of the development of cancer. Consequently, a treatment was developed in which estrogen was combined with a form of progesterone in an effort to reduce the risk of uterine cancer and other diseases. Today, the most widely used regimen calls for estrogen in the lowest effective dose. A form of progesterone called progestin is added to this therapy, and then both hormones are stopped. Uterine bleeding, similar to that of a menstrual period, may occur, allowing the progesterone to break down any excess buildup of cells in the endometrium.

In the past, a number of women were given hormone therapy to alleviate menopausal symptoms, and they may have received longer-term therapy with the intention of preventing cardiac disease and osteoporosis. Some clinicians prescribed estrogen therapy for women with severe symptoms after a surgical menopause.

In the early twenty-first century, however, the use of hormone therapy—either long-term or short-term—was questioned. A study called the Women's Health Initiative, funded by the NIH, compared thousands of women who took combination hormone therapy to women who were given placebos. Those on the combination treatment had an increased risk for heart disease, stroke, and blood clots in the lungs. As a result, organizations such as the American Heart Association, the American College of Obstetricians and Gynecologists, and the North American Menopause Society recommended that combination therapy not be used for the prevention of cardiac disease, osteoporosis, or dementia. Today, combination hormone therapy is offered only to women with vasomotor symptoms (hot flashes and associated discomforts) that are severe enough to negatively impact life, and dosages are intended to be the lowest possible dose for the shortest period of time. Other drugs can be used to prevent or treat osteoporosis, drugs such as bisphosphonates and estrogen agonists/ antagonists, which do not carry the same risks as hormone therapy.

Anecdotal evidence and some research studies suggest that stress reduction and exercise can relieve some of the symptoms of the menopause, including hot flashes and mood swings. In addition, a host of herbal remedies on the market claim to improve menopausal symptoms, although caution should be used in choosing these products. A double-blind pilot study of women using soy as a natural estrogen replacement

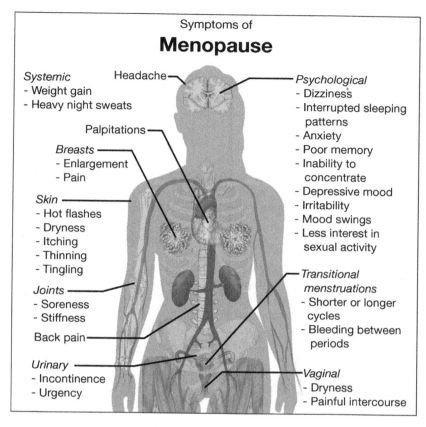

Symptoms of
Menopause

Systemic
- Weight gain
- Heavy night sweats

Headache

Palpitations

Breasts
- Enlargement
- Pain

Skin
- Hot flashes
- Dryness
- Itching
- Thinning
- Tingling

Joints
- Soreness
- Stiffness

Back pain

Urinary
- Incontinence
- Urgency

Psychological
- Dizziness
- Interrupted sleeping patterns
- Anxiety
- Poor memory
- Inability to concentrate
- Depressive mood
- Irritability
- Mood swings
- Less interest in sexual activity

Transitional menstruations
- Shorter or longer cycles
- Bleeding between periods

Vaginal
- Dryness
- Painful intercourse

(Mikael Häggström via Wikimedia Commons)

therapy turned out positive; hot flashes decreased significantly in women taking soy powder for six weeks. The isoflavones in soy are chemically similar to estrogens. However, other studies involving the effects of soy have been inconsistent. Vitamin E, which is structurally similar to estrogen at the molecular level, decreases hot flashes in some women. Evidence of this is anecdotal, however, as no large studies have been conducted that prove the claim. Black cohosh is the best documented of all the herbal remedies.

Studies suggest that it can relieve menopause-related headaches, depression, anxiety, hot flashes, night sweats, heart palpitations, and vaginal dryness and thinning. Black cohosh suppresses the secretion of luteinizing hormone, a hormone that is believed to be at the root of many menopausal symptoms. One European study of eighty women found that black cohosh relieved menopausal symptoms more effectively than estrogen replacement therapy. Other studies had mixed results.

PERSPECTIVE AND PROSPECTS

The menopause, in various guises, was referred to in many early cultures and texts. Initially, an association was made between age and the loss of fertility. By the sixth century, written records on the cessation of menstruation were well documented. At that time, it was believed that menstruation does not cease before the age of thirty-five, nor does it usually continue after the age of fifty. It was thought that obese women cease menstruation very early and that periods remain normal or abnormal and increase in flow or become diminished depending on age, the season of the year, the habits and peculiar traits of women, the types of food eaten, and complicating diseases. Similar descriptions of menstrual cessation and its age of onset continued for another thousand years. It was not until the late eighteenth and early nineteenth centuries, however, that much advancement in the knowledge of the topic took place.

John Leake, influenced by William Harvey's historic description of the circulatory system, made one of the first reasonable attempts to explain the etiology of the menopause in his 1777 book *Medical Instructions Towards the Prevention and Cure of Chronic or Slow Diseases Peculiar to Women*. He believed that as long as the "prime of life" continues, along with the circulating force of the blood being more than equal to the resistance of the uterine vessels, the menses will continue to flow. When these vessels become firm from the effect of age, however, the diminished current of blood is insufficient to force the uterine vessels open, and then periodic discharge will cease.

A later development in the history of menstruation studies was to link menstruation with all sorts of other problems, both emotional and organic. In Leake's work he comments that at the time of cessation of menses, women are often afflicted by various chronic diseases. He adds that some women are prone to pain and light-headedness, others are plagued by an intolerable itching at the neck of the bladder, and some are affected by low spirits and melancholy. Leake thought, because it seemed extraordinary that so many disorders should result from such a natural occurrence in a woman's life, that these symptoms can be explained away by indulgence in excesses, luxury, and an "irregularity" in the passions. Laying the blame for complications with the menopause on societal (in particular, female) excesses continued for some time.

Specific disease associations were also made; in 1814, John Burns announced that the cessation of menses seems to cause cancer of the breast in some women. Edward John Tilt, a British physician, wrote one of the first full-length books on *The Change of Life in Health and Disease* (1857). Some of his views were that women should adhere to a strict code of hygiene during menstruation because they are often afflicted with cancer, gout, rheumatism, and nervous disorders. These beliefs reflect a tendency from the mid-nineteenth century onward for medical literature to associate the menopause with many negative sociological features. For example, Colombat de l'Isère, in his book *Traité des maladies des femmes et de l'hygiène spéciale de leur sexe* (1838; *A Treatise on the Diseases and Special Hygiene of Females*, 1845), expresses his belief that during the menopause women cease to live for the species and live only for themselves. He thought it prudent for men to avoid having erotic thoughts about women in whom these feelings ought to be extinct; he believed that after the menopause sexual enjoyment for women is ended forever.

Not all physicians, however, took such a negative attitude. Some believed that examining this phase in a woman's life presents a challenge. They believed that the boundaries between the physiological and the pathological in this field of study are ill-defined and that it is in the interest of the male gender to conduct more research into this stage of a woman's life. The narrow boundary between normal physiology and pathology was still not fully defined nearly a hundred years later, nor did the many negative and unsubstantiated theories cease. Well into the 1960s, the menopause was still considered "abnormal" and a "negative" state by some physicians.

Three major milestones exist in the history of menopause research in the twentieth century. The first event was the achievement of Adolf Butenandt, who won the Nobel Prize in Chemistry. He succeeded in 1929 in isolating and obtaining, in pure form, a hormone from the urine of pregnant women that was eventually called estrone. The second development was the publication of *Feminine Forever* in 1966, which became an instant best seller. As a result of the book's publication, physicians were prompted to take sides in a heated and continuing debate. The third landmark was the publication of an editorial and two original articles in *The New England Journal of Medicine* of December 4, 1975, claiming an association between exogenous estrogens and endometrial cancer. This claim brought about legal action by initiating, at least in the United States, a series of health administration inquiries.

—*Genevieve Slomski, Ph.D.;*
Updated by Karen E. Kalumuck, Ph.D.

FOR FURTHER INFORMATION

Corio, Laura E., and Linda G. Kahn. *The Change Before the Change: Everything You Need to Know to Stay Healthy in the Decade Before Menopause.* 2d ed. London: Piatkus Books, 2005.

Edelman, Julia Schlam. *Menopause Matters: Your Guide to a Long and Healthy Life.* Baltimore, Maryland: Johns Hopkins University Press, 2010.

"FAQs: Menopause Basics." *North American Menopause Society*, 2013.

"Hormone Replacement Therapy." *MedlinePlus*, June 27, 2013.

Love, Susan, and Karen Lindsey. *Dr. Susan Love's Menopause and Hormone Book: Making Informed Choices.* Rev. ed. New York: Three Rivers Press, 2003.

"Menopause." *MedlinePlus*, July 1, 2013.

"Osteoporosis." *MedlinePlus*, June 4, 2013.

Sheehy, Gail. *The Silent Passage: Menopause.* Rev. ed. New York: Pocket Books, 1998.

Stoppard, Miriam. *Menopause.* 2d ed. London: DK, 2002.

Menopause and colorectal cancer

CATEGORY: Biology
Disease/Disorder

WHAT WE KNOW

Age is the central risk factor for colorectal cancer in women. An individual with a lack of iron, with or without anemia, and unusually elevated concentrations of iron are associated with increased risk of colorectal cancer in menopausal and postmenopausal women

Causes that decrease iron levels include hormone replacement therapy (HRT), aspirin, supplemental calcium, coffee, gastrointestinal ulcers, and daily physical activity

Reasons that iron levels increase include obesity, body mass index (BMI) > 25, supplemental iron, red meat intake, alcohol consumption of greater than 30 g/day, alcohol-induced chronic liver damage and inflammation, and high intake of vitamin C

HRT use in menopausal women is connected with reduced risk of colorectal cancer possibly due to gene regulation in the colon; however, some conflicting findings have been reported

In the California Teachers Study, researchers found that individuals who used HRT were at a 36 percent lower risk of colon cancer compared to women who never used HRT. Women who used HRT for 5–15 years had the lowest risk of colon cancer; increasingly lower risk was not detected among women who used HRT for less than 15 years

HRT provided the greatest risk reduction among women with first-degree family history of colorectal cancer

In the Women's Health Initiative study in the United States, investigators reported that people who used HRT with estrogen-progestin had a 38 percent lower risk of colon cancer; no reduction in risk was found for HRT users who used estrogen alone

Researchers found that HRT seemed to be either a protective factor or have no result on colorectal cancer except for the age group of 70 to 79-year olds. In this group, there were a considerably higher number of cases of colorectal cancer among people who received a form of HRT that was combined equine estrogen versus women who had the placebo

A study in Nordic countries did not show a protective effect of HRT on colon cancer among postmenopausal women

Research has not found that the following interventions and lifestyle factors have an impact on the risk of colorectal cancer in postmenopausal women: a) calcium supplementation combined with vitamin D supplementation; or b) low-fat diet (less than or equal to 20 percent of calories from fat) with greater than or equal to 5 servings of fruits and vegetables and greater than or equal to 6 servings of grains per day.

It is suggested that dietary changes made well before menopause may have an effect on the risk of colorectal cancer after menopause

WHAT CAN BE DONE

Learn about the latest research on the risk for colorectal cancer in menopausal and postmenopausal women so we can accurately assess individual personal characteristics and health education needs.

Encourage people to ask their primary clinician for an individual risk assessment for colorectal cancer and a risk/benefit analysis for taking HRT

Address any anxiety people may have regarding their risk of colorectal cancer and/or having a colorectal cancer screening

Discuss the importance of annual lab work and age-appropriate disease screening with our individuals, including colorectal cancer screening and testing for serum iron levels; encourage people to ask their primary clinician for a referral to a gastrointestinal specialist for a colonoscopy if they identify symptoms of concern

Try to find a "peer coach" for people to discuss their colonoscopy screening

Research has shown a two-fold increase in attendance at a scheduled colonoscopy if the individual had a phone call beforehand from someone who had gone through the process

—*Darlene Strayer, RN, MBA, and Sharon Richman, MSPT*

FOR FURTHER INFORMATION

Bassuk, S. S., & Manson, J. E. (2015). Oral contraceptives and menopausal hormone therapy: Relative and attributable risks of cardiovascular disease, cancer, and other health outcomes. *Annals of Epidemiology, 25*(3), 193-200. doi:10.1016/j. annepidem.2014.11.004

"Cancer Facts and Figures 2017." American Cancer Society. https://www.cancer.org/content/dam/cancer-org/research/cancer-facts-and-statistics/annual-cancer-facts-and-figures/2017/cancer-facts-and-figures-2017.pdf. Accessed March 8, 2019.

Manson, J. E., Chlebowski, R. T., Stefanick, M. L., Aragaki, A. K., Rossouw, J. E., Prentice, R. L., & Wallace, R. B. (2013). Menopausal hormone therapy and health outcomes during the intervention and extended post-stopping phases of the Women's Health Initiative randomized trials. *JAMA: The*

Journal of the American Medical Association, 310(13), 1353-1368. doi:10.1001/jama.2013.278040

Prentice, R. L., Pettinger, M. B., Jackson, R. D., Wactawski-Wende, J., LaCroix, A. Z., Anderson, G. L., & Rossouw, J. E. (2013). Health risks and benefits from calcium and vitamin D supplementation: Women's Health Initiative clinical trial and cohort study. *Osteoporosis Internati-onal, 24*(2), 567-580. doi:10.1007/s00198-012-2224-2

Thomson, C. A., Van Horn, L., Caan, B. J., Aragaki, A. K., Chlebowski, R. T., Manson, J. E., & Prentice, R. L. (2014). Cancer incidence and mortality during the intervention and postintervention periods of the Women's Health Initiative dietary modification trial. *Cancer Epidemiology, Biomarkers & Prevention, 23*(12), 2924-2935. doi:10.1158/1055-9965.EPI-14-0922

Menopause and depression

CATEGORY: Biology
Disease/Disorder

WHAT WE KNOW

There is accumulating evidence that fluctuations in sex hormone levels, symptoms associated with menopause (e.g., hot flashes, difficulty focusing, insomnia, headaches), and other factors such as the presence of stressful life events, comorbid conditions (e.g., cardiovascular disease), and lack of social support increase the vulnerability of women to depression during the menopausal transition.

Menopause is when a woman's ovaries stop producing the hormones estrogen and progesterone, resulting in the cessation of the menstrual period. Perimenopause is the transition period into menopause; it is a time in which hormone levels can fluctuate and menstrual periods may stop and start. The median age in the United States of transition to menopause is 47.5 years.

Although the physiologic process is not completely understood, it is believed that estrogen levels affect the functioning of the neurotransmitters serotonin, norepinephrine, and dopamine in regions of the brain involved in mood regulation. When estrogen levels decline during the menopausal transition, the levels of these neurotransmitters may also decrease, predisposing women to changes in mood, cognition, and libido.

Approximately 20 percent of women experience depression at some point during menopause. Although neurobiologic changes occur in all women during the menopausal transition, not all women report an increase in symptoms of depression. Researchers theorize that a combination of biologic and psychosocial factors are involved in menopause-related depression.

Although depression is more common in women, especially during periods of change in reproductive hormones, there is conflicting evidence regarding the association between menopause and depression. Depression occurs frequently during the menopausal transition, but other factors may be involved, including:

1. major life events (e.g., children leaving the family home, resulting in empty-nest syndrome; parental illness; loss of loved ones).
2. aging and age-related health changes in addition to the menopausal process. (Women who perceive their overall level of health as poor or who maintain a negative attitude toward aging report more depressive symptoms at perimenopause.)
3. a high level of menopause-related symptoms, especially vasomotor symptoms (e.g., hot flashes) and poor quality of sleep. (More than 80 percent of perimenopausal women with depression experience vasomotor symptoms, compared with 49 percent of those without depression. Poor sleep quality is associated with depression independent of life stage, including menopause.)
4. attitudes about menopause, which vary greatly worldwide according to cultural values and beliefs. (Women with negative beliefs about menopause are more likely to experience depression. Women who are from cultures that value having a positive attitude, having a strong sense of community, and providing social support during life transitions experience depression less frequently.
5. marital discord or the absence of a life partner.
6. low socioeconomic status and/or low level of educational attainment.
7. unhealthy behaviors (e.g., cigarette smoking, lack of exercise).
8. sexual changes and decreased libido.

The link between menopause and depression is uncertain in part because the symptoms of perimenopause and depression, including fatigue, poor concentration, sleep disturbance, weight changes, and libido changes, overlap.

Women are especially at risk for depression during perimenopause, which typically lasts 2-8 years, during which estrogen levels fluctuate and ultimately decline and levels of follicle-stimulating hormone (FSH) and luteinizing hormone (LH) increase. Some women (e.g., those with a history of a mood disorder, premenstrual dysphoric disorder, or postpartum depression) are predisposed to depression during perimenopause.

The menopause transition most often occurs in midlife, which is a time of change and transition for women anyway both socially and personally. Women at this time face role changes at home and work and may also face declines in their physical well-being, libido, and ability to have children. The biopsychosocial-spiritual needs that are present highlight the need for a biopsychosocial-spiritual theoretical approach.

The age of menarche (i.e., onset of first period) may act as a risk factor for depression with menopause. Researchers found that women with a later onset for menarche also presented with an increased likelihood of experiencing depression with menopause. A longer interval between menarche and menopause seems to be a protective factor, with subjects with later menarche and earlier menopause having the highest incidence of depression with menopause.

Women with a history of depression are up to 5 times more likely to experience depression during perimenopause, although even women without prior depression are at increased risk.

Women with no history of depression are twice as likely to experience depression during perimenopause as they are during premenopause (i.e., the period before noticeable symptoms of menopause begin, usually age 35–40).

It is unclear whether women who experience sudden menopause as a result of surgery or chemotherapy have a higher incidence of depression than women who transition naturally into menopause; however, younger women who have had hysterectomies may be at greater risk for depression than older women who have had hysterectomies.

Several protective factors have been identified that reduce the risk of depression; these might help social workers plan interventions with clients. Women who have social supports in place, women who have higher education and employment satisfaction, and women who exercise have recorded lower rates of depression.

Psychotherapy, group therapy, and client education may be effective in treating depression during perimenopause and menopause.

Perimenopausal women can benefit from cognitive behavioral therapy (CBT), which focuses on discussion of negative thoughts or behaviors and introduces new ways of thinking.

Group therapy involves educating women about what to expect during menopause and how to manage symptoms and promotes contact with others who face similar health challenges.

Educating women that symptoms of depression typically abate after menopause can relieve distress over depressive symptoms.

—*Jan Wagstaff, MA, MSW*

FOR FURTHER INFORMATION

Brandon, A. R., Minhajuddin, A., Thase, M. E., & Jarret, R. B. (2013). Impact of reproductive status and age on response of depressed women and cognitive therapy. *Journal of Women's Health, 22*(1), 58-66. doi:10.1089/jwh.2011.3427

Gibbs, Z., Le, S., & Kulkarni, J. (2012). What factors determine whether a woman becomes depressed during the perimenopause? *Archives of Women's Mental Health, 15*(5), 323-332. doi:10.1007/ s00939-012-0304-0

Gibson, C. J., Joffe, H., Bromberger, J. T., Thurston, R. C., Lewis, T. T., Khalil, N., & Matthews, K. A. (2012). Mood symptoms after natural menopause and hysterectomy with and without bilateral oophorectomy among women in midlife. *Obstetrics & Gynecology, 119*(5), 935-941. doi:10.1097/ AOG.0b0-13e318-24f9c14

Gramann, S. B. (2015, November). Menopause and mood disorders. *Medscape*. Retrieved November 28, 2015, from http://emedicine.medscape.com/ article/295382-overview

Jung, S. J., Shin, A., & Kang, D. (2015). Menarche age, menopause age, and other reproductive factors in association with post-menopausal onset depression: Results from Health

Examinees Study (HEXA). *Journal of Affective Disorders*, *187*, 127-135. doi:10.1016/j.jad.2015.08.047\

"Menopause Basics." *Office of Women's Health. US Department of Health and Human Services.* May 22, 2018. https://www.womenshealth.gov/menopause/menopause-basics/. Accessed March 8, 2019.

Sandilyan, M. B., & Dening, T. (2011). Mental health around and after the menopause. *Menopause International, 17*(4), 142-147. doi:10.1258/mi.2011.011102

Vivian-Taylor, J., & Hickey, M. (2014). Menopause and depression: Is there a link? *Maturitas, 79*(2), 142-146. doi:10.1016/j.maturi-tas.2014.05.014

Menopause and endometrial cancer

CATEGORY: Biology
Disease/Disorder

WHAT WE KNOW

Endometrial cancer (EC; also called *uterine cancer*) is the fourth most common cancer in women in the United States and usually occurs in menopausal women (i.e., during and after menopause). There are two types of EC: adenocarcinoma, which begins in glandular tissue and causes most cases, and uterine sarcoma, which begins in the connective tissue or muscle of the uterus and is more common among women 40–69 years of age. The most common appearance of EC includes abnormal vaginal bleeding, pelvic pain, and unexplained weight loss; a swelling or mass in the pelvic area may develop, indicating advanced EC.

In 2016 there were 60,050 new cases of endometrial cancer in the United States and 10,470 deaths from EC.

The risk for EC in menopausal women under the age of 50 who experience abnormal vaginal bleeding is low.

In approximately 25 percent of women, EC is diagnosed before menopause. The risk for EC increases considerably until the age of 55, after which it increases moderately.

Researchers report that although women with recurrent postmenopausal bleeding (PMB) are no more likely to have EC than all women who present for initial evaluation of PMB, women with recurrent PMB should be reevaluated every 6 months.

The cause of EC remains unclear; risk factors for the development of EC in menopausal women include:

1. Older age
2. Obesity and/or adult weight gain
3. Never having been pregnant; women who have never been pregnant have a risk that is 2–3 times higher than that of women who has been pregnant
4. Early menarche (i.e., menstruation/period beginning before age 12 years)
5. Late menopause (i.e., cessation of menstruation/period after age 52 years)
6. High levels of unchallenged estrogen (i.e., an imbalance between estrogen and progesterone) in the body (e.g., as a result of polycystic ovarian disease)
7. Use of tamoxifen (i.e., a medication used to prevent and treat breast cancer)
8. Hypertension
9. Race: Though EC is more common in white women, black women are more likely to die from the disease

Receiving hormone replacement therapy (HRT) that contains estrogen only (referred to as *estrogen replacement therapy* [ERT]) in menopausal women who have an intact uterus, which increases the risk for endometrial hyperplasia (i.e., excessive and abnormal uterine cell growth) by approximately 20 percent after 1 year of use; the risk may increase up to 62 percent after 3 years.

The risk for progression of endometrial hyperplasia to EC is approximately 29 percent.

Higher doses of ERT are connected with greater risk for EC compared with lower doses of ERT.

Certain types of estrogen (e.g., estriol) are connected with a greater risk for EC than other types of estrogen.

ERT is appropriate for women who have had a hysterectomy and request estrogen as treatment for menopausal symptoms (e.g., hot flashes); ERT use does not increase risk for EC in this population.

Diabetes has not been shown to be a risk factor for EC when obesity is not present, so obesity is most likely the factor responsible in the increased risk for EC.

Caffeinated coffee consumption lowers the risk for EC in obese postmenopausal women. The role of decaffeinated coffee consumption remains unclear in the risk for EC.

Researchers in a study in Norway, a country with high coffee consumption, found that women who consumed 8 cups of coffee a day or more had a significant decrease in risk for EC.

Women who have Lynch syndrome, an autosomal-dominant inherited susceptibility syndrome, are at increased risk for the development of EC.

Postmenopausal bleeding patterns can indicate endometrial cancer, with the specific limits including the person being age 55 or older, the person having a history of recurrent bleeding, and the person's bleeding exceeding five pads a day.

Researchers found that EC was diagnosed in 12.7 percent of female subjects with postmenopausal bleeding.

Various treatments have been introduced to reduce risk for EC among menopausal women.

The addition of progestin to the estrogen (in a formulation of HRT that is prescribed for women with an intact uterus to relieve menopausal symptoms and to treat atypical hyperplasia) reduces the relative risk for EC in women who have an intact uterus compared with the use of ERT alone.

HRT should include progestin for a minimum of 12–14 days per cycle

Historically, it has been considered practical to remove asymptomatic polyps in postmenopausal women because it was assumed that removal prevented development of EC; statistics showed that atypical hyperplasia progresses to EC in about 50 percent of all cases even after the addition of progestin for treatment.

In a systematic review and meta-analysis, researchers reported that in women with endometrial polyps, postmenopausal status and abnormal vaginal bleeding are related with increased risk for endometrial cancer.

However, a 2009 study showed that the risk for EC in postmenopausal women with atrophic endometrium is less than 1 in 1,000, and another 2009 study revealed that the occurrence of precancerous and cancerous endometrial polyps is about 3 percent.

Pairing selective estrogen receptor modulators (SERMs [e.g., bazedoxifene]; also called *tissue-selective estrogen complex* [TSEC]) with conjugated estrogens protects the uterus from EC while treating menopausal symptoms. Bazedoxifene is a SERM that does not stimulate the endometrium.

There is large evidence that women who have used combination estrogen/progesterone oral contraceptive pills (OCPs) have a reduced risk of developing EC. The risk is reduced depending on the duration of OCP use: 20 percent with 1 year of use, 40 percent with 2 years of use, and 60 percent with 4 or more years of use. This protection was most evident in women who have never been pregnant.

Researchers found that participants who took conjugated equine estrogen with medroxyprogesterone acetate (MPA) had a reduced risk for EC immediately post-HRT treatment when compared to women who received the placebo, and this effect was still present during cumulative follow-ups.

The 5-year survival rate for women who develop EC is 82 percent for white women and 62 percent for black women.

—*Darlene Strayer, RN, MBA, and Sharon Richman, MSPT*

FOR FURTHER INFORMATION

"Cancer Facts and Figures 2017." *American Cancer Society.* https://www.cancer.org/content/dam/cancer-org/research/cancer-facts-and-statistics/annual-cancer-facts-and-figures/2017/cancer-facts-and-figures-2017.pdf.

Bregar, A., Taylor, K., & Stuckey, A. (2014). Hormone therapy in survivors of gynecological and breast cancer. *Obstetrician & Gynecologist, 16*(4), 251-258. doi:10.1111/tog.12146

Hackethal, V. (2015). Guidance issued for endometrial cancer, hints for diagnosis. Retrieved from http://www.medscape.com/viewarticle/842241

Hilliker, B., & Hopkins, M. P. (2015). Endometrial cancer and uterine sarcoma. In *The 5-minute clinical consult standard 2015* (23rd ed., pp. 397-399). Philadelphia, PA: Wolters Kluwer Health/Lippincott Williams & Wilkins.

Salmon, M. C., Bozdag, G., Dogan, S., & Yuce, K. (2013). Role of postmenopausal bleeding pattern and women's age in the prediction of endometrial cancer. *Australian & New Zealand Journal of Obstetrics & Gynaecology, 53*(5), 484-488. doi:10.1111/ajo.12113

Menopause and gallbladder disease

CATEGORY: Biology

Disease/Disorder

WHAT WE KNOW

Gallbladder disease is common in menopausal and postmenopausal women. Hormonal changes result in decreased levels of estrogen and progesterone, which slows the gallbladder's ability to drain bile, resulting in small, rock-like deposits.

An unfavorable effect of hormone replacement therapy (HRT; composed of estrogen alone or estrogen plus progesterone) for menopausal symptoms is an increased risk for gallbladder disease (GD) during and after menopause.

Randomized clinical trials and observational studies have linked HRT with increased risk for cholelithiasis (i.e., gallstones), cholecystitis (i.e., inflammation of the gallbladder), and cholecystectomy (i.e., surgical gallbladder removal).

HRT can double the risk for GD. After HRT is discontinued, HRT-associated increased risk for GD slowly decreases over time; however, risk is still slightly raised 10 years after HRT has stopped

Cholesterol gallstones, which account for two thirds of gallstone cases, occur more frequently in women than in men (ratio of 2–3:1).

The gender difference in the creation of gallstone is thought to be caused by estrogen, with gender difference starting at puberty and diminishing after menopause.

HRT containing estrogen increases risk for cholesterol gallstones. HRT alters the composition of bile (i.e., a digestive fluid stored in the gallbladder and elsewhere) and prevents normal bile synthesis; dietary cholesterol is redirected from the liver to the stored bile, increasing its cholesterol saturation and cholesterol stone formation.

Risk for GD in general is dose related; lower-dose HRT causes a smaller risk increase compared to higher doses of HRT.

Oral HRT is associated with higher risk for GD than transdermal (i.e., skin patch).

When administered orally, estrogen is absorbed in the stomach and absorbed in the liver before entering the systemic circulation; metabolites are excreted in bile and urine.

Transdermal HRT contains lower doses and is absorbed through the skin directly into the circulation, bypassing the liver.

The type/formulation of estrogen used affects risk; equine estrogen (i.e., derived from the urine of pregnant mares) imparts a slightly higher risk for GD compared with estradiol (i.e., steroid and female sex hormone derived from cholesterol), possibly because equine preparations consist largely of conjugated estrogens, which are absorbed differently from the way estradiol is.

Presence or absence of progestogens does not seem to influence degree of HRT-associated increased GD risk.

A study using subjects from the Women's Health Initiative found that 1.64 percent of women with a previous hysterectomy who were using conjugated equine estrogen had gallbladder disease, compared to 1 percent of women who were taking a placebo.

GD can be extremely painful and may require surgery to remove the gallstones or the gallbladder.

A blocked bile duct may cause jaundice (i.e., yellowing) of the skin and whites of the eyes.

Risk for gallstones and GD in menopausal women is increased by obesity, unhealthy dietary patterns, physical inactivity, and history of GD or gallstones, whether or not they are receiving HRT.

It is common for women experiencing menopause to report a lower health-related quality of life, having issues with work, and have higher use of healthcare as a result of symptoms and additional disease processes that were triggered by menopause or HRT.

Researchers found that depression and anxiety were the most commonly reported mental health symptoms; insomnia, forgetfulness, and a decreased interest in sex were also reported in large percentages of the people whom participated in the study. These are all symptoms that might need to be addressed in counseling or other alternative therapies.

A possible alternative therapy is exercise. Aerobic exercise in women who were previously inactive can have a positive effect on menopausal symptoms (e.g., night sweats, mood swings, irritability).

WHAT CAN BE DONE

Learn about research findings on increased risk for GD in menopausal women receiving estrogen-containing HRT so you can educate yourself.

If you are menopausal and are requesting or already receiving HRT for other GD risk factors and talk with your healthcare provider about your individualized risks.

Recognize the impact of menopause symptoms on your quality of life and seek help in order to decrease these symptoms.

It is important to engage in aerobic exercise to potentially decrease menopausal symptoms such as night sweats, mood swings, and irritability.

Equally important is to speak with your healthcare professional regarding a low-fat diet and increase in dietary fiber especially for women with GD risk factors who choose to receive HRT. It is also helpful to increase your physical activity.

It maybe appropriate to ask your healthcare professional for referrals to an appropriate weight-loss or exercise program to help you achieve success.

Lastly, if you noticed that you are filling any emotional needs with food seek counsel from a mental health professional whom can assist you in making the mental adjustments needed for success.

—Darlene Strayer, RN, MBA,
and Sharon Richman, MSPT

FOR FURTHER INFORMATION

Menopause Health Matters. (2015). Gallbladder disease. http://menopausehealthmatters.com/menopause-and-weight-gain/gallbladder-disease/

Moilanen, J. M., Mikkola, T. S., Raitanen, J. A., Heinonen, R. H., El Tomas, N. C. H., & Luoto, R. M. (2012). Effect of aerobic training on menopausal symptoms – a randomized controlled trial. *Menopause, 19*(6), 691-696. doi:10.1097/ gme.0b013e3-1823cc5f7

Whiteley, J., DiBonaventura, M. D., Wagner, J. S., Alvir, J., & Shah, S. (2013). The impact of menopausal symptoms on quality of life, productivity, and economic outcomes. *Journal of Women's Health, 22*(11), 983-990. doi:10.1089/jwh.2-012.3719

Menopause and hormone replacement therapy: Risk for cardiovascular disease

CATEGORY: Biology

Disease/Disorder

WHAT WE KNOW

Cardiovascular disease is a leading cause of death in postmenopausal women in the United States Although nearly 30 years of observed information had suggested that hormone replacement therapy (HRT, with estrogen/progesterone combined) and estrogen replacement therapy (ERT, with estrogen only) benefited the cardiovascular systems of menopausal women. subsequent randomized, double-blind, placebo-controlled clinical trials have not confirmed these benefits; researchers are now suggesting that exogenous (i.e., originating outside the body) HRT or ERT may be harmful to some postmenopausal women who receive it.

In a review of studies, the United States Preventive Services Task Force did not find cardio protective results and in fact found increased risk for cardiovascular events of death or heart attack in women using hormone therapy.

The American College of Obstetricians and Gynecologists also states that HRT should not be used for primary or secondary prevention of coronary heart disease.

Results from two trials that included 22,300 healthy postmenopausal women showed that use of HRT is associated with increased risk for cardiovascular disease, including heart attack and stroke.

HRT is also connected with increased risk for blood clots, embolism, breast cancer, and abnormal mammograms, particularly false positives.

Results from a Danish study suggested that when started early in menopause, there was a decreased risk for death, heart failure, or heart attack in women who received HRT.

Although use of ERT in postmenopausal women is not linked with an increased risk for heart disease or breast cancer, ERT therapy is connected to an increased risk for stroke, blood clots in the legs, and mammography abnormalities.

Among postmenopausal women who experience heart attack, HRT use is not related with mortality benefit within 30 days.

The increased risk for complications is highest in the first few years of HRT/ERT use.

Researchers have found that progestin has a role in the development of vascular disease, but this does not indicate that all HRT or ERT should be stopped because of the risk of cardiovascular issues.

HRT can be useful for vasomotor symptoms (e.g., hot flashes).

HRT should not be used to simply reduce cardiovascular risk. However, HRT can be appropriate and well tolerated if used in the early years after menopause if menopause began at a normal age.

The risks of HRT and ERT may be greater than the potential benefits for women who already have at-risk plaque; therefore, timing of treatment is critical.

Simultaneous factors that further increase the risk for cardiovascular events in postmenopausal women receiving HRT or ERT include: a) hip or lower-extremity fracture; b) inflammatory conditions such as cancer, diabetes mellitus, or hypertension; c) obesity and android pattern weight distribution (i.e., weight gain distributed around the waist); d) use during late menopause (e.g., over age 62), because risk for cardiovascular disease is higher in women of older age; e) smoking.

Compared to postmenopausal women who are college graduates and earn > $50,000/year, postmenopausal women who are not high school graduates and earn < $20,000/year have a greater occurrence of hospitalization for heart failure.

Physical exercise, especially aerobic exercise, has positive results on the cardiovascular autonomic nervous system while also having a positive impact on quality of life.

A client's obstetric history can influence whether she will experience a cardio protective result from HRT and if the estrogen deficiency present in menopause will cause extra physical stress.

Recurrent miscarriage, intrauterine growth restriction, preterm labor, preeclampsia, and gestational diabetes are all pregnancy complications that can result in cardiovascular changes and influence reaction to estrogen deficiency later in life.

HRT is currently recommended only for a limited duration (i.e., a few years) as treatment for menopausal symptoms in women who do not have additional risk factors for cardiovascular disease.

Women using short-term HRT should not expect it to provide cardio protection. Women who initiate HRT within 10 years after menopause do not experience a reduction in coronary heart disease within the first 2 years; a cardio protective result may emerge after 6 years of HRT.

It is recommended that if a patient needs HRT, it should be given for the shortest period of time and be closely monitored. The professional providing the medical care should review the treatment plan on a regular basis to discuss the risks and benefits of continuation.

—*Jessica Therivel, LMSW-IPR*

FOR FURTHER INFORMATION

Abernathy, K. (2015). Making sense of hormone replacement therapy. *Nurse Prescribing, 13*(9), 452-456.

Bakour, S., & Williamson, J. (2015). Latest evidence on using hormone replacement therapy in the menopause. *Obstetrician & Gynaecologist, 17*(1), 20-28.

Bluming, Avrum, and Tavris, Carol. *Estrogen Matters: Why Taking Hormones in Menopause Can Improve Women's Well-Being and Lengthen Their Lives – Without Raising the Risk of Breast Cancer.* New York: Little, Brown Spark, 2018.

Faubion, Stephanie S. *Mayo Clinic, The Menopause Solution.* Birmingham, AL: Oxmoor House, 2016.

Kantrowitz, Barbara, and Wingert, Pat. *The Menopause Book.* New York: Workman Publishing Company, 2018.

Mahendru, A. A., & Morris, E. (2013). Cardiovascular disease in menopause: Does the obstetric history have any bearing? *Menopause International, 19*(3), 115-120. doi:10.1177/1754045313495675

Nkonde-Price, C., & Bender, J. (2015). Menopause and the heart. *Endocrinology & Metabolism Clinics of North America, 44*(3), 559-564. doi:10.1016/j.ecl.2015.05.005

Menopause and hot flashes

CATEGORY: Biology

WHAT WE KNOW

Menopause is a gradual process and is defined as the absence of menstrual periods for 12 months. Hot flashes are the most common symptom reported in up to 85 percent of women undergoing menopause. Hot flashes may occur as a natural part of the aging process, as a result of declining ovarian function, as a result of hormonal fluctuation, or secondary to oophorectomy (i.e., surgical removal of the ovaries), radiation therapy, or chemotherapy

Hot flashes are transient periods of flashing and sweating, periods of intense heat in the face, neck, body, and upper arms, and are often accompanied by palpitations and feelings of anxiety followed by the chills. Hot flashes occur at unpredictable intervals and usually last 3-4 minutes

The pathophysiology of hot flashes continues to be the subject of debate among researchers, but it is generally thought that alterations in how the brain controls body temperature result in a release of the neurotransmitter norepinephrine, which causes vasodilation of superficial blood vessels in the skin, similar to the response to heat stress

Up to one third of women continue to experience hot flashes 10 years or more after menopause, but moderate to severe hot flashes occur for an average of 5 years after menopause

Hot flashes usually are treated with hormone therapy (HT) but can reappear after cessation of treatment with HT and persist for many years beyond the onset of menopause. Hot flashes can significantly decrease quality of life because they can lead to severe sleep disturbances, fatigue, embarrassment and social anxiety, depression, anger, irritability, and frustration, decreased energy levels, difficulty concentrating, changes in personal relationships, acute physical discomfort.

Lifestyle and other factors are being studied as potential risk predictors of more severe or more frequent hot flashes. Research findings vary and include the following: a) Cigarette smoking is associated with hot flashes (Compared with women who never smoked, women who smoke have significantly higher levels of and androstenedione and a higher androgen-to-estrogen ratio, which may contribute to hot flashes; b) Compared with women who never smoked, former and current cigarette smokers have significantly lower progesterone levels, which may contribute to hot flashes

Women who are obese may be at increased risk for hot flashes during menopause because of hormonal abnormalities and a reduced ability to dissipate heat

Compared with middle-aged women of normal weight, middle-aged women who are obese have: a) lower estradiol, estrone, progesterone, and sex hormone-binding globulin (SHBG) levels; b) higher testosterone levels and follicle-stimulating hormone (FSH) levels.

Obesity may increase the risk for hot flashes because body fat acts as an insulator that restricts dissipation of body heat

Acupuncture can have a positive effect on hot flashes by reducing severity and reducing the number of incidents of hot flashes for some women

Women who engage in higher levels of physical activity experience less severe menopausal symptoms, including hot flashes

Exercise can help counter the weight gain and muscle loss attributed to menopause. In a systematic review of studies examining the effects of exercise on hot flashes, some studies showed a positive effect but not all studies found a significant impact

Some women may be genetically predisposed to hot flashes because of variation in the genes involved in the metabolism of sex hormones

In the United States, differences in the incidence of hot flashes within various racial/ethnic groups are reported, which could be related to cultural differences in diet, activity level, and cultural expectations regarding expression of discomfort

Black American women report the highest incidence of hot flashes, followed by white American women. Japanese women report the lowest incidence of all symptoms of menopause, including hot flashes

Some researchers postulate that hot flash frequency does not actually differ significantly among women of various demographic groups but that sociocultural attitudes about menopause and bodily changes affect how hot flashes and other symptoms of menopause are perceived and reported

WHAT CAN BE DONE

Learn about the latest research on potential risk factors for hot flashes so you can accurately assess your clients' personal characteristics and their health education needs; share this information with your colleagues

Develop an awareness of your own cultural values, beliefs, and biases and develop knowledge about the histories, traditions, and values of your clients. Adopt treatment methodologies that reflect the cultural needs of the client

Encourage your clients to adopt a healthy lifestyle (e.g., dietary restriction of sodium, fats, cholesterol, caffeine, and alcohol; avoidance of trigger foods such as spicy foods and hot beverages; weight loss, if overweight; smoking cessation, if applicable; stress management; and regular aerobic exercise [at least 30 minutes per day]).

Assist your clients in accessing smoking cessation, alcohol reduction, acupuncture, or weight loss programs

To help with stress management, counsel on stress reduction and relaxation techniques

Refer to menopause support group if appropriate

Other management strategies include dressing in layers so that layers can be removed when warm, products that may help with coolness at night, including wicking sheets and sleepwear, fans, and cooling pillows.

Provide information on early menopause and the resulting symptoms to all your female clients undergoing oophorectomy, tubal ligation, hysterectomy, radiation therapy, or chemotherapy

Provide referrals to a mental health clinician for women who become distressed over their hot flash symptoms

—*Tanja Schub, BS, and Jessica Therivel, LMSW-IPR*

FOR FURTHER INFORMATION

Faubion, Stephanie S. *Mayo Clinic, The Menopause Solution*. Birmingham, AL: Oxmoor House, 2016.

Faubion, S., Sood, R., Thelen, J., & Shuster, L. (2015). Caffeine and menopausal symptoms: What is the association? *Menopause, 22*(2), 155- 158. doi:10.10.1097/GME/0000000000000301

Kantrowitz, Barbara, and Wingert, Pat. *The Menopause Book*. New York: Workman Publishing Company, 2018.

Lorenz, T. K., et al. "Presence of young children at home may moderate development of hot flashes during the menopausal transition." *Menopause*, 22, no 4, 2015, 448-482. doi:10.1097/GME.00000000-00000334

MedicineNet.com. (2015). What are the symptoms of hot flashes? *MedicineNet.com.*. Retrieved November 1, 2015, from http://www.medicinenet. com/hot_flashes/page2.htm

Menopause and obesity

CATEGORY: Biology

WHAT WE KNOW

The risk for weight gain and obesity is increased in women once they reach menopause, likely due to a combination of factors including changes in levels of reproductive hormones and age-related changes in body composition and metabolism of carbohydrates and lipids (i.e., fats).

Multiple factors influence the development of obesity in adults, including the amount of energy intake, eating behavior, and the level of energy expenditure and physical activity. Hormones that modify energy expenditure/intake, as well as glucose and lipid levels, include estradiol, testosterone, and inhibin B, an ovarian hormone that controls follicle-stimulating hormone (FSH) secretion.

Although the role of estrogens in the development of obesity is not well understood, there is evidence that metabolic changes that occur during midlife and menopause are associated with obesity and metabolic syndrome.

Low levels of estradiol, the main sex hormone produced by ovaries, and sex hormone binding globulin (SHBG), a protein that binds sex hormones, have been found in obese premenopausal women.

Although estradiol may be synthesized by adipose (i.e., fatty) tissue, where it may play a important role in the development of obesity in postmenopausal women, total levels of circulating estradiol remain low after menopause.

Menopausal women have increased risk of developing metabolic syndrome, a condition characterized by insulin resistance, hyperglycemia (i.e., high blood sugar), and dyslipidemia (i.e., high cholesterol), which are risk factors for cardiovascular diseases.

Results from a study of Tunisian women indicated that postmenopausal women had higher average values of waist circumference, blood pressure, plasma lipids, and fasting glucose than premenopausal women. The percentage of women with metabolic syndrome was much higher among postmenopausal women (45.7 percent) than premenopausal women (25.6 percent)

Obesity may increase the severity of symptoms linked with menopause.

Additional factors that have been connected with weight gain in menopausal women include:

1. Menstruation that began in the early teenage years, late maternal age at first birth, low number of births, high weight gain during pregnancies, and/or a short duration of breastfeeding.
2. Aging process, which induces lower basal metabolic rate and sympathetic nervous system activity and reduced levels of human growth hormone.
3. Changing lifestyle factors that affect energy balance (i.e., the equilibrium between energy expenditure and energy intake), which may include a decrease in physical activity or a change in diet that increases the amount of fat eaten, carbohydrates, and/or protein.
4. Genetic susceptibility for weight gain.
5. Difficulty maintaining healthy weight in childhood or adolescence.
6. Race/ethnicity, with Chinese and Japanese women relatively protected from menopause-related weight gain compared with White, Black, and Hispanic women.

Surgical menopause (i.e., menopause secondary to surgical removal of the ovaries), which is linked with a 78 percent increased risk of obesity and a 500 percent increased risk of severe obesity compared with natural menopause.

Changes in body composition in menopausal women include weight gain and buildup of central/abdominal fat due to decreased energy expenditure and a decline in levels of estrogen, which normally promote fat removal in the gluteofemoral region of the body (i.e., lower body, hips, and thighs).

Abdominal or central obesity refers to a concentration of fat in the abdominal wall (subcutaneous fat) and surrounding the abdominal organs (visceral fat). It is defined by a waist-to-hip ratio > 0.85 for women (defined as > 0.9 for men).

Weight gain and abdominal obesity have been linked with increased risk of cardiovascular diseases, diabetes mellitus, sleep apnea, hypertension, and several forms of cancer, and have been linked to:

1. Atherosclerosis and resulting cardiovascular and cerebrovascular disease.
2. Diabetes mellitus, type 2 (DM2). Obesity is the most predictive risk factor for developing DM2 because it is connected with hyperinsulinemia, a result of impaired insulin resistance and a precursor to DM.
3. Poor sleep quality and sleep-disordered breathing (i.e., sleep apnea), along with complications of sleep-disordered breathing (e.g., respiratory insufficiency, chronic hypoxia[i.e., oxygen depletion], hypertension).
4. Increased risk of hypertension and coronary heart disease.
5. Increased risk of depression and anxiety.
6. Increased risk of endometrial, breast, and renal cancers. Cancer risk is related with increased extra ovarian estrogen. Progesterone is often prescribed to reduce the risk of cancer when using estrogen supplements.

Among menopausal and postmenopausal women, weight gain is linked to increased severity of hot flashes.

It is common for women experiencing menopause to report a lower health-related quality of life, poorer performance at work, and higher use of healthcare as a result of symptoms and additional disease processes that were triggered by menopause or hormone replacement therapy.

In a study, researchers found that depression and anxiety were the most commonly reported mental health symptoms in menopausal women; additionally, insomnia, forgetfulness, and a decreased interest in sex were also reported in large percentages of individuals whom participated in the study. These are all symptoms that may need to be addressed within counseling for successful client attempts at weight loss

Treatment for obesity varies according to the underlying cause. Significant reduction in weight can be achieved through changes in lifestyle, including:

1. Putting into action dietary changes to improve nutrition and reduce caloric intake; e.g., reducing dietary amounts of fats eaten, increasing intake of fruits, vegetables, and whole grains;
2. Increasing physical activity, especially aerobic exercise. Brisk walking 3 days per week may be the best plan because of its accessibility and low risk; physical exercise has positive results on the cardiovascular autonomic nervous system as well as a positive impact on quality of life;
3. In women who previously were inactive, aerobic exercise can alleviate menopausal symptoms

(e.g., night sweats, mood swings, irritability) and lead to weight loss; and

4. Participating in counseling (e.g., individual or group therapy) for resolution of emotional issues related to eating, if appropriate.

An important component of counseling is determining if the individual is ready to lose weight using the stages of change model and then moving forward with either cognitive-behavioral therapy or motivational interviewing. Counseling should include engaging in lifestyle modification along with behavior modification to assist the individual in achieving long-term success.

For people who are unable to achieve weight loss with conventional treatments, bariatric surgery, for clients with BMI > 40 or BMI of 35–40 with obesity-related complications, may be appropriate.

—*Darlene Strayer, RN, MBA,*
and Sharon Richman, MSPT

FURTHER READING

Healy, L. A., Ryan, A. M., Carroll, P., Ennis, D., Crowley, V., Boyle, T., & Reynolds, J. V. (2010). Metabolic syndrome, central obesity and insulin resistance are associated with adverse pathological features in postmenopausal breast cancer. *Clinical Oncology,* 22(4), 281-288. doi:10.1016/j. clon.2010.02.001

Keller, C., Larkey, L., Distefano, J. K., Boehm-Smith, E., Records, K., Robillard, A., & O'Brian, A. -M. (2010). Perimenopausal obesity. *Journal of Women's Health,* 19(5), 987-996. doi:10.1089/jwh.2009.1547

Mastorakos, G., Valsamakis, G., Paltoglou, G., & Creatsas, G. (2010). Management of obesity in menopause: Diet, exercise, pharmacotherapy and bariatric surgery. *Maturitas,* 65(3), 219-224. doi:10.1016/j. maturitas.2009.12.003

Moilanen, J. M., Mikkola, T. S., Raitanen, J. A., Heinonen, R. H., El Tomas, N. C. H., & Luoto, R. M. (2012). Effect of aerobic training on menopausal symptoms – a randomized controlled trial. *Menopause,* 19(6), 691-696. doi:10.1097/ gme.0b013e31-823cc5f7

"Overweight and Obesity." *Center for Disease Control and Prevention.* September 17, 2018. https://www.cdc.gov/obesity/.

Souza, H. C., & Tezini, G. C. (2013). Autonomic cardiovascular damage during post-menopause: The role of physical training. *Aging and Disease,* 4(6), 320-328. doi:10.14336/AD.2013.0400320

Menopause and oral conditions

CATEGORY: Biology

Disease/Disorder

WHAT WE KNOW

Menopause is a gradual process and is defined as the absence of menstrual periods for 12 months. Symptoms of menopause can include hot flashes, night sweats, urologic disorders, joint and muscle pain, insomnia, dizziness, and mood and skin changes. Complications that may develop during menopause include osteoporosis and cardiovascular disease as well as an increased risk for chronic oral conditions.

Oral discomfort, greater sensitivity to hot and cold, altered taste, and decreased salivary flow can occur as a consequence of hormonal variation resulting from menopause.

Menopause has been found to have an effect on oral tissues, which has been attributed to the effects of decreased estrogen levels on mucosa.

The main oral symptoms experienced by some women during the perimenopausal, menopausal, and postmenopausal periods (collectively called menopausal unless otherwise specified below) are xerostomia (i.e., dry mouth) and burning mouth syndrome (BMS).

Xerostomia is described as oral mucosal dryness that interferes with swallowing, speech, denture retention, and adequate oral hygiene; xerostomia may be present without a measurable decrease in salivary flow.

Although some researchers have found that decreased production of salvia is associated with menopause, others have not found changes in amount of saliva or composition in menopausal women.

Despite finding no significant differences in stimulated whole saliva flow rate between menopausal women with and menopausal women without xerostomia, authors of a recent study found that salivary calcium concentration and output may be higher in menopausal women with xerostomia.

Decreased production of saliva or lack of saliva may result from taking certain medications (e.g., diuretics, antidepressants, antihistamines, anticholinergics), dehydration, anxiety, or Sjögren's syndrome (i.e., an autoimmune disease of the salivary glands); smoking and depression are both risk factors for xerostomia.

Xerostomia is linked with increased risk for dental caries, taste alterations, and dental plaque.

Diagnosis is made following a complete history, a physical examination, laboratory tests, and the exclusion of other diagnostic possibilities; the underlying cause is frequently not identified.

Treatment is based on the cause, if identified; hormone replacement therapy (HRT) decreases symptoms in some women.

BMS (also called glossodynia, glossopyrosis, glossalgia, stomatodynia, and stomatopyrosis) is characterized by an oral burning sensation, dysgeusia (i.e., alterations in taste), dry mouth, increased thirst, swallowing difficulties, and intense pain; generally, there are no lesions seen.

Most clients with BMS are menopausal women. Other causes may be infection (e.g., with *Candida albicans*, staphylococci, streptococci, or anaerobes), vitamin B or estrogen deficiency, medication reactions, neuropathy, decreased salivary production, chronic irritation from dentures or abnormal oral practices, and psychological disorders (e.g., depression, anxiety, phobias).

A connection exists between BMS and vulvodynia (i.e., vulvar pain) as a symptom of vulvostomatodynia, a rare condition characterized by a burning sensation of the tongue, lips, vestibule, and other genital and nongenital mucosal sites. Diagnosis is typically made following otherwise normal physical examination and lab tests, reviewing client history, and excluding alternative diagnostic possibilities; the underlying cause is frequently not identified. Treatment depends on the cause but is often complicated by the lack of a known causal factor; HRT improves symptoms in some women

Oral conditions less commonly associated with menopause include:

A. Mucosal disorders such as lichen planus;
B. Sjögren's syndrome and pemphigus vulgaris, autoimmune diseases characterized by salivary gland inflammation and mucosal erosion, respectively;
C. Sticky saliva and taste alterations;
D. Periodontal disease and dental caries;
E. Tooth loss and edentulism (i.e., lack of teeth);
F. Osteoporosis of the jaw.

Scientific evidence of a connection between female sex hormone levels and symptoms of oral conditions is weak; most information are from studies on oral contraceptives and pregnancy. Estrogen and progesterone receptors have been detected in the oral mucosa and salivary glands.

Researchers report that moderate alcohol intake might reduce the risk of oral cancer in nonsmoking postmenopausal women. Research findings are conflicting regarding the effectiveness of HRT or selective estrogen receptor modulator (SERM) therapy in the treatment or prevention of oral conditions in menopausal women. Some studies have found that estrogen supplementation improves oral health and reduces the incidence of adverse dental outcomes, whereas others have found no connection with the development of oral symptoms after controlling for variables

WHAT CAN BE DONE

Learn about the oral conditions associated with menopause so you can assess and educate yourself.

Identify dental professionals who are familiar with the systemic and oral problems that occur in menopausal women.

Ask your primary care provider for help in order to access professionals and ask that they advocate for insurance coverage and/or find low-cost options for uninsured people.

If you are menopausal, educate yourself about good dental hygiene and symptom prevention strategies, including: a) control of bacterial plaque, either by mechanical means or through the use of pharmacologic products such as chlorhexidine, or both; b) prevention of dental caries by using fluoride toothpaste, gel, or tablets; and c) use of saliva flow stimulators or saliva substitutes, which may relieve dry mouth.

It is important the diagnosis and treatment of oral conditions is usually by trial and error and may take a long time, and that these conditions may become chronic.

Talk with their primary care provider, specialty, or dental clinician about the latest research results on HRT and SERM treatment for oral conditions.

Ask for referrals to a mental health clinician if you are feeling distressed over your oral symptoms.

—Darlene Strayer, RN, MBA,
and Sharon Richman, MSPT

FOR FURTHER INFORMATION

Grover, C. M., More, V. P., Singh, N., & Grover, S. (2014). Crosstalk between hormones and oral health in the mid-life of women: A comprehensive review. *Journal of International Society of Preventative & Community Dentistry*, *4*(Suppl 1), S5-S10. doi:10.4103/2231-0762.144559

Saluja, P., Shetty, V., Dave, A., Aror, M., Hans, V., & Madan, A. (2014). Comparative evaluation of the effect of menstruation and pregnancy on salivary flow rate, pH and gustatory function. *Journal of Clinical and Diagnostic Research: JCDR*, *8*(10), 81-85. doi:10.7860/JCDR/2014/9935.5071

Suri, V., & Suri, V. (2014). Menopause and oral health. *Journal of Mid-Life Health*, *5*(3), 115-120. doi:10.4103/0976-7800.141187

Menopause and sexual dysfunction

CATEGORY: Biology
Disease/Disorder

WHAT WE KNOW

Sexual dysfunction is an umbrella term for a range of symptoms that prevent women who seek sexual pleasure from attaining it. The *Diagnostic and Statistical Manual of Mental Disorders, Fourth Edition* (*DSM-IV*) contained four categories of female sexual dysfunction: sexual arousal disorder, sexual desire disorder, orgasmic disorder, and sexual pain disorder. The updated *DSM-5* describes three disorders: female orgasmic disorder, genito-pelvic pain/penetration disorder, and female sexual interest/arousal disorder. The latter diagnosis collapses the distinction between sexual desire and physical arousal.

Sexual dysfunction is more prevalent among women than men; 43 percent of women experience sexual dysfunction at some time in their lives, compared to 31 percent of men. The percentage of menopausal women (those whose menstrual cycle is in the process of stopping, typically between ages 40 and 55) who report sexual dysfunction ranges from 31 percent to 88 percent.

The causes of sexual dysfunction can result from multiple etiologies, including physical (e.g., heart disease, diabetes), biological (e.g., aging, hormonal changes), psychological (e.g., depression, anxiety), and sociocultural (e.g., relationship tension; conflict with religious, personal, or family values), and may impair quality of life.

Symptoms of sexual dysfunction among menopausal women include reduced sexual responsivity, low libido, lack of pleasure, difficulty achieving orgasm, inhibition, anxiety, and physical pain.

Menopause may cause genital pain, termed vaginal dyspareunia, which can occur before, during, and after intercourse. Menopause may also cause inflammation, sometimes described as atrophic vaginitis, which happens when reduced levels of estrogen cause the walls of the vagina to become thin and dry. These physical conditions can be the cause of sexual dysfunction among women experiencing menopause.

Reduced androgen (testosterone) production in menopausal women is associated with reduced libido.

Low sexual desire is the most commonly reported symptom by menopausal women: half of postmenopausal women in one study indicated low libido compared to a third of premenopausal women.

Desire or libido may be affected by many factors. To plan treatment for clients experiencing lowered sexual desire (i.e., low libido), the social worker needs to determine if the issue concerns sex drive (i.e., has a physiological basis), expectations or wishes (i.e., is based in values and beliefs), or motivation (i.e., has a psychological/relationship basis).

A 2013 analysis of 27 studies on the use of hormone replacement therapy (HRT) to help with sexual dysfunction in menopausal women indicated uncertain, small, or moderate improvements in sexual functioning. The most commonly reported improvement was a reduction in physical pain experienced during vaginal intercourse.

Some postmenopausal women report that HRT increases sexual desire, vaginal lubrication, and satisfaction and reduces symptoms of depression.

The relationship between menopause, sexual dysfunction, and depression is not clear. Some studies indicate increased frequency of onset of depression during menopause and then link menopause with sexual dysfunction. Other studies have associated depression in women with high rates of sexual dysfunction. Some report high rates of depression for younger women and older, menopausal women.

In a 2011 study of 27,000 women, researchers found that gynecological conditions were unrelated to reduced sexual activity among postmenopausal women. Depression, poor health, dissatisfaction with life, and adverse life events, such as partner death or illness, were predominant conditions in the lives of older women reporting less sexual activity.

Histories of sexual victimization, unsatisfactory relationships, lower education attainment, poverty, negative attitudes, poor health, and stressful life events have all been shown to predict sexual dysfunction among women.

In a 2010 study of midlife women, researchers reported that poor sleep was significantly associated with sexual dysfunction.

In a 2010 study, researchers found that a woman's culture influences the reporting of menopausal symptoms. The researchers suggest that different levels of acculturation and different attitudes toward menopause and aging may increase or decrease the likelihood that a woman will report menopausal symptoms.

A 2012 study linked the use of antidepressants by midlife women with sexual dysfunction.

In a 2014 study, researchers found that social and personal characteristics (e.g., age, marital status, relationship status) influenced sexual function, but that age at onset of menopause was not significantly related to sexual function.

An individual's beliefs about sexuality may inform and shape her experience of sexual functioning. For example, in a 2006 study, researchers found that women with sexual dysfunction were more likely to believe that after menopause women lost their sexual desire, that older women experienced less sexual pleasure, and that being physically attractive was necessary for sexual satisfaction.

In a 2014 attitudinal study, researchers found that 67 percent of postmenopausal women who were experiencing low sexual desire were not aware that it could be a treatable medical condition and 81 percent had never mentioned this issue to a healthcare provider.

During client assessment, clinicians are advised not to consider the frequency of sexual activity as a measure of sexual well-being because women may participate in sexual activity that is not driven by their own desire.

It's worth noting that researchers in a 2011 study reported that while both sexual function and activity decreased with age, sexual satisfaction was not reduced.

The research on sexual dysfunction in menopausal women suggests complex biopsychosocial interplay of causes; therefore, treatment of sexual dysfunction should be individualized. Women are likely to require more than one type of intervention (e.g., counseling, use of a lubricant, hormone treatment).

It's recommended that therapy focusing on lifestyle and psychosocial education be used prior to the use of pharmacological approaches such as HRT.

WHAT CAN BE DONE

Learn about sexual dysfunction so we can accurately assess our clients' personal characteristics and health education needs; share this information with our colleagues.

Learn about the impact of culture on our clients' experiences of menopause by exploring their experiences of menopause to improve our evaluations and better assess our clients' health education needs.

Develop an awareness of our own cultural values, beliefs, and biases, and develop knowledge about the histories, traditions, and values of our clients. Adopt treatment methodologies that reflect the cultural needs of the client.

Determine which components of sexual desire are involved when clients express a decrease in sexual desire in order to frame appropriate treatment.

Increase client awareness that sexual dysfunction is a treatable condition.

Educate clients regarding the physical changes associated with menopause and aging.

Become knowledgeable about sexual counseling services and ensure that clients are aware of potential sexual problems during menopause and have information about sex after menopause.

Provide referral(s) for comprehensive medical evaluation/treatment, sexual health education, sex therapist, and/or group cognitive behavioral therapy, as indicated.

—*Darlene Strayer, RN, MBA, and Sharon Richman, MSPT*

FOR FURTHER INFORMATION

Albaugh, J. (2014). Female sexual dysfunction. *International Journal of Urological Nursing, 8*(1), 38-43. doi:10.1111/ijun.12027

Chedraui, P., & Perez-Lopez, F. R. (2015). Assessing sexual problems in women at midlife using the short version of the female sexual function index.

Maturitas, 82(3), 299-303. doi:10.1016/j. maturitas.2015.07.005

Kingsberg, S. A. (2014). Attitudinal survey of women living with low sexual desire. *Journal of Women's Health, 23*(10), 817-823. doi:10.1089/ jwh.2014.4743

Nastri, C. O., Lara, L. A., Ferriani, R. A., Rosa-e-Silva, A. C. J. S., Figueredo, J. B. P., & Martins, W. P. (2013). Hormone therapy for sexual function in perimenopausal and postmenopausal women (review). *Cochrane Database of Systematic Reviews, Issue 6.* Art. No.: CD009672. doi:10.1002/-14651858. CD009672.pub2

Thornton, K., Chervenak, J., & Neal-Perry, G. (2015). Menopause and sexuality. *Endocrinology & Metabolism Clinics of North America, 44*(3), 649-661. doi:10.1016/j.ecl.2015.05.009

Tierney, D. K., Palesh, O., & Johnston, L. (2015). Sexuality, menopausal symptoms, and quality of life in premenopausal women in the first year following hematopoietic cell transplantation. *Oncology Nursing Forum, 42*(5), 488-497. doi:10.1188/15. onf.488-497

Topatan, S., & Yildiz, H. (2012). Symptoms experienced by women who enter into natural and surgical menopause and their relation to sexual functions. *Health Care for Women International, 33*(6), 525-539. doi:10.1080/07399332.2011. 64-6374

Yücel, C., & Eroğlu, K. (2013). Sexual problems in postmenopausal women and coping methods. *Sexuality & Disability, 31*(3), 217-228. doi:10.1007/ s11195-013-9306-8

Menorrhagia

CATEGORY: Disease/Disorder

KEY TERMS:

menorrhagia: excessive uttering bleeding that lasts more than 7 days or loss of more than 80 mL of blood per cycle

leiomyomas: also known as fibroids, benign smooth muscle tumor occurring frequently in the uterus

adenomyosis: condition in which endometrial tissues grows into the uterine wall

hysterectomy: surgical removal of the uterus

CAUSES AND SYMPTOMS

Menorrhagia can be caused by many disorders: anatomic abnormalities of the uterus, hormonal imbalances, certain medical conditions, medications, and malignancy. Common anatomic causes are uterine fibroids and adenomyosis. Irregular menstrual cycles resulting from hormonal imbalances can be associated with menorrhagia. Medical conditions such as blood clotting disorders and liver or thyroid disease contribute to menorrhagia. Medications that prevent blood clotting, such as warfarin or heparin, can lead to increased menstrual flow. Uterine and other reproductive tract cancers can also result in unusually heavy menstrual flow.

Symptoms of menorrhagia are uterine bleeding that is excessive (more than 80 milliliters per cycle) and/or bleeding that lasts for more than seven days. Unlike metrorrhagia, menorrhagia occurs at regular intervals. Menorrhagia can cause a patient to become anemic and exhibit symptoms of either acute or chronic blood loss. Obvious findings such as large palpable fibroids, evidence of hypothyroidism, or liver disease may be some of the signs and symptoms of the cause of menorrhagia.

TREATMENT AND THERAPY

Menorrhagia can be treated via a medical or a surgical approach. The selection of treatment often depends on the cause and severity of the menorrhagia. If menorrhagia is the result of an underlying medical condition (such as thyroid disorder), then treatment and control of these conditions may decrease the bleeding. If the patient has irregular cycles (for example, because of lack of ovulation), then medications such as hormonal oral contraceptive pills or injected medroxyprogesterone may be used to regulate the cycles and decrease menstrual flow. A patient who is nearing menopause can receive hormone injections that place her into an earlier artificial menopause, and hence eliminate menstrual bleeding altogether. If the patient encounters acute and profuse bleeding, then high-dose estrogens may be given.

If menorrhagia is resistant to medical management, then surgical treatment may be necessary. Examples of procedural treatments for menorrhagia are dilation and curettage (D & C), thermal ablation of the endometrial lining, hysteroscopy with resection of endometrial polyps or fibroids, and placement of a progesterone-impregnated intrauterine device (IUD). Hysterectomy is the definitive surgery for menorrhagia, no matter what the cause, since menstrual bleeding cannot occur after the uterus is removed. Patients with large fibroids or adenomyosis are often not responsive to medical management and may be candidates for hysterectomy. In patients with large fibroids and menorrhagia who wish to retain childbearing potential, a myomectomy, surgical removal of fibroids, may be performed instead of hysterectomy. If a patient is suspected or known to have a malignancy of the reproductive tract that is causing menorrhagia, then surgical management is the appropriate treatment.

Finally, patients can become severely anemic from menorrhagia, and blood transfusion may be necessary for symptomatic anemia. Mild anemia can be treated with iron supplementation.

—Anne Lynn S. Chang, MD
Updated by Christine Gamble, MD

For Further Information

Apgar B. S., et al. "Treatment of Menorrhagia." *American Family Physician*, vol. 75, 2007, 1813–1819,1820. http://www.aafp.org/afp/20070615/1813.html

Badash, Michelle. "Heavy Menstrual Bleeding." *Health Library*, September 27, 2012.

"Heavy Menstrual Bleeding." *Centers for Disease Control and Prevention*, December 20, 2017.

Icon Health. *Menorrhagia: A Medical Dictionary, Bibliography, and Annotated Research Guide to Internet References*. San Diego, Calif.: Author, 2004.

Kasper, Dennis L., et al., editors. *Harrison's Principles of Internal Medicine*. 16th ed. New York: McGraw-Hill, 2005.

"Menorrhagia (Heavy Menstrual Bleeding)." *Mayo Clinic*, July 15, 2017. https://www.mayoclinic.org/diseases-conditions/menorrhagia/symptoms-causes/syc-20352829

O'Donovan, Peter, Paul McGurgan, and Walter Prendiville, eds. *Conservative Surgery for Menorrhagia*. San Francisco: Greenwich Medical Media, 2003.

Stenchever, Morton A., et al. *Comprehensive Gynecology*. 4th ed. St. Louis, Mo.: Mosby/Elsevier, 2006.

Tierney, Lawrence M., Stephen J. McPhee, and Maxine A. Papadakis, eds. *Current Medical Diagnosis and Treatment 2017*. New York: McGraw-Hill Medical, 2017.

Menstruation

Category: Biology

Key Terms:

endometrium: the layer of cells lining the inner cavity of the uterus; the source of menstrual discharge

feedback: a system in which two parts of the body communicate and control each other, often through hormones; can be either negative (inhibitory) or positive (stimulatory)

follicle: a spherical structure within the ovary that contains a developing ovum and that produces hormones; each ovary contains thousands of follicles

hormone: a chemical signal produced in some part of the body that is carried in the blood to another body part, where it has some observable effect

menstrual cycle: the cycle of hormone production, ovulation, menstruation, and other changes that occurs on an approximately monthly schedule in women

ovary: the organ that produces ova and hormones; the two ovaries lie on either side of the uterus, within the abdominal cavity

ovulation: the process by which an ovum is released from its follicle in the ovary; occurs in the middle of each menstrual cycle ovum (*pl. ova*): the egg or reproductive cell produced by the female, which when fertilized by a sperm from the male will develop into an embryo

prostaglandins: chemical signals that have local effects on the organ that produces them

uterus: the organ that nourishes and supports the developing embryo; also called the womb

Process and Effects

Menstruation is the monthly discharge of bloody fluid from the uterus. It occurs in humans and in other primates (apes and monkeys), but not in all mammals; for example, horses, cats, and dogs do not menstruate. The menstrual fluid consists of blood, cells, and debris from the endometrial lining of the uterus, and mucus and other fluids. The color of the discharge varies from dark brown to bright red during the period of flow. The menstrual discharge does not normally clot after leaving the uterus, but it may contain endometrial debris that resembles blood clots. The flow lasts from four to five days in most women, with spotting (the discharge of scant fluid) possibly continuing for another day or two. The volume of fluid lost ranges from ten to eighty milliliters, with a median of about forty milliliters. The blood in the menstrual discharge amounts to only a small fraction of the body's total blood volume of about five thousand milliliters, so normal physiological functioning is not usually impaired by the blood loss that occurs during menstruation.

The first menstruation (menarche) typically begins between the ages of eleven and fourteen, when a girl goes through puberty; the last episodes of menstruation occur some forty years later at the time of menopause. Menstruation does not occur during the months of pregnancy or for the first few months after a woman has given birth.

Menstruation is the most visible event of the woman's monthly menstrual cycle. The average length of the menstrual cycle in the population is about 29.1 days, but it may vary from sixteen to thirty-five days, with variation occurring between different individuals and in one individual from month to month. Girls who have just gone through puberty and women who are approaching the menopause tend to have more variation in their cycles than do women in the middle of their reproductive years. There is also an age-related change in cycle length: Cycles tend to be relatively long in teenagers, then decrease in length until a woman is about forty years old, after which cycles tend to lengthen and become irregular.

Hormones cause menstruation to be coordinated with other events in the menstrual cycle. Uterine function is regulated by two hormones, estrogen and progesterone, which are produced in the ovaries. In turn, the production of estrogen and progesterone is controlled by follicle-stimulating hormone (FSH) and luteinizing hormone (LH), both of which are produced in the pituitary gland. The hormones from the ovaries and from the pituitary have mutual control over each other: they participate in a feedback relationship. The fact that females produce ova only once a month, in a cycle rather than continuously, is the result of a change in the feedback relationships between the ovarian and pituitary hormones as the menstrual cycle proceeds.

In the first half of the cycle, the follicular phase, a predominant negative feedback effect keeps pituitary hormone levels low while allowing estrogen to increase. Day one of the menstrual cycle is defined as the day of the onset of the menstrual flow. During the days of menstrual bleeding, levels of estrogen and progesterone are low, but FSH levels are high enough to cause the growth of follicles in the ovary. As the follicles start to grow, they secrete estrogen, and increasing amounts are secreted as the follicles continue to enlarge over the next five to ten days. The estrogen exerts negative feedback control over the pituitary: FSH and LH production is inhibited by estrogen, so levels of these hormones remain low during the follicular phase. Besides producing estrogen, the growing follicles contain ova that are maturing and preparing for ovulation. Meanwhile, estrogen acts on the uterus to cause the growth of the endometrial lining. The lining becomes thicker and its blood supply increases; glands located in the lining also grow and mature. These uterine changes are known as endometrial proliferation.

As the woman nears the middle of her cycle, a dramatic change in hormonal feedback occurs. The increasing secretion of estrogen shifts the hormonal system into a positive feedback mode, whereby an increase in estrogen stimulates the release of LH and FSH from the pituitary instead of inhibiting it. Thus, at the middle of the cycle (around day fourteen), simultaneous peaks in levels of estrogen, LH, and FSH occur. The peak in LH triggers ovulation by causing changes in the wall of the follicle, allowing it to break open to release its ovum. Although a group of follicles has matured up to this point, usually only the largest one ovulates, and the remainder in the group die and cease hormone production.

Following ovulation, negative feedback is reestablished. The follicle that just ovulated remains as a functional part of the ovary; it becomes transformed into the corpus luteum, a structure that produces estrogen and progesterone throughout most of the second half of the cycle, the luteal phase. During this phase, the combined presence of estrogen and progesterone reestablishes negative feedback over the pituitary, and LH and FSH levels decline. A second ovulation is prevented because a LH peak is not possible at this time. The combined action of estrogen and progesterone causes the uterus to enter its secretory phase during the second half of the cycle: The glands in the thickened endometrium secrete nutrients that will support an embryo if the woman becomes pregnant, and the ample blood supply to the endometrium can supply the embryo with other nutrients and oxygen. If the woman does in fact become pregnant, the embryo will secrete a hormone that will ensure the continued production of estrogen and progesterone, and because of these hormones, the uterus will remain in the secretory condition throughout pregnancy. Menstruation does not occur during pregnancy because of the high levels of estrogen and progesterone, which continually support the uterus.

If the woman does not become pregnant, the corpus luteum automatically degenerates, starting at about the twenty-fourth day of the menstrual cycle. As the corpus luteum dies, it fails to produce estrogen and progesterone, so levels of these hormones decrease. As the amounts of estrogen and progesterone drop, the uterus begins to produce prostaglandins, chemicals that act as local signals within the uterus. The prostaglandins cause a number of changes in uterine function: blood flow to the endometrium is temporarily cut off, causing the endometrial tissue to die, and the uterine muscle begins to contract, causing further changes in blood flow. The decreased blood flow and the muscle contractions contribute to the cramping pain that many women feel just before and at the time of menstrual bleeding. Menstrual bleeding starts when the blood flow to the endometrium is reestablished and the dead tissue is sloughed off and washed out of the uterus. This event signals the start of a new menstrual cycle.

COMPLICATIONS AND DISORDERS

Many disorders involving menstruation exist. Toxic shock syndrome is a disease that, while not caused directly by menstruation, sometimes occurs during menstruation in women who use tampons to absorb the menstrual flow. The symptoms of toxic shock syndrome—fever, rash, a drop in blood pressure, diarrhea, vomiting, and fainting—are caused by toxins produced by the bacterium *Staphylococcus aureus*. This bacterium is normally present in limited numbers within the vagina, but the use of high-absorbency tampons is associated with a higher-than-normal bacterial growth and toxin production. Toxic shock syndrome requires immediate medical attention, since it may be fatal if left untreated. Women can reduce the risk of toxic shock syndrome by changing tampons often, using lower-absorbency types, and alternating the use of tampons and sanitary napkins.

Amenorrhea is defined as the absence of menstruation. It is usually, but not always, coincident with a lack of ovulation. Amenorrhea may be primary (the

woman has never menstruated) or secondary (menstrual cycles that were once normal have stopped). The condition is usually associated with abnormal patterns of hormone secretion, but the problem in hormone secretion may itself be merely the symptom of some other underlying disorder. One of the most common situations leading to both primary and secondary amenorrhea is low body weight, caused by malnutrition, eating disorders, or sustained exercise. Body fat has two roles in reproduction: it provides energy needed for tissue growth and cell functions, and it contributes to circulating estrogen levels. Loss of body fat may create a situation in which the reproductive system ceases to function because of low estrogen levels and because of lack of needed energy. The result is seen as amenorrhea.

Emotional or physical stress may also cause amenorrhea, because stress results in the release of hormones that interfere with the reproductive hormones. Ideally, amenorrhea is treated by removing its cause; for example, a special diet or a change in an exercise program can bring about an increase in body fat stores, or stress levels can be reduced through changes in lifestyle or with counseling. Ironically, sometimes birth control pills are prescribed for women with amenorrhea. The pills do not cure the amenorrhea, but they can counteract some of the long-term problems associated with it, such as changes in the endometrial lining and loss of bone density.

Dysmenorrhea refers to abnormally intense uterine pain associated with menstruation. It is estimated that 5 to 10 percent of women experience pain intense enough to interfere with their school or work schedules. Dysmenorrhea may be primary (occurring in women with no known disease) or secondary (caused by a disease condition such as a tumor or infection). Studies have shown uterine prostaglandin levels to be correlated with the degree of pain perceived in primary dysmenorrhea, and drugs that interfere with prostaglandins offer an effective treatment for this condition. These drugs include aspirin, acetaminophen, ibuprofen, and naproxen; some formulas are available without a doctor's prescription, but the stronger drugs require one. Secondary dysmenorrhea is best managed by removing the underlying cause; if this is not possible, the antiprostaglandin drugs may be useful in controlling the pain.

Menorrhagia is excessive menstrual blood loss, usually defined as more than eighty milliliters of fluid

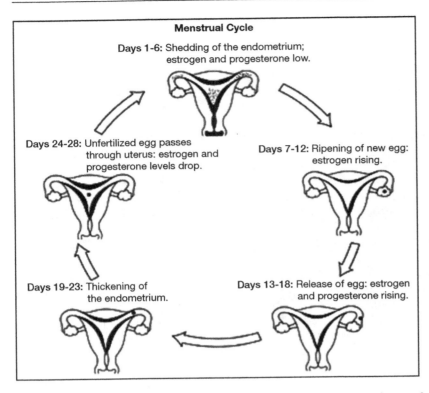

Menstrual Cycle

Days 1-6: Shedding of the endometrium; estrogen and progesterone low.

Days 24-28: Unfertilized egg passes through uterus: estrogen and progesterone levels drop.

Days 7-12: Ripening of new egg: estrogen rising.

Days 19-23: Thickening of the endometrium.

Days 13-18: Release of egg: estrogen and progesterone rising.

Exact timing varies from woman to woman; day 1 is defined as the day of onset of menstrual flow; ovulation occurs in mid-cycle (around day 14). Hormonal levels are rising and falling throughout the cycle. © *EBSCO*

lost per cycle. This condition can have serious health consequences because of the loss of red blood cells, which are essential for carrying oxygen to tissues. Women who have given birth to several children are more likely to suffer from menorrhagia, possibly because of enlargement of the uterine cavity and interference with the mechanisms that limit menstrual blood flow. Women who have diseases that interfere with blood clotting may also have menorrhagia. Although the menstrual discharge itself does not usually form clots after it leaves the uterus, clots do form within the uterine endometrium; these clots normally prevent excessive blood loss. Treatment for menorrhagia may begin with iron and vitamin supplements to induce increased red blood cell production, or transfusions may be used to replace the lost red blood cells. If this is unsuccessful, treatment with birth control pills, destruction of the endometrium by laser surgery, or a hysterectomy (surgical removal of the uterus) may be necessary.

Endometriosis is a condition in which endometrial cells from the uterus become misplaced within the abdominal cavity, adhering to and growing on the surface of internal organs. The outside of the uterus, the oviducts (fallopian tubes), the surface of the ovaries, and the outer surface of the intestines can all support the growth of endometrial tissue.

Endometriosis is thought to arise during menstruation, when endometrial tissue enters the oviducts instead of being carried outward through the cervix and vagina. Through the oviducts, the endometrial tissue has access to the abdominal cavity. Since the misplaced endometrial tissue responds to hormones in the same way that the normal endometrium does, it undergoes cyclic changes in thickness and attempts to shed at the time of menstruation. Endometriosis results in intense pain during menstruation and can cause infertility because of interference with ovulation, ovum or sperm transport, or uterine function. Endometriosis is treated with birth control pills or with drugs that suppress menstrual cycles, or the endometrial tissue may be removed surgically.

Premenstrual syndrome (PMS) is a set of symptoms that occurs in some women in the week before the start of menstruation, with the symptoms disappearing once menstruation begins. Researchers and physicians who study PMS have struggled to devise a standard definition for the disorder, but the list of possible symptoms is lengthy and varies from woman to woman and even within one woman from month to month. The possible symptoms include both psychological and physical changes: irritability, nervous tension, anxiety, moodiness, depression, lethargy, insomnia, confusion, crying, food cravings, fatigue, weight gain, swelling and bloating, breast tenderness, backache, headache, dizziness, muscle stiffness, and abdominal cramps. A diagnosis of PMS requires that the symptoms show a clear relation to the timing of menstruation and that they recur during most menstrual cycles. Researchers estimate that 3 to 5 percent of women have PMS symptoms that are so severe that they are incapacitating, but that milder symptoms occur in about 50 percent of all women.

Because of the variability in symptoms between women, some researchers believe that there are several subtypes of PMS, each with its own cluster of symptoms. It is possible that each subtype has a unique cause. Suggested causes of PMS include an imbalance in the ratio of estrogen to progesterone following ovulation; changes in the hormones that control salt and water balance (the renin-angiotensin-aldosterone system); increased levels of prolactin (a hormone that acts on the breast); changes in amounts of brain chemicals; altered functioning of the biological clock that determines daily rhythms; poor diet or sensitivity to certain foods; and psychological factors such as attitude toward menstruation, stresses of family or professional life, and underlying personality disorders. Studies evaluating these theories have yielded contradictory results, so that no one cause of PMS has yet been found. Current treatments for PMS include dietary therapy, hormone administration, and psychological counseling, but no treatment has been found effective in all PMS patients.

An interesting phenomenon associated with menstruation is menstrual synchrony, also known as the "dormitory effect." Among women who live together, menstrual cycles gradually become synchronized, so that the women begin to menstruate within a few days of one another. Researchers have found that this phenomenon probably occurs because of pheromones, chemical signals that are produced by an individual and that have an effect on another individual. Pheromones act on the brain through the sense of smell, even though there may not be an odor that is consciously perceived.

PERSPECTIVE AND PROSPECTS

Early beliefs about menstruation were based on folk magic and superstition rather than on scientific evidence. Even today, some cultures persist in believing that menstruating women possess deleterious powers: that the presence of a menstruating woman can cause crops to fail, farm animals to die, or beer, bread, jam, and other foods to be spoiled. Some people believe that these incidents will occur even if the menstruating woman has no evil intention. Because of the possibility of these events, some cultures prohibit menstruating women from interacting with others.

In the most rigorous example of such a taboo, some societies require that menstruating women live in special huts for the duration of the bleeding period.

Folk beliefs about menstruating women have been bolstered by religious views of menstruating women as "unclean" and in need of purification. In Orthodox Judaism, there are detailed proscriptions to be observed by a menstruating woman, including the avoidance of sexual intercourse. Seven days after her menstrual flow has stopped, the Orthodox Jewish woman undergoes a ritual purification, after which she may resume sexual relations with her husband. Early Christians absorbed the Jewish belief in the uncleanliness of a menstruating woman and prohibited her from entering church or receiving the sacraments. These injunctions were lifted by the seventh century, but the view of women as spiritually and bodily impure persists in some Christian groups to this day.

Many couples abstain from intercourse during the woman's menstrual period. There is no medical justification for this behavior; in fact, research has demonstrated that intercourse can alleviate menstrual cramping, at least temporarily. Still, surveys have shown that a majority of both men and women think that it is wrong for a woman to have intercourse while menstruating.

There are also persistent beliefs that women's physical and mental abilities suffer during menstruation. In fact, this was the predominant medical opinion up through the nineteenth and early twentieth centuries. Medical writings from this time are filled with injunctions for women to rest and to refrain from exercise and intellectual strain while menstruating. It was a common belief that education could actually cause physical harm to women. Some men used this advice as justification for excluding women from equal opportunities in education and employment. Starting in the late nineteenth century, however, scientific studies clearly demonstrated that education has no harmful effects and that there is no diminution of intellectual or physical performance during menstruation. Nevertheless, the latter finding has been one that the general population finds difficult to accept.

The latest view of menstruation is that, far from being harmful, menstrual bleeding is directly beneficial to a woman's health. Margie Profet, an evolutionary biologist at the University of California, theorized that menstruation evolved as a means of periodically removing disease-causing bacteria and viruses from the woman's uterus. These organisms might enter the uterus along with sperm after sexual activity. In Profet's view, the energetic cost of replacing the blood and tissue lost through menstruation is more than outweighed by the protective benefits of menstruation. Her theory implies that treatments that suppress menstruation, as birth control drugs sometimes do, are not always advantageous.

The suppression of menstruation through extended or continuous cycling with combined hormonal contraception has recently been reexamined for various benefits, including increased contraceptive efficacy. Some clinicians and consumers have embraced this concept, which can be done with any continuous (no placebo or no-pill interval) use of a monophasic combined oral contraceptive pill, the *Ortho Evra* patch, or *NuvaRing*. New formulations of combined oral contraceptives include *Seasonale* and *Seasonique*, both of which result in menstrual bleeding every three months, and *Lybrel*, which eliminates cycles for one year. Other formulations have shortened the one-week pill-free interval, resulting in shorter and lighter menses.

—*Marcia Watson-Whitmyre, Ph.D.*

FOR FURTHER INFORMATION

Ammer, Christine. *The Encyclopedia of Women's Health*. 6th ed. New York: Facts on File, 2009.

Berek, Jonathan S., and Emil Novak, editors. *Berek and Novak's Gynecology*. 15th ed. Philadelphia: Lippincott Williams & Wilkins, 2012.

Loulan, JoAnne, and Bonnie Worthen. *Period: A Girl's Guide to Menstruation*. Rev. ed. Minnetonka, Minn.: Book Peddlers, 2001.

"Menopause." *MedlinePlus*, July 1, 2013.

"Menstrual Cycle." Womenshealth.gov, Office on Women's Health, 2017, www.womenshealth.gov/menstrual-cycle.

"Menstruation." *MedlinePlus*, May 28, 2013.

"Premenstrual Syndrome." *MedlinePlus*, April 29, 2013.

Quilligan, Edward J., and Frederick P. Zuspan, editors. *Current Therapy in Obstetrics and Gynecology*. 5th ed. Philadelphia: W. B. Saunders, 2000.

Rako, Susan. *No More Periods? The Risks of Menstrual Suppression and Other Cutting-Edge Issues in Women's Reproductive Health*. New York: Harmony Books, 2003.

Weschler, Toni. *Taking Charge of Your Fertility*. Rev. ed. New York: Collins, 2006.

Migraine headache

CATEGORY: Disease/Disorder

KEY TERMS:

common migraine: Migraine without an aura. Classically described as a throbbing, pounding headache associated with nausea, vomiting, or photophobia

classic migraine: Migraine with an aura. An aura is a sensation prior to a seizure or a migraine that manifests as flashes of light, shimmering shapes, strange visual sensations, odd smells, or tingling in the hands and feet

complex migraine: Migraine with other, non-aura neurological complications. An example is migraine plus complete loss of strength in one arm

trigeminal nerve: The trigeminal nerve is the nerve responsible for the sensations of light touch, pain, and temperature in the face

CAUSES AND SYMPTOMS

Migraines are a common disorder caused by a combination of neural and vascular changes. There are three major types of migraines (3 C's): common, classic, and complex. Common migraines account for 80% of migraines while classic and complex migraines account for the remaining 20%. Other migraine types may include retinal migraines (attacks of blindness and vision loss), menstrual migraines (occurring during menstruation), and abdominal migraines (severe abdominal pain). Patients suffering from migraines often experience severe, throbbing pain, typically on one side of the head. Symptoms may also include nausea, vomiting, and photophobia (light sensitivity). Attacks may be preceded by changes in mood or energy and are often followed by fatigue and apprehension. Patients with migraines often find relief by avoiding lights and sounds and lying down in a dark, quiet room.

Migraine headaches may occur spontaneously or be triggered by personal, lifestyle, or environmental factors. Triggers include emotional stress, hormone imbalances, weather changes, lights/sounds/smells, alcohol or tobacco, exercise and sexual activity, medications, and sleep disturbances.

The exact cause of migraine headaches is currently unclear. Previously, migraines were thought to be associated with widening, or dilation, of blood vessels feeding the brain. This theory was supported by the efficacy of medications and drugs such as caffeine that cause constriction of blood vessels. However, recent research points away from vasodilation as a cause of migraines. Current leading hypotheses suggest that neural dysfunction leads to irritation of outer layers of the brain and pain. This theory, called "cortical spreading depression," suggests that neurons in one area of the brain activate a domino-like cascade of activity that spreads in a wave across the surface of the brain. This wave of spreading electrical activity may simultaneously a) cause the classic migraine aura by triggering specific areas of the brain, b) activate the trigeminal nerve and induce pain, and c) cause vascular changes that cause inflammation of the highly sensitive outer layers of the brain.

Migraines may affect up to 12% of the population. Women are more likely than men to have migraines (17% vs. 6%) and patients are typically middle-aged (30-39). Migraines likely have a genetic link, as they have also been shown to run in families.

Treatment and Therapy

Migraines may be triggered by a variety of factors. Avoiding triggers may significantly reduce the requency of migraine episodes. Patients are recommended to use a diary to record foods eaten, daily activities, and timing of migraines to help identify triggers.

The American Migraine Foundation recommends an approach called "Headache Hygiene" to reduce the incidence of migraines. This approach focuses on maintaining regular sleep patterns, regular exercise (at least 30 minutes, three times weekly), eating regular meals, and avoiding known triggers such as drinking alcohol and smoking. While sudden changes in lifestyle may act as triggers for migraine headaches, regular exercise and lifestyle changes reduces the incidence of migraine headaches in the long term.

Prophylactic treatments aim to prevent or reduce the incidence of migraines. Examples of prophylactic medications include anti-hypertensives (beta blockers, calcium channel blockers, ACE inhibitors, and angiotensin receptor blockers), anti-depressants (serotonin-noradrenergic reuptake inhibitors, tricyclic antidepressants), and anti-seizure medications (topiramate, valproate). There are also several anti-inflammatory medications, vitamins, and minerals that have been suggested to reduce the frequency of migraine headaches. Patients who continue to have migraines despite treatment may also benefit from injections of botulinum toxin (Botox), nerve stimulation, and acupuncture.

Abortive treatments aim to reduce the duration or intensity of migraines. Common abortive therapies include non-steroidal anti-inflammatory drugs (NSAI-Ds) and acetaminophen (Tylenol), triptans (Sumatriptan), anti-nausea medications, and ergots. Mild to moderate migraines are often treated with weaker medications, such as NSAIDs or acetaminophen. Moderate to severe migraines may benefit from more aggressive therapy with triptans, which may also be used in emergency situations. Finally, opioids have been suggested as treatment options for migraines but should be avoided due to side effects and risk of addiction.

Summary

Migraines are incredibly common headaches that can be debilitating. While a variety of treatments are now available for management of migraines, little is known about the pathophysiology of migraines and a cure has yet to be developed. Individuals who suffer from migraines should learn about their migraine triggers and how to avoid them. Patients are also encouraged to lead healthy lifestyles, which have been shown to reduce the frequency and intensity of migraine headaches, and to follow prescribed prophylactic treatment regimens and continue medical surveillance to monitor health status.

—*Cherie Marcel, BS*
Updated by Derrick Cheng, BSc, BA, and Carol Shi, BA

For Further Information

Aminoff, M. J., and Kerchner, G. A. "Nervous system disorders." *2014 Current Medical Diagnosis & Treatment*, 53rd ed., edited by M. A. Papadakis, S. J. McPhee, & M.W. Rabo, New York, NY: McGraw-Hill Medical, 2014, 928-929.

Ratini, Melinda. *Fighting Food-Related Headaches*. WebMD, 19 Sept. 2014, www.webmd.com/migraines-headaches/guide/triggers-specific-foods.

Finocchi, C., & Sivori, G. "Food as a trigger and aggravating factor of migraine." *Neurological Sciences*, vol. 33, no. Suppl 1, 2012, S77-S80.

Marcus, D. A. Chronic headache: The importance of trigger identification. *Headache & Pain: Diagnostic Challenges, Current Therapy*, vol. 14, no. 3, 2003, 139-144.

Mayo Clinic Staff. "Meniere's Disease." *Mayo Clinic,* Mayo Foundation for Medical Education and Research, 8 Dec. 2018, www.mayoclinic.org/diseases-conditions/menieres-disease/basics/definition/con-20028251.

Niklasch, D. M., & Starkweather, A. (2010). Neurologic disorders. In *Lippincott manual of nursing practice* (9th ed., pp. 571-573). Ambler, PA: Wolters Kluwer Health/Lippincott Williams & Wilkins.

Miscarriage

CATEGORY: Disease/Disorder
Also known as: Spontaneous abortion

KEY TERMS:

abortion: the medical term for intended and unintended pregnancy loss

blighted ovum: a condition in which the gestational sac and placenta grow without a developing child inside

ectopic pregnancy: a pregnancy in which the implantation of the fertilized egg occurs anywhere outside the uterus, usually in the Fallopian tube

human chorionic gonadotropin (hCG): the hormone, produced only in pregnancy, that makes the uterine lining receptive for the developing embryo or fetus; pregnancy tests determine its presence

molar pregnancy: abnormal, cyst-like placental tissue that grows either in place of the developing child (complete mole) or in addition to the developing child (partial mole)

recurrent miscarriage: a condition in which a woman experiences three consecutive miscarriages

threatened abortion: when the symptoms of a miscarriage first occur

CAUSES AND SYMPTOMS

Approximately 15 to 20 percent of all known pregnancies end in miscarriage. Furthermore, it is estimated that 50 to 75 percent of all fertilized eggs fail to implant in the uterus— a situation generally unknown to the woman. The likelihood of a miscarriage drops during the pregnancy's duration: approximately 10 percent in the first four weeks after implantation, 5 percent for the next six weeks, and 3 percent for the following eight weeks. (The stillbirth rate is approximately 1 percent.)

The symptoms of a threatened loss of pregnancy may include spotting of blood, which may turn into heavier bleeding; cramping, possibly accompanied by lower back pain and vaginal discharge of tissue, clots, or pinkish fluid. A completed miscarriage may also demonstrate changes in pregnancy signs, such as nausea and breast sensitivity. A hormonal sign of a threatened abortion is the failure of human chorionic gonadotropin (hCG) levels to double every two days.

There are three conditions where a woman experiences a miscarriage and the developing child is missing in the sac. About 30 percent of miscarriages before the eighth gestational week are blighted ova, as an embryo has failed to develop. Complete molar pregnancies arise when a sperm (or two) fertilize an egg that has lost its genes. The resulting development of pregnancy tissues—absent the developing child—usually leads to the symptoms of a miscarriage in the first several gestational weeks, but expulsion of the placenta may not occur. Because of the higher likelihood of residual disease (including cancer) in the abnormal tissue if any is left behind, surgical removal of the molar tissue is often warranted.

Women who have aborted a molar pregnancy are advised to not get pregnant again for a year, and then they must be closely monitored for subsequent pregnancies, as they are at increased risk for further abnormalities that can become malignant. Finally, a woman may have a recognized pregnancy yet not realize that she was actually pregnant with twins and that one died. This "vanishing twin syndrome" occurs in an estimated 3.5 percent of all twin pregnancies.

Analyses reveal the probability of the most common causes of miscarriages: 50 to 60 percent, genetic abnormalities; 10 to 15 percent, defects in the uterus (such as double or septal uterus) or the cervix (such as incomplete closure); and 10 to 15 percent, hormonal (such as low progesterone or thyroxin) and/or immune disorders (such as lupus or antiphospholipid antibody syndrome). A woman's poor health, history of disease (such as endometriosis), history of miscarriages, and advanced age (a 75 percent miscarriage rate for women forty-five and older) also increase the probability of a miscarriage. Recent studies have indicated that the presence of bacterial vaginosis is associated with late-onset miscarriages and preterm deliveries. The presence of the bacteria known as beta strep in the mother's birth canal is tied to preterm labor when it goes untreated. Lifestyle choices that can compromise a successful pregnancy may involve the abuse of substances such as large amounts of caffeine, cocaine, or nicotine; the contraction of sexually transmitted diseases (STDs), such as chlamydia, human immunodeficiency virus (HIV); or exposure to harmful agents, such as radiation.

TREATMENT, THERAPY AND IMPACT ON WOMEN

Little can be done to stop a miscarriage in the first two months of pregnancy, though some effective interventions are possible in later gestational periods. Magnesium sulfate is effective in combating preeclampsia (high blood pressure during pregnancy) and premature labor contractions. A cervical stitch (cerclage) can rectify an incompetent cervix (premature dilation). Most medical efforts, however, are directed toward the prevention of future miscarriages—the treatment of disease, lifestyle changes, RhoGAM shots for Rh problems—and recovery from the present miscarriage. For example, medications to reduce the risk of miscarriage include antibiotics, which treat or prevent infections, and aspirin and similar medications that treat blood-clotting issues. Surgical procedures are also used to prevent miscarriages by treating certain uterine problems, such as uterine fibroids and a weakened cervix.

There are two aspects of recovery from a miscarriage. The physical part involves the natural or artificial removal of pregnancy tissue—either chemically, as with *Pitocin*, or surgically, as with dilation and curettage (D & C)—and the establishment of a new menstrual cycle. A typical physical recovery ranges from a few days to a few weeks for the miscarriage itself and one to two months after the miscarriage for the next period. Women are usually advised to wait one to two normal periods before trying to conceive again. Approximately 60 percent of women trying to conceive will be successful within six months of the miscarriage.

The psychological recovery may take longer than the physical recovery. Unfortunately for women, miscarriage has historically not been openly discussed, despite its common occurrence. This has caused women to feel increase guilt, shame and self-blame when they experience this loss of pregnancy. Although more often than not, the women's behavior and actions have no impact on the miscarriage at all. Taking on responsibility for miscarriage and feeling alone in the experience increase negative emotional

---

Information on Miscarriage

Causes: Genetic abnormalities, uterine or cervical defects, hormonal or immune disorders; risks increase with poor health, history of reproductive tract disease or miscarriage, age over forty-five, certain substances (caffeine, cocaine, nicotine), radiation exposure, STDs

Symptoms: Spotting that turns into heavier bleeding; cramping and lower back pain; vaginal discharge (tissue, clots, pinkish fluid); nausea; loss of pregnancy signs

Duration: Acute

Treatments: None in first two months of pregnancy; later, magnesium sulfate for preeclampsia or premature contractions, cervical stitch for incompetent cervix

---

struggles. Increasing knowledge about the frequency of miscarriage can normalize the experience, decrease self-blame and therefore helping the women cope with this loss. Social support, good mental health prior to the miscarriage, religious faith, and successful grieving (mourning, not denying, the loss and then moving forward in life) are some of the factors correlated with a better psychological recovery. Support groups exist for individuals who have suffered miscarriage, stillbirth, or infant death. Similar groups exist to provide support to individuals who are pregnant after the loss of an earlier pregnancy. Such support is essential in decreasing anxiety and depressive symptoms. Individual therapy may also be necessary if the woman continues to struggle with this loss. It is common to see increased anxiety in the next pregnancy with a woman who has experienced a miscarriage. Finding support through family, friends, support groups, religion or individual therapy can help the woman and her family move forward in healing from the loss and help reduce stress in further pregnancies, and parenthood.

PERSPECTIVE AND PROSPECTS

Until the latter half of the twentieth century, miscarrying women received little satisfaction from the medical community. In fact, many of the drugs introduced in the mid-twentieth century, such as diethylstilbestrol (DES) and its numerous estrogenic cousins, caused more harm than good. However, by the latter part of the twentieth century significant progress was made in diagnosing and preventing miscarriages.

In the early twenty-first century, three avenues of research appear to be promising. Studies are revealing certain genetic predispositions for miscarriages, such as the low production of nitric oxide, resulting in less blood to the uterus. Miscarriages are also being linked to autoimmune disorders and hormonal deficiencies. Use of hormone injections to women who are found to have a hormonal imbalance can help to prevent miscarriage. Finally, assisted reproductive technologies offer intriguing possibilities, such as the ethically controversial opportunity to screen preimplantation embryos for chromosomal abnormalities. In these and other areas of research, new hopes are being raised for old griefs.

—*Paul J. Chara, Jr., Ph.D., and Kathleen A. Chara, M.S.;*
Updated by Robin Kamienny Montvilo, R.N., Ph.D.
and Kimberly Ortiz-Hartman, Psy.D., LMFT

FOR FURTHER INFORMATION

Eisenberg, Arlene, Heidi E. Murkoff, and Sandee E. Hathaway. *What to Expect When You're Expecting.* 4th ed. New York: Workman, 2009.

Jutel, A. "What's in a Name? Death Before Birth." *Perspectives in Biology and Medicine*, vol. 49, no. 3, 2006, 425–434.

Larsen, E. C. "New Insights into Mechanisms behind Miscarriage." *BMC Medicine*, vol. 11, no. 1, 2013, 154.

Tranquilli, A. L. "Miscarriages: Causes, Symptoms and Prevention." *Obstetrics and Gynecology Advances.* New York: Nova, 2012.

Wood, Deborah. "Miscarriage." *Health Library*, September 10, 2012.

Miscarriage, stillbirth, perinatal death risk factors

CATEGORY: Disease/Disorder

WHAT WE KNOW

Miscarriage refers to a pregnancy loss before 20 weeks of gestation; stillbirth refers to a pregnancy loss after 20 weeks of gestation; and perinatal death includes pregnancy loss after 20 weeks of gestation and neonatal death in the first 28 days after delivery.

In the United States, approximately 8–20 percent of all clinically recognized pregnancies (a "clinically recognized" pregnancy means that the pregnancy has been visualized on an ultrasound or that pregnancy tissue was identified after a pregnancy loss) result in miscarriage, with 80 percent of miscarriages occurring in the first 12 weeks.

The miscarriage rate increases to nearly 50 percent when both clinically recognized pregnancies (e.g., live births, induced abortions, ectopic pregnancies) and biochemically recognized pregnancies (i.e., pregnancies detected by urinary hormone assay) are counted together.

The stillbirth rate for all pregnancies is approximately 4.91 per 1,000. The perinatal mortality rate for all pregnancies is approximately 6.26 per 1,000.

In England and Wales, there were 3,558 stillbirths in 2012, the perinatal mortality rate is 7 deaths per 1,000 births.

Worldwide, the stillbirth rate, which varies significantly by country, is approximately 18.9 percent. Pakistan has one of the highest rates of stillbirth at 47 percent, and the perinatal death rate is 8.4 percent.

Although miscarriage, stillbirth, or perinatal death may occur in the absence of identifiable risk factors, numerous fetal, maternal, and environmental factors have been linked with increased risk of these adverse pregnancy outcomes.

Fetal factors that increase the risk of miscarriage and stillbirth include genetic abnormalities, growth abnormalities, and viral, bacterial, fungal, and infections.

Chromosomal abnormalities (e.g., such as Down syndrome, Edwards syndrome) are responsible for 50–65 percent of first-trimester miscarriages.

Congenital anomalies increase the risk of stillbirth 15-fold (e.g., heart problems, neural tube defects).

Stillbirth is more common in fetuses that are either abnormally large for gestational age or abnormally small for gestational age.

Demographic factors, including low socioeconomic status, and inadequate prenatal care are associated with increased risk of stillbirth.

In the United States the risk of stillbirth is increased for women under the age of 20 and over the age of 34. In the United States stillbirth is twice as common in black women as in white women, however this may be due to socioeconomic factors rather than racial differences.

Maternal systemic diseases associated with increased risk of miscarriage and stillbirth include blood clotting disorders, diabetes mellitus, systemic lupus erythematosus, hypertension, thyroid disease, polycystic ovarian syndrome, congenital heart defects, obesity, diabetes, and kidney disease.

As maternal body mass index (BMI) increases, rates of miscarriage, stillbirth, and perinatal deaths increase. Women with either type 1 or type 2 diabetes have a higher risk of stillbirth after 32 weeks gestation.

Research confirms that the age of the mother is a risk factor for miscarriage, stillbirth, and perinatal death. Neonatal death is higher among women over age 40 and under age 25. Stillbirth rates increase with advancing maternal age.

Uterine factors that increase risk for miscarriage include uterine leiomyomas (i.e., fibroids), intrauterine synechiae (i.e., Asherman syndrome, a condition characterized by destruction and scarring of the endometrium subsequent to uterine curettage), abnormally shaped uterus and cervical incompetence (e.g., due to in utero exposure to diethylstilbestrol [DES]), and abnormal placentation (i.e., abnormal growth of the placenta inside the uterus).

Exposure to environmental toxins, cigarette smoking, cocaine use, and alcohol consumption increase the risk of miscarriage and stillbirth.

Moderate to heavy levels of alcohol use during pregnancy are associated with increased risk of miscarriage, stillbirth, and sudden infant death syndrome (SIDS); there is no consistent evidence regarding the effects of lower levels of alcohol use on these pregnancy outcomes.

Exposure to air pollution is associated with increased rates of stillbirth.

The risk for miscarriage increases by 1 percent for each cigarette smoked by the mother per day, and secondhand smoke exposure increases the risk of miscarriage by 11 percent.

Trauma and intimate partner abuse increase the risk of miscarriage. The miscarriage rate is 38.7 percent in women who experienced at least one life-threatening domestic violence event in the previous year and 13.3 percent in those who experienced non-life-threatening domestic violence in the previous year.

Multiple gestation (e.g., twins, triplets), fetal growth restriction, and placental abnormalities increase the risk of stillbirth.

WHAT CAN BE DONE

Become knowledgeable regarding risk factors for miscarriage, stillbirth, and perinatal death so that you can educate yourself.

Work to maintain good health and become educated regarding the details of positive lifestyle changes, including: a) how to initiate and maintain a regular exercise program, as approved by your doctor; b) the components of good nutrition and a healthy diet; and c) the importance of vitamin supplements with folic acid.

Educate yourself on the benefit of a folic acid supplement, as it prevents neural tube defects and may decrease the risk of spontaneous abortion and stillbirth.

Stop smoking when you find out you are pregnant and avoid alcohol during pregnancy and preconception.

Find information regarding quitting smoking and weight management programs, if applicable.

Become knowledgeable on the child welfare laws in your state to know if prenatal drug and alcohol use is considered a reportable situation.

If you or someone you know is struggling with drug use while they are pregnant refer them to seek treatment and prenatal care.

Make sure that you approach drug and alcohol abuse by pregnant clients as a health problem that needs a solution, not a legal situation; offer empowering strategies.

If you or someone you know has experienced a miscarriage, stillbirth, or perinatal death, request referral to a mental health clinician, as appropriate, for grief counseling or other psychological support.

Remember that it is important to recognize and acknowledge the emotional impact of a miscarriage or stillbirth, if you or someone you know has experienced these make sure to assess the person's needs, provide information and support and refer to mental health professional for individual, family and local support groups.

—Tanja Schub, BS, and Laura McLuckey, MSW, LCSW

FURTHER READING

Aune, D., Tonstad, S., Saugstad, O. D., & Henriksen, T. (2014). Maternal body mass index and the risk of fetal death, stillbirth, and infant death: A systematic review and meta-analysis. *Jama, 311*(15), 1536-1546. doi:10.1001/ jama.20-14.2269

Gregory, E. C. W., MacDormand, M. F., & Martin, J. A. (2014, November). Trends in fetal and perinatal mortality in the united states, 2006-2012. *ational Center for Health Statistics (NCHS)*. Retrieved from http://www.cdc.gov/nchs/data/databriefs/ db169.pdf

Holman, N., Bell, R., Murphy, H., & Maresh, M. (2014). Women with pre-gestational diabetes have a higher risk of stillbirth at all gestations after 32 weeks. *Diabetic Medicine, 31*(9), 1129-1132.

Moraitis, A. A., Wood, A. M., Fleming, M., & Smith, G. C. (2014). Birth weight percentile and the risk of term perinatal death. *Obstetrics and Gynecology, 124*(2), 274-283. doi:10.1097/ AOG.000000000000-0388

Patton, E. W., & Aronson, P. K. (2012). Abortion, spontaneous (miscarriage). In F. J. Domino (Ed.), *The 5-minute clinical consult 2012* (20th ed., pp. 4-5). Philadelphia, PA: Wolters Kluwer Health/ Lippincott Williams & Wilkins.

Pineles, B. L., Park, E., & Samet, J. M. (2014). Systematic review and meta-analysis of miscarriage and maternal exposure to tobacco smoke during pregnancy. *American Journal of Epidemiology, 179*(7), 807-823. doi:10.1093/aje/kwt334

Multiple births

CATEGORY: Biology

KEY TERMS:

chromosomes: the rod-shaped structures in the nucleus of a cell that carry genes

concordance: the condition among twins of having the same physical or psychological trait

dizygotes: fraternal twins; born from two ova separately fertilized by two sperm

embryo: the cells growing after conception until the eighth week of pregnancy

monozygotes: identical twins; born of a single ovum that divides after a single sperm fertilizes it

ovum: the egg cell released from the ovaries during ovulation

placenta: the membrane sac developed from the uterine wall that passes nutrients to the fetus through interconnected blood vessels

ultrasonography: an imaging technique that uses high-frequency sound waves to view fetuses in the womb, as well as other internal structures

zygote: a fertilized ovum before multicellular development begins

INTRODUCTION

Multiple births have historically been rare events, but the incidence is increasing with assisted reproductive technologies. The most common multiple births are twins; this occurs in approximately one of every eighty complete pregnancies. Twins can come from a single egg or from two different eggs. Triplets occur in approximately one in every eight hundred completed pregnancies. Quadruplets occur in one in every eight thousand completed pregnancies. Quintuplets occur naturally in approximately one of every eighty thousand completed pregnancies.

As the number of fetuses increases, the chances that all will survive decreases. Multiple births are most commonly combinations of twins and single eggs. By reviewing the mechanics of twin formation, greater multiples can be understood.

THE DIFFERENT TYPES OF TWINS

Two types of twins are well known: fraternal twins and identical twins. Behind these general terms, however, lies considerable variation. This variation is based on the many changes that a human ovum can undergo after it is released by the ovary, is fertilized, travels along the Fallopian tube to the uterus, and implants there to develop into an embryo. Fraternal twins are also known as dizygotic or binovular twins. In a normal menstrual cycle, only a single egg is released.

When a sperm penetrates an ovum, the fertilized egg releases a chemical that prevents other sperm from penetrating the same egg. If a second egg has been released, however, it can also be fertilized. Upon completion of fertilization, the egg is transformed into a zygote. If both zygotes succeed in attaching to the uterine walls, a twin pregnancy begins. Usually, this dual insemination occurs during a single release of semen in a single copulation, so that the embryos have the same father. Occasionally, the two eggs may be fertilized in separate copulations during the same ovulation, a phenomenon called superfecundation. It is then possible for dizygotic twins to have different fathers. This possibility seems to have long been recognized. The Greek myth of Leda and the Swan derives from such a pregnancy.

Fraternal twins have separate placentas and membranes in the womb. The placenta comprises maternal and fetal tissues interconnected by blood vessels. Nutrients pass from the mother to the fetus through the placenta. Waste products are removed from the fetus by a reverse process. Sometimes, the placentas press against each other in the womb and fuse. Having had separate placentas or one fused together, however, does not affect the nature of the twins after birth. Fraternal twins, even though they share the same birthday, are no more similar in appearance or manner than two siblings from separate births.

Identical twins are the result of different initial events. They are also called monozygotic or mon-ovular twins. Identical or look-alike twins originate when a single egg spontaneously divides after penetration by a sperm cell. Each half develops separately. The reason for this division is not known. One theory holds that sometimes the fertilized ovum does not implant in the uterus right away as is normally the case. During the delay, the chromosomes double and the zygote halves, with each half then implanting and becoming a separate embryo.

Another theory suggests that early in the pregnancy, a genetic mutation occurs in one of the cells. Later, while the embryo is still no more than a few hundred cells, the normal cells recognize the genetic difference and reject the mutant cells, much as the immune system rejects substances foreign to it. The rejected group of cells develops separately. If this theory proves to be true, identical twins must not be completely identical after all. Cases in which one identical twin has a genetic disease and the other remains healthy appear to support this theory, although mutation in one twin may occur after splitting rather than causing the splitting.

Variation sometimes appears after birth in monozygotic siblings. Twins can vary in birth weight greatly (one may weigh twice as much), develop at different rates, and die from unrelated natural causes. As a rule, however, identical twins share an overwhelming majority of traits. When two (or more) siblings share a trait, they are considered to be concordant for that trait. Typically, body structures and coloration will be

strikingly concordant. Features such as facial shape, hair texture and color, eye color, and height are typical examples of concordance. "Mirror" twins are an uncommon phenomenon. They show mirror-image symmetry in some traits.

For example, one may be left-handed while the other is righthanded. Whorls on the scalp may also occur as mirror images. In very rare cases, one mirror twin will have situs inversus: the placement of all internal organs is reversed. An individual with situs inversus will have the liver and appendix on the left side of the abdomen and the spleen on the right.

Genetic variation may account for the subtle variations in even the most concordant of twins. The internal environment of the womb also has an effect. Most identical twin fetuses share the same placenta but have different inner or chorionic sacs. They may have separate placentas (and separate chorions) depending on when the initial splitting of the zygote took place. Usually, those sharing a single placenta have separate chorions. In the rarest variation, the fetuses also share the same amnion. The degree of separation or number of barriers can influence the amount of oxygen or nutrients that each twin receives. Relatively minor differences can affect development.

A third type of twin is theoretically possible. During maturation and before becoming fertilized, the mature ovum could divide into a secondary oocyte (the cell to be fertilized) and a much smaller polar body. It is possible for the ovum to divide into roughly equal portions, both of which are viable and contain the same genetic material. If separate sperm then fertilize these ova, they would become two zygotes. Such twins would have exactly the same maternal genes, but a portion of the paternal genes would differ. They would be less identical than monozygotes but more so than dizygotes. Although this type of twinning has been described in rats and mice, no human case has been indisputably identified and reported.

A fourth variant of twinning is conjoined twins, popularly called Siamese twins. Conjoined twins share some tissue. This can range from simple joining of skin on the head or shoulders to having one heart or kidney or two torsos and a single pair of legs. Conjoined twins are identical (or monozygotic) twins created by incomplete cell division during early fetal life. The portions of cells that divide normally continue to develop in a normal fashion. The cells that did not divide completely also develop normally. The result is a portion of the body that is duplicated and a portion that is not. If the incomplete division occurred early in fetal development, the amount of shared tissue is likely to be greater than with an incomplete division that occurred later in fetal development.

About one-third of all twin births result in identical twins. The proportion of males and females is approximately equal. The incidence of identical twins remains constant throughout the world's diverse ethnic populations. Fraternal twins, however, show different proportions and distributions. About half the pairs have the same gender (with a nearly equal number of male-male and female-female pairs); about half are male-female pairs. Fraternal twin births occur most frequently among rural Nigerians (45 pairs per 1,000 births) and least frequently among Chinese and Japanese parents (4 pairs per 1,000 births). European and American rates, for both blacks and whites, are approximately halfway between these extremes.

Evidence suggests that women inherit a tendency to conceive fraternal twins from their mothers. There is little scientific evidence to support the belief that fathers possess a gene for monozygotic twins. Physiological factors can increase the likelihood of a woman having fraternal twins. Women who are tall and heavy and who have previously given birth to children have more twins than small women or those who have not been pregnant before. Women between thirty-five and forty years of age are the most likely to have twins, but the chances decrease thereafter.

Naturally occurring multiple pregnancies (triplets and more) are usually combinations of twins. Identical triplets do rarely occur, but triplets consisting of two identical and one fraternal sibling are the norm. Naturally occurring multiple births of four or more infants are almost always combinations of twins. Physicians can ascertain the status of multiple birth siblings by examining placentas and chorionic sacs.

POSSIBLE COMPLICATIONS

Multiple births create special problems for mothers. Specifically, they are more difficult to carry in the womb and to nurture through infancy than singletons. Multiples are smaller, so that vaginal deliveries have the potential to be easier. Many physicians, however, recommend birth by cesarean section to manage complications better. Most twins are born healthy, but they must be monitored carefully. As the number of fetuses increases, their size decreases. Because they are not fully mature, this increases the chances for medical problems.

Positively identifying multiple fetuses in the womb is not always an easy task, even though medical science has developed a variety of techniques. The traditional signs of considerable fetal movement, multiple heartbeats, and a large weight gain by the mother can be inaccurate and contradictory. Tests for the human chorionic gonadotropin hormone in the mother's blood or urine or alpha-fetoprotein in the blood may suggest the presence of multiple fetuses if the hormone or protein levels are unusually elevated. Nevertheless, imaging technologies provide the most reliable test.

Ultrasonography has supplanted X-rays, which declined in use because of the radiation hazard to fetuses. The images produced by ultrasonography can usually resolve multiple fetuses early in the pregnancy.

A multiple pregnancy itself strains the mother's body and is particularly subject to medical complications. Typically, a mother carrying multiple fetuses gains from 30 to 80 pounds, about twice the weight of a single pregnancy. The added weight can cause skeletal and muscular problems. The fetuses' demands on the mother's body may also worsen pre-existing medical conditions, such as heart or kidney disease. As the multiple fetuses develop, their size stretches the uterus, which can initiate early labor. For this reason, the premature birth rate is higher for multiple fetuses than for single fetuses. Twins occasionally reach full term; triplets and greater multiples do not.

Similarly, multiple pregnancies miscarry at more than three times the rate of singletons. Occasionally, one fetus will develop at the expense of the other by drawing a disproportionate amount of nutrients from the mother, a condition called twin transfusion syndrome. In cases of identical (monozygotic) twins who share a single placenta, a phenomenon known as a twin-twin transfusion can occur. When this occurs, one twin receives most of the blood, nutrients, and oxygen, in turn becoming much larger than the other twin. In some instances, the smaller twin (the donor) perishes due to lack of these vital substances. In other cases, the larger twin (the recipient) succumbs to heart failure as a result of having to pump the increased blood flow. A new surgical technique (ablation) is currently being used in the third trimester to sever the connection,

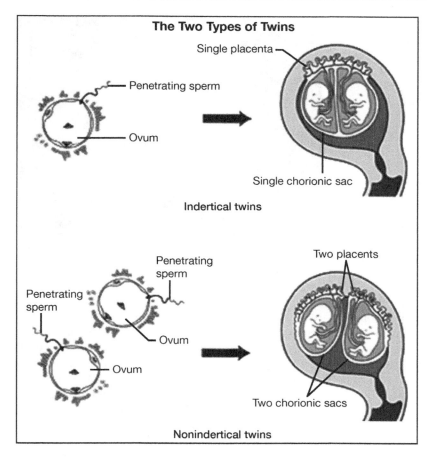

The Two Types of Twins

Single placenta

Penetrating sperm

Ovum

Single chorionic sac

Indertical twins

Penetrating sperm

Penetrating sperm

Ovum

Ovum

Two placents

Two chorionic sacs

Nonindertical twins

© *EBSCO*

stopping the twin-twin transfusion. If one fetus dies for any reason, then the mother's body may reabsorb it partially or completely, a phenomenon known as the vanishing twin. Some doctors believe that because of unobserved vanishing twins, miscarriages, and induced abortions, the number of twin conceptions has been underestimated.

Doctors carefully monitor the fetal development of multiple fetuses to ensure their health and, especially, to prepare for delivering them. Amniocentesis and genetic tests detect potential biochemical defects, genetic anomalies, and diseases. Ultrasonography allows doctors to identify defects in shape and the relative position of the fetuses in the womb.

Their position is important during labor. Normally, babies are born head-first. In multiples, one of the fetuses frequently lies crosswise or feet-first. These positions greatly lengthen and complicate

delivery, so that the second fetus runs a higher risk of dying during labor. Moreover, the mother's over distended uterus, unable to contract properly after delivery, might begin to bleed. If labor lasts too long it could result in dangerous maternal exhaustion. Because of such problems, many obstetricians recommend delivery by cesarean section-that is, by cutting a passage through the abdomen into the uterus-at the first sign of trouble to either mother or fetuses.

The prematurity and low birth weight common in multiple infants mean that many are placed on life support. Studies have found that multiple infants suffer congenital defects as much as three times more often than singletons. Identical siblings are the most likely of all to have abnormalities. Heart malformations are most common. According to some studies, closed esophagus, clubfeet, excess fingers or toes, and forms of mental retardation such as Down syndrome occur at a slightly higher rate.

Conjoined twins are relatively rare, appearing approximately once in a hundred thousand pregnancies. Most are attached at the back, or at the back of the head or neck. In an extreme rarity, one identical twin has a full set of chromosomes while the other has only the X chromosome from the mother; in this case the twin will be a female with a condition called Turner Syndrome. Therefore, identical twins will be of opposite gender if the first twin has the XY chromosomes that define a male and the other is a female with Turner Syndrome.

That multiple birth siblings develop in the same environment and from a common origin allows researchers to trace the genetic and environmental influences on human development in general. Most of this research has been conducted on twins because of the relative rarity of triplets or larger groups of siblings. The reasoning is straightforward. In the case of identical twins, either their genetic heritage (nature) or the environment (nurture) dominates in determining how they grow mentally and physically.

Researchers have tested the idea by tracking down identical twins that were separated while young, usually at birth, and reared separately. If genetics control development, then the separated twins should still look and behave similarly. If environment predominates, then separated twins should show variations in appearance and temperament.

The reported research results have been mixed. Some separated twins do not look or act any more alike than siblings born separately. Others show an uncanny degree of similarity throughout their lives-dressing the same way, marrying in the same year, having the same number of children, and dying nearly at the same time of the same disease. Their intelligence, which many scientists believe is heavily influenced by environment, nevertheless shows high concordance.

PERSPECTIVE AND PROSPECTS

Worldwide, superstitions and a strong moral overtone have traditionally accompanied multiple births. Some societies view one twin as automatically good and the other evil and treat them accordingly as they mature. Others believe twins are shameful, a sign of corruption or promiscuity in the mother. These babies might be killed at birth or separated because of it. An African curse reflects the deep suspicion that some societies have held for twins: "May you be the mother of twins." On the other hand, some nations believed that twins have divine origin or power over the elements or special talents for prophecy and telepathy.

Multiple siblings enjoy a special advantage: They are rarely lonely. Some twins even share their own private language, a phenomenon known as idioglossia. Their common development means increased requirements of time and money for their families. It also provides continuous opportunities for sharing and relying on each other. The many national and international organizations created by and for twins and other multiple birth siblings reflect their pride in their status.

Triplets have historically had a reasonable chance for survival. Before the advent of support equipment for premature babies, lung immaturity was the factor that usually determined life or death. Surfactant is a chemical that is secreted in the seventh month of pregnancy. Without surfactant, lung tissues stick together, and infants cannot breathe. Because of the combined size of all fetuses, many multiple infants

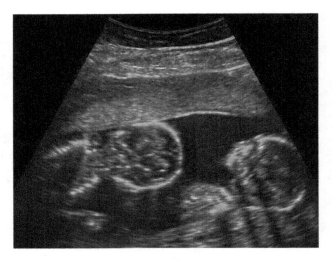

Identical twins sharing a womb. (Mikael Häggström via Wikimedia Commons)

are born before the seventh month of gestation. The Dionne quintuplets, who were born in the 1930s, were unusual in that for the first time in history, all five survived into adulthood. Modern support technology has helped several sets of sextuplets (six infants) to survive. In 1997, the same technology permitted all the McCaughey sextuplets (seven infants) to survive. This was the first time such an event had occurred. Incidentally, the chances of naturally conceiving sextuplets are one in eight to ten million conceptions. In 2009, controversy erupted when Nadya Suleman gave birth to octuplets (eight infants), all of whom survived. A fertility doctor (who later had his medical license revoked for this procedure) had implanted eight embryos into Suleman, a single mother who already had six children conceived through artificial insemination.

Advances in the field of assisted reproduction have increased the odds of multiple pregnancies. Women who have difficulty conceiving are initially treated with drugs that cause more than one egg to be released during ovulation. This increases the chance of pregnancy but also increases the chance of carrying multiple fetuses. Couples who seek medical assistance to achieve pregnancy routinely use fertility drugs. A woman will have several eggs or zygotes implanted to improve the odds of successfully initiating a pregnancy. The result of this approach is an increased number of multiple births. In 1988, twelve fetuses, which were miscarried, resulted from a fertility drug. Artificially induced pregnancies have posed ethical dilemmas for many who believe that scientists should not manipulate human biological processes.

Multiple births raise other moral and ethical questions as well. Genetic tests can now identify potential fetal defects in the womb early enough that surgeons can remove a defective fetus without harming the healthy fetus, a procedure called selective birth, selective abortion, or selective feticide. Those who hold abortions to be immoral have reservations about selective feticide even when the defective fetus has little chance of surviving and may threaten the lives of the remaining healthy fetuses. That selective feticide may be used simply because a mother does not want to rear more than one child has caused far greater concern. Since the procedure is tricky to perform and can result in the death of all fetuses, most doctors find selective feticide for nonmedical reasons to be ethically indefensible.

Twin births bear witness to the successes of modern health care. In the United States, incidents of multiple births, both fraternal and identical, have increased since the 1970s, and more multiples are surviving to adulthood. Fertility drugs may account for part of the increase, as does the trend among American women to delay childbearing until their thirties or forties. Nevertheless, prenatal care, better diet, improvements in neonatal intensive care, and education about pregnancy and birth are as important.

IMPACT ON WOMEN

Recent research has suggested that mothers of multiples have a 43% higher chance of experiencing a Perinatal Mood Disorder (Postpartum Depression/ Anxiety/ Psychosis). Based on all the above discussed information, many factors may lead to the increased struggles. Starting in pregnancy, carrying multiples can cause increased stress on the mother's body and health concerns in pregnancy, and higher emotional stress coming from increased likelihood of pregnancy loss, premature birth and possible birth or health risks for the infant. Increased likelihood of caesarian section, medical intervention at birth and Neonatal Intensive Care Unit (NICU) stay for infants may also lead to postpartum struggles. Lastly, caring for more than one infant at a time creates greater difficulty, lack of sleep, and more trouble seeking support and help (due to difficulty managing multiple babies at once and the increased cost of childcare). Support groups for mothers with multiples are common. Women may find these very helpful in learning to manage the increased demand on her and connect with other mothers who also have multiples.

—*Roger Smith, Ph.D., and L. Fleming Fallon, Jr., M.D., Ph.D., M.P.H.; Updated by Samar Aslam, M.D. and Kimberly Ortiz-Hartman, Psy.D., LMFT*

FOR FURTHER INFORMATION

Cunningham, F. Gary, et al., eds. *Williams Obstetrics.* 24th ed. New York: McGraw-Hill, 2014.

Luke, Barbara, and Tamara Eberliein. *What to Expect When You're Expecting Twins, Triplets, or Quads: A Complete Resource.* 3rd ed. New York: HarperCollins, 2013.

Malmstrom, Patricia Maxwell, and Janet Poland. *The Art of Parenting Twins.* New York: Random House International, 2000.

Malone, J.A., S.P. Margevicius, and E.G. Damato. "Multiple Gestation: Side Effects of Antepartum Bed Rest." *Biological Research in Nursing,* vol. 8, no. 2, 2006, 115-128.

Noble, Elizabeth. *Having Twins and More: A Parent's Guide to Pregnancy, Birth, and Early Childhood.* 3rd ed. New York: Houghton- Mifflin, 2003.

Rand, L., K.A. Eddleman, and J. Stone. "Long-Term Outcomes in Multiple Gestations." *Clinical Perinatology,* vol. 32, no. 2, 2005, 495-513

Multiple sclerosis

CATEGORY: Disease/Disorder

KEY TERMS:

autoimmunity: a condition in which the immune system fails to recognize its own tissues as "self" and mounts an immune response against its own cells

demyelination: the destruction of myelin

disseminated sclerosis: another name for multiple sclerosis (MS)

myelin: a fatty substance wrapping nerves as a sheath that accelerates electric impulse propagation

primary progressive MS: the most aggressive form of MS, characterized by the absence of remissions and continual decline *relapsing-remitting MS:* the most common form of MS, characterized by unpredictable attacks (relapses) followed by periods free of symptoms (remission)

remyelination: the repair of myelin

sclerosis: a process of hardening of tissues

secondary progressive MS: a form that occurs in patients who initially had relapsing-remitting MS and transition to a more aggressive MS

CAUSES AND SYMPTOMS

Multiple sclerosis (MS) is a chronic and disabling disease of the nervous system. Symptoms can range from mild (limb numbness) to severe (paralysis and loss of vision). Disease progression and severity are difficult to predict, with substantial person-to-person variation.

Multiple sclerosis is caused by degeneration of the nervous system. A fatty substance called myelin surrounds and protects many nerve fibers of the brain and spinal cord. Myelin is important because it speeds up signals propagating along the nerve fibers. In MS, the body attacks its own tissues through an autoimmune reaction, and a breakdown in the myelin layer along the nerves ensues. When any part of the myelin sheathing is destroyed, nerve impulses to and from the brain are slowed, distorted, or interrupted. The disease is termed "multiple" because it affects many areas of the brain. Scleroids are hardened, scarred patches that form over the damaged areas of myelin.

The initial symptoms of MS may include tingling, numbness, slurred speech, blurred or double vision, loss of coordination, and muscle weakness. Later manifestations include unusual fatigue, muscle tightness, loss of bowel and bladder control, sexual dysfunction, and paralysis. Cognitive dysfunction can also occur, affecting short-term memory, abstract reasoning, verbal fluency, and speed of information processing. All the mental and physical symptoms listed may come or go ("relapse and remit") in any combination. The symptoms may also vary from mild to severe in intensity throughout the course of the disease.

The symptoms of MS not only vary from person to person but also may periodically vary within the same person. This makes the prognosis of the disease difficult to foresee. Although the general course of the disease may be anticipated, the symptoms and their severity seem to be quite unpredictable in most individuals. In the "classic" course of MS, as time progresses, chronic problems gradually accumulate over many years, slowly worsening the sufferer's quality of life.

The typical pattern of MS (accounting for 85% of cases) is marked by active periods of the disease during which the nerves are being ravaged by the immune system. These periods are called attacks, relapses, or exacerbations. The active periods of the disease are followed by calm periods called remissions. The cycle of attack and remission will differ from sufferer to sufferer. Most people with MS have what is known as the relapsing-remitting form of the disease. They suffer many attacks over time, and these attacks occur unpredictably; the attacks are then followed by complete remission which may last months or years. Again, the injuries may take many years to accumulate to complete disability.

The more aggressive form of the disease is primary progressive MS. In this type of MS, the disease follows a rapid course that steadily worsens from its first onset. Although there are still attacks and partial remission, the attacks are quite severe and occur more regularly in time. Typically presenting as gait dysfunction, this form of MS may result in full paralysis within three to five years. Secondary progressive MS occurs in patients who initially have the relapsing-remitting type and later develop the more aggressive form.

Both genetic and environmental factors have been implicated in inducing the onset of MS. Viral infection has been suggested as a cause, but no single virus has ever been shown to be associated with MS. Although infections such as the common cold, flu, and gastroenteritis increase the risk of relapse, flu vaccination is safe in patients with MS. Risk may be conferred by exposure to a specific environment during adolescence, but that environment and the genetic risk factors have not yet been characterized. The support for the genetic component comes from identical twin studies. The likelihood of MS in the second identical twin, when the first twin has MS, is 30 percent. Researchers Sharon Lynch and John Rose suggested that certain racial and geographic populations are less susceptible than others to the disease. MS is uncommon in Japanese people as well as among American Indians. The disease is more common among Northern European Caucasians as well as among North Americans of higher latitudes.

There is an additional sexual dimorphism in the epidemiology of MS; the disease is found more frequently in women, by a ratio of nearly 3:1. Women of child-bearing age are particularly prone to developing the disease. Interestingly, pregnancy has shown to have a potential protective effect in the setting of MS; some sources cite a 70% decrease in relapse rates during the third trimester of pregnancy. This is presumed to be largely hormonally-mediated, through hormones such as estriol and estradiol.

Still, certain considerations must be taken into account. For one, women in the postpartum period are at higher risk of relapse, particularly in those with a history of active relapsing MS shortly before pregnancy. Moreover, women with highly active MS must take extra precautions with regard to family planning, pregnancy, and breastfeeding, should they choose to become pregnant. For instance, certain treatment options may reduce fertility and viability, as well as compromising the health of the child during breastfeeding. Prospective parents may also consider that the risk of MS in a child increases ten-fold (though at a fairly low 2-3%) when one of the parents has MS. Nevertheless, given the growing abundance of treatment options, most women with MS who wish to have children can safely become pregnant and breastfeed their children without significant concern over harming themselves or their children.

The disease usually begins its first manifestations in late adolescence (around age eighteen) to early middle age (around age thirty-five). It is not clear how the interaction between the genetics of the sufferer and the environment may trigger onset. The progressive type of MS is more common over the age of forty, so those with late-onset MS often have the quickest deterioration of motor function. The reason that an older age predisposes someone to primary chronic progressive MS is still not clear.

Studies by Swiss researcher Avinoam Safran have shown that occasionally MS manifests after the age of fifty. This condition has been named late-onset multiple sclerosis. Late-onset MS is not rare, with nearly 10 percent of MS patients demonstrating their first symptom after the age of fifty. This type of MS often goes undetected by physicians, who do not expect to see MS in the aged.

TREATMENT AND THERAPY

Scientists have been encouraged by advancements in MS diagnosis using the MRI brain scan. In 2002 they announced that these scans appear to detect damage around nerve fibers in patients with possible early signs of MS. This detection helps doctors predict those who will eventually develop MS and how severe one's experience with the disease might be. In turn, this allows for prompt initiation of a drug regimen. New research has found that putting patients on MS drugs at the first sign of nerve inflammation drastically slows the chances of developing MS within a few years, though most will eventually still develop the disease.

While there is no tried-and-true cure for MS, there are many effective disease-modifying therapies, of which ten are approved for MS relapses. In most cases, steroidal drugs are used to treat relapses or attacks of the disease. Corticotropin was the first steroidal immunosuppressant of widespread use in MS treatment. The primary effect of the drug is to shorten the duration of an attack, though it does not appear to reduce the severity of the attack. Although it is still used with patients who respond well to it, corticotropin has been supplanted by other drugs. Methylprednisolone is one such immunosuppressant and steroid. It has been shown to control the inflammation that accompanies demyelination. These steroids seem to work by sealing leaking blood vessels in the brain and reducing the responsiveness of the white blood cells of the immune system, such that they cannot attack the myelin as easily. Certain steroids (such as Solu-Medrol) appear to be safer options for treating MS relapses in pregnancy (particularly during the second and third trimesters). Intravenous immunoglobulins similarly represent a safer treatment option for pregnant or nursing mothers.

Several federally approved drugs can slow the rate of attacks. *Avonex*, *Rebif*, and *Betaseron* are preparations of interferon- (proteins regulating the immune system). Interferon injections (given subcutaneously or intramuscularly) can reduce clinical relapse rates of MS by 30-35 percent. *Copaxone* (glatiramer acetate, also marketed as a generic drug called *Glatopa*) is a mixture of small synthetic peptides (injected subcutaneously) that protects myelin. Glatiramer acetate reduces clinical relapse rates by 30 percent. It is the best tolerated of all the available drugs to treat MS and is also safe for pregnant women.

The most effective drug for treating MS is natalizumab (*Tysabri*). Natalizumab is a monoclonal antibody that is also used to treat Crohn disease, and prevents immune cells from crossing the blood-brain barrier and attacking myelinated axons. This drug is given by infusion every four weeks and reduce clinical relapse rates by 68 percent. Unfortunately, natalizumab can cause a severe neurological condition called progressive multifocal leukoencephalopathy (PML) in some patients. It appears that some patients are infected by a virus called the JC virus that our immune system normally keeps at bay. Administration of natalizumab can potentially activate the JC virus, which may lead to a potentially fatal infection in about 0.2 percent of patients. However, prescreening patients for JC virus infections can greatly lower the risk of PML.

Alemtuzumab (*Lemtrada*) is a humanized monoclonal antibody against the lymphocyte cell surface protein CD52 that depletes CD52-positive lymphocytes. This drug is infused once a day for 5 successive days, and then not again until a year later, which makes this drug highly convenient. Alemtuzumab reduces clinical relapse rates by 50-55 percent. Unfortunately, alemtuzumab increases the risk of cancer and autoimmune conditions, and is usually reserved for patients who have failed other drugs.

Oral agents to treat MS include fingolimod (*Gilenya*), which prevents the egress of lymphocytes from lymph nodes. It can reduce clinical relapse rates by 55 percent, but it can cause the signs of liver damage and increases the tendency to acquire severe viral and fungal infections. Another oral drug for MS is dimethyl fumarate (*Tecfidera*), which blocks cytokine production by lymphocytes and reduces clinical relapse rates by 50 percent. This drug can also decrease white blood cell counts and induce the signs of liver damage. Patients on dimethyl fumarate have also suffered from PML. Once again, prescreening the patient is important before starting them on this drug. The third oral drug for MS is teriflunomide (*Aubagio*), which reduces white blood cell proliferation. This drug is not as effective as either fingolimod or dimethyl fumarate and is also poorly tolerated. None of the oral drugs for MS are safe for pregnant women.

Although these drugs do not stop MS entirely, they limit the level of myelin destruction, as observed in magnetic resonance imaging (MRI) scans of the brain. *Avonex* slows the rate of progression to disability.

In the News:
New Drug Treatments for Multiple Sclerosis

The neurodegeneration that characterizes multiple sclerosis (MS) results from the destruction of myelin that surrounds and protects nerves by the immune system. Myelin-specific T cells are required for this attack. Corticosteroids have been used as therapy because of their known immunosuppressive properties. They have proved to be effective against the symptoms of MS episodes, but they have serious side effects and can be taken only for short times. Because they suppress the immune system in a general, nonspecific way, they inhibit not only the destruction of myelin but also the body's ability to fight infection. This problem has led to the deaths of some MS patients. In addition, corticosteroids do not delay the long-term progression of MS. More recently, interferon-_ has been used to treat MS. Although interferon-_ therapy can be given for long periods and has been shown to reduce the frequency of relapses and to slow the progression of the disease, why it works is not known. One theory is that it reduces inflammation. New drugs on the horizon aim to stop the progression of MS and eliminate all relapses. The theory behind them is that a drug should targeted to inhibit only the components of the immune system that destroy myelin. Such drugs, unlike the drugs currently available, would be attacking the underlying cause of MS, rather than its symptoms, and would be expected to cause few or no side effects.

Two of these new drugs, *Tovaxin* from Opexa Therapeutics and a not-yet named candidate, now called RTL1000, from Artielle Immuno-Therapeutics, act by specifically inactivating the patient's own myelin-specific T cells, while not interacting with other immune system cells. Myelin-specific T cells are required for the destruction of myelin, and when a large number of them are inactivated, myelin destruction slows down. Another approach is being developed by Immune Response. Their drug *NeuroVax* acts by specifically stimulating patients' cells that down-regulate myelin-specific T cells. Clinical trials of *NeuroVax* are underway.

—*Lorraine Lica, Ph.D.*

During the 1990s, in a study supported by the National Institutes of Health and conducted at the Mayo Clinic, plasma exchange, also called plasmapheresis, was proven to be an effective treatment for certain patients suffering from severe symptoms of multiple sclerosis who were not responsive to conventional methods of treatment. Plasma exchange involves the removal of the patient's blood; the elimination of the plasma-containing antibodies that target myelin, which is then replaced by a fluid with similar properties, usually containing albumin; and its subsequent return to the patient. This procedure has been successfully used for treatment of other autoimmune diseases such as myasthenia gravis and Guillain-Barré syndrome. Plasmapheresis is typically reserved for severe, acute attacks that are unresponsive to high-dose steroids. Since the vast majority (90 percent) of people experiencing acute attacks respond well to the standard steroid treatment, plasma exchange would be considered a treatment alternative only for the approximately 10 percent who do not.

As additional therapy, patients with MS should participate in a regular exercise program. Exercise is vital to the maintenance of functional ability in MS sufferers. It strengthens muscles, benefits gait, and generally improves coordination. The best type of exercise is aquatic in nature. Sufferers are often heat-intolerant, and participation in a regular aerobic program would be unpleasant. Also, aquatic exercise is a low-impact activity that puts less stress on chronically sore muscles. Exercise programs also encourage socialization of patients and engender peer support. The efficacy of aquatic exercise has been tested and confirmed in recent study of female participants; in this randomized controlled trial, significant improvements in fatigue severity, perception of physical fatigue, and quality of life were reported.

Perspective and Prospects

The first written report of MS was published in 1400 when the famed Dutch skater Lydwina of Schieden was diagnosed. It was recognized initially as a wasting disease of unknown origin. The disease was described clinically by Jean-Martin Charcot in 1877. Charcot initially characterized the clinical signs and symptoms of MS. He recognized that the disease affects the nervous system and tried many remedies, without success. In 1890, the cause of MS was thought to be suppression of sweat; the treatment was electrical stimulation and bed rest. At the time, life expectancy for a sufferer was five years after diagnosis. By 1910, MS was thought to be caused by toxins in the blood, and purgatives were alleged the best treatment. In the 1930s, poor circulation was believed to cause MS, and blood-thinning agents became the treatment of choice. In the 1950s through the 1970s, MS was thought to be caused by severe allergies; treatments included antihistamines. Not until the 1980s was the basis of MS understood and effective treatment developed.

By the early twenty-first century, it was estimated that thousands of people had this disorder of the brain and spinal cord, which causes disruption in the smooth flow of electrical messages from brain and nerves to the body. The progress of the disease is slow and may take decades to achieve complete nerve degeneration and paralysis. Although often considered a disease of youth, MS has the potential to become an increasing problem in aging populations. More cases of late-onset MS have come to light in individuals over forty years of age, including such celebrities as comedian Richard Pryor, entertainer Annette Funicello, and talk-show host Montel Williams. Several novel therapies that have been under investigation are sphingosine receptor modulator (fingolimod), vitamin D, inosine (*Axosine*), and antimicrobial agents. Various combinations of drugs are also being examined. Current clinical trials are likely to reveal treatment strategies that will further facilitate controlling of the symptoms and progression of MS.

—James J. Campanella, Ph.D.;
Updated by W. Michael Zawada, Ph.D.
and Ariel Choi, ScB

For Further Information

"About MS." *National Multiple Sclerosis Society*, 2013.

Alan, Rick, and Rimas Lukas. "Multiple Sclerosis-Adult." *Health Library*, Sept. 30, 2012.

Alan, Rick, Rebecca Stahl, and Kari Kassir. "Multiple Sclerosis- Child." *Health Library*, June 6, 2012.

"Drugs for Multiple Sclerosis." *The Medical Letter on Drugs and Therapeutics*, vol. 58, no. 1496, 2016, 71-74.

Holmoy, T., and Oivind Torkildsen. "Family planning, pregnancy and breastfeeding in multiple sclerosis." *Tidsskriftet*. vol. 136, no. 20, 2016, 1726-1729.

Kalb, Rosalind, ed. *Multiple Sclerosis: The Questions You Have, the Answers You Need*. 5th ed. New York: Demos Vermande, 2012.

Kooshiar, H., et al. "Fatigue and quality of life of women with multiple sclerosis: a randomized controlled clinical trial." *The Journal of Sports Medicine and Physical Fitness*, vol. 55, no. 6, 2015, 668-674.

"Multiple Sclerosis." *MedlinePlus*, May 7, 2013.

"NINDS Multiple Sclerosis Information Page." *National Institute of Neurological Disorders and Stroke*, Aug. 14, 2012.

Wingerchuk, D.M., and J.L. Carter. "Multiple sclerosis: current and emerging disease-modifying therapies and treatment strategies." *Mayo Clinic Proceedings*, vol. 89, no. 2, 2014, 225-240.

Myomectomy

CATEGORY: Procedure

KEY TERMS:

hysteroscope: a thin, lighted tube that is inserted into the vagina to examine the cervix and inside of the uterus

laproscopy: a surgical diagnostic procedure used to examine the organs inside the abdomen

uterine fibroid: benign smooth muscle tumors of the uterus

vasoconstrictive: the narrowing of the blood vessels resulting from contraction of the muscular wall of the vessels

INDICATIONS AND PROCEDURES

The most common indication for a myomectomy is the need to remove a symptomatic uterine fibroid. In many cases, these fibroids are large (greater than 8 centimeters).A myomectomy is chosen over a hysterectomy (removal of the uterus) if the patient desires future childbearing and if there is no evidence of malignancy of the uterus. A myomectomy can be performed using abdominal, laparoscopic, vaginal, or hysteroscopic approaches. The choice of approach depends on the location and size of the fibroids, as well as on the experience of the surgeon.

The most common type is abdominal myomectomy. This procedure is performed in the operating room with the patient under general anesthesia. The abdomen is incised and entry into the pelvic cavity is obtained. The uterus is then identified and inspected for fibroids. Some surgeons apply a tourniquet to the uterine arteries for hemostasis. A vasoconstrictive agent is injected into the myometrium surrounding the fibroid to minimize blood loss. The myometrium over the fibroid is then incised, and the fibroid is dissected out. Finally, the myometrial defect is closed with a suture to stop blood flow. In patients desiring fertility, care is taken to minimize entry into the endometrial cavity, as the procedure may increase the risk of uterine rupture with pregnancy.

In laparoscopic and vaginal myomectomies, access to the fibroids is obtained using endoscopic instruments and through an incision in the vagina, respectively. In hysteroscopic myomectomies, access to fibroids in the endometrial cavity is obtained using a hysteroscope inserted through the cervical canal. The hysteroscope holds an instrument that shaves away fibroids in the endometrial cavity.

USES AND COMPLICATIONS

The primary use of myomectomy is the relief of symptoms caused by fibroids. These symptoms can be any of the following: pressure sensation, pelvic pain, dyspareunia (painful intercourse), menorrhagia (excessive menstruation), dysmenorrhea (painful menstruation), urinary urgency or frequency, urinary incontinence, and constipation.

The short-term risks of abdominal myomectomies are the same as those for most pelvic surgeries. These risks are small but include infection, damage to internal organs such as the bowel or bladder, blood loss requiring transfusion, and complications from anesthesia. Long-term consequences include an increased risk of uterine rupture with future pregnancy, the recurrence of fibroid growth, and pelvic adhesion (scar tissue) formation. Laparoscopic myomectomies are less invasive than abdominal myomectomies, but the same short-term and long-term risks are present. Hysteroscopic myomectomies carry less risks than abdominal procedures, since no incision is made on the abdomen and there is no entry into the pelvic cavity, but the risks unique to hysteroscopy exist, such as uterine perforation and fluid overload.

—*Anne Lynn S. Chang, M.D.*

FOR FURTHER INFORMATION

DeCherney, Alan H., et al. *Current Diagnosis and Treatment: Obstetrics and Gynecology, 12ᵗʰ ed.,*. New York: McGraw-Hill Medical, 2019.

Falcone, T., and M. A. Bedaiwy. "Minimally Invasive Management of Uterine Fibroids." *Current Opinion in Obstetrics and Gynecology*, vol. 14, no. 4, 2002, 401–07.

Hoffman, Barbara L., et al. *Williams Gynecology*. New York: McGraw-Hill Medical, 2012.

Rock, John A., and Howard W. Jones III, eds. *Te Linde's Operative Gynecology*. 10th ed. Philadelphia: Wolters Kluwer/Lippincott Williams & Wilkins, 2008.

Stenchever, Morton A., et al. *Comprehensive Gynecology*. 4th ed. St. Louis, Mo.: Mosby/Elsevier, 2006.

Tulandi, Togas, ed. *Uterine Fibroids: Embolization and Other Treatments*. New York: Cambridge University Press, 2003.

Youngkin, Ellis Quinn, et al. *Women's Health: A Primary Care Clinical Guide*. Boston: Pearson, 2013.

N

Nails

CATEGORY: Anatomy

KEY TERMS:

cuticle: cutaneous or skin tissue that surrounds the nail plate on its proximal sides and provides a protective barrier to the nail bed; it is attached to the proximal nail fold and to the nail plate

hyponychium: cutaneous tissue underlying the free nail at its point of separation from the nail bed; structurally similar to the cuticle

keratinocytes: matrix basal epithelial cells that differentiate, fill with keratin, and form the dead horny substance making up the nail plate

lunula: a white, crescent-shaped area at the end of the proximal nail fold that marks the end of the nail matrix and is the site of nail growth

nail plate: The keratinized structure that serves as the visible nail unit extending from the skin outwards.

nail bed: The soft tissue directly beneath the nail unit that acts as a barrier between the nail plate and underlying soft tissue and osseous structures

onychomycosis: common nail disorder in which fungal organisms invade the nail bed causing progressive changes in the color, texture, and structure of the nail

STRUCTURE AND FUNCTIONS

Nails function to protect fingers and toes against bumps and trauma, and can help with grabbing as was their historic function as a vestigial claw. They also aid in fine touch and skillful manipulation of small objects. Nails can be important social communicators of beauty and sexuality and hence are the focus of a major cosmetic industry in many cultures.

Biologically, nails are characterized as plates of tightly packed, hard epidermal cells filled with a protein called keratin. Nails are normally seen on the dorsal side (the side opposite the palm or sole) of all fingers and toes. The anatomy of the normal nail consists of a nail plate, proximal nail fold, nail bed, matrix, and hyponychium. These components are epithelial-derived structures, like skin and hair, which emerge from the live germinative zone of the epidermis. In nails, these cells differentiate and form a keratinized layer.

The nail plate is a relatively hard, transparent, and flattened structure that is rectangular in shape. It rests on the underlying nail bed and typically extends beyond the bed as an unattached, free-growing edge reaching toward or beyond the tip of the finger or toe. On the fingers, the thickness of the plate in adults increases from about 0.7 millimeters at the proximal edge to about 1.6 millimeters at the distal edge. The terminal tip thickness varies considerably between people and age groups. Normally, a pinkish nail bed is seen through the transparent nail plate. Frequently in the thumbnail and sometimes in the other fingernails, a whitish, semilunar-shaped structure called the lunula is seen that extends under the proximal nail fold. The borders of the nail plate are covered by skin structures: two lateral folds and a single proximal fold.

The proximal nail fold is the cutaneous, or skin, structure that is in continuity with the visible border of the nail and overlies part of the nail root. The ventral side (underside) of the proximal nail fold provides physical protection to the germinative zone of the nail and aids in the physical attachment of the nail plate. About a fourth of the total surface area of the nail plate is located under the proximal fold. The cuticle is a layer of epidermis extending from the proximal nail fold and attached to the dorsal side of the nail. The cuticle functions to provide a physical barrier against microbes and chemical irritants, which may otherwise enter the nail fold and affect nail production or cause infection.

The nail bed is the portion of the digit upon which the nail rests. The nail bed is highly vascular, with numerous capillaries. It consists of epithelial tissue and extends from the lunula to the point where the bed separates from the nail. A series of fine longitudinal folds in the nail bed corresponds to the undersurface structure of the nail which enhances the adherence of the nail plate to the nail bed.

The nail matrix is generally considered the most proximal part of the nail unit and is bordered by the surrounding nail folds. On the distal end, it is bordered by the distal margin of the lunula. The nail matrix epithelium cells consist predominantly of keratinocytes in both a basal and a spinous layer. Melanocytes and langerhans cells are intermingled with keratinocytes. It is within the matrix that the germinating center of nail growth is found. Basal epithelial cells increase in number through mitosis, or cell division, and differentiate into keratinocytes. These are epithelial cells filled with keratin protein. These keratinocytes condense their cytoplasm, lose their nucleus, and form flat cells. As further cell division occurs in the nail matrix, more distal keratinocytes are pushed out to form the nail plate. The hyponychium consists of epidermis tissue that underlies the edge of the nail plate and extends from the nail bed to the distal groove. It functions to provide a defense against entry of bacteria under the free edge of the nail plate. Excessively vigorous cleaning may damage the hyponychium and allow for bacteria to enter more readily under the nail plate.

The turnover rate of matrix cells determines the growth rate of the nail. This rate varies with age, environmental conditions, nutritional status, and the specific digit. The growth rate proportionately increases with the length of the digit; thus, the middle finger nail grows the fastest while the growth rate in the little finger is the slowest. Fingernails grow three times as rapidly as toenails. The growth rate is more rapid in the winter than in the summer. Furthermore, nails grow faster in young children than in adults. It takes about six months for a fingernail to completely grow in. Male nails grow faster than female nails, and nails on the dominant hand grow faster than those on the other hand.

If nails are protected and untrimmed, they can grow to considerable lengths. Such long nails were prized by the wealthy classes in imperial Chinese culture as an indication of status. The practice of painting toenails red may have originated in the Ottoman Seraglio, where it was a signal of menstrual status.

Nails continue to grow throughout life without a resting phase. Contrary to folk belief, nails cease growing when an individual dies. The matrix cells stop dividing soon after death, and thus the nail bed cannot grow longer. The appearance of nail growth after death is due to a retraction or shrinkage of nail matrix tissue, resulting in the apparent lengthening of the nail plate.

Professional grooming of the finger nails for both men and women is termed a manicure. Manicure procedures include cutting the nails according to fashion standards to improve their cosmetic appearance. A pedicure is the term applied to grooming the toenails. Typically, the nails are first soaked in a soapy solution to soften the nail plate and to remove dirt and debris. It is often fashionable to trim the nails to a delicate arc whose apex is at the middle of the fingertip. The corners of the nail are typically filed. While this shape is attractive in creating the illusion of longer, slender fingers, it heightens the probability of nail plate fractures, hangnails, or ingrown nails. The cuticle, considered to be unattractive by manicurists, is typically minimized, partially removed, or traumatized. This may increase the incidence of fungal invasion and disease. Most of the problems associated with a manicure or pedicure arise from excessive manipulation of the cuticle.

Nail polish typically consists of pigments suspended in a volatile solvent that also contains a film-forming agent. When the polish is applied to the finger, a covering film develops over the nail. The film is permeable to oxygen, which allows gas exchange to occur between the atmosphere and the nail plate. Resins and plasticizers are added to the polish to increase the flexibility of the film and to minimize chipping. The variety in nail polish color is due to the addition of coloring agents. Deep red nail polishes have been found to cause a temporary yellowish staining of the nail plate.

Nail adornments are sometimes used as well. Frequently, small nail jewels or ribbons are applied to the fingernails immediately before the nail polish dries, allowing the decoration to adhere. People can develop contact dermatitis from application of different accessories due to the presence of nickel and are advised to use gold or nickel-free jewels as an alternative. Artificial nail tips made of plastic may be glued to the nail tip to create the illusion of an elongated natural nail tip. The gluing may cause nail problems, since a portion of the natural nail is occluded by the glue. This occlusion inhibits oxygen transfer and stresses the nail plate. Frequently, the nail may thin and be unable to support its own weight after the plastic tip is removed, resulting in easily cracked or pitted nails.

DISORDERS AND DISEASES

Nails are useful indicators of skin disease and internal disorders. An abnormally pigmented band in the nail may indicate a malignant melanoma. A yellow nail may indicate psoriasis or a fungal infection. Pulmonary disease or smoking may also cause yellow or brownish nails. Antimalarial drugs may cause the nail to darken in appearance. Frequently, psoriasis causes pitting of nails and an acceleration in their growth rate.

Chronic chest disease or a cyanotic congenital heart disorder is frequently associated with club-shaped deformity of the nail plate. Beau's lines, which are transverse depressions in the nail plates, are associated with illnesses such as coronary thrombosis, pneumonia, and severe injuries. Drug treatment may cause nail breakdown, destruction, or complete shedding of the nail plate.

An unexplained aspect of nail physiology is its relationship to lung physiology. Hippocrates first described a connection between lung parenchymal disorders and an edema in the connective tissue beneath the lunula that results in clubbing. The relationship has long been recognized, but the causal link is remains unknown.

An ingrown nail results when a deformed nail grows improperly into the skin or when the skin around the nails engulfs part of the nail. Wearing narrow, tight shoes can cause or worsen this pathology. Initially, symptoms may be slight or mild, but may increase in pain over time. The affected area becomes reddish and, if not treated, may become infected. If infected, the area becomes swollen, inflamed, and painful. Treatment involves trimming away the nail from the infected area to allow the inflammation to recede.

Clubbing is a disorder characterized by a bulb-like enlargement of the nail with increased horizontal and longitudinal curvatures. Clubbing involves both fingers and toes and commonly begins at puberty. The disorder may be genetically inherited or acquired. Clubbed nails often have a spongy feel when pressure is placed on the proximal nail fold. This is due to the expanded soft tissue that underlies the nail. Acquired clubbing is often associated with another clinical pathology, most commonly pulmonary or cardiovascular disease. It may also be associated with gastrointestinal inflammatory disease or cystic fibrosis.

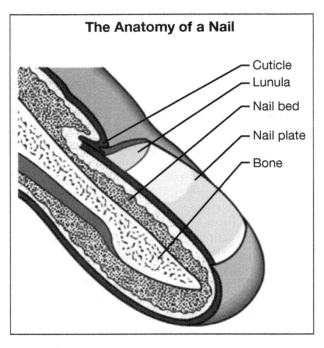

The Anatomy of a Nail

- Cuticle
- Lunula
- Nail bed
- Nail plate
- Bone

© EBSCO

A fungal infection is the cause of onychomycosis, which is the most common nail disorder. About half of all nail problems can be linked to this disease, which affects as many as 15 to 20 percent of people in North America. It is uncommon in children and more frequently seen in aged adults. There is a genetic component related to people's predispositions for contracting onychomycosis, but the direct link has not been determined. Several fungi may cause onychomycosis, although most belong to the group called dermatophytes. The fungi are present in soil, and indirect transmission to humans frequently occurs through public swimming pools, shower floors, and dirt. Some yeasts and molds can also cause this clinical condition. In addition, this infection is associated with athlete's foot infection and often relates to the same causative organism. Typically, this condition is found in toenails. The presence of the fungus is further evidenced by scaling on the plantar surface of the foot, where it is often harbored.

In onychomycosis, the fungal organism invades the nail bed and nail matrix, causing a progressive change in the color, texture, and structure of the nail. The nail may turn different colors, thicken, and even

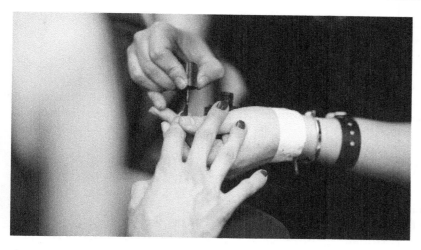

A woman getting her nails painted by a beautician. (Kris Atomic via Wikimedia Commons)

detach from the nail bed. Debris from the infected nail often collects under its free edge. If untreated, the pathology may involve the entire nail plate, and rarely will the nail unit spontaneously heal itself. An infected nail can also lead to adjacent fungal infection of the surrounding soft tissues.

Since several organisms may induce the pathology, effective treatment depends on matching the curative with the causal agent. Topically applied antifungals are seldom effective because most cannot penetrate the nail-plate barrier to reach the causal organism. Systemically (orally) administered antifungal therapy frequently uses one of several drugs such as terbinafine, griseofulvin, thiabendazole, or ketoconazole. These drugs are generally effective in halting further invasion of the fungus. Once administered, normal nail will eventually push out the infected nail and will appear to "clear" in a proximal-to-distal direction.

More than seventy tumors have been associated with parts of the nail. They may originate from the epidermis, dermis, subcutaneous tissues, or bone, and may be found in the nail bed, nail matrix, hyponychium, or nail fold. The tumors may take various forms, including warts, erosion or ulceration of the nail bed, malignant neoplasms from underlying melanocytes, benign fibromas of the connective tissue, or squamous cell carcinomas. Diagnosis usually is made by taking a biopsy of the affected area. Treatment typically involves surgical removal of the tumor with it's directly underlying tissue.

PERSPECTIVE AND PROSPECTS

The earliest cellular growth leading to nail formation can be seen histologically at eight weeks of human development, at the end of the embryonic period. Microscopically, the cells forming the proximal edge of the nail fold and the future matrix can be distinguished at this time. The earliest gross anatomical appearance of nails is seen on the finger digit surface at about nine weeks of development during the early fetal stages. By eleven weeks of age, the nail fold is seen clearly on the hand digits of the fetus. By twenty weeks of age, the fetus shows a nail plate and bed as well as a proximal cuticle. By thirty-two weeks, the third trimester of pregnancy, adult-type nail structures are visible in the fetus, including a nail plate, matrix, and bed.

Aging results in changes and disorders in nails. When people get older, the color, contour, growth rate, surface texture, and thickness of the nail plate change. Some disorders are more prevalent with aging, such as brittle nails, splitting or fissuring of the nail plate, and an increased risk of infection. Aged nails appear dull and opaque, with their color varying from yellow to gray. Frequently in older persons, the lunula is decreased in size or is absent. The growth rate of nails decreases with aging. The most rapid period of growth is during the first thirty years, after which the rate steadily declines. Nail plate thickness frequently increases with advanced age, in combination with discoloration and loss of translucency of the nail plate.

For many years, blood and urine specimens have been used to detect and measure body concentrations of therapeutic drugs or drugs of abuse. During the past decade, alternative biological specimens such as nails and hair have been frequently used as the basis for drug detection. The basis for drug detection in nail clippings is that the dividing epidermal cells that form the nail plate also incorporate drugs from the systemic circulation. The subsequent cornification of these cells traps the drug within the forming nail plate. Drug-detection methods involve taking a sample of nail and extracting drug molecules via immunochemical or chromatographic techniques. These techniques are extremely sensitive and capable of detecting minute quantities of drug; as little as ten milligrams of nail sample is required to detect the presence of a drug. Twenty-first century drug-screening methods have detected amphetamines and cocaine in nail samples. Using nail samples for drug analysis and screening provides a long-term measure of drug exposure that may potentially represent months or even years of drug use. Furthermore, nail samples are relatively easy to collect and involve a noninvasive procedure.

Modern medicine in the early twenty-first century still lacks adequate descriptive science as well as understanding of the molecular mechanisms that control nail development and growth. To date, the specific genes or gene products that initiate nail growth have yet to be identified. The molecular basis for brittle nails, clubbing, and other nail pathologies is not known, only hypothesized. Molecular control of nail pathology remains understudied and will likely see advances within the near future as medical interests concerning nail physiology are piqued.

—*Roman J. Miller, PhD*
Updated by Zachary Sax, DPM

FOR FURTHER INFORMATION

myVMC. (2019). "What are nails made of? Nail anatomy information." myVMC, 2019, https://www.myvmc.com/anatomy/nails/. Accessed 2 Feb. 2019.

Baran, R., et al., editors. *Baran and Dawber's Diseases of the Nails and Their Management.* 3d ed. Malden, Mass.: Blackwell Science, 2001.

Du Vivier, Anthony. *Atlas of Clinical Dermatology.* 4th ed. Edinburgh: Churchill Livingstone, 2012.

Hordinsky, Maria K., Marty E. Sawaya, and Richard K. Scher, editors. *Atlas of Hair and Nails.* Philadelphia: Churchill Livingstone, 2000.

Mix, Godfrey F. *The Salon Professional's Guide to Foot Care.* Albany: Milady SalonOvations, 1999.

Porter, Robert S., et al., eds. *The Merck Manual Home Health Handbook.* Whitehouse Station, N.J.: Merck Research Laboratories, 2009.

Standring, Susan, et al., editors. *Gray's Anatomy.* 40th ed. New York: Churchill Livingstone/Elsevier, 2008.

Zaias, Nardo. *The Nail in Health and Disease.* 2d ed. Norwalk, Conn.: Appleton & Lange, 1992.

Nail removal

CATEGORY: Procedure

KEY TERMS:

cauterization: burning the skin or flesh of a wound with a heated instrument or caustic substance, typically to stop bleeding or prevent the wound from becoming infected

tourniquet: a device for stopping the flow of blood through a vein or artery, typically by compressing a limb with a cord or tight bandage

INDICATIONS AND PROCEDURES

Invasive nail procedures should be performed by a physician in either an office or operative setting.

The patient's foot or hand is first cleansed with antiseptic solution and draped. Sterile techniques are used throughout the procedure. Patients undergoing partial or total nail removal require adequate anesthesia, which is usually done through a digital block via local anesthetic. This serves to numb the entire digit. This procedure is performed at the base of the digit with lidocaine or a similar anesthetic to numb the entire finger or toe. A tourniquet may be applied to minimize bleeding and enhance anesthesia. An instrument is then used to separate the nail from the nail bed, with care to preserve healthy soft tissue deep to the nail plate. In a complete removal, the nail is gently pulled away from the nail bed once fully separated. In a partial removal, scissors or specialized instrumentation are used to cut the desired amount of nail away from the intact nail. Once an adequate amount of nail has been removed, the physician may choose to chemically destroy the nail matrix if clinically indicated. This will prevent future growth, and as such, is often done to a small portion of the nail matrix to allow for a cosmetically anatomic nail unit.

Following the procedure, a topical antibiotic ointment may be applied with gauze along with a light compressive dressing. The patient may also receive a special shoe or flip-flop to prevent direct pressure to the toe, although. When a toenail is removed, patients may walk immediately after the procedure and resume any activity as tolerated. Local wound care instructions are given, and if the procedure is performed secondary to an infected digit, oral antibiotics may be ordered. Daily cleansing with soap and water along with dressing changes for approximately two weeks are advised. The procedure usually takes approximately fifteen minutes to complete.

USES AND COMPLICATIONS

Partial nail removal or trimming may also be performed in diabetic patients or those unable to perform routine nail care. Fungal infections cannot be cured with nail removal alone, though in severe or painful cases, the procedure may be performed in conjunction with the administration of antifungal agents.

Pain is one of the most common complications of the procedure, especially if the digit was already infected. Bacterial infection may also occur after the procedure without proper wound care. Adequate compression or cautery usually stops any continued bleeding after the procedure, although slight bleeding can occur following the procedure and is remedies with regular dressing changes. Patients must also be warned that the nail may not grow back with the same shape prior to removal. Nails should be cut straight across without curvature to prevent any ingrown nail recurrence. If done properly, partial or complete nail removal can be a very helpful procedure for painful or misshapen nails.

—*Jeffrey R. Bytomski, D.O.*
Updated by Zachary Sax, DPM

FOR FURTHER INFORMATION

Mayoclinic.org. (2019). *Ingrown toenails - Diagnosis and treatment - Mayo Clinic.* https://www.mayoclinic.org/diseases-conditions/ingrown-toenails/diagnosis-treatment/drc-20355908. Accessed March 15, 2019.

Clark, Robert E., and Whitney D. Tope. "Nail Surgery." Roland G. Wheeland, editor, *Cutaneous Surgery,* Philadelphia: W. B. Saunders, 1994.

"Nail Diseases." *MedlinePlus,* April 11, 2013.

Woods, Michael, et al. "Ingrown Toenail Removal." *Health Library,* May 2, 2013.

Zuber, Thomas J. "Ingrown Toenail Removal." *American Family Physician,* vol. 65, no. 12, 2002, 2547–2554.

Neonatal brachial plexus palsy

CATEGORY: Disease/Disorder

Also known as: Erb's palsy, obstetric brachial plexus palsy, birth brachial plexus palsy

KEY TERMS:

brachial plexus: complex of nerves that carry motor and sensory function to the arm

contractures: permanent shorting of muscles or joints

Erb's palsy: stereotyped clinical presentation of neonatal brachial plexus palsy resulting from injury to the C5, C6, and sometimes C7 spinal nerve roots

Horner's syndrome: ptosis (eyelid drooping), miosis (abnormal constriction of the pupil of the eye), and anhydrosis (decreased sweating on the face)

incidence: the rate at which a certain event occurs or the number of new cases of a specific disorder occurring during a certain period in a population at risk

pan-plexopathy: a form of neonatal brachial plexus palsy comprising of injury to all of the spinal nerve roots manifesting as a flaccid arm

perinatal period: the period immediately before and after birth, commencing at 20 weeks of gestation and ending at 28 weeks after birth (140 days total)

range of motion: movement of a joint from full flexion to full extension

shoulder dystocia: diagnosed when the delivery of the fetal head is not followed by the emergence of the shoulder due to impaction of the fetus' shoulder in the birth canal

CAUSES AND SYMPTOMS

Children with neonatal brachial plexus palsy (NBPP) may have a weak or paralyzed arm, and their passive range of motion is greater than their active range of motion. NBPP becomes evident early in life and usually results from stretching or compression of the nerves of the brachial plexus during the perinatal period. NBPP occurs with an incidence of 1.5 cases per 1000 live births, with or without shoulder dystocia at the time of both vaginal and cesarean delivery. Risk factors for NBPP include abnormal positioning of the fetus, labor abnormalities, artificial labor induction, large fetus, and shoulder dystocia. However, except for shoulder dystocia, none of these risk factors are statistically significant clinical predictors for the occurrence of NBPP.

Compression or stretching of the nerves of the brachial plexus can occur during development in the uterus or during the descent and emergence of the fetus from the uterus and pelvis with maternal pushing and naturally expulsive forces. Biomechanically, nerve injury can result from forces applied by clinicians, or natural physical events that move the fetus from the uterus through the birth canal and out of the mother's pelvis. No one force or factor seems to be solely responsible for NBPP, but the available data do suggest that the occurrence of NBPP may be a multifactorial event.

The brachial plexus is a very complex structure that connects the spinal nerves in the neck to their terminal branches in the arm and is divided into 5 zones: (1) C5 through T1 spinal nerve roots; (2) upper, middle, and lower trunks; (3) anterior and posterior divisions of each trunk; (4) lateral, posterior, and medial cords; and (5) terminal branches. These nerves carry the signals necessary for the normal movement and sensation in the entire arm. The brachial plexus is analogous to a set of intersecting highways with overpasses, underpasses, and multiple merging traffic intersections, with several roads leading into (analogous to the spinal nerve roots) and out of (analogous to the terminal branches) the intersections. However, for simplicity, the nerve roots can be indexed to the muscles in the following fashion: C5-shoulder movement, C6-elbow flexion, C7-elbow extension, C8/T1-hand and finger movement.

Not all cases of NBPP are the same, and the symptoms may be radically different depending on which parts of the brachial plexus are injured. The intricate intersecting nature of the brachial plexus implies that thousands of potentially different palsies can ensue, but in reality, only a few variations actually occur. The most useful classification scheme for clinical presentation of NBPP is the Narakas Grade system that represents the extent of the spinal nerve root injury: only C5 and C6 nerve roots are injured in Grade 1, C5, C6, C7 nerve roots in Grade 2, and C5 through T1 injured in Grade 3 (without Horner's syndrome) and Grade 4 (with Horner's syndrome). When this classification system is used in 2-4-week-old affected babies, it may guide the prognosis for spontaneous recovery, since up to 90 percent of the patients with Grade 1 NBPP regain functional use of the affected arm, but less than 5 percent of the patients with Grade 4 NBPP regain functional use without medical and/or surgical intervention.

Other classification systems are based on the clinical manifestations of NBPP. Erb's palsy, the most common type of NBPP, is synonymous with an "upper" plexus palsy that specifically results from damage to C5, C6, and sometimes C7 spinal nerve roots. Patients with Erb's palsy present a "waiter's tip" posture when their affected arm is pulled toward the midline of the body, an internally rotated shoulder, flexed wrist, extended fingers that result from loss of both shoulder control and elbow bending. Contrastingly, the extremely rare Klumpke's palsy is synonymous with a "lower" plexus palsy characterized by a flaccid hand attached to an otherwise active arm. Total plexus palsy or pan-plexopathy is equivalent to Narakas Grade 3 and 4 and is recognized by loss of total function of the arm.

TREATMENT AND THERAPY

Lack of normal arm movement observed during the perinatal period warrants confirmation of the diagnosis of NBPP by a specialist. Possible skeletal injuries or fractures should be confirmed by clinical and radiographic evaluation since these injuries may preclude early occupational/physical therapy. Immobilization of the arm is not recommended except in the case of skeletal injuries.

With regard to the specific motor function of the affected arm, the treating physician assesses the passive and active range of motion of the affected arm. Available assessment scales of motor function in NBPP are used to determine the extent and severity of nerve injury, to prognosticate potential functional recovery, and to guide and assess the outcomes from further treatment. Traditional scales focus only upon the affected arm, but more recently, assessment methods are focusing upon the overall function of the child. Supplementing the physical examination with electro-diagnostic / electro-myographic (EMG) and radiographic (magnetic resonance imaging, MRI) findings are helpful to decide whether surgical nerve reconstruction will be beneficial.

Early referral of those babies with severe or extensive NBPP to interdisciplinary specialty clinics can improve overall functional outcomes as the baby

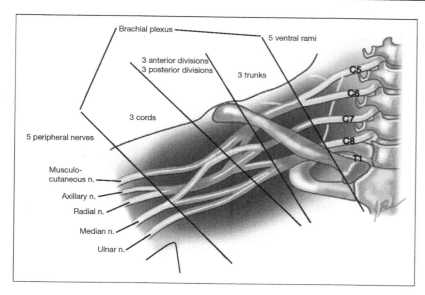

Nerves of the brachial plexus, cervical and thoracic spinal nerves and the major nerves of the upper arm.
(http://www.backpain-guide.com)

grows. Regardless of the need for surgical intervention, rehabilitation management is critical. Occupational/physical therapy to maintain the normal passive range of motion in all upper extremity joints (especially shoulder external rotation and forearm rotation) is necessary to facilitate successful functional recovery. Parents and caregivers should consider themselves to be the patient's primary therapist by performing range of motion exercises regularly, with multimedia assistance if available (e.g., during every diaper change). Reinforced use of the affected arm while constraining the normal arm (similar to patching a lazy eye) can aid the child's recognition of the arm and strengthen the arm through increased arm use during age-appropriate activities. Normal childhood developmental milestones must be encouraged, including crawling. Splinting may be used during sleep to avoid contractures or to protect floppy joints. As the child grows, recreational activities like swimming, dance, sports, and potentially therapist-designed video game platforms can help to sustain the goals of formal occupational/physical therapy.

For NBPP patients who do not recover with conservative management, surgical nerve reconstruction may be an option, usually occurring between 3-9 months of age. Although the indications and timing for nerve reconstruction have not been absolutely established, most practitioners agree that babies with the extensive total brachial plexus palsy and those with the severe Erb's palsy will benefit from nerve surgery. The goal of nerve reconstruction is not to regain a normal arm, but surgical intervention is a step towards a functional arm with adequate movement, if not power. Nerve repair using autologous nerve graft and/or nerve transfer (using a good nerve to re-innervate an injured one) constitute the primary options for reconstructing the function of the brachial plexus. As nerve repair and transfer rely upon regrowth of the normal portions of the nerve through the residual pathways after injured nerve is cleared away (Wallerian degeneration), and as this nerve regeneration is very slow, the ultimate functional outcome from nerve reconstruction surgery may not be apparent for 1-3 years.

Toddlers and older children with incomplete recovery following neurosurgical or conservative treatment may have functional limitations because of residual muscle weakness and soft tissue contractures, especially around the shoulder and elbow. MRI imaging can guide the decision to pursue orthopedic intervention. Internal rotation contracture of the shoulder is most common and can be associated with progressive shoulder joint deformity and instability. Indications for surgical intervention include persistent internal rotation contracture despite aggressive nonsurgical therapy, progressive joint deformity, and obvious joint dislocation. Surgical options include muscle lengthening combined with tendon transfers, corrective bone surgery (osteotomies), and open or arthroscopic reduction of the shoulder joint.

For children with residual elbow, forearm, and hand problems, secondary procedures by a hand surgeon may be appropriate. These procedures include soft tissue releases, joint fusions, muscle transfers, and corrective osteotomies. The usual age for secondary reconstruction of the elbow/forearm function is 4-6 years of age, and for wrist/hand function is 6-13 years of age.

Information on Neonatal Brachial Plexus Palsy

Causes: Damage to the nerves of the brachial plexus during or after birth

Symptoms: One of the arms does not move normally

Duration: Depends on the severity; some children recover completely, others only partially, while some are permanently affected

Treatments: Physical and occupational therapy, exercises, orthopedic or neural surgery

For all surgical interventions, the most important factor in producing the optimal result is a cooperative child with intense investment from assertive parents/caretakers. The parents must understand the objectives of the surgical procedure and work hard with their children in postoperative rehabilitation- and maintenance of function by being their children's primary therapists. Surgery alone without subsequent rehabilitation management and therapy is unlikely to yield the desired outcome.

PERSPECTIVE AND PROSPECTS

Overall, the majority of infants with NBPP have a good prognosis for recovering adequate functional use of the affected arm-with rehabilitation management and therapy, supplemented with surgical intervention when and where appropriate and so desired by the patient and parents/caretakers. Early occupational/ physical therapy can support the spontaneous recovery of function and minimize consequent musculoskeletal comorbidities along with more efficient recovery of function after surgery. Despite the similar incidence of NBPP to cerebral palsy, public awareness of this perinatal disorder and its lifelong implications (medical and psychosocial) for the more extensively/severely affected children are significantly lacking.

Similarly, published research studies regarding NBPP number only a fraction of that regarding cerebral palsy. Therefore, current efforts exist not only to find new medical treatment techniques but also to increase awareness, to address and improve the quality of life for patients with NBPP via traditional and recent technology-assisted modalities. Early referral to an interdisciplinary specialty brachial plexus clinic can avail the patient of the most current treatment paradigms to achieve the optimal outcome.

—*Lynda J. S. Yang, M.D., Ph.D., F.A.A.N.S.*
Updated by Christine Gamble, M.D.

FOR FURTHER INFORMATION

Bowerson, M., V. S. Nelson, and L.J. Yang. "Diaphragmatic Paralysis Associated with Neonatal Brachial Plexus Palsy." *Pediatric Neurology* vol. 42, no. 3, 2010, 234-236. Case study of a NBPP baby whose diaphragm was also paralyzed.

Chung, Kevin C., Lynda J.-S. Yang, and John E. McGillicuddy, editors. *Practical Management of Pediatric and Adult Brachial Plexus Palsies*. London: Elsevier, 2011. Extensive overview of the medical and surgical techniques for managing disorders of the brachial plexus. Presents a multidisciplinary approach to pediatric brachial plexus palsy treatment and rehabilitation, obstetric considerations, and other timely topics in the field (includes DVD).

Mehta, S.H., and B. Gonik. "Neonatal Brachial Plexus Injury: Obstetrical Factors and Neonatal Management." *Journal of Pediatric Rehabilitation Medicine* vol. 4, no. 2, 2011, 113-118. A review of the potential causes of and risk factors for NBPP.

Murphy, K.M., et al. "An Assessment of the Compliance and Utility of a Home Exercise DVD for Caregivers of Children and Adolescents with Brachial Plexus Palsy: A Pilot Study." *PM & R* vol. 4, no. 3, 2012, 190-197. Small, initial study of the efficacy of home exercises for NBPP children.

Piatt, J.H., Jr. "Birth Injuries of the Brachial Plexus." *Clinical Perinatology* vol. 32, no. 1, 2005, 39-59. Excellent summary of the classification of various types of NBPP.

Squitieri, L.. et al. "Medical Decision-Making among Adolescents with Neonatal Brachial Plexus Palsy and Their Families: A Qualitative Study." *Plastic and Reconstructive Surgery* vol. 131, no. 6, 2013, 880e-887e. A study that examines why patients make particular treatment choices and stresses the need for proper patient education.

Sutcliffe, Trenna, L. "Brachial Plexus Injury in the Newborn." *NeoReviews*, vol. 8, no. 6, 2007, e239-e246. A summary of the types of injuries that occur during birth that can damage the nerve of the brachial plexus and affect the functionality of the upper limbs.

Neonatology

CATEGORY: Specialty

KEY TERMS:

congenital disorders: abnormalities present at birth that occurred during fetal development as a result of genetic errors, exposure to toxins and microorganisms, or maternal illness

incubator: in the nursery, a Plexiglas unit that encloses the premature or sick infant to allow strict temperature regulation

intrauterine growth retardation: the condition of infants who are born significantly smaller than the standard for the number of weeks that they have spent in the uterus

neonatal intensive care unit: a hospital nursery with advanced equipment and specially trained staff to maintain the vital functions of sick newborns and to monitor their progress closely

neonatal period: the first month of life; derived from the Greek *neo* (meaning "new") and the Latin *natum* (meaning "birth")

prematurity: strictly defined, birth before a full-term pregnancy (thirty-eight weeks); more commonly associated with birth before thirty-five weeks

respirator: a machine that inflates and deflates the lungs, imitating normal breathing; connected to the patient through a tube placed into the windpipe (endotracheal tube)

respiratory distress syndrome: a life-threatening illness primarily of premature infants; immature lungs lack surfactant, a vital substance that keeps the tiny air sacs (alveoli) from collapsing upon exhalation

SCIENCE AND PROFESSION

Neonatology has grown dramatically since its beginnings in the late 1960s, and neonatologists have become an integral part of the obstetric-pediatric team at major medical centers throughout the world. In addition to being cared for by physicians who specialize in neonatology, some neonatal infants, in particular those who are critically ill or premature, are cared for by nurse practitioners with the specialty certification of neonatal nurse practitioner (NNP). In large part because of an ever-expanding technological base and marked advances in scientific research, these health care professionals have changed the outlook for premature and sick newborns.

As a subspecialty of pediatrics, neonatology is concerned with the most critical time of transition and adjustment—the first four weeks of life, or the neonatal period—whether the infant is healthy (a normal birth) or sick (as a result of genetic problems, obstetric complications, or medical illness). By the early 1970s, it became increasingly clear to health administrators that hospitals throughout the United States had varying abilities to care for medical and pediatric cases requiring the most sophisticated staff and equipment. Consequently, they developed a system that designated hospitals as either level I (small, community hospitals), level II (larger hospitals), or level III (major regional medical centers, also called tertiary care centers). It was in the last group that the most advanced neonatal care could be delivered. In these major centers, there are two types of nurseries, separating the normal healthy infant from the sick or high-risk infant: the routine nursery and the neonatal intensive care unit (NICU).

Routine nurseries are the temporary home of the vast majority of newborns. The services of the neonatologist are rarely needed here, and the general pediatrician or family practitioner observes and examines the infant for twenty-four to forty-eight hours to be sure that it has made a smooth transition from intrauterine to extrauterine life. These babies soon leave the hospital for their homes. Those neonates with minor problems arising from multiple births, difficult deliveries, mild prematurity, and minor illness are easily managed by a primary care physician in consultation with a neonatologist, perhaps at another hospital. It is in the neonatal intensive care unit, however, that the most difficult situations present themselves. Here several teams of pediatric subspecialists—surgeons, cardiologists, anesthesiologists, and highly trained nurses, along with many other health professionals—are led by a neonatologist, who coordinates the team's efforts. These newborns have life threatening conditions, often as a result of extreme prematurity (more than six weeks earlier than the expected date of delivery), major birth defects (genetic or developmental), severe illness (such as overwhelming infections), or being born to drug or alcohol-addicted mothers. They require the most advanced technological and medical interventions, often to sustain life artificially until the underlying problem is corrected. It is in this setting that the most dramatic successes of neonatology are found.

After hours of being inside a forcefully contracting uterus and sustaining the stress of passing through a narrow birth canal, the newborn emerges into a dry, cold, and hostile environment. The umbilical cord, which has provided oxygen and nutrients, is clamped and cut; the fluid-filled lungs must now exchange air instead, and the respiratory center of the infant's brain begins a lifetime of spontaneous breathing, usually heralded by crying. The vast majority of neonates make this extraordinary adjustment to extrauterine life without difficulty.

At one minute and again at five minutes, the newborn is evaluated and scored on five physical signs: heart rate, breathing, muscle tone, reflexes, and skin tone. The healthy infant is vigorously moving, crying, and pink regardless of race. These Apgar scores, named for neonatology pioneer Virginia Apgar, evaluate the need for immediate resuscitation. A brief physical examination follows, which can identify other life-threatening abnormalities.

It is essential to remember that the medical history of a neonate is in fact the medical and obstetric history of its mother, and seemingly normal infants may develop problems shortly after birth. Risk factors include very young or middle-aged mothers; difficult deliveries; babies with Rh-negative blood types; mothers with diabetes mellitus, kidney disease, or heart disease; and concurrent infections in either the mother or the baby. Anticipating these problems of the healthy newborn by using the Apgar scores and the results of the physical examination allows the proper assignment of the infant to the nursery or NICU.

The NICU is a daunting place containing high-tech equipment, a tangle of wires and tubes, the sounds of beeps and alarms, and tiny, fragile infants. All this technology serves two simple purposes: to monitor vital functions and to sustain malfunctioning or nonfunctioning organ systems. Looked at individually, however, the machines and attachments become much more understandable. The incubator, perhaps the most common device, maintains a warm, moist environment of constant temperature at 37 degrees Celsius (98.6 degrees Fahrenheit). Small portholes with rubber gloves allow people to touch the child safely. Generally, the infants will have small electrodes taped on their chests, connected to video monitors that record the heart and breathing rates and that will sound alarms if significant deviations occur. These monitors will also record blood pressure through an arm or thigh cuff. To ensure immediate access to the blood, for delivering medications and taking blood for testing, catheters (plastic tubes) are placed into larger arteries or veins near the umbilicus, neck, or thigh (in adults, intravenous access is found in the arms).

The remaining equipment is used for the very serious business of life support, in particular the support of the respiratory system. Maintaining adequate oxygenation is critical and can be accomplished in several ways, depending on the baby's needs. The least stressful are tubes placed in the nostrils or a face mask, but these methods require that breathing be spontaneous although inadequate. More often, unfortunately, neonates with the types of problems that bring them to an intensive care unit cannot breathe on their own. In these cases, a tube must be connected from the artificial respirator into the windpipe (the endotracheal tube). Warm, moistened, oxygen rich air is delivered under pressure and removed from the lungs rhythmically to simulate breathing. Tranquilizers and paralytic agents are used to calm and immobilize the infant. Sick or premature infants are also generally unable to feed or nurse naturally, by mouth. Again, several methods of feeding can be employed, depending on the problems and the length of time that such feedings will be needed. For the first few days, simple solutions of water, sugar, and protein can be given through the intravenous catheters. These lines, because of the very small, fragile blood vessels of the newborn, are seldom able to carry more complex solutions. A second method, known as gavage feeding, employs tubing that is inserted through the nose directly into the stomach. Through that tube, infant formula (water, sugar, protein, fat, vitamins, and minerals) and, if available, breast milk can be given.

As the underlying problems are resolved, the infant is slowly weaned, first feeding orally and then breathing naturally. Next, the infant will be placed in an open crib, and gradually the tangled web of tubes and wires will clear. With approval from the neonatologist, the baby is transferred to the routine nursery, a transitional home until discharge from the hospital is advisable.

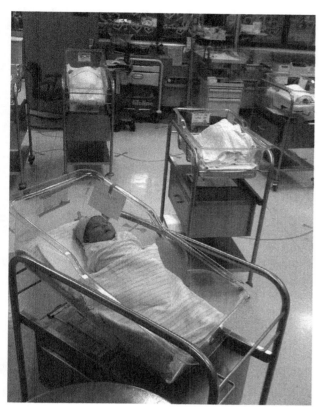

A neonatal ward where nurses can monitor the health of the babies. (Wikimedia Commons)

DIAGNOSTIC AND TREATMENT TECHNIQUES

Neonatology has amassed an enormous body of knowledge about normal neonatal anatomy and physiology, disease processes, and, most important, how to manage the wide variety of complications that can occur. Specific treatment protocols have been developed that are practiced uniformly in all neonatal intensive care units. Short-term stays (twenty-four to forty-eight hours) are meant to observe and monitor the infant with respiratory distress at birth that required immediate intervention. Long-term stays, lasting from several weeks to months, are the case for the sickest newborns, most commonly those with severe prematurity and low birth weight (less than 1,500 grams), respiratory distress syndrome (also known as hyaline membrane disease), congenital defects, and drug or alcohol addictions.

Infants born prematurely make up the major proportion of all infants at high risk for disability and death, and each passing decade has seen younger and younger babies being kept alive. While many maternal factors can lead to preterm delivery, often no explanation can be found. The main problem of prematurity lies in the functional and structural immaturity of vital organs. Weak sucking, swallowing, and coughing reflexes lead to an inability to feed and to the danger of choking. Lungs that lack surfactant, a substance that coats the millions of tiny air sacs (alveoli) in each lung to keep them from collapsing and sticking together after air is exhaled, cause severe breathing difficulty as the infant struggles to reinflate the lungs. When premature delivery is inevitable but not immediate, lung maturity can be increased by administration of steroids to the mother. An immature immune system cannot protect the newborn from the many viruses, bacteria, and other microorganisms that exist. Inadequate metabolism causes low body temperature and inadequate use of food or medications. Neurological immaturity can lead to mental retardation, blindness, and deafness.

Aggressive management of the preterm baby begins in the delivery room, with close cooperation between the obstetrician and the neonatologist. Severely preterm infants, some born after only twenty weeks of pregnancy, require immediate respiratory and cardiac support. Placement of the endotracheal tube, assisted ventilation with a handheld bag, and delicate chest compressions similar to the cardiopulmonary resuscitation (CPR) performed on adults to stimulate the heartbeat are each accomplished quickly. Once the respiratory and circulatory systems have been stabilized, excess fluid will be suctioned, while a brief physical examination is performed to note any abnormalities that require immediate attention. As soon as transport is considered safe, the newborn is sent to the NICU. If the infant has been delivered at a small community hospital, this may involve ambulance or even helicopter transport to the nearest tertiary care center.

Once in the unit, the neonate will be placed in an incubator and attached to video monitors that record heart rate, breathing, and blood pressure. The endotracheal tube can now be attached to the respirator machine, and intravenous or intra-arterial catheters will be placed to allow the fluid and medication infusions and the blood drawing for the battery of tests that the neonatologist requires. Feeding methods can be set up as soon as the infant has stabilized. Shortly after delivery, the premature newborn has a flurry of activity about it and is surrounded by the most sophisticated equipment and staff available. Supporting the immature organs becomes the first priority, although the ethical issues of saving very sick infants must soon be addressed as complications begin to occur. Nearly 15 percent of surviving preterm infants whose birth weights were less than 2,000 grams have serious physical and mental disabilities after discharge. The majority, however, grow to lead normal, healthy lives.

Congenital defects are common, and it is estimated that the majority of miscarriages are a direct result of congenital defects that are incompatible with life. Many infants that do survive development and delivery die shortly after birth despite the most sophisticated and heroic attempts to intervene. The causes of such defects are arbitrarily assigned to two broad categories, although a combination of these factors is the most likely explanation: genetic errors (such as breaks, doubling, and mutations) and environmental insults (such as chemicals, drugs, viruses, radiation, and malnutrition). In the United States, among the most common birth defects that require immediate intervention are heart problems, spina bifida (an open spine), and tracheoesophageal fistulas and esophageal atresias (wrongly connected or incomplete wind and food pipes).

The birth of a malformed infant is rarely expected, and the neonatologist's team plays a key role in its survival. Congenital heart disease is the most prevalent life-threatening defect. During development in utero, the umbilical cord supplies the necessary oxygen; it is not until birth, when that lifeline is cut, that the neonate's circulatory and respiratory systems acquire full responsibility. At delivery, all may appear normal, and the one-minute Apgar score may be high. Several minutes later, however, the pink skin color may begin to darken to a purplish blue (cyanosis), indicating that insufficient oxygen is being extracted from the air. Immediately, the infant receives rescue breathing from the bag mask. Upon admission to the neonatal unit, the source of the cyanosis must be determined. A chest x-ray may provide significant information about the anatomy of the heart and lungs, but special tests are usually needed to pinpoint the problem. Catheters that are threaded from neck or leg vessels into the heart can reveal the pressure and oxygen content of each chamber in the heart and across its four valves. Echocardiograms, video pictures similar to sonograms generated by sound waves passing through the chest, enhance the data provided by the x-rays and catheterizations, and a diagnosis is made. Based on the physical signs and symptoms of the newborn, a treatment plan is devised.

Because of the nature of congenital defects and structural abnormalities, their correction generally requires surgery. Openings between the heart's chambers (septal defects), valves that are too narrow or do not close properly, and blood vessels that leave or enter the heart incorrectly are all common defects treated by the pediatric heart surgeon. Because of the delicacy of the operation and the vulnerability of the newborn, surgery may be postponed until the baby is larger and stronger while it is provided with supplemental oxygen and nutrients. The risk of such operations is high, and depending on the degree of abnormality, several operations may be required. Another group of infants who have benefited from advances in neonatology are those born to drug-addicted women. The lives of these infants are often complicated by congenital defects and life-threatening withdrawal symptoms.

For example, heroin-addicted babies are quite small, are extremely irritable and hyperactive, and develop tremors, vomiting, diarrhea, and seizures. The newborn must be carefully monitored in the unit, and sedatives and anti-seizure medications are given, sometimes for as long as six weeks. Cocaine and its derivatives frequently cause premature labor, fetal death, and maternal hemorrhaging during delivery. Infants that do survive often have serious congenital defects and suffer withdrawal symptoms. The risk of acquired immunodeficiency syndrome (AIDS) adds another dimension to an already complicated picture.

PERSPECTIVE AND PROSPECTS

Throughout human history, maternal and neonatal deaths have been staggering in number. Ignorance and unsanitary conditions frequently resulted in uterine hemorrhaging and overwhelming infection, killing both mother and baby. Highly inaccurate records at the beginning of the twentieth century in New York City show maternal death averaging 2 percent; in fact, the rate was probably greater, since most births occurred at home. Neonatal deaths from respiratory failure, congenital defects, prematurity, and infection loom large in these medical records. The expansion of medical, obstetric, and pediatric knowledge and technology that began after World War II has dramatically lowered maternal and infant mortality. It should not be forgotten, however, that non-industrialized nations, the majority in the world, remain devastated by the neonatal problems that have plagued civilization for thousands of years.

Ironically, the problems associated with neonatology in Western nations are now at the other end of the spectrum: saving and prolonging life beyond what is natural or "reasonable." As neonatology advanced scientifically and technically, saving life took precedence over ethical issues. The famous and poignant story of Baby Doe in the early 1980s illustrates the dilemmas that occur daily in neonatal intensive care units. Baby Doe was a six-pound, full-term male born with Down syndrome and severe congenital defects of the heart, trachea, and esophagus. These malformations were deemed surgically correctable, although the underlying problem of Down syndrome, a disease characterized by intellectual disabilities and particular facial and body features, would remain. The parents did not agree to any operations and requested that all treatment be withheld. Baby Doe was given only medication for sedation and died within a few days. The case was later related by the attending physician in a letter to *The New England Journal of Medicine*, sparking enormous controversy. On July 5, 1983, a law was passed in effect stating that all newborns with disabilities, no matter how seriously afflicted, should receive all possible life-sustaining treatment, unless it is unequivocally clear that imminent death is inevitable or that the risks of treatment cannot be justified by its benefit. The legislators believed that Baby Doe had been allowed to die because of his underlying condition of Down syndrome.

Since then, attorneys, ethicists, juries, and courts have used the example of Baby Doe, and the law that grew from it, to interpret many cases that have come to light. Life-and death decisions are made on a daily basis in the neonatal care unit. They are always difficult, but they usually remain a private matter between the parents and the neonatologist. These cases become public matters, however, when the family disagrees with the medical staff. Then the question of what is in the best interest of the child is compounded by who will pay for the treatments and who will care for the baby after it is discharged.

Such ethical dilemmas will continue as expertise and technology grow. A multitude of questions, previously relegated to philosophy and religion, will arise, and the benefits of saving a life will have to be weighed against its quality and the resources necessary to maintain it.

—*Connie Rizzo, M.D., Ph.D.;*
Updated by Alexander Sandra, M.D.

FOR FURTHER INFORMATION

Behrman, Richard E., Robert M. Kliegman, and Hal B. Jenson, editors. *Nelson Textbook of Pediatrics.* 18th ed. Philadelphia: Saunders/ Elsevier, 2007.

Bradford, Nikki. *Your Premature Baby: The First Five Years.* Toronto, Ont.: Firefly Books, 2003.

Crisp, Stuart, and Jo Rainbow, editors. *Emergencies in Paediatrics and Neonatology.* 2d ed. Oxford: Oxford University Press, 2013.

MacDonald, Mhairi G., Mary M. K. Seshia, and Martha D. Mullett, editors. *Avery's Neonatology: Pathophysiology and Management of the Newborn.* 6th ed. Philadelphia: Lippincott Williams & Wilkins, 2005.

Martin, Richard J., Avroy A. Fanaroff, and Michele C. Walsh, editors. *Fanaroff and Martin's Neonatal-Perinatal Medicine: Diseases of the Fetus and Infant.* 2 vols. 8th ed. Philadelphia: Mosby/Elsevier, 2006.

Meeks, Maggie, Maggie Hallsworth, and Helen Yeo, editors. *Nursing the Neonate.* 2d ed. Malden: Wiley-Blackwell, 2013.

Moore, Keith L., and T. V. N. Persaud. *The Developing Human.* 8th ed. Philadelphia: Saunders/Elsevier, 2008.

Ruhlman, Michael. *Walk on Water: Inside an Elite Pediatric Surgery Unit.* New York: Viking-Penguin, 2003.

Sadler, T.W. *Langman's Medical Embryology.* 11th ed. Philadelphia: Lippincott Williams & Wilkins, 2009.

Sinha, Sunil, Lawrence Miall, and Luke Jardine. *Essential Neonatal Medicine.* 5th ed. Malden: Wiley-Blackwell, 2012.

Woolf, Alan D., et al., editors. *The Children's Hospital Guide to Your Child's Health and Development.* Cambridge, Mass.: Perseus, 2002.

Nursing

CATEGORY: Specialty

KEY TERMS:

assessment: the systematic process of collecting, validating, and communicating patient data; these data will include information gathered from the patient's history and from physical examination and laboratory test results

healing: the restoration to a normal physical, mental, or spiritual condition

health: a condition in which all functions of the body, mind, and spirit are normally active

holistic: the philosophy that individuals function as complete units or integrated systems and are not understood merely through their parts

illness: the condition of being sick or diseased

nurture: the act or process of raising or promoting development and well-being

service: work done or duty performed for another or others

treatment: any specific procedure used for the cure or improvement of a disease or pathological condition

THE ROLE OF NURSING

It is difficult at times to distinguish nursing from medicine, since there are so many ways in which they interrelate. Whereas some people think that nursing began with Florence Nightingale (1820–1910), nursing is as old as medicine itself. Throughout history, there have been periods when the two fields functioned interdependently and times when they were practiced separately from each other. It seems likely that the role of the mother-nurse would have preceded the magician-priest or medicine-man. Even the seeds of medical knowledge were sown by the natural remedies used by the mother.

Over the course of human history, the words *nurse* and *nursing* have had many meanings, and the connotations have changed as tribes became highly developed and sophisticated nations. The word *nurse* comes from the Latin *nutrix,* which means "nursing mother." The word *nursing* originated from the Latin *nutrire,* meaning "to nourish." The word *nurse* as a noun was first used in the English language in the thirteenth century, being spelled "norrice," then evolving to "nurice" or "nourice," and finally to the present "nurse." The word *nurse* as a verb meant to suckle and to nourish. The meanings of both the noun and the verb have expanded to include more and more functions related to the care of all human beings. In the sixteenth century, the meaning of the noun included "a person, but usually a woman, who waits upon or tends the sick." By the nineteenth century, the meaning of the verb included "the training of those who tend the sick and the carrying out of such duties under the supervision of a physician."

With the origin of nursing as mother care came the idea that nursing was a woman's role. Suckling and nurturing were associated with maternal instincts. Ill or helpless children were also cared for by their mothers. The image of the nurse as a loving and caring mother remains popular. The true spirit of nursing, however, has no gender barriers, though men only make up 12% of the nursing workforce. Nursing statistics show that men earn more that $6,000 more annually than their female counterparts, considering total hours worked, years of nursing experience, age, educational level and certification status. This is no surprise: all across the healthcare industry, men earn nearly 18% more than women.

In history, the role of nursing developed with the culture and society of a given age. Tribal women practiced nursing as they cared for the members of their own tribes. As tribes developed into civilizations, nursing began to be practiced outside the home. As cultures developed, nursing care became more complex, and qualities other than a nurturing instinct were needed to do the work of a nurse. Members of religious orders, primarily those composed of women, responded by devoting their lives to study, service, and self-sacrifice in caring for the needs of the sick. These individuals were among the educated people of their time, and they helped set the stage for nursing to become an art and a science.

It was not until the nineteenth century that the basis of nursing as a profession was established. The beliefs and examples of Florence Nightingale laid that foundation. Nightingale was born in Italy in 1820, but she grew up in England. Unlike many of the children of her time, she was educated by governesses and by her father. Against the wishes of her family, she trained to be a nurse at the age of thirty-one. Amid enormous difficulties and prejudices, she organized and managed the nursing care for a military hospital in Turkey during the Crimean War. She returned to England after the war, where she established a school, the Nightingale Training School for Nurses, to train nurses. Again, she encountered great opposition, as nurses were considered little more than housemaids by the physicians of the time. Because of her efforts, the status of nurses was raised to a respected occupation, and the basis for professional nursing in general was established.

Nightingale's contributions are noteworthy. She recognized that nutrition is an important part of nursing care. She instituted occupational and recreational therapy for the sick and identified the personal needs of the patient and the role of the nurse in meeting those needs. Nightingale established standards for hospital management and a system of nursing education, making nursing a respected occupation for women. She recognized the two components of nursing: promoting health and treating illness. Nightingale believed that nursing is separate and distinct from medicine as a profession.

Nightingale's methods and the response of nursing to American Civil War casualties in the 1860s pointed out the need for nursing education in the United States. Schools of nursing were established, based on the values of Nightingale, but they operated more like apprenticeships than educational programs. The schools were also controlled by hospital administrators and physicians.

In 1896, nurses in the United States banded together to seek standardization of educational programs, to establish laws to ensure the competency of nurses, and to promote the general welfare of nurses. The outcome of their efforts was the American Nurses Association. In 1900, the first nursing journal, the *American Journal of Nursing*, was founded. The effects of World War II also made clear the need to base schools of nursing on educational objectives. Many women had responded to the need for nurses during the war. A great expansion in medical knowledge and technology had taken place, and the roles of nurses were expanding as well. Nursing programs developed in colleges and universities and offered degrees in nursing to both women and men. While there were impressive changes in the expectations and styles with which nursing care has been delivered from ancient times into the twenty-first century, the role and function of the nurse have been and continue to be diverse. The nurse is a caregiver, providing care to patients based on knowledge and skill. Consideration is given to physical, emotional, psychological, socioeconomic, and spiritual needs. The role of the nurse-caregiver is holistic and integrated into all other roles that the nurse fulfills, thus maintaining and promoting health and well-being.

The nurse is a communicator. Using effective and therapeutic communication skills, the nurse strives to establish relationships to assist patients of all ages to manage and become responsible for their own health needs. In this way, the nurse is also a teacher who assists patients and families to meet their learning needs. Individualized teaching plans are developed and used to accomplish set goals.

The nurse is a leader. Based on the self-confidence gained from a nursing education and experience, the nurse is able to be assertive in meeting the needs of patients. The nurse facilitates change to improve care for patients, whether individually or in general. The nurse is also an advocate. Based on the belief that patients have a right to make their own decisions about health and life, the nurse strives to protect their human and legal rights in making those choices.

The nurse is a counselor. By effectively using communication skills, the nurse provides information, listens, facilitates problem-solving and decision-making abilities, and makes appropriate referrals for patients.

Finally, the nurse is a planner, a task that calls forth qualities far beyond nurturing and caring. In an age confronted with controversial topics such as abortion, organ transplants, the allocation of limited resources, and medical research, the role of nurses will continue to expand to meet these challenges in the spirit that allowed nursing to evolve and become a respected profession.

SCIENCE AND PROFESSION

While the nurse-mother of ancient times functioned within a very limited framework, the modern nurse has the choice of many careers within the nursing role. The knowledge explosion of the last century created many job specialties from which nurses can choose a career. The clinical nurse specialist is a nurse with experience, education, or an advanced degree in a specialized area of nursing. Some examples are enterostomal therapy, geriatrics, infection control, oncology, orthopedics, emergency room care, operating room care, intensive and coronary care, quality assurance, and community health. Nurses who function in such specialties carry out direct patient care; teach patients, families, and staff members; act as consultants; and sometimes conduct research to improve methods of care.

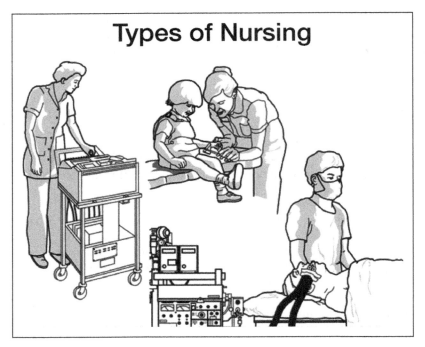

Types of Nursing

Nurses may become involved in many areas of health care, including the administration of diagnostic tests, the performance of physical examinations, and assistance during surgical procedures. © EBSCO

The nurse practitioner is a nurse with an advanced degree who is certified to work in a specific aspect of patient care. Nurse practitioners work in a variety of settings or in independent practice. They perform health assessments and give primary care to their patients.

The nurse anesthetist is a nurse who has also successfully completed a course of study in anesthesia. Nurse anesthetists make preoperative visits and assess patients prior to surgery, administer and monitor anesthesia during surgery, and evaluate the postoperative condition of patients. The nurse midwife is a nurse who has successfully completed a midwifery program. The nurse midwife provides prenatal care to expectant mothers, delivers babies, and provides postnatal care after the birth.

The nurse administrator functions at various levels of management in the health care field. Depending on the position held, advanced education may be in business or hospital administration. The administrator is directly responsible for the operation and management of resources and is indirectly responsible for the personnel who give patient care. The

nurse educator is a nurse, with a master's or doctoral degree, who teaches or instructs in clinical or educational settings. This nurse can teach both theory and clinical skills.

The nurse researcher usually has an advanced degree and conducts special studies that involve the collection and evaluation of data in order to report on and promote the improvement of nursing care and education.

DUTIES AND PROCEDURES

Creativity and education are the keys to keeping pace with continued changes and progress in the nursing profession. Nurses are expected to play many roles, function in a variety of settings, and strive for excellence in the performance of their duties. A service must be provided that contributes to the health and well-being of people. The following examples of nursing— an operating room nurse and a home health nurse— provide a limited portrait of how nurses function and what roles they play in health care.

Operating room nurses function both directly and indirectly in patient care and render services in a number of ways. Operating room nurses, usually known as circulating nurses, briefly interview patients upon their arrival at the operating room. They accompany patients to specific surgery rooms and assist in preparing them for surgical procedures. They are responsible for seeing that surgeons correctly identify patients prior to anesthesia. They are also directly attentive to patients when anesthesia is first administered.

Circulating nurses perform the presurgical scrub, which is a cleansing of the skin with a specified solution for a given number of minutes. It is their overall responsibility to monitor aseptic (sterile) techniques in certain areas of the operating room and to deal with the situation immediately if aseptic techniques are broken. They count the surgical sponges with surgical technologists before the first incision is made, throughout the procedure as necessary, and again before the incision is closed. They secure needed items requested by surgical technologists, surgeons, or anesthesia personnel: medications, blood, additional sterile instruments, or more sponges. At times, they prepare and assist with the operation of equipment used for surgeries, such as lasers, insufflators (used for laparoscopic surgery), and blood saver and reinfuser machines. They arrange for the transportation of specimens to the laboratory. They may also be instrumental in sending communications to waiting family members when the surgery takes longer than anticipated. When the surgery is completed, they accompany patients to the recovery room with the anesthesia personnel.

Home health nurses, on the other hand, function in a very different manner. This type of nurse usually works for a private home health services agency, or as part of an outreach program for home services through a hospital. Referrals come to the agency or program via the physician, through the physician's office, by way of the social services department in a hospital, or by an individual requesting skilled services through the physician.

Since nursing remains a female dominated profession women's health is important to nurses both as they care for themselves and to their patients. There are many areas of practice in which nurse's care for various women's health care needs. Some of the most common areas of nursing intervention center around breast health, cervical cancer screenings, menopause, pregnancy, and women's mental health issues.

PERSPECTIVE AND PROSPECTS

From the beginning of time, nursing and the role of the nurse have been defined by the people and the society of a particular age. Nursing as it is known today is still influenced by what occurred over the centuries.

In primitive times, people believed that illness was supernatural, caused by evil gods. The roles of the physician and the nurse were separate and unrelated. The physician was a medicine man, sometimes called a shaman or a witch doctor, who treated disease by ritualistic chants, by fear or shock techniques, or by boring holes into a person's skull with a sharp stone to allow the evil spirit or demon an escape. The nurse, on the other hand, was usually the mother who tended to family members and provided for their physical needs, using herbal remedies when they were ill.

As tribes evolved, the centers for medical care were temples. Some tribes believed that illness was caused by sin and the displeasure of gods. The physician of this age was a priest and was held in high regard. The nurse was a woman, seen as a slave, who performed menial tasks ordered by the priestphysician. Living in the same era were Hebrew tribes who used the Ten Commandments and the Mosaic Health Code to develop standards for ethical human relationships, mental health treatment, and disease control. Nurses visited the sick in their homes, practiced as midwives, and provided for the physical and spiritual needs of family members who cared for the ill.

These nurses provided a family-centered approach to care. With the advent of Christianity, the value of the individual was emphasized, and the responsibility for recognizing the needs of each individual emerged. Nursing gained an elevated position in society. A spiritual foundation for nursing was established as well. The first organized visiting of the sick was done by deaconesses and Christian Roman matrons of the time. Members of male religious orders also cared for the sick and buried the dead.

The worst era in nursing history was probably from 1500 to 1860. Nursing at this time was not a respected profession. Women who had committed a crime were sent into nursing as an alternative to serving a jail term. Nurses received poor wages and worked long hours under deplorable conditions. Changes in the Reformation and the Renaissance did little or nothing to improve the care of the sick. The attitude prevailed that nursing was a religious and not an intellectual occupation. Charles Dickens quite aptly portrayed the nurse and nursing conditions of the time through his caricatures of Sairey Gamp and Betsey Prig in *Martin Chuzzlewit* (1843–1844).

It was not until the middle of the nineteenth century that this situation began to change. Through Nightingale's efforts, nursing became a respected occupation once more. The quality of nursing care improved tremendously, and the foundation was laid for modern nursing education. As innovations in health care have an impact on nursing, nurses' roles will continue to expand in the future. Nursing can also be a background from which both men and women begin to bridge gaps of service where other affiliations are needed: computer science, medical-legal issues, health insurance agencies, and bioethics, to name a few. The words of Florence Nightingale still echo as a challenge to the nursing profession:

> *May the methods by which every infant, every human being will have the best chance of health, the methods by which every sick person will have the best chance of recovery, be learned and practiced! Hospitals are only an intermediate state of civilization never intended, at all events, to take in the whole sick population.*

Nursing will continue to meet this challenge to improve the quality of health care around the world.
—*Karen A. Mattern*
Updated by Mary Dietmann Ed. D. APRN CNS

For Further Information

American Nurses Association. *Nursing World*, 2013.

Delaune, Sue C., and Patricia K. Ladner, eds. *Fundamentals of Nursing: Standards and Practices*. 4th ed. Albany, N.Y.: Delmar Thomson Learning, 2011.

Donahue, M. Patricia. *Nursing: The Finest Art*. 3d ed. Maryland Heights: Mosby Elsevier, 2011.

Kozier, Barbara, et al. *Fundamentals of Nursing: Concepts, Process, and Practice*. 2nd ed. Harlow, England; New York: Pearson, 2012.

Legasse, Jeff. "Male Nurses Still Earn More than $6,000 Annually More than Women, New Survey Shows." Healthcare Finance News, 18 June 2018, www.healthcarefinancenews.com/news/male-nurses-earn-6000-more-women-annually-new-survey-shows.

MedlinePlus. "Health Occupations." *MedlinePlus*, August 29, 2013.

Park, Melissa, et al. "Nurse Practitioners, Certified Nurse Midwives, and Physician Assistants in Physician Offices." *Centers for Disease Control and Prevention: NCHS Databrief*, August 17, 2011.

United States Department of Labor. "Licensed Practical and Licensed Vocational Nurses." *Bureau of Labor Statistics: Occupational Outlook Handbook*, March 29, 2012.

———. "Registered Nurses." *Bureau of Labor Statistics: Occupational Outlook Handbook*, March 29, 2012.

Vorvick, Linda J. "Types of Health Care Providers." *MedlinePlus*, August 14, 2012.

"Women's Health." *ANA*, American Nurses Association, www.nursingworld.org/practice-policy/work-environment/health-safety/healthy-nurse-healthy-nation/womens-health/

O

Obstetrics

CATEGORY: Specialty

KEY TERMS:

amniocentesis: a technique by which a fine needle is inserted through a pregnant woman's abdomen and into the uterus and amniotic sac in order to collect fetal amniotic cells for biochemical and genetic analysis

birth defect: a genetic or developmental abnormality which occurs in utero that leads to anatomic or functional problems after birth; the defect can be serious, with potentially significant consequences for the fetus or mother, or the defect can be minor

cesarean section: a surgical procedure whereby the infant is delivered through an incision on the mother's abdomen

forceps: curved metal blades that are carefully placed around the fetal head through the vagina to facilitate delivery

gestation: the period from conception to birth, in which the fetus reaches full development in order to survive outside the mother's body

placenta: an organ in the uterus through which the fetus receives its oxygen and nutrients and removes its waste products; it serves as a blood barrier between the mother's circulatory system and the fetal circulatory system

Rh0(D) immune globulin: also known as RhoGAM; a type of gamma globulin protein injected into Rh-negative mothers who may have an Rh-positive fetus to protect the fetus from an immune reaction called isoimmunization

trimester: one of three periods of time in pregnancy, each period lasting three months; the first trimester is zero to twelve weeks of gestational age, the second trimester is thirteen to twenty-four weeks of gestational age, and the third trimester is twenty-five to thirty-seven weeks of gestational age

ultrasonography: an imaging modality in which sound waves penetrate bodily tissues in order to generate an image; in obstetrics, this technique is commonly used to assess the fetus, amniotic fluid, and uterus and ovaries

vacuum: a device with a suction cup that is applied to the fetal head through the vagina to assist in delivery of the infant

SCIENCE AND PROFESSION

Obstetrics is the branch of medical science dealing with pregnancy and childbirth in women. Once conception has occurred and a woman is pregnant, major physiological changes occur within her body as well as within the body of the developing embryo or fetus. Obstetrics deals with these changes leading up to and including childbirth. As such, obstetrics is a critical branch of medicine, for it involves the complex physiological events by which every person comes into existence.

The professional obstetrician is a licensed medical doctor whose area of expertise is pregnancy and childbirth. Often, the obstetrician is also a specialist in the closely related science of gynecology, the study of diseases and conditions that specifically affect women, particularly non-pregnant women. The obstetrician is especially knowledgeable in female anatomy and physiology, including the major bodily changes that occur during and following pregnancies. Obstetricians also have a detailed understanding of the necessary diagnostic procedures for monitoring fetal and maternal health, and they are educated in the latest technologies for facilitating a successful pregnancy and childbirth with minimal complications. Obstetrical care is also provided by certified nurse midwives (CNMs) and by nurse practitioners, particularly those with certification in women's health (women's health care nurse practitioners).

Broadly, the diseases and conditions managed by the clinicians in this field include preconception counseling, normal prenatal care, and the management of pregnancy-specific problems such as preeclampsia, gestational diabetes, premature labor, premature rupture of membranes, multiple gestations, fetal growth problems, and isoimmunization. In addition, obstetricians manage medical problems that can occur in any woman but that take on special importance in pregnancy, such as thyroid disorders or infections. Obstetricians make assessments and decisions regarding when a baby is best delivered, particularly if there are in utero conditions that make it safer for the baby to be born immediately, even if prematurely.

Obstetricians manage both normal and abnormal labors. They are able to assess the progress and position of the infant as it makes its way down the birth canal. They are knowledgeable about pain control options during labor and make decisions regarding when a cesarean section is indicated. Obstetricians assist with normal vaginal deliveries, either spontaneous or induced, and sometimes use special instruments such as forceps or vacuum-suction devices. They also perform cesarean sections. Obstetricians are trained in appropriate postpartum care for the mother and infant.

In natural, spontaneous fertilization, pregnancy begins with the fertilization of a woman's egg by a man's sperm following sexual intercourse, the chances of which are highest if intercourse takes place during a two-day period following ovulation. Ovulation is the release of an unfertilized egg from the woman's ovarian follicle, which occurs roughly halfway between successive periods during her menstrual cycle. Fertilization usually occurs in the upper one-third of one of the woman's fallopian tubes connecting the ovary to the uterus; upon entering the woman's vagina, sperm must travel through her cervix to the uterus and up the fallopian tubes, only one of which contains a released egg following ovulation.

Once fertilization has occurred, the first cell of the new individual, called a zygote, is slowly pushed by cilia down the fallopian tube and into the uterus. Along the way, the zygote undergoes several mitotic cellular divisions to begin the newly formed embryo, which at this point is a bundle of undifferentiated cells. Upon reaching the uterus, the embryo implants in the lining of the uterus. Hormonal changes occur in the woman's body to maintain the pregnancy. One of these hormones is human chorionic gonadotropin, which is the chemical detected by most pregnancy tests. Failure of the embryo to be implanted in the endometrium and subsequent lack of hormone production (specifically the hormone progesterone) will cause release of the endometrium as a bloody discharge; the woman will menstruate, and there will be no pregnancy. Therefore, menstrual cycles do not occur during a pregnancy. The embryo will grow and develop over the next nine to ten months of gestation. The heart forms and begins beating at roughly five and one-half weeks following conception.

Over the next several weeks and months, major organ systems begin to organize and develop. By the end of the first three months of the pregnancy, the developing human is considered to be a fetus. All the major organ systems have formed, although not all systems can function yet. The fetus is surrounded by a watery amniotic fluid within an amniotic sac. The fetus receives oxygen and nutrients from the mother and excretes waste products into the maternal circulation through the placenta. The fetus is connected to the placenta via the umbilical cord. During the second and third trimesters, full organ system development; massive cell divisions of certain tissues such as nervous, circulatory, and skeletal tissue; and preparation of the fetus for survival as an independent organism occur. The fetus cannot survive outside the mother's body, however, until the third trimester.

Changes also occur in the mother. Increased levels of the female steroid hormone estrogen create increased skin vascularization (that is, more blood vessels near the skin) and the deposition of fat throughout her body, especially in the breasts and the buttocks. The growing fetus and stretching uterus press on surrounding abdominal muscles, often creating abdominal and back discomfort. Reasonable exercise is important for the mother to stay healthy and to deliver the baby with relative ease. A balanced diet also is important for the nourishment of her body and that of the fetus.

Late in the pregnancy, the protein hormones prolactin and oxytocin will be produced by the woman's pituitary gland. Prolactin activates milk production in the breasts. Oxytocin causes muscular contractions, particularly in the breasts and in the uterus during labor. Near the time of birth, drastically elevated levels of the hormones estrogen and oxytocin will cause progressively stronger contractions (labor pains) until the baby is forced through the vagina and out of the woman's body to begin its independent physical existence. The placenta, or afterbirth, is discharged shortly thereafter.

DIAGNOSTIC AND TREATMENT TECHNIQUES

The role of the obstetrician is to monitor the health of the mother and unborn fetus during the course of the pregnancy and to deliver the baby successfully at the time of birth. Once the fact of the pregnancy is established, the obstetrician is trained to identify specific developmental changes in the fetus over time in order to ensure that the pregnancy is proceeding smoothly.

The mainstay of diagnosis is the physical examination during prenatal visits. Early in the pregnancy, prenatal visits occur monthly, but they become more frequent as the pregnancy progresses. During these visits, the woman may receive counseling regarding a balanced diet, folic acid and iron supplementation, and substances or foods to avoid that may pose a risk to the pregnancy. The woman's growing uterus is measured to confirm proper growth, and, if indicated, a vaginal or cervical examination may be performed. After ten weeks of gestational age, fetal heart tones are also assessed at every prenatal visit using a simplified ultrasonic technique, to ensure that they are within the normal number of beats per minute. Fetal heart tones that are abnormally slow may indicate a fetus in jeopardy.

The other main component of diagnosis is through laboratory tests. Early in the pregnancy, the woman will receive a Pap test to screen for cervical cancer. Blood tests will be ordered to determine whether the mother is a carrier of the human immunodeficiency virus (HIV) or hepatitis or C viruses, which can be transmitted to the fetus. In addition, the mother is checked for anemia, and the blood type of the mother is assessed. If the mother's blood type indicates that she is Rh negative, she will receive RhoGAM in the third trimester to prevent the development of a disease called isoimmunization, a condition that could be fatal to the fetus. An additional diagnostic test performed routinely during pregnancy is a screening test for diabetes, which pregnant women are at increased risk for.

Another important method of diagnosis in obstetrics is ultrasonography. Ultrasonography early in pregnancy can determine the gestational age of a pregnancy in cases in which a woman's last menstrual period is unverified. The correct development of the fetus and the presence of any birth defects can be assessed using this procedure. Ultrasound can also determine whether the placenta is growing in a safe location and whether the proper amount of amniotic fluid is found in the amniotic sac. Toward the end of pregnancy, ultrasound is an invaluable diagnostic tool for determining fetal well-being and the position of the infant in the uterus in preparation for delivery. Ultrasound is also a useful tool in guiding diagnostic procedures. For instance, amniocentesis can be extremely safe when performed under ultrasound guidance. Finally, one of the main methods of diagnosis in the third trimester is fetal heart monitoring. This technique involves following the heartbeat of the infant while in utero.

The heart rate of the infant is typically followed for twenty to thirty minutes. Any concerning dips in the heart rate may be indicative of a poor fetal state and a cause for increased monitoring or, in extreme cases, delivery of the infant. Obstetricians have at their disposal a variety of treatment modalities. They are trained to turn manually fetuses that are in a breech (feet-first) position, a procedure called external cephalic version. In cases where the artificial induction of labor is desirable, the obstetrician may employ mechanical or hormonal means of cervical dilation, followed by infusions of a hormone called *Pitocin* to stimulate contractions or the artificial rupture of the amniotic sac to promote natural contractions. When immediate delivery of the infant is needed and the chances of it emerging via the vaginal route are remote, then the obstetrician may perform a cesarean section. Common indications for cesarean section include fetal distress and lack of progress in labor.

Other treatments commonly used by obstetricians include the use of medications such as magnesium to relax the uterus in cases of premature labor and maternal steroid injections to induce fetal lung maturity when the fetus is premature, but delivery is anticipated. When a woman experiences difficulty in the final stages of labor and the fetal head has descended almost to the vaginal opening, the obstetrician may employ forceps or vacuum devices to facilitate the delivery, particularly in cases of fetal distress. Obstetricians also treat the complications associated with childbirth, including postsurgical care after a cesarean section and repair of any lacerations of the vagina, cervix, or rectum after vaginal delivery.

PERSPECTIVE AND PROSPECTS

Obstetrics is central to medicine because it deals with the very process by which all humans come to exist. The health of the fetus and its mother in pregnancy is of primary concern to these doctors. The field of obstetrics has blossomed as a sophisticated specialty, more likely to be practiced by obstetricians, certified nurse midwives, and specially trained and certified nurse practitioners, rather than the general practitioners who used to provide this care.

Advances in medical technology have enabled more precise analysis and monitoring of the fetus inside the mother's uterus, and obstetrics has therefore become a complex specialty in its own right. Technology such as ultrasonography and fetal heart rate monitoring, among other techniques, allows the obstetrician to collect a much larger supply of fetal data than was available to the general practitioner of the 1960s. Increased data availability enables the obstetrician to monitor the pregnancy closely and to identify any problems earlier.

New advances in product development continue to improve the diagnostic ability of obstetricians. One example is the development of a test for fetal fibronectin, which enables obstetricians to predict which patients are at low risk of premature delivery. This test involves a simple swab of the upper vagina. When negative, this test is highly reliable and allows the pregnant patient to leave the hospital and avoid prolonged and unnecessary hospitalization.

Advances in prenatal diagnosis and basic science have made it possible for parents to obtain information about their fetuses down to the molecular level. Through techniques such as amniocentesis and chorionic villus sampling (in which a small sample of placental cells is obtained early in pregnancy), genetic analysis has enabled the detection of chromosomal defects responsible for mental retardation and single-gene defects responsible for inherited diseases (such as cystic fibrosis). Amniocentesis has also made it possible to detect biochemical changes that may be indicative of major structural defects in the fetus, as well as to assess the developmental maturity of organs such as the lungs.

Advances in medical practice have dramatically decreased the morbidity and mortality of premature birth. For instance, with the introduction and widespread use of maternal steroid injections, the severity of serious diseases of prematurity, such as respiratory distress syndrome, has been dramatically reduced. The development of drugs against HIV has prevented the transmission of the virus from mother to infant in many cases. The medical science of obstetrics continues to advance.

There is ongoing research into the physiology and basic science of preeclampsia and eclampsia, common and potentially dangerous diseases peculiar to pregnancy. Fetal surgery programs at academic centers open the possibility that serious birth defects may be correctable while the fetus is in utero. Although many controversies currently exist in the field of obstetrics, an increased push toward medical practice grounded in scientific evidence promises many exciting advances in the future. It is hoped that many of these advances will result in improved outcomes and quality of life for patients.

—*David Wason Hollar, Jr., Ph.D.;*
Updated by Anne Lynn S. Chang, M.D.

FOR FURTHER INFORMATION

American College of Obstetricians and Gynecologists. *American College of Obstetricians and Gynecologists*, 2013.

Cohen, Barbara J. *Memmler's The Human Body in Health and Disease.* 11th ed. Philadelphia: Wolters Kluwer Health/Lippincott Williams & Wilkins, 2009.

Doyle, Kathryn. "Midwife-Led Care Linked to Fewer Premature Births." Reuters Health Information. *MedlinePlus*, August 28, 2013.

Gabbe, Steven G., Jennifer R. Niebyl, and Joe Leigh Simpson, editors. *Obstetrics: Normal and Problem Pregnancies.* 6th ed. Philadelphia: Saunders, 2012.

Limmer, Daniel, et al. *Emergenc yCare.* 12th ed. Boston: Brady, 2012.

MedlinePlus. "Childbirth." *MedlinePlus*, August 13, 2013.

MedlinePlus. "Pregnancy." *MedlinePlus*, August 29, 2013.

Vorvick, Linda J. "Certified Nurse-Midwife." *MedlinePlus*, September 12, 2011.

———. "Choosing the Right Health Care Provider for Pregnancy and Childbirth." *MedlinePlus*, August 23, 2012.

Opportunistic infections

CATEGORY: Disease/Disorder

KEY TERMS:

CD4: a type of white blood cell (specifically a type of T-cell) that is affected by the human immunodeficiency virus (HIV)

encephalitis: inflammation of the brain

immunocompromised: the state of having a weakened immune system

lumbar puncture: also known as a spinal tap; a procedure that involves insertion of a needle into the lumbar spinal column

pneumonia: infection of the lung

prophylaxis: a method of preventing a disease

CAUSES AND SYMPTOMS

Opportunistic infections (OI) can be caused by various microorganisms, including viruses, bacteria, fungi, and protozoa. They may be transmitted through the air, bodily fluids, or in through contaminated water or food. While they are capable of infecting healthy individuals, the infection is either without symptoms or the disease is mild. Individuals with a weakened immune system are the most susceptible to OI and they can result in detrimental infections. For example, acquired immunodeficiency syndrome (AIDS), resulting from human immunodeficiency virus (HIV), is a widely known disease that weakens the immune system.

Other situations where the immune system can be compromised and become susceptible to opportunistic infections are: being on chronic glucocorticoid therapy, taking immunosuppressive medications after organ transplantation, undergoing chemotherapy for cancer, being malnourished, or having a genetic predisposition. Below are some examples of opportunistic infections that can manifest as a result of a weakened immune system.

Pneumocystis jirovecii is a fungus capable of causing life-threatening pneumonia in the immunocompromised. In those with HIV, the majority of *Pneumocystis* pneumonia develops in those with a very low CD4 cell count. Common symptoms include high fever, dry cough, progressive difficulty breathing (especially with exertion), fatigue, chills, chest pain, and weight loss.

Toxoplasmosis is a ubiquitous infection caused by the intracellular protozoan parasite *Toxoplasma gondii.* The parasite can be carried by warm-blooded animals including: rodents, birds, and cats. Transmission is via ingestion of contaminated soil or undercooked meats, usually red meats and pork, that contain the protozoan oocyte. Infection in the healthy person is usually asymptomatic, but the organism can remain dormant in the host indefinitely. In immunocompromised patients such as those with very low CD4 cell count,

the organism reactivates and causes active infection. Infection by *T. gondii* may occur in the brain, testes, heart, pancreas, liver, colon, lungs, and retina. The principal site of involvement is the central nervous system. *T. gondii* can cause encephalitis and masses within the brain. Symptoms may include confusion, fever, seizures, and headache. *T. gondii* can also cause pneumonia accompanied by difficulty breathing, fever, and cough. Pregnant women who have an active infection can pass it to their offspring, leading to infantile neurological deficits, mental retardation, and eye infections.

Mycobacterium avium complex (MAC) usually causes widespread disease in the immunocompromised and is due to several nontuberculous species, *M. avium, M. kansasii,* and *M. intracellulare.* These organisms are ubiquitous in the environment such as in soil, with transmission typically through inhalation or ingestion. Acquisition of infection typically takes place when the CD4 count is extreme low. Symptoms include fever, night sweats, abdominal pain, diarrhea, weight loss, weakness, and wasting.

Cytomegalovirus (CMV) is a herpes virus found worldwide. It is commonly transmitted via feces, saliva, breast milk, urine, and genital secretions. In immunocompetent individuals, the virus remains latent and usually does not cause any severe disease. In the immunocompromised, however, the dormant virus reactivates, and infection occurs. Symptoms generally include fever, night sweats, chills, fatigue, and muscle and joint aches. Other symptoms depend on the organ system affected: Gastrointestinal involvement typically produces symptoms of colitis (inflammation of the colon), such as abdominal pain and bloody diarrhea; lung involvement produces a pneumonitis (inflammation of the lung) with cough and difficulty breathing; encephalitis of the brain, and eye involvement (retinitis) is an emergency and can lead to blindness. The adrenal gland and the nervous system can also be affected.

Another opportunistic fungus associated with immunocompromised hosts is *Cryptococcus neoformans,* which causes cryptococcosis. The organism is normally found in soil contaminated with pigeon droppings, and transmission is usually through inhalation. The initial site of infection is in the lungs where it subsequently spreads to the brain, causing what is known as meningoencephalitis (inflammation of the brain and its surrounding protective tissues).

Meningoencephalitis is the most common clinical syndrome in immunocompromised patients, developing slowly over one to two weeks with fever, malaise, headache, stiff neck, photophobia (aversion to bright lights), and vomiting. Disseminated rash is another symptom occurring in those with a weakened immune system.

There are many other causes of opportunistic infections, including the viruses *Varicella* and herpes simplex; the bacteria *Nocardia*, *Listeria*, and the less common *Mycobacterium* species; the protozoans *Cryptosporidium*, *Isospora*, *Microsporidia*, and *Cyclospora*; and the fungi *Coccidioides*, *Candida*, *Histoplasma*, and *Aspergillus*. While all these organisms are capable of causing disease in the healthy, their impact on the immunocompromised is much more severe.

TREATMENT AND THERAPY

Treatment involves addressing the specific infection that resulted from a compromised immune system. The best way to avoid opportunistic infections is to correct the underlying problem that is causing the weakened immune system. In some cases, this may not be possible, such as in those who require immunosuppressive therapy after organ transplantation or those undergoing chemotherapy for cancer. However, advances in HIV therapy with the implementation of highly active antiretroviral therapy (HAART) as well as institution of prophylaxis against opportunistic infections have dramatically decreased the mortality rate in these patients.

Treatment of *Pneumocystis* pneumonia requires the demonstration of organisms from respiratory specimens. Treatment is with anti-*Pneumocystis* regimens typically for twenty-one days, with or without corticosteroids. The latter is used in severe cases when oxygenation becomes problematic. Symptoms typically worsen after two to three days of therapy as a result of increased inflammation in response to dying microorganisms. After initial therapy, prophylactic therapy against future infections is instituted.

Treatment of toxoplasmosis requires antiprotozoan medications for at least six weeks. Prophylaxis against future infection is also required, which is the same medication as that used for *Pneumocystis* prophylaxis. In high-risk persons, as a means of prevention it is important to avoid undercooked meats and cat litter boxes. For pregnant women, food should be cooked to safe temperatures and measured for their internal heat with a food thermometer. The USDA recommends whole cuts of non-poultry meat to be cooked to at least 145° F (63° C) and a rest time of 3 minutes before consuming. Non-poultry ground meat should be cooked to at least 160° F (71° C). All poultry products should be cooked to at least 165 ° F (74° C). Other recommendations of safe handling of food include: thoroughly wash and peel fruits, avoid drinking untreated water and unpasteurized goat's milk, avoid eating raw or undercooked shellfish, and wash cutting boards, dishes, counters, utensils and hands with warm soapy water after they come into contact with raw meat or unwashed fruits or vegetables.

Treatment of MAC involves combination antibiotics for at least twelve months, with subsequent prophylaxis.

Cytomegalovirus infection is treated with antiviral agents. Immunoglobulin may be used to reduce the risk of infection in certain transplant recipients. If the eye is involved, then a pellet that releases an antiviral agent may be implanted into the eye with surgery. While not curative, this treatment may hinder the progression of the eye disease.

The treatment of cryptococcosis is with antifungal agents, initially with combination medications for what is known as induction therapy, followed by consolidation therapy, and finally maintenance therapy. Because the disease can also cause an increased pressure surrounding the brain, frequent lumbar punctures are sometimes required to relieve this pressure, or if severe enough, a drain placed in the spinal cord may be necessary to continuously relieve the pressure. While prophylactic therapy is needed when the CD4 cell count is low, it may be withdrawn when the CD4 cells improve.

PERSPECTIVE AND PROSPECTS

Pneumocystis was originally identified by the Brazilian physician Carlos Chagas in 1909. Chagas was also the discoverer of the protozoan *Trypanosoma cruzi*, the organism that causes trypanosomiasis, or Chagas" disease. Initially, he mistakenly thought that the *Pneumocystis* cysts from the lungs of rats were part of the *Trypanosoma* life cycle. It was in 1910 that the Italian physician Antonio Carini discovered that these cysts were also present in lungs without *T. cruzi* infection, and he thus concluded that these cysts were a different type of infection. In 1912, Pierre and Marie Delanoe at the Pasteur Institute also confirmed that these cysts were present in the absence of *T. cruzi* infection, and they subsequently named these cyst-like organisms *Pneumocystis carinii*, after Carini. Because these infections appeared to affect only rats, however, the organism did not become a major issue at that time.

It was not until the 1940s that *P. carinii* was found to cause pneumonia in human infants and adults. However, these patients all had some type of immune system compromise, such as malnutrition, genetic immune deficiency, or immunosuppressive medications. Before the AIDS epidemic, there were fewer than one hundred confirmed cases per year in the United States. It was later determined that there were several species of *Pneumocystis*, one of which causes disease in rats and another in humans. It was in 1999 when the specific epithet *P. jirovecii* (named after the Czech parasitologist Otto Jiroveci) was officially coined to refer to the disease occurring in humans. *P. carinii* still refers to the disease in rats. It was also in 1999 that *Pneumocystis* was recognized as a fungus rather than a protozoan, as previously thought.

In late 1980 to early 1981, the Centers for Disease Control and Prevention (CDC) described a cluster of five cases of *Pneumocystis* pneumonia in young gay men. Since then, the cases of *Pneumocystis* pneumonia increased, as did the cases of Kaposi's sarcoma (rare HIV-related skin cancer). It was soon realized that both of these illnesses were not exclusive to gay males; they also affected heterosexuals, intravenous drug users, and others who were immunocompromised. In 1982, the CDC officially coined the term "acquired immunodeficiency syndrome," or AIDS, for this syndrome. In 1983, Luc Montagnier and his team from the Pasteur Institute isolated a virus that was thought to be the causative agent of AIDS, which they termed lymphadenopathy-associated virus. In 1984, Robert Gallo and his team from the United States also isolated a virus presumptive to cause AIDS; they named it human T lymphotropic virus type III (HTLV-III). Later, it was recognized that both viruses were the same, and the virus was officially termed human immunodeficiency virus (HIV) in 1986.

In the beginning of the AIDS epidemic, death was certain. Treatment of HIV did not begin until 1986, when the Food and Drug Administration (FDA) approved the first antiviral agent, zidovudine, a nucleoside reverse transcriptase inhibitor (NRTI)—an agent

---

> ## Information on Opportunistic Infections
>
> **Causes:** Viruses, bacteria, fungi, protozoa
> **Symptoms:** Fever, weakness, lack of appetite, rash, cough, difficulty breathing, confusion, headache, blurry vision, chest pain, weight loss, night sweats
> **Duration:** Acute to chronic
> **Treatments:** Antibiotics, antiviral medications, antifungal medications, antiprotozoan medications

---

that inhibits viral replication. However, single agent therapy did not prove to be as effective due to drug resistance. In 1995, newer classes of antiviral medications were approved—non-nucleoside reverse transcriptase inhibitor (NNRTI) and protease inhibitors (PI)—and began the trend of combination therapy of what is now known as highly active antiretroviral therapy (HAART). The thought behind combination therapy is that if the virus develops a genetic mutation and becomes resistant to one drug, the other two would still be active against it. However, while successful, even this powerful combination of drugs is still not adequate enough to achieve a complete cure since the virus is capable of remaining dormant inside cells and becoming resistant to medications even after a brief episode of missed doses.

In 2007, the FDA approved two new classes of antiretroviral therapy, integrase inhibitors and CCR5 co-receptor antagonists, which are used for advanced stages of HIV infection.

As of 2013, there are currently no available vaccines effective against HIV, although there are vaccines in various stages of clinical trial. A report in 2009 of a study of healthy volunteers with an experimental HIV vaccine in Thailand showed only a modest success rate (about 31 percent) in the prevention of HIV. In 2013, however, a two-year-old child was declared "functionally cured" of HIV infection, but further research will be conducted to determine if the results can be replicated in clinical trials involving other HIV-infected children.

While there are still obstacles to conquer in the fight against HIV, the battle against opportunistic infections has made great strides with the introduction of HAART and prophylactic medications.

—*Andrew Ren, M.D.*
Updated by Shirley Kuan, BS, RN

FOR FURTHER INFORMATION

"AIDs and Opportunistic Infections." *Centers for Disease Control and Prevention,* March 5, 2019

Fauci, Anthony, editors. *Harrison's Principles of Internal Medicine.* 17th ed. New York: McGraw-Hill, 2008.

Mandell, Gerald, et al., editors. *Mandell, Douglas, and Bennett's Principles and Practice of Infectious Diseases.* 7th ed. Philadelphia: Churchill Livingstone/Elsevier, 2010.

Mathis, Diane J., and Alexander Y. Rudensky, editors. *Immune Tolerance.* Cold Spring Harbor, N.Y.: Cold Spring Harbor Laboratory Press, 2013.

"Opportunistic Infections and Their Relationship to HIV/AIDS." *AIDS.gov,* November 16, 2011.

Rubin, Robert, eds. *Clinical Approach to Infection in the Compromised Host.* 4th ed. New York: Kluwer Academic, 2002.

St. Georgiev, Vassil. *Opportunistic Infections: Treatment and Prophylaxis.* Totowa, N.J.: Humana Press, 2003.

Stine, Gerald James. *AIDS Update 2013: An Annual Overview of Acquired Immune Deficiency Syndrome.* New York: McGraw-Hill, 2013.

"Surveillance for Norovirus Outbreaks." *Centers for Disease Control and Prevention,* January 28, 2013.

"Toddler 'Functionally Cured' of HIV Infection, NIH-Supported Investigators Report." *National Institutes of Health,* March 4, 2013.

Orthorexia nervosa

CATEGORY: Disease/Disorder

KEY TERMS:

cognitive behavioral therapy: a type of psychotherapy in which people learn to recognize and change negative and self-defeating patterns of thinking and behavior

Diagnostic and Statistical Manual of Mental Disorders: the handbook the American Psychiatric Society uses to categorize and diagnose mental disorders

BACKGROUND

As more information about nutritional research is released to the public, it generally results in a healthier population. However, some individuals take this information as absolute fact, without understanding that research is a work in progress. They develop an unhealthy obsession with applying the knowledge at a level that most in the population do not. This obsession is most commonly focused on types of foods purported to be best for perfect health, how they should be prepared, and when and how much should be eaten.

The term orthorexia nervosa was coined by Steven Bratman, an American physician, in 1997. The term means "correct diet," and denotes an unhealthy fixation with eating food that is optimally healthy, "clean," "pure," and "correct." This obsession goes well beyond the desire to eat a healthy diet and extends to rituals involving eating the exact amount of "correctly" prepared food at the specific times during the day or allowing certain foods to be eaten only during certain seasons. This obsession can interfere with social relationships (e.g., the refusal to eat at friends' houses or in restaurants) and may result in nutritional deficits.

Orthorexia nervosa is not considered an official psychiatric disorder like anorexia nervosa or bulimia. It does not have an official diagnosis in the *Diagnostic and Statistical Manual of Mental Disorders;* however, it shares many characteristics with obsessive-compulsive disorders and anorexia nervosa. Ursula Philpot, chair of the British Dietetic Association, stated that individuals who have this condition are only concerned about the quality of food they consume, and only eat what they perceive to be "pure" food. When these individuals experience intense feelings of hunger and cravings, they punish themselves for being weak. The deprivation can be so severe that it results in death.

Physicians and eating disorder specialists often fail to distinguish between orthorexia nervosa and anorexia nervosa. It is important to understand the difference; anorexia nervosa is an eating disorder that results from the fear of being overweight, whereas in orthorexia nervosa, the goal is to achieve perfect health by controlling diet, not necessarily to lose weight. Still, both disorders can lead to malnutrition and health problems.

Even though increased attention is being given to better understanding the risk factors, behavior, and outcomes of therapy, there remains much to be learned. As of 2015, only one study has addressed the overlap of orthorexia, or other obsessive-compulsive disorders, with another type of eating disorder, including bulimia and anorexia. It appears that the longer a person is preoccupied with healthy eating, the higher the likelihood that he or she will develop a clinical eating disorder (up to 53 percent three years after diagnosis). Orthorexia can also develop in an individual recovering from another eating disorder.

OVERVIEW

Individuals with orthorexia nervosa are preoccupied with eating healthy foods, and avoid those high in fat, preservatives, animal products, or pesticides. Many of these individuals become malnourished because they avoid sources of necessary nutrition in favor of a small number of "safe" foods. One example of dietary restriction is the raw food diet. Individuals who follow this and similarly restrictive diets (i.e., veganism or fruitarianism) have an elevated risk of becoming emaciated and can develop nutritional deficiencies if they do not sufficiently vary their diet to ensure adequate intake of vitamins, minerals, proteins, fiber, and other nutritional requirements found in food.

Orthorexia disorders are similar to and potentially overlap other psychiatric disorders such as obsessive-compulsive disorders, somatic symptom disorder, hypochondria, and psychotic spectrum disorders. Individuals are generally more concerned about the quality of the food opposed to the amount of food in hopes of obtaining an ideal body appearance. One interesting overlap between orthorexia and other eating disorders is the displeasure with eating and the trading of control over one's life for control over diet.

It is not clear what demographic group is more susceptible to developing the disorder. In one 2008 study in Germany, nutrition students were investigated for developing the disorder because of their in-depth knowledge of nutrition and how to achieve optimal health. It was found that nutrition students did not have higher orthorexic tendencies than non-nutrition students. In a similar study in Portugal, it was found that orthorexic tendencies measured by a diagnostic questionnaire decreased as a nutrition student progressed through their education. The orthorexia questionnaire measured eating behaviors and attitudes toward nutrition. The students did have higher scores in regard to having more restrictive eating behaviors than non-nutrition students, but this is unsurprising given their education about healthy eating; however, it did not indicate that these students had unhealthy attitudes towards eating. In a study of adults in the general population in the U.S in 2011, it was found that there is a 57.6% prevalence of orthorexia nervosa in the sample taken and a female/male ratio of 2:1.

Symptoms of orthorexia nervosa include obsessive concern about one's diet, spending excessive amounts of time analyzing the source of a food for pesticides, worrying about whether milk or meat contains growth hormones or antibiotics, worrying about the safety of genetically modified foods (GMOs), overcooking food (thus losing nutrition) or eating only raw food, and avoiding packaged food. These individuals spend a lot of time planning menus, measuring portions, and obsessing about health and diet. Orthorexic individuals develop nutritional deficiencies because they tend to omit entire food groups. Nutritional deficiencies can lead to medical complications such as anemia, osteopenia, and metabolic, hormonal, neurological and blood deficiencies. There is also an associated risk of developing anorexia nervosa as a result of some restrictive diet like veganism or rawfoodism.

Diagnosis of orthorexia nervosa is performed using a fifteen-point questionnaire, called ORTO-15. This questionnaire assesses the beliefs of patients about their perception of eating healthy, food selection attitudes, food consumption habits, and the extent that food concerns affect daily life. Responses are scored using a four-point scale; a score below 40 is considered diagnostic of orthorexia whereas a score higher than 40 indicates a healthy view of eating. In addition, blood samples are drawn to assess for nutritional deficiencies.

Treatment for orthorexia nervosa has not been standardized. After a diagnosis has been made, the patient is referred to psychotherapists and dietitians, and sometimes prescribed medication (often antidepressants) and behavioral therapy. Medication may pose as a challenge to orthorexia nervosa with their belief that medication is unnatural. Psychotherapists focus their therapy according to the patient's needs. Among the varied approaches, patients undergo cognitive behavioral therapy to restructure their thoughts and reprogram their minds to avoid obsessive behavior and attitudes toward their diet. It appears that patients who undergo these therapies have some success in changing their attitudes towards food, with correct education about nutrition.

– Mandy M. McBroom, M.P.H.
Updated by Tish Davidson, M.A.
and Shirley Kuan, BS, RN-BC

FOR FURTHER INFORMATION

Bratman, Steven. "The Authorized Orthorexia Self-Test." http://www.orthorexia.com.

Brytek-Matera, Anna, et al. "Predictors of Orthorexic Behaviours in Patients with Eating Disorders: A Preliminary Study." *BMC Psychiatry* 15. (2015): 1–8. https://bmcpsychiatry.biomedcentral.com/articles/10.1186/s12888-015-0628-1.

Ramacciotti, Carla E.,et al. "Orthorexia nervosa in the general population: A preliminary screening using a self-administered questionnaire (ORTHO-15)." *EWD* vol. 16., 2011: e127-e130.

Kratina, Karin. "Orthorexia Nervosa." National Eating Disorders Association. https://www.nationaleatingdisorders.org/orthorexia-nervosa.

Reddy, Sumathi. "When Healthy Eating Calls for Treatment." *Wall Street Journal - Eastern Edition* 11 Nov. 2014: D1+. https://www.wsj.com/articles/when-healthy-eating-calls-for-treatment-1415654737.

Osteoarthritis

CATEGORY: Disease/Disorder

KEY TERMS:

Bouchard's nodes: osteophytes or bony spurs that develop as a result of destruction of joint cartilage in proximal interphalangeal joints

cartilage: a smooth material covering the ends of bone joints that cushions the bone, allowing the joint to move easily

collagen: a fibrous protein substance in connective tissue, bone, tendons, and cartilage

crepitus: the scraping or grinding sound heard or felt when bone rubs over bone in joint spaces

degenerative: marked by progression to a state below what is considered normal or desirable

distal: away from the point of origin

distal interphalangeal joints: the distal joints of the fingers

Herberden's nodes: osteophytes or bony spurs that develop as a result of destruction of joint cartilage in distal interphalangeal joints

inflammatory: irritation that causes swelling, heat, and discomfort

joints: the junctions at the ends of bones that allow for movement

proximal: toward the point of origin

proximal interphalangeal joints: the proximal joints in the fingers

synovial fluid: fluid contained in the synovium of joint margins that reduces friction during movement of the joints

synovium: fluid-filled sacs in joint margins

CAUSES AND SYMPTOMS

Arthritis is defined as inflammation of one or more joints in the body. Osteoarthritis (OA) is the most common form of arthritis, affecting more than 240 million people worldwide and over 30 million people in the United States of America. The number one symptom associated with OA is pain and it develops due to the combination of mechanical, cellular, and biomechanical factors on synovial joints.

Overall, women have a higher prevalence and severity of OA when compared to men, especially regarding the knees and hands. There are several reasons why some researchers think that women have an increased risk of developing OA. There is mounting evidence that estrogen plays a protective effect on the articular cartilage and prevents its degradation within joints. After menopause, when estrogen levels equalize that of men's, there is an increased risk of developing OA. Women are also at a higher risk of developing OA due to the alignment of their joints. Regarding the joints of the lower body, the anatomical shape of the female pelvis can put a strain on the hip joint and increase the risk of developing OA. There is also a genetic component to OA, with up to thirty percent of cases of OA being hereditary. However, as of now, there is no single identifiable gene that is associated with OA, but a combination of traits that might lead to the development of this condition depending on the activation of these genes. Scientists have not found a difference in the incidence of these genes among gender. Lastly, lifestyle factors such as weight and occupation can lead to OA through increased strain on joints, but studies show that this is a factor across populations, not sexes.

Cartilage containing synovial fluid and elastic tissue reduces friction as joints move. Osteoarthritis develops when the cartilage wears away and bone rubs against bone. The most prominent symptom of osteoarthritis is joint pain. Other symptoms include morning stiffness or stiffness after long periods of immobility. Early in the disease, individuals may

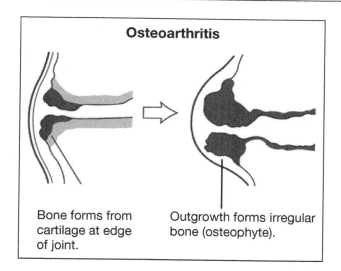

Osteoarthritis

Bone forms from cartilage at edge of joint.

Outgrowth forms irregular bone (osteophyte).

Osteoarthritis results when irregular bone growth occurs at the edge of a joint, causing impaired movement of the joint and pressure on nerves in the area. © EBSCO

experience joint pain after strenuous exercise. As the disease progresses, joints stiffen and diminished joint mobility is experienced even with slight activity. As joint mobility decreases, the muscles surrounding the joint weaken, thereby increasing the likelihood of further injury to the joint. As the cartilage wears away, crepitus can often be heard as bone moves against bone. The development of Herberden's nodes on the distal interphalangeal joints and Bouchard's nodes on the proximal interphalangeal joints of the hands is not uncommon.

Confirmation of osteoarthritis is based on a history of joint pain and physical findings that indicate arthritic changes in the joints. An x-ray shows a loss of joint space, osteophytes, bone cysts, and sclerosis of subchondral bone. Sometimes, a computed tomography (CT) scan or magnetic resonance imaging (MRI) may be helpful in confirming the presence of osteoarthritis.

Treatment and Therapy

The goal of treatment for OA is to preserve physical function and reduce pain. Education, physical therapy, and occupational therapy are instrumental in maintaining independence and improving muscle strength around affected joints. Pacing activities to avoid overexertion of the affected joints is an effective means to prevent further pain and injury. Heat

therapies such as warm soaks, paraffin, and mud treatments may help to lessen the discomfort in tender joints. Moderate exercise such as walking, swimming, strength training, and stretching all may help to maintain mobility in arthritic joints and to improve posture and balance. Relaxation techniques, stress reduction activities, and biofeedback may also be helpful.

Topical analgesic ointments may help to reduce joint swelling and pain. Acetaminophen is very effective for controlling OA pain. However, persons who take blood-thinning medicines, have liver disease, or consume large amounts of alcohol should use acetaminophen with caution. Non-steroidal anti-inflammatory drugs (NSAIDs) such as ibuprofen and naproxen are also effective for pain relief, but they may cause gastrointestinal bleeding. COX-2 selective inhibitors are the most recently introduced NSAIDs. This class of drugs selectively blocks the enzyme COX-2, thus controlling the production of prostaglandins, natural chemicals that contribute to body inflammation and cause the pain and swelling of arthritis. Since they do not block the COX-1 enzyme cyclooxygenase-1, which is present in the stomach and inflammation sites, the natural mucous linings of the stomach and intestine are protected, thereby reducing the incidence of upset, ulceration, or bleeding. This feature of blocking COX-2 but not COX-1 makes these drugs unique among traditional NSAIDs. COX-2 selective inhibitors include Celebrex (celecoxib), Vioxx (rofecoxib), and Bextra (valdecoxib); the latter two are no longer on the market, however. Other COX-2 inhibitors sold outside the United States include Prexige (lumiracoxib) and Arcoxia (etoricoxib). Any medication used to treat OA should be taken under the direction of a health care provider.

Glucosamine and chondroitin naturally occur in the body. Both have been promoted for the treatment of OA. Glucosamine may promote the formation and repair of cartilage, while chondroitin may promote water retention and elasticity in cartilage and prevent cartilage breakdown. However, recent studies indicate that taking glucosamine for arthritis may increase a patient's risk of developing glaucoma.

When interventions to relieve symptoms of OA no longer work, an orthopedic surgeon may inject cortisone or hyaluronic acid into joint spaces such as the knee. Hyaluronic acid is used to replace the synovial fluid that a joint has lost in order to maintain knee

Information on Osteoarthritis

Causes: Traumatic injuries, joint overuse, obesity, genetic or metabolic diseases

Symptoms: Joint pain (commonly in hands, hips, knees, spine); stiffness in morning or after long periods of immobility; development of nodes

Duration: Chronic and progressive

Treatments: Occupational therapy; physical therapy; moderate exercise; heat therapy (warm soaks, paraffin, mud treatments); pain medications such as topical analgesic ointments, acetaminophen, NSAIDs (ibuprofen, naproxyn); COX-2 inhibitors; glucosamine; chondroitin; injections of cortisone or hyaluronic acid; surgery in severe cases

movement without pain. Cortisone may be injected into affected joint spaces to provide temporary relief of joint pain. Surgical intervention to trim torn and damaged cartilage from joint spaces, to partially or totally replace severely damaged joints in the knees and hips, or to fuse bones together are effective treatments in the most severe, debilitating stages of OA. Realignment of a joint (osteotomy) is another possible procedure.

—Sharon W. Stark, R.N., A.P.R.N., D.N.Sc.;
Updated by Victoria Price, Ph.D.
and Nicholas Feo

FOR FURTHER INFORMATION

Ali, Naheed. *Arthritis and You: A Comprehensive Digest for Patients and Caregivers.* Lanham, Md.: Rowman and Littlefield, 2013.

Atukorala, I., Makovey, J., Lawler, L., Messier, S. P., Bennell, K. and Hunter, D. J. (2016), "Is There a Dose-Response Relationship Between Weight Loss and Symptom Improvement in Persons With Knee Osteoarthritis?" *Arthritis Care & Research*, 68: 1106-1114. doi:10.1002/acr.22805

Brower, Anne C. *Arthritis in Black and White.* Philadelphia: Elsevier Saunders, 2012.

Gebhart, J J et al. "Relationship between pelvic incidence and osteoarthritis of the hip" *Bone & Joint Research*. vol. 5,2 (2016): 66-72.

"Osteoarthritis (OA) | Basics | Arthritis | CDC." Centers for Disease Control and Prevention, Centers for Disease Control and Prevention, 10 Jan. 2019, www.cdc.gov/arthritis/basics/osteoarthritis.htm.

Tanamas, S., Hanna, F. S., Cicuttini, F. M., Wluka, A. E., Berry, P. and Urquhart, D. M. (2009), "Does knee malalignment increase the risk of development and progression of knee osteoarthritis? A systematic review." *Arthritis & Rheumatism*, 61: 459-467. doi:10.1002/art.24336

Ovarian cysts

CATEGORY: Disease/Disorder

KEY TERMS:

androgen: a hormone producing or stimulating the development of male characteristics

bimanual examination: an internal exam of the pelvis conducted by a medical professional, often with a supervising "chaperone" in the room

follicle: a small, spherical, secretory structure in the ovary that releases the ovum or "egg"

laparoscopy: a minimally invasive surgery technique that utilizes small incisions through the skin to pass a camera and other surgical instruments into the abdomen or pelvis; typically results in decreased postoperative pain and length of recovery compared to traditional open procedures

polycystic ovary: an ovary containing multiple cysts, may occur as part of a hormonal condition known as polycystic ovary syndrome (PCOS)

torsion: "twisting", as in the case of an ovary twisting around itself and cutting off the blood supply

ultrasound: a non-invasive, diagnostic imaging modality that uses high-frequency sound waves to produce images that are interpreted by a physician; does not result in radiation exposure as in the case of X-ray or computed tomography (CT)

CAUSES AND SYMPTOMS

One or more ovarian cysts may develop at any age on one or both ovaries. The cyst consists of a thin, transparent outer wall enclosing one or more chambers filled with clear fluids or old blood that presents as thick brownish or jellylike material; in some cases tissue material may be present as well. Such cysts range in size from that of a raisin to that of a large orange. The normal ovary measures 3 centimeters by 2 centimeters;

the cystic ovary requiring investigation is one which is enlarged to more than twice its normal size.

Large cysts may cause a feeling of fullness in the abdominal area, cramping pain with various levels of severity, or pain during vaginal intercourse. Often, however, there are no apparent symptoms, and the cyst is discovered only during a routine gynecologic examination when the clinician, on bimanual examination, discovers that one ovary is considerably enlarged. At this point, it is important to rule out malignancy, because ovarian cancers in their early stages often exhibit similar or no warning symptoms, and may also occur at any age.

Polycystic ovaries causing significant enlargement occur in a variety of conditions. For example, polycystic ovaries can result from an enzyme deficiency in the ovaries that interferes with the normal biosynthesis of hormones, resulting in the release of an abnormal amount of androgens.

More than half of all ovarian cysts are functional; that is, they arise out of the normal functions of the ovary during the menstrual cycle. These cysts are relatively common. A cyst can form when a follicle has grown in preparation for ovulation but fails to rupture and release an egg; this type is called a follicular cyst. Sometimes the structure formed from the follicle after ovulation, the corpus luteum, fails to shrink and forms a cyst; this is called a corpus luteum cyst. Another type of ovarian cyst, most often found in younger women, is the dermoid cyst, which contains particles of teeth, hair, or calcium-containing tissue that are thought to be an embryologic remnant; such cysts usually do not cause menstrual irregularity and are very common. Dermoids are bilateral in 25 percent of cases, making careful examination of both ovaries mandatory. The cyst has a thickened, white, opaque wall and is more buoyant than other types of cysts.

Ovarian cysts cause problems when they become very large, when they rupture and cause severe internal bleeding, or when a cyst's pedicle suddenly twists and cuts off its blood supply, creating severe pain and possibly infection. Rupture of a cyst is followed by the acute onset of severe lower abdominal pain radiating to the vagina and lower back. The most severe symptoms of pain and collapse are associated with rupture of a dermoid cyst, as the cyst contents are extremely irritating.

Torsion of a cyst may occur at any age but most often in the twenties; it may be associated with pregnancy. A twisted dermoid cyst is the most common, probably because of its increased weight. The onset of pain often occurs in the umbilical region and radiates to one or the other side of the pelvis. Pain on the right is frequently confused with appendicitis. Hemorrhage may sometimes occur from a vessel in the wall of the cyst or within the capsule.

TREATMENT AND THERAPY
The diagnosis of an ovarian cyst is made with consideration of the patient's age, medical and family history, symptoms, and the size of the enlarged ovary. In women under the age of thirty, clinicians, after a manual examination, will usually wait to see if the ovary will return to its normal size. If pregnancy has been ruled out and the ovary does not return to its normal size, then a pelvic X-ray and/or an ultrasound may be used to determine the exact size of the ovaries and distinguish between a cyst and a solid tumor. In women age forty and older, X-rays and ultrasounds may be done sooner due to increased risk of malignancy as compared to younger women. If uncertainty still exists, the physician may recommend laparoscopy,

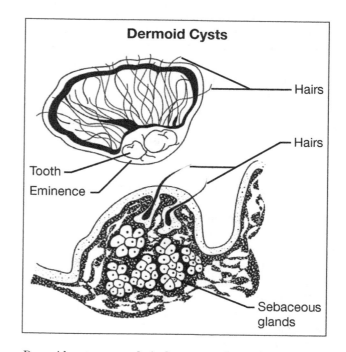

Dermoid cysts are a relatively common form of ovarian cyst often found in younger women. © EBSCO

Information on Ovarian Cysts

Causes: Depends on type; may include functional disorders involving follicles or corpus luteum, hormonal imbalance, embryological remnants

Symptoms: Often asymptomatic; with large cysts, may include feeling of fullness in abdomen, pain with intercourse, compromised fertility; if rupture occurs, severe internal bleeding and intense lower abdominal pain; if cyst becomes twisted, severe pain and possibly gangrene

Duration: Acute to chronic

Treatments: Oral contraceptives, surgery

the visual examination of the abdominal cavity using a device consisting of a tube and optical system inserted through a small incision. The physician may also suggest the option of a larger incision and a biopsy.

In the case of the functional ovarian cyst, if no severe pain or swelling is present, the clinician may adopt a "watchful waiting" approach for one or two more menstrual cycles, during the course of which this type of cyst frequently disappears on its own accord. Sometimes this process is hastened by administering oral contraceptives for several months, which establishes a regular menstrual cycle. Women already taking oral contraceptives rarely develop ovarian cysts.

In the case of torsion or rupture, surgical treatment is indicated, preferably the removal of the cyst only and preservation of as much of the normal ovarian tissue as possible. Sometimes, with a very large cyst, the ovary cannot be saved and must be removed, a procedure called oophorectomy or ovariectomy.

—*Genevieve Slomski, Ph.D.*
Updated by Thomas J. Martin, M.D. Candidate

FOR FURTHER INFORMATION

Kovacs, Gabor T., and Robert Norman, eds. *Polycystic Ovary Syndrome.* 2d ed. New York: Cambridge University Press, 2012.

Leung, Peter C. K., and Eli Y. Adashi, eds. *The Ovary.* 2d ed. San Diego, Calif.: Academic Press, 2004.

"Ovarian Cyst." *Family Doctor*, August 2010.

Rosenblum, Laurie. "Ovarian Cyst." *Health Library*, September 10, 2012.

Vorvick, Linda J., Susan Storck, and David Zieve. "Ovarian Cysts." *Medline Plus*, February 26, 2012.

Ovaries

CATEGORY: Anatomy

KEY TERMS:

atresia: the programmed process of cell death

corpus luteum: the structure that develops from an emptied ovarian follicle after ovulation

Fallopian tubes or oviducts: tubular structures attached at their lower ends to the uterus; the passageways for ova following ovulation

follicle: a structure composed of an oocyte and surrounding granulosa cells

hormone: a chemical messenger secreted by one cell type and acting on another to cause a predictable response

oocyte: a female germ cell that differentiates to become a mature ova

ovum (pl. ova): an egg cell

STRUCTURE AND FUNCTIONS

Ovaries develop from undifferentiated gonadal tissue in the absence of a Y chromosome. They are ductless glands located in the female pelvis, attached on either side of the uterus by the ovarian ligaments. Each is a flattened lumpy oval about 5 centimeters (cm) in length, 2.5 cm wide, and less than 1 cm in thickness. They are often described as being about the size and shape of an almond. There are three regions to each ovary: An outer cortex contains the developing oocytes, an inner medulla produces steroid hormones, and the hilum serves as the point of attachment and entry of blood vessels and nerves.

A principal function of the ovaries is gametogenesis, the production of ova through meiosis. This process begins during fetal life, and about 1 to 2 million immature oocytes are present in the cortex of the ovaries at birth. By puberty, this number has been reduced to about 300,000 through the process of atresia, and only about 400 mature ova are actually ovulated during life. The number of lifetime ovulated oocytes are reduced if oral contraceptives are used. Recent research has found that it may be possible to increase oocyte numbers during life through the implantation of stem cells that are capable of mitosis. These stem cells can be isolated from the ovaries of reproductive age women. Studies done on mice have isolated germline stem cells from ovaries that can actively divide and produce oocytes when implanted in a human body.

Within the mature ovarian cortex are many follicles, each containing an oocyte. At any given time, there are oocytes in all stages of development, and only a small percentage of available oocytes ever undergo ovulation; the rest undergo atresia and are recycled by the body. This occurs because groups of oocytes are activated during ovulation, and only one makes it to the luteal stage, while the others undergo atresia.

Immature oocytes remain dormant until puberty. During this time, the hypothalamus region of the brain releases a surge of hormone, the Ganadotropin-releasing hormone, that initiates the release of hormones from the pituitary, which will drive the process of ovulation. During puberty, eggs mature successively, and one breaks through the ovarian wall each cycle in the process of ovulation. This continues until menopause, or cessation of reproductive functioning in the female. After release from the ovary, the ovum passes through the Fallopian tube and into the uterus. If the ovum is fertilized, then pregnancy ensues and the ovum (now a blastocyst) implants in the uterine lining.

Following ovulation, the empty follicle left in the ovary becomes the corpus luteum. It appears as a yellow body (because of lipid droplets in the cells) on the surface of the ovary and secretes progesterone to prepare the uterine lining for implantation. The corpus luteum deteriorates after ten to twelve days if conception does not occur, and the decrease in progesterone allows deterioration of the uterine lining, and thus, menstruation begins.

The ovarian medulla is also responsible for hormonogenesis. The primary steroids produced here are estradiol (estrogen) and progesterone. Androgens (particularly androstenedione and testosterone) are also secreted, but most of them are converted to estradiol within the ovary. Estrogens are essential for the development of ova and female body characteristics (including breasts, body shape, fat deposition, and body hair distribution) and for implantation and pregnancy maintenance. They also initiate mammary gland maturation and contribute to bone mineralization. Progesterone prepares the uterine lining for implantation and pregnancy, regulates the release of luteinizing hormone (LH) from the pituitary, and contributes to the maturation of mammary gland alveoli.

In addition to the steroid hormones, peptide hormones are produced by the ovaries. Relaxin is secreted from the corpus luteum and induces relaxation of the pelvic bones and ligaments, inhibits myometrial motility, softens the cervix, and induces uterine growth. Activins stimulate the release of follicle stimulating hormone (FSH) from the pituitary, and inhibin causes decreasing FSH output, although the mechanism is not yet understood. The ovary has been found to produce a variety of neuropeptides such as b-endorphin, adrenocorticotropin, -melanocyte-stimulating hormone, vasopressin, and oxytocin. The physiologic roles that these peptides may play in the ovary are uncertain.

Human ovaries display a regular cycle in reproductively mature females. This cycle, known as menstruation, includes a follicular phase, during which FSH promotes growth and maturation of the granulosa cells, partial maturation of oocytes, synthesis of proteins, and estrogen secretion. Next is the ovulatory phase, during which one mature oocyte and the surrounding cells are discharged. Lastly is the luteal phase, in which progesterone is secreted. The average ovarian cycle is twenty-eight days, with a normal range between twenty-four and thirty-two days in length.

DISORDERS AND DISEASES

Polycystic ovary syndrome (PCOS), or Stein-Leventhal syndrome, is the most common ovarian disorder, affecting 6 to 10 percent of all women. The ovarian stroma becomes enlarged and produces excessive amounts of androgens. Atretic follicles accumulate and large numbers of cysts (fluid-filled sacs) may form; most are harmless and require no treatment. Ovarian follicle development is incomplete, and menstrual cycles are usually irregular. Symptoms can be alleviated with combination contraceptives and anti-androgens. Ovulation can sometimes be induced by clomiphene.

Ovulatory dysfunction is one of the causes of infertility. Most often this is hormonal in nature, and many cases of infertility can be overcome by hormone treatments.

Ovarian cancer is a major cause of death in females and comes in a variety of forms. The lifetime risk is about 1.6 percent, but it increases with age and in women with relatives who have had reproductive cancers. In women with an altered BRCA1 or BRCA2 gene, the risk is 25 to 60 percent, depending on the specific mutation. Pregnancy decreases the overall risk, as do oral contraceptives. Surgery is the treatment of choice, often followed by chemotherapy. Prognosis is poor overall, mostly due to the lack of clear symptoms that would lead to early diagnosis.

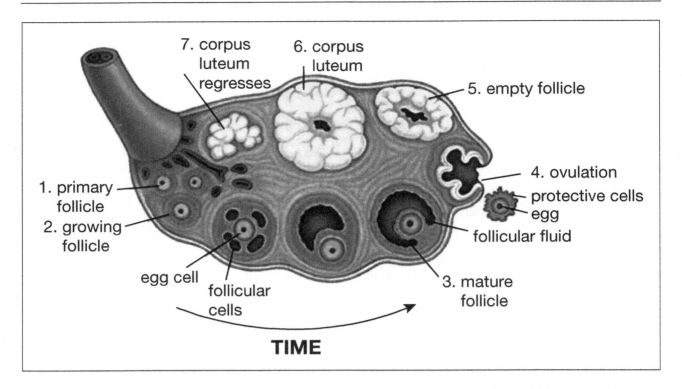

The anatomy of the internal structures of the ovary, showing the life cycle of the ovum. (Kimanh Nguyen via Wikimedia Commons)

PERSPECTIVE AND PROSPECTS

The human ovary was first described by Renier De Graaf in 1672. In 1701, the first surgery to remove an ovarian tumor was performed by Robert Houston, and in 1809 the first known ovary removal (ovariectomy or oophorectomy) was performed by Ephraim McDowell. Throughout the nineteenth and early twentieth centuries, study of the ovaries centered on their anatomy and physiology, while during the latter part of the twentieth century studies turned to their endocrine functions.

Many postulated ovarian hormones are still being searched and studied for their effects. They include transforming growth factor beta (TGF-β), anti-Mullerian hormone (AMH), folliculostatins, and many other peptides involved in the control of growth and differentiation. Gonadotropin surge attenuating factor (GnSAF) has also been hypothesized to be physiologically involved in the control of LH secretion during the menstrual cycle.

—*Kerry L. Cheesman, Ph.D.;*
Updated by Catherine Avelar

FOR FURTHER INFORMATION

Futterweit, Walter, and George Ryan. *A Patient's Guide to PCOS: Understanding-and Reversing-Polycystic Ovary Syndrome.* New York: Holt, 2006.

Johnson, J., J. Canning, T. Kaneko, J.K. Pru, and J.L. Tilly. "Germline Stem Cells and Follicular Renewal in the Postnatal Mammalian Ovary." *Nature* 428, no. 6979 (2004): 145-150.

Kaipia, Antti, and Aaron Hsueh. "Regulation of Ovarian Follicle Atresia." *Annual Review of Physiology* 59 (1997): 349-363.

Moore, K.L., T.V.N. Persaud, M.G. Torchia, and T.V.N. Persaud. *The Developing Human: Clinically Oriented Embryology.* Philadelphia: Saunders/Elsevier, 2008.

Plourde, Elizabeth. *Your Guide to Hysterectomy, Ovary Removal, and Hormone Replacement: What All Women Need to Know.* Ashland, OH: New Voice/ Atlas Books, 2002.

P

Pap test

CATEGORY: Procedure

Also known as: Pap sampling, Pap smear, Papanicolaou test

KEY TERMS:

cytobrush: a long cotton swab with a conical head used to collect cervical cell samples

Ayre spatula: a wooden spatula with U shaped openings on one side and a flat surface on another

speculum: a metal or plastic instrument that is used to dilate the vaginal canal

INDICATIONS AND PROCEDURES

Pap testing guidelines have recently changed. Formerly, the procedure was recommended for all women over the age of eighteen or for women who are sexually active. Revised guidelines have been issued by the American Cancer Society, the American College of Obstetricians and Gynecologists, and the Preventive Services Task Force, part of the US Department of Health and Human Services. These updated guidelines all stipulate that Pap tests should begin in women aged twenty-one and older. Updated guidelines have been issued as well for human papillomavirus (HPV) testing, which frequently accompanies the procedure; it is now recommended that HPV testing be done in women aged thirty and older because HPV in younger women is usually a transient infection that will clear without need for intervention.

For women ages 21-65 with no history of abnormal pap test it is recommended they get this test done every three years. The guidelines also recommend less frequent Pap testing for women who have had three consecutive negative tests; the guidelines also call for a cutoff to Pap testing in older women without abnormalities. More frequent testing is recommended for women who have tested positive for HPV or have had abnormal results for other reasons. Pap testing guidelines for women who have had a hysterectomy (with sampling of the vaginal cuff) vary depending on whether the hysterectomy was done for benign or malignant causes. The guidelines recommend that only women who have had malignant disease continue Pap testing.

A Pap test is performed easily in an office visit. Generally, the patient lies on her back with legs flexed and knees apart, although alternative positions can be utilized for women with limited mobility or with disabilities. A speculum is then carefully inserted into the vagina, and the cervix is visualized. An Ayre spatula is used to gently scrape off cells from the transition zone of the cervix. A cytobrush samples cells from the cervical canal. These cells are then placed in a preservative and sent to a pathology laboratory for analysis. The term "Pap smear" derives from the fact that before the advent of liquid preservative methods of collecting samples, samples were "smeared" on a glass slide and then sent to a laboratory for analysis.

USES AND COMPLICATIONS

The main use of Pap testing is to identify asymptomatic cases of dysplasia (abnormal growth) of the cervix and vagina. With early treatment of dysplasia, the incidence of and number of deaths from cervical cancer have decreased dramatically. Although cancer screening is the primary purpose and use of Pap testing, incidental findings may include vaginal infections of bacteria, fungi, or parasites. In rare cases, Pap tests may also detect abnormal cells shed from the endometrium. There are no serious risks from the procedure. Women may see a small amount of spotting after the procedure as a result of abrasions from the spatula or cytobrush.

PERSPECTIVE AND PROSPECTS

The Pap test was introduced in 1943 by George N. Papanicolaou and Herbert F. Traut. Since then, the incidence of invasive cervical cancer has dramatically, although cervical cancer remains the second most prevalent malignancy among women worldwide, according to the World Health Organization.

A screening test analogous to cervical Pap sampling, called the anal cytology, or "anal Pap test," has been developed to screen for anal dysplasia and cancer. It has been used primarily on high-risk patients, such as those with human immunodeficiency virus (HIV), women who have had cervical or vulvar cancer, and HIV-negative men who have sex with men.

—Clair Kaplan, A.P.R.N./M.S.N.;
additional material by Anne Lynn S. Chang, M.D.

For Further Information

A.D.A.M. Medical Encyclopedia. "Pap Smear." *MedlinePlus*, February 26, 2012.

"Cervical Cancer Screening." *Centers for Disease Control and Prevention,* June 13, 2013.

Kumar, Vinay, et al., eds. *Robbins Basic Pathology.* 9th ed. Philadelphia: Saunders/Elsevier, 2013.

Lentz, Gretchen M., et al. *Comprehensive Gynecology.* 6th ed. Philadelphia: Mosby/Elsevier, 2012.

National Cancer Institute. "Cervical Cancer Screening." *National Institutes of Health, US Department of Health and Human Services,* July 19, 2012.

"Pap Test." *Health Library,* March 15, 2013.

Wright, Thomas C., Jr., et al. "2001 Consensus Guidelines for the Management of Women with Cervical Cytological Abnormalities." *Journal of the American Medical Association* 287, no. 16 (April, 2002): 2120–2129.

Pediatrics

Category: Specialty

Key Terms:

acute: referring to a short and sharp disease process

chronic: referring to a lingering disease process

congenital: inborn, inherited

full-term: referring to a gestation period of a full nine months

premature: referring to a birth that is less than full term

puberty: the time of hormonal change when a child begins the physical process of becoming an adult

Science and Profession

The practice of pediatrics begins with birth. Most babies are born healthy and require only routine medical attention. Many hospitals, however, have a neonatology unit for babies who are born prematurely, who have disease conditions or birth defects, or who weigh less than 5.5 pounds (even though they may be full-term babies). All these infants may require short-term or prolonged care by pediatricians in the neonatology unit.

The problems of premature babies usually center on the fact that they have not fully developed physically, although other factors may also be involved, such as the health and age of the mother, undernourishment during pregnancy, lack of prenatal care, anemia, abnormalities in the mother's genital organs, and infectious disease. A past record of infertility, stillbirths, abortions, and other premature births may indicate that a pregnancy will not go to full term.

Low birth weight in both premature and full-term babies is directly related to the incidence of disease and congenital defects and may be indicative of a low intelligence quotient (IQ). Between 50 and 75 percent of babies weighing under 3 pounds, 5 ounces are mentally disabled or have defects in vision or hearing. Recent studies also indicate an increase in neurological problems such as attention-deficit hyperactivity disorder and autism in these children.

Because the lungs are among the organs that develop late in pregnancy, many premature infants are unable to breathe on their own. Some premature babies are born before they have developed the sucking reflex, so they cannot feed on their own.

Hundreds of congenital diseases can be present in the neonate. Some are apparent at birth; some become evident in later years. Some may be life-threatening to the infant or become life-threatening in later years. Others may be harmless. The child may be born with an infection passed on from the mother, such as rubella (German measles) or human immunodeficiency virus (HIV), the virus that causes acquired immunodeficiency syndrome (AIDS). Rubella may also infect the child in the womb, causing severe physical deformities, heart defects, mental disability, deafness, and other conditions.

Genital herpes affects about 1,500 newborns in the United States each year and may cause serious complications. Aherpes infection during the second or third trimester of a woman's pregnancy may increase the chance of preterm delivery or cesarean section. Group beta strep (GBS) infections are another serious problem for one of every 2,000 newborns in the

United States. GBS may cause sepsis (blood infection), meningitis, and pneumonia.

Among the most prevalent congenital birth defects is cleft lip, which occurs when the upper lip does not fuse together, leaving a visible gap that can extend from the lip to the nose. Cleft palate occurs when the gap reaches into the roof of the mouth.

Various abnormalities may be present in the hands and feet of neonates. These can be caused by congenital defects or by medications given to the pregnant mother. Arms, legs, fingers, and toes may fail to develop fully or may be missing entirely. Some children are born with extra fingers or toes. In some children, fingers or toes may be webbed or fused together. Clubfoot is relatively common. In this condition, the foot is twisted, usually downward and inward. Many congenital heart defects can afflict the child, including septal defects (openings in the septum, the wall that separates the right and left sides of the heart), the transposition of blood vessels, the constriction of blood vessels, and valve disorders.

Congenital disorders of the central nervous system include spina bifida, hydrocephalus, cerebral palsy, and Down syndrome. Spina bifida is a condition in which part of a vertebra (a bone in the spinal column) fails to fuse. As a result, nerves of the spinal cord may protrude through the spinal column. This condition varies considerably in severity; mild forms can cause no significant problems, while severe forms can be crippling or life-threatening. In hydrocephalus, sometimes called "water on the brain," fluid accumulates in the infant's cranium, causing the head to enlarge and putting great pressure on the brain. This disorder, too, can be life-threatening.

Cerebral palsy is caused by damage to brain cells that control motor function in the body. This damage can occur before, during, or after birth. It may or may not be accompanied by mental disability. Many children with cerebral palsy appear to be mentally disabled because they have difficulty speaking, but, in fact, their intelligence may be normal or above normal. Down syndrome is one of the most common congenital birth defects, affecting 1 in 200 infants born to mothers over age thirty-five. It is caused by an extra chromosome passed on to the child. The distinct physical characteristics of Down syndrome include a small body, a small and rounded head, oval ears, and an enlarged tongue. Mortality is high in the first year of life because of infection or other disease.

Cystic fibrosis is one of the most serious congenital diseases of Caucasian children. Because the lungs of children with this disease cannot expel mucus efficiently, it thickens and collects, clogging air passages. The mucus also becomes a breeding ground for bacteria and infection. Other parts of the body, such as the pancreas, the digestive system, and sweat glands, can also be impaired. A common congenital disorder among African American children is sickle cell disease. It causes deformities in red blood cells that clog blood vessels, impair circulation, and increase susceptibility to infection.

One of the major problems of infancy is sudden infant death syndrome (SIDS), in which a baby that is perfectly healthy, or only slightly ill, is discovered dead in its crib. In 2010 in the United States, over 2,000 infant deaths were reported as SIDS. The cause is not known. The child usually shows no symptoms of disease, and autopsies reveal no evidence of smothering, choking, or strangulation. Research indicates that rebreathing of carbon dioxide as well as exposure to secondhand cigarette smoke and other forms of indoor air pollution may greatly increase the risk of SIDS. Infectious diseases are more prevalent in childhood than in later years. Among the major diseases of children (and often adults) throughout the centuries have been smallpox, malaria, diphtheria, typhus, typhoid fever, tuberculosis, measles, mumps, rubella, varicella (chickenpox), scarlet fever, pneumonia, meningitis, and pertussis (whooping cough). In more recent years, AIDS and hepatitis have become significant threats to the young.

Certain skin diseases are common in infants and young children, such as diaper rash, impetigo, neonatal acne, and seborrheic dermatitis, among a wide variety of disorders. Fungal diseases of the skin occur often in the young, usually because of close contact with other youngsters. For example, tinea pedis (athlete's foot), tinea cruris (jock itch), and tinea corporis (a fungal infection that occurs on nonhairy areas of the body) are spread by contact with an infected playmate or by the touching of surfaces that harbor the organism. Similarly, parasitic diseases such as head lice, body lice, crabs, or scabies are easily spread among playmates. Some skin conditions are congenital. Between 20 and 40 percent of infants are born with, or soon develop, skin lesions called hemangiomas. They may be barely perceptible or quite unsightly; they generally resolve by the age of seven.

One form of diabetes mellitus arises in childhood, insulindependent diabetes mellitus (IDDM) or type 1. In the healthy individual, the pancreas produces insulin, a hormone that is responsible for the metabolism of blood sugar, or glucose. In some children, the pancreas loses the ability to produce insulin, causing blood sugar to rise. When this happens, a cascade of events causes harmful effects throughout the body. In the short term, these symptoms include rapid breathing, rapid heartbeat, extreme thirst, vomiting, fever, chemical imbalances in the blood, and coma. In the long term, diabetes mellitus contributes to heart disease, atherosclerosis, kidney damage, blindness, gangrene, and a host of other conditions.

Cancer can afflict children. One of the most serious forms is acute lymphocytic leukemia. Its peak incidence is between three and five years of age, although it can also occur later in life. Leukemic conditions are characterized by the overproduction of white blood cells (leukocytes). In acute lymphocytic leukemia, the production of lymphoblasts, immature cells that ordinarily would develop into infection-fighting lymphocytes, is greatly increased. This abnormal proliferation of immature cells interferes with the normal production of blood cells, increasing the child's susceptibility to infection. Before current treatment modalities, the prognosis for children with acute lymphocytic leukemia was death within four or five months after diagnosis.

In addition to the wide range of diseases that can beset the infant and growing child, there are many other problems of childhood that the parent and the pediatrician must face. These problems may involve physical and behavioral development, nutrition, and relationships with parents and other children.

Both parents and pediatricians must be alert to a child's rate of growth and mental development. Failure to gain weight in infancy may indicate a range of physical problems, such as gastrointestinal, endocrine, and other internal disorders. In three-quarters of these cases, however, the cause is not a physical disorder. The child may simply be underfed because of the mother's negligence. The vital process of bonding between mother and child may not have taken place; the child is not held close and cuddled, is not shown affection, and thus feels unwanted and unloved. This is seen often in babies who are reared in institutions where the nursing staff does not have time to caress and comfort infants individually. Similarly,

later in childhood, failure to grow at a normal rate can be caused by malnutrition or psychological factors. It could also be attributable to a deficiency in a hormone that is the body's natural regulator of growth. If this hormone is not released in adequate supply, the child's growth is stunted. An excess of this hormone may cause the child to grow too rapidly. Failure to grow normally may also indicate an underlying disease condition, such as heart dysfunction and malabsorption problems, in which the child does not get the necessary nutrition from food.

The parent and pediatrician must also ensure that the child is developing acceptably in other areas. Speech and language skills, teething, bone development, walking and other motor skills, toilet habits, sleep patterns, eye development, and hearing have to be evaluated regularly. Profound mental disability is usually evident early in life, but mild to moderate disability may not be apparent until the child starts school. Slowness in learning may be indicative of mental disability, but this judgment should be carefully weighed, because the real reason may be impaired hearing or vision or an underlying disease condition. The diagnosis of neurological disorders, such as autism and attention-deficit hyperactivity disorder (ADHD), has greatly increased in recent years and poses a special challenge to both parents and pediatricians.

The battery of diseases and other disorders that may beset a child remains more or less constant throughout childhood. Puberty, however, begins hormonal changes that trigger new disease threats and vast psychological upheaval. As early as eight years of age in girls and after ten or eleven years of age in boys, the body begins a prolonged metamorphosis that changes the child into an adult. Hormones that were previously released in minimal amounts course throughout the body in great quantities.

In boys, the sex hormones are called androgens. Chief among them is testosterone, which is secreted primarily by the testicles. It causes the sexual organs to mature and promotes the growth of hair in the genital area and armpits and on the chest. Testosterone also enlarges the larynx (voicebox), causing the voice to deepen.

Girls also produce some testosterone, but estrogens and other female sex hormones are the major hormones involved in puberty. They cause the sexual organs to mature, the hips to enlarge and become rounded, hair to grow in the genital area and armpits, the breasts to enlarge, and menstruation to begin. Many disease conditions can arise in association with the hormonal changes that occur during puberty, such as breast abnormalities and genital infections. Far and away the most common medical disorder at this time, however, is acne. Acne is a direct result of the rise in testosterone that occurs during puberty. About 85 percent of teenagers experience some degree of acne, and about 12 percent of these will develop severe, deep acne, a serious condition that can leave lifelong scars.

Important psychological changes also occur during puberty. The personality can be altered as the developing child begins to crave independence. Ties to the family weaken, and the teenager becomes closer to his or her peer group. Sexual feelings can be strong and difficult to repress. In modern Western society, this is usually the time when the teenager may begin to experiment with tobacco, alcohol, drugs, or other means of achieving a "high," although in some groups the use of these substances begins much earlier. Substance abuse is a major problem throughout society, but it is particularly devastating among young people.

Sexual activity among teenagers is widespread and, combined with inadequate education about health issues and limited access to care, has led to significant medical problems. The incidence of sexually transmitted infections (STIs) is higher among teenagers than any other group. Teenage pregnancy is one of the most challenging issues in modern society. If the pregnant teenager who continues her pregnancy is from a disadvantaged family background, she is even more likely than other teen mothers to receive little or no prenatal care. Risks of delayed or absent prenatal care can include a fetus that is not properly nourished. Additional risks can arise from a mother who smokes, drinks alcohol, or takes drugs throughout the pregnancy. In these cases, the child often may be born prematurely, with all the physical problems that premature birth involves. Hospital care of these infants is extremely costly, as is the maintenance of the mother and child if the baby survives.

Another important issue of teenage sexuality is the rapid spread of HIV, both as a sexually transmitted infection and as an infection passed from mother to baby.

DIAGNOSTIC AND TREATMENT TECHNIQUES

Pediatrics is one of the widest-ranging medical specialties, embracing virtually all major medical disciplines. Some pediatricians are generalists, and others specialize in certain disease areas, such as heart disease, kidney disease, liver disease, or skin problems.

Doctors and nurses specializing in neonatology, including advanced practice nurse practitioners with specialty certification in pediatrics or neonatology, have radically improved the survival rates of premature and low-weight babies. In neonatal care of the premature, the infant may have to be helped to breathe, fed through tubes, and otherwise maintained to allow it to develop.

Infectious diseases passed from the mother to the newborn child are a particular challenge. In some cases, such as with GBS and herpes infections, appropriate antibiotics and antiviral agents can be given. In others, such as with babies born with HIV, support measures and medications that help prevent the progress of the disease are the only procedures available.

Many birth defects and deformities can be repaired or at least ameliorated. Disorders such as cleft lip or palate, deformities of the skeletal system, heart defects, and other physical abnormalities often can be remedied by surgery. Certain structural malformations may require prosthetic devices and/ or physical therapy.

The treatment of spina bifida depends on the seriousness of the condition; surgery may be required. With hydrocephalus, medication may be helpful, but most often a permanent shunt is implanted to drain fluids from the cranium. Before this technique was developed, the prognosis for babies with hydrocephalus was poor: More than half died, and a great many suffered from mental disability and physical impairment. Today, 70 percent or more live through infancy. Of these, about 40 percent have normal intelligence; the others are mentally disabled and may also have serious physical impairment.

There are no cures for cerebral palsy, but various procedures can improve the child's quality of life, exercise and counseling among them. Neither is there a cure for Down syndrome. If mental disability is profound, the child may have to be institutionalized. When a child with Down syndrome can be cared for at home in a loving family, his or her life can be improved.

SIDS continues to be a problem both in hospitals and in the home. The American Academy of Pediatrics" Back to Sleep campaign, in which parents are encouraged to place babies on their backs for sleeping, has been extremely successful, however, and has resulted in a decrease in the incidence of SIDS by 70 to 80 percent.

Managing the infectious diseases of childhood is one of the major concerns of pediatric providers, who are often called on to treat infections, for which they have a wide variety of antibiotics and other agents. Pediatric providers also seek to prevent infectious diseases through immunization. Medical authorities now recommend routine vaccination of all children in the United States against diphtheria, tetanus, pertussis, measles, mumps, rubella, poliomyelitis, pneumococcal pneumonia, *Hemophilus influenzae*, varicella, and hepatitis A and B. Vaccines are also available against rabies, influenza, cholera, typhoid fever, plague, and yellow fever; these vaccines can be given to the child if there is a danger of infection. Vaccines for diphtheria, tetanus, and pertussis are generally given together in a combination called DTaP. Measles, mumps, and rubella vaccines are also given together as MMR. Repeated doses of some vaccines are necessary to ensure and maintain immunity.

Skin disorders of childhood, including teenage acne, are usually treated successfully at home with over-the-counter remedies. As with any disease, however, a severe skin disorder requires the attention of a trained provider.

Patients with diabetes mellitus type 1 are dependent on insulin throughout life. It is necessary for the pediatrician or attending nurse to teach both the parent and the patient how to inject insulin regularly, often several times a day. Furthermore, patients must monitor their blood and urine constantly to determine blood sugar levels. They must also adhere to stringent dietary regulations. This regimen of diet, insulin, and constant monitoring is often difficult for the child to learn and accept, but strict adherence is vital if the patient is to fare well and avoid the wide range of complications associated with diabetes.

Other serious conditions are now considered to be treatable. Modern pharmacology has greatly improved the prognosis of children with leukemia. Similarly, many children with growth disorders can be helped by treatments of growth hormone. Medications and other treatment modalities for the mental disorders of childhood have improved in recent years. Mentally disabled children can often be taught to care for themselves, and some even grow up to live independently. Children with behavioral problems may be helped by clinicians specializing in child psychology or psychiatry.

The problems of sexuality, sexually transmitted infections, and pregnancy among teenagers have provoked a nationwide response in the United States among medical and sociological professionals. Safersex programs have been launched, and clinics specializing in counseling for teenage girls are in operation to stem the rise in teenage pregnancies.

PERSPECTIVE AND PROSPECTS

Pediatrics affects virtually every member of society. Diseases that once raged through populations of all ages are now being controlled through the mass immunization of children. Some diseases of childhood are not yet controllable by vaccines, but research in this area is ongoing.

Childhood health is directly related to economics. Middleclass and upper-class children have ready access to professional care for any problems that may arise. The medical and psychological needs of disadvantaged children, however, especially those who live in inner cities, are often neglected. Many of these children are not being immunized fully and remain susceptible to diseases that are no longer a problem among the middle and upper classes.

In an effort to improve the medical care of disadvantaged children, some vaccines are being made available at low or no cost to inner-city families. Programs educate parents and teachers about the need for a child to receive the full dosage of vaccine. Computerized records allow authorities to keep track of the immunization status of individual children and to alert their parents when a follow-up inoculation is due.

The psychological problems of inner-city children, as well as children who live in disadvantaged rural areas, are at least as serious as the bodily diseases that threaten them. They may live in a universe of violence, deprivation, and drug addiction, and they might lack a stable family environment and opportunities for advancement. Pediatric providers at all levels can advocate for these youth by becoming involved in medical, psychological, and sociological outreach programs to help disadvantaged children.

—*C. Richard Falcon;*
Updated by Lenela Glass-Godwin, M.W.S.

FOR FURTHER INFORMATION

American Academy of Pediatrics. http://www.aap.org.

Doyle, Barbara T., and E. D. Iland. *Autism Spectrum Disorders from A to Z.* Arlington, Tex.: Future Horizons, 2004.

Hay, William W., Jr., et al., eds. *Current Diagnosis and Treatment: Pediatrics.* 21st ed. New York: Lange Medical Books/McGraw-Hill, 2012.

Kimball, Chad T. *Childhood Diseases and Disorders Sourcebook: Basic Consumer Health Information About Medical Problems Often Encountered in Pre-adolescent Children.* Detroit, Mich.: Omnigraphics, 2003.

Kliegman, Robert M., andWaldo E. Nelson, eds. *Nelson Textbook of Pediatrics.* 19th ed. Philadelphia: Saunders/Elsevier, 2011.

Litin, Scott C., ed. *Mayo Clinic Family Health Book.* 4th ed. New York: HarperResource, 2009.

Middlemiss, Prisca. *What's That Rash? How to Identify and Treat Childhood Rashes.* London: Hamlyn, 2002.

Nathanson, LauraWalther. *The Portable Pediatrician: A Practicing Pediatrician's Guide to Your Child's Growth, Development, Health, and Behavior from Birth to Age Five.* 2d ed. New York: HarperCollins, 2002.

Sanghavi, Darshak. *A Map of the Child: A Pediatrician's Tour of the Body.* New York: Henry Holt, 2003.

Pelvic inflammatory disease (PID)

CATEGORY: Disease/Disorder

KEY TERMS:

contact tracing: also known as partner referral; a process that involves identifying the sexual partners of infected patients, informing the partners of their exposure to disease, and offering resources for counseling and treatment

ectopic pregnancy: a pregnancy that occurs anywhere other than in the uterus; ectopic pregnancies can be life-threatening, since they can rupture and bleed profusely

laparoscopy: a minimally invasive surgical procedure performed through small incisions in the abdomen

polymicrobial infection: an infection caused by multiple microorganisms such as bacteria and viruses

sexually transmitted disease (STD): an infection caused by organisms transferred through sexual contact (genital-genital, oral-genital, oral-anal, or anal-genital); the transmission of infection occurs through exposure to lesions or secretions that contain the organisms

CAUSES AND SYMPTOMS

Pelvic inflammatory disease (PID) is a polymicrobial infection of the upper genital tract. The infectious microbes may be sexually transmitted organisms (such as *Neisseria gonorrhea, Chlamydia trachomatis,* and *Mycoplasma genitalium*) and/or endogenous bacteria found in the vagina (e.g., staphylococci, streptococci, enteric bacteria, such as *Klebsiella* species, *Escherichia coli* or *Proteus* species, or anaerobic bacteria like *Bacteroides* species). These microorganisms can travel from the lower genital tract (vagina, cervix) into the upper genital tract (uterus, Fallopian tubes, ovaries, and pelvic cavity) and establish infection there. Occasionally, PID can occur via another mechanism, such as any infection and rupture of the appendix or lower gastrointestinal tract that causes spillage of bacteria into the pelvic cavity.

85 percent of PID cases are caused by sexually transmitter microorganisms or by bacteria that cause infections of the birth canal (vaginosis). The remaining PID cases are caused by normal microbial residents of the lower reproductive tract of females.

Approximately 106,000 outpatient visits and 60,000 hospitalizations each year are due to PID. Each female PID patient costs around $2,000 to treat, and this number can rise to $6,000 if she develops chronic pelvic pain.

Most cases of PID are asymptomatic. In cases where symptoms occur, the patient has lower abdominal or pelvic pain. The Centers for Disease Control and Prevention (CDC) stipulates the diagnostic criteria for PID, noting that the diagnosis is made on clinical findings rather than on laboratory evidence. During abdominal examination, the lower abdomen is tender to palpation. Upon pelvic examination, either the cervix is tender upon movement by the examiner or one or both ovaries or the Fallopian tubes are tender to palpation; both of these symptoms can be present as well. Other symptoms and signs of PID include fever and abnormal cervical discharge.

Laboratory tests can be helpful in establishing a diagnosis when clinical symptoms are ambiguous and in emphasizing the need for partner treatment. Tests include blood tests that suggest systemic inflammation (such as the erythrocyte sedimentation rate) and cultures or nucleic acid amplification tests for *N. gonorrhea* or *C. trachomatis*. With ultrasound or other imaging techniques, fluid collections associated with the Fallopian tubes, ovaries, or elsewhere in the pelvic cavity can be identified as consistent with PID. On rare occasions, PID can spread to the upper abdomen, leading to pain and tenderness in that area. In particular, the infection can affect the region surrounding the liver, leading to Fitz-Hugh Curtis syndrome.

Long-term consequences of PID can be significant and can occur in asymptomatic as well as symptomatic patients. PID can cause scarring of the reproductive tract leading to infertility. Damaged fallopian tubes can fill with fluid (hydrosalpinx) and cause pain and infertility. PID increases the risk for ectopic pregnancy, a potentially life-threatening condition. If the infection spreads beyond the reproductive tract, then organs such as the bowels may become involved in the infection as well. Any organs involved in the infection run the risk of becoming damaged and scarred and might abnormally adhere to other organs. In addition to the acute pain of PID, the disease can also lead to chronic pelvic pain, which can be difficult to treat. Women with a history of PID have an almost two-fold increase in the risk of ovarian cancer.

TREATMENT AND THERAPY

Pelvic inflammatory disease is usually treated in an outpatient setting, although severe cases require hospitalization and intravenous medications. Antibiotics are the first-line treatment for PID, which is most commonly treated empirically based on clinical suspicion. Because PID is polymicrobial, combinations of antibiotics, each targeted at different bacteria, are given simultaneously. Drug regimens differ according to the severity of the disease. For severe PID, patients are usually treated in the hospital with cefotetan or cefoxitin combined with doxycycline, or clindamycin plus gentamicin. For mild to moderate PID, outpatient therapy is preferred and first-line treatments typically consist of ceftriaxone or cefoxitin/probenecid or cefotaxime plus doxycycline. Metronidazole

---

> ### Information on Pelvic Inflammatory Disease (PID)
>
> **Causes:** Bacterial infection transmitted through sexual contact or from other areas of body
> **Symptoms:** Usually asymptomatic; may involve lower abdominal or pelvic pain, fever, abnormal cervical or vaginal discharge; can lead to scarring, infertility, ectopic pregnancy
> **Duration:** Chronic
> **Treatments:** Antibiotics, abscess drainage if needed

---

is sometimes added to regimens as a third drug to cover anaerobic organisms and is always included if infection with the protozoan *Trichomonas vaginalis* is suspected. Unfortunately, the stomach discomfort caused by metronidazole can cause patients to stop taking it prematurely. Infections with *C. trachomitis* may warrant the inclusion of azithromycin, and for *N. gonorrhea* infections, ceftriaxone and doxycycline are particularly effective. Because of resistance, fluoroquinolone antibiotics (e.g., ciprofloxacin, moxifloxacin) are no longer used to treat gonorrhea infections. Patients are normally treated for 14 days.

Since PID is usually sexually transmitted, therapy involves counseling regarding the prevention of sexually transmitted infections (STIs) and safer sexual techniques. Condoms and other barrier techniques decrease the spread of STIs. Anal penetration followed by vaginal penetration during intercourse may increase the risk of infection of the female reproductive tract. Testing for other STIs, such as hepatitis B and C and syphilis; wet prep testing for bacterial vaginosis and trichomonas; and screening for human immunodeficiency virus (HIV) are all encouraged, since the risk factors for PID and other STIs are similar. Contact tracing is offered to notify sexual partners of their possible exposure to STIs and to encourage them to seek medical attention. Treatment of these partners can decrease reinfection of the patient from subsequent sexual encounters and prevent the partners from spreading infection to others. Having multiple sex partners is a risk factor for PID.

PERSPECTIVE AND PROSPECTS

One of the first reports of PID was from ancient Greece and involved a case in which pus from the pelvis was drained through the vagina. However, it was not until the 1880s that the sequence of events starting with the ascension of lower genital tract infection to cause upper tract disease was recognized. With the widespread use of laparoscopy in the 1960s, a more accurate diagnosis of PID could be made, allowing clinicians to recognize that PID has many clinical presentations. Future prospects focus primarily on the prevention of PID, since treatment does not prevent many of the long-term effects. Prevention involves continued widespread screening of asymptomatic men and women at risk for STDs, as well as partner referral and safer-sex education. Studies have shown that the screening and treatment of asymptomatic women for STDs has reduced the prevalence of these infections in the general population in the United States, thus translating into a reduction in the incidence of PID. With these prevention techniques, there is hope that the morbidity and serious sequelae of PID will be reduced.

—*Anne Lynn S. Chang, M.D.*
Updated by Michael A. Buratovich Ph.D.

FOR FURTHER INFORMATION

Handsfield, Hunter H. *Color Atlas & Synopsis of Sexually Transmitted Diseases.* 3rd ed., New York: McGraw-Hill, 2011.

Jameson, Larry J. et al. (Eds.). *Harrison's Principles of Internal Medicine.* 20th ed., New York: McGraw-Hill, 2018.

"Pelvic Inflammatory Disease (PID) Treatment." *Centers for Disease Control and Prevention,* March 1, 2013.

Schuiling, Kerri Durnell, and Frances E. Likis. *Women's Gynecologic Health,* 3rd ed., Burlington, MA: Jones and Bartlett Learning, 2016.

Sutton, Amy L. *Sexually Transmitted Diseases Sourcebook.* Detroit, Mich.: 2013.

Stewart, Miranda. *Pelvic Inflammatory Disease: A Step by Step Guide to Detect and Treat.* Seattle, WA: Amazon Digital Services LLC, 2016.

Vorvick, Linda J. "Pelvic Inflammatory Disease (PID)." *MedlinePlus,* September 12, 2011.

Workowski, Kimberly A., and Bolan, Gail A. "Sexually Transmitted Diseases Treatment Guidelines 2015." Morbidity and Mortality Weekly Report, *Centers for Disease Control and Prevention,* 64(RR3), 1-137.

Perinatology

CATEGORY: Specialty

KEY TERMS:

amniotic fluid: fluid within the amniotic cavity produced by the amnion during the early embryonic period (two to eight weeks) and later by the lungs and kidneys

cesarean section: an incision made through the abdominal and uterine walls for the delivery of a fetus

fetus: the unborn offspring in the postembryonic period, from nine weeks after fertilization until birth

infant: a young child from birth to twelve months of age

ischemia: a local anemia or area of diminished or insufficient blood supply as a result of mechanical obstruction of the blood supply (commonly narrowing of an artery)

fetal macrosomia: a newborn who's significantly larger than average

placenta: a fetomaternal organ that joins mother and offspring; it secretes endocrine hormones and selectively exchanges soluble, blood-borne substances through its interior structures

Rh: a human blood factor, originally identified in rhesus monkeys, that can be either positive (present) or negative (absent)

SCIENCE AND PROFESSION

Practitioners of perinatal medicine include physicians and advanced practice nurses with a specialty in perinatology (neonatal and pediatric nurse practitioners). They then complete additional training specifically related to the perinatal period (defined variously as beginning from twenty to twenty-eight weeks of gestation and ending one to four weeks after birth). The emphasis of perinatology is on a time period rather than on a specific organ system. The principal event of the perinatal period is birth. Prior to delivery, the perinatologist is concerned with the physiological status and well-being of both mother and fetus. Immediately after delivery, the perinatologist strives to maximize the newborn's chances for survival.

DIAGNOSTIC AND TREATMENT TECHNIQUES

Prior to the birth, several diagnostic procedures are commonly employed by the perinatologist: ultrasonography, the measurement of fetal activity, and the evaluation of fetal lung maturity. Ultrasonography uses sound waves to create images. Sound waves are transmitted from a transducer that has been placed on the skin. Waves that are sent into the body reflect off internal tissues and structures, and the reflections are received by a microphone. Sound travels through tissues with different densities at different rates, which are characteristic for each tissue. Computers interpret the reflected sounds and convert them into an image that can be viewed. The images must be interpreted or read by someone with specialized training, usually a radiologist. Ultrasound does not involve radiation; thus it is not harmful to the fetus. Because sound waves are longer than radiation, the image generated is not as clear as that obtained with electromagnetic waves.

The measurement of fetal activity is important in evaluating fetal health. Fetal movement is normal; the earliest movement felt by the mother is called quickening. The diminution or cessation of fetal movement is indicative of fetal distress. Accordingly, movement is monitored by reports from the mother, palpation by the clinician, and ultrasound: Mothers report movements, individuals examining pregnant women can apply their hands to the abdomen and feel fetal movements, and ultrasonography can show breathing and other movements in real time using continuous video records of fetal movements.

Fetal lung maturity is assessed by measuring the relative amounts of lecithin and sphingomyelin in amniotic fluid. The concentration of lecithin increases late in fetal development, while sphingomyelin decreases. A lecithin-sphingomyelin ratio that is greater than two indicates sufficient fetal lung maturity to ensure survival after birth.

Labor and delivery are the primary events of the perinatal period. Factors that can lead to difficulties include abnormalities of the placenta and prematurity. The placenta can be abnormally located (placenta previa) or can separate prematurely (placenta abruptio). Normally, the placenta is located on the lateral wall of the uterus. Placenta previa is defined as a placenta located in the lower portion of the uterus. The placenta is compressed by the fetus during passage through the birth canal. This compression compromises the blood supply to the fetus, which causes ischemia and can lead to brain or other tissue damage or to death. This condition is usually managed by a cesarean section. Placenta abruptio refers to a normal placenta that separates prior to fetal delivery. This condition is potentially life-threatening to both mother and fetus; immediate hospitalization is indicated.

Prematurity is defined as delivery before the fetus is able to survive without unusual support. Premature infants are placed in incubators. A lack of body fat in the infant leads to difficulty in maintaining a normal body temperature; special heating is provided to offset the problem. Lung immaturity may require mechanical assistance from a respirator. An immature immune system makes premature infants especially susceptible to infections; strict isolation precautions and prophylactic antibiotic therapy address this problem.

Many factors contribute to increasing the risks normally associated with pregnancy and delivery: maternal size and age; drug, tobacco, or alcohol use; infection; medical conditions such as diabetes mellitus and hypertension; and multiple gestations. A woman with a small pelvic opening may be unable to deliver her child normally; the solution in this case is a cesarean section. The risk of genetic abnormalities increases with advancing maternal (and, to a lesser degree, paternal) age. Counseling prior to conception is indicated. Once an older woman becomes pregnant, amniotic fluid should be obtained to test for genetic abnormalities. The degree of surveillance is dependent on maternal age: The recommended frequency of medical checks increases for older women.

Alcohol intake during pregnancy can result in an infant who is both developmentally disabled and mentally retarded; smoking during pregnancy frequently leads to an infant with a low birth weight. Drug usage during pregnancy can lead to anatomic or mental impairment. Avoiding the use of all substances is the easiest way to eliminate problems completely; any drug should be used only under the guidance of a physician. Some viral infections such as German measles (rubella) early in pregnancy can cause birth defects. Immunization prior to conception will avoid these problems.

Diabetes mellitus can cause abnormally large intrauterine growth and babies (frequently more than 10 pounds and referred to as macrosomic) who are too large for normal delivery. Diabetes that commonly develops during pregnancy is called gestational diabetes. Medical monitoring to detect diabetes early is prudent. Appropriate medical management of preexisting diabetes minimizes problems associated with pregnancy. A macrosomic infant must be delivered with a cesarean section. Hypertension can also develop during pregnancy. Like diabetes, it can compromise both mother and fetus. Appropriate and aggressive medical management, sometimes including complete bed rest, is needed to control high blood pressure during pregnancy. Multiple gestations (such as twins or triplets) strain the supply of maternal nutrients to the developing fetuses. Because space is limited, multiple fetuses are usually smaller than normal at birth.

Rhesus disease, also known as Rh incompatibility, can complicate pregnancy. It can occur only in the child of a father whose blood type is Rh-positive and a mother whose blood type is Rh-negative, and it affects the blood supply of a fetus. The treatment includes the identification of both maternal and paternal blood types and the administration of Rho(D) immune globulin to the mother at twenty-six weeks of gestation and again immediately after birth. An affected infant may require blood transfusions; in a severe case, transfusions may be needed during pregnancy.

PERSPECTIVE AND PROSPECTS

Management of a pregnancy requires specialized skills. As the number of risk factors related to either mother or fetus increases, the problems associated with pregnancy also increase. The care of a pregnant woman and her fetus requires input from many individuals with specialized training. Consequently, perinatology is very much a team effort. Together, the team members can ensure a safe journey through the perinatal period for a pregnant woman and a healthy transition to life outside the womb for a newborn infant.

—*L. Fleming Fallon, Jr., M.D., Ph.D., M.P.H.*

FOR FURTHER INFORMATION

Cunningham, F. Gary, et al., eds. *Williams Obstetrics.* 23d ed. New York: McGraw-Hill, 2010.

Martin, Richard J., Avroy A. Fanaroff, and Michele C. Walsh, eds. *Fanaroff and Martin's Neonatal-Perinatal Medicine: Diseases of the Fetus and Infant.* 2 vols. 9th ed. Philadelphia: Mosby/Elsevier, 2011.

Moore, Keith L., and T. V. N. Persaud. *The Developing Human.* 9th ed. Philadelphia: Saunders/Elsevier, 2013.

"Pregnancy and Perinatology Branch (PPB)." *National Institute of Child Health and Human Development,* November 30, 2012.

Ruhlman, Michael. *Walk on Water: Inside an Elite Pediatric Surgery Unit.* New York: Viking-Penguin, 2003.

Sadler, T.W. *Langman's Medical Embryology.* 12th ed. Philadelphia: Lippincott Williams & Wilkins, 2012

Pituitary gland

CATEGORY: Anatomy

KEY TERMS:

adenohypophysis: another name for the anterior lobe of the pituitary gland

estrogen:

negative feedback: a common physiological process by which the product of a process feeds back to inhibit further stimulation (or reverse) the process

neurohypophysis: another name for the posterior lobe of the pituitary gland

positive feedback: a physiological process in which a product feeds back to stimulate the process, resulting in additional production or the continuation of that process

progesterone:

STRUCTURE AND FUNCTIONS

The pituitary gland is similar in size to a pea and has two lobes, the anterior (adenohypophysis) and the posterior (neurohypophysis). The anterior lobe accounts for a greater proportion of the total weight, approximately 80%. The pituitary gland is involved in the release of numerous hormones that have a multitude of effects throughout the body; as a result, it is often referred to as the "master" gland. The functions of the hormones released from the pituitary gland include reproductive functions (including childbirth and lactation), bone growth and development, and regulation of metabolic processes, body temperature, water balance, circulation, and blood pressure. Therefore, a normally functioning pituitary gland is essential to the health and maintenance of homeostasis in humans.

Hormones released from the anterior lobe of the pituitary gland include thyroid-stimulating hormone

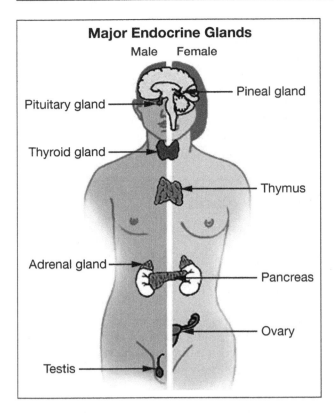

Major Endocrine Glands

Male   Female

Pituitary gland

Thyroid gland

Adrenal gland

Testis

Pineal gland

Thymus

Pancreas

Ovary

The endocrine system in both sexes, controlled by the pituitary gland. (Wikimedia Commons)

(TSH) or thyrotropin, growth hormone (GH), adrenocorticotropic hormone (ACTH), follicle-stimulating hormone (FSH), luteinizing hormone (LH), prolactin (PRL), and oxytocin. The hypothalamus, which is located just superior to the pituitary gland, regulates the release of hormones from the anterior pituitary gland by releasing hormones that travel through a blood network called the hypophyseal portal system to the anterior pituitary. For example, the hypothalamus releases growth-hormone- releasing hormone (GHRH), which travels to the anterior pituitary and stimulates the release of growth hormone.

Alternatively, if the body wants to decrease the secretion of GH, the hypothalamus may do so by releasing growth hormone-inhibiting hormone (GHIH), also known as growth hormone-release-inhibiting hormone (GHRIH) or somatostatin. Another common inhibiting hormone released from the hypothalamus is prolactin-inhibiting hormone

(PIH), which reduces the release of PRL from the anterior pituitary.

In contrast to the anterior lobe, the posterior lobe of the pituitary gland releases two hormones: oxytocin and antidiuretic hormone (ADH), which is commonly referred to as vasopressin. The release of these hormones is influenced by blood pressure, osmolarity of the blood, and other inputs, such as those from the nervous and reproductive systems. Several hormones released by the pituitary gland stimulate other organs or tissues directly, resulting in changes in overall physiologic function. For example, GH increases protein synthesis and the related growth of muscles, bones, and tissues. GH also increases the release of glucose and fat breakdown to fuel these anabolic processes. Finally, ADH causes the kidneys to reabsorb or retain water, aiding in the body's ability to regulate water balance and hydration levels.

Other hormones released by the pituitary gland stimulate the release of still other hormones from subsequent endocrine glands. These include TSH, which stimulates the thyroid gland to release thyroid hormones; ACTH, which stimulates the cortex of the adrenal glands to release cortisol; and the sex hormones FSH and LH, also called gonadotrophs, which stimulate the sex organs to release hormones involved in the ovaries' production of estrogen and progesterone and the function of the menstrual cycle.

The release of most hormones from the pituitary gland is controlled by classic negative-feedback loops. In these systems, an increase in product feeds back to inhibit further stimulation of that system. Using the thyroid hormones as an example, the hypothalamus releases thyrotropin-releasing hormone (TRH), which stimulates the anterior pituitary to release TSH, which then causes the thyroid gland to release thyroid hormones. When circulating levels of thyroid hormones are higher than normal or necessary, they feed back to inhibit or slow the release of TRH from the hypothalamus and TSH from the anterior pituitary. Conversely, when circulating levels of thyroid hormones are low, they feed back to increase the release of TRH and TSH, which will ultimately increase the release of thyroid hormones from the thyroid gland. Therefore, there are several sites of control involved in the release of products from the pituitary gland.

A notable exception to this trend is the presence of a positive-feedback process involving the pituitary gland and the hormone oxytocin. In this system, the stretching of the cervix during labor causes the release of oxytocin, which increases contractions in the uterus to assist with the progression of labor and eventual childbirth. The oxytocin feeds back in a positive fashion by increasing the stretching of the cervix, which then leads to the release of even more oxytocin. This cycle continues until the child is born, at which time the stimulus of cervical stretch and the related oxytocin release both cease.

DISORDERS AND DISEASES

Pituitary dysfunction is typically characterized by an oversecretion or undersecretion of pituitary hormones. An overactive pituitary gland is an endocrine defect characterized by excessive growth in stature and mass, plus a variety of other symptoms, depending on which hormones are elevated. The increased hormone release from the pituitary gland is often attributed to a pituitary tumor. If this is the case, then the tumor may be treated with radiation therapy, surgical removal, or the use of an antagonist to decrease the release of pituitary hormones.

Individuals with underactive pituitary glands, or hypopituitarism, experience symptoms such as short stature, low body mass, infertility or reproductive difficulties (including the inability of women to lactate following childbirth), low energy levels, perpetual feeling of cold due to an inability to regulate body temperature, and fatigue. Hypopituitarism may also be caused by a pituitary tumor, as well as injury to or infection of the hypothalamus or pituitary gland. The treatment for hypopituitarism involves stimulating the release of hormones from the target organs or tissues, rather than stimulating the pituitary gland itself.

—*Kristin S. Ondrak, Ph.D.*

FOR FURTHER INFORMATION

Freeman, Susan, L. "The Anterior Pituitary." In *Endocrine Pathophysiology*, edited by Catherine B. Niewoehner. 2d ed. Hayes Barton Press, 2004.

Klibanski, Anne, and Nicholas Tritos, editors. "Pituitary Disorders." *Hormone Health Network*, May 2013.

Mayo Clinic Staff. "Pituitary Tumors." *Mayo Clinic*, Mayo Foundation for Medical Education and Research, 2018, www.mayoclinic.org/diseases-conditions/pituitary-tumors/symptoms-causes/syc-20350548.

"Pituitary Disorders." *MedlinePlus*, July 11, 2013.

Placenta

CATEGORY: Biology

KEY TERMS:

afterbirth: the placenta and fetal membranes discharged from the uterus after birth

placenta abruption: when the placenta separates early from the uterus

placenta previa: a condition in which the placenta partially or wholly blocks the neck of the uterus

trophoblasts: cells forming the outer layer of a blastocyst, which provide nutrients to the embryo and develop into a large part of the placenta

STRUCTURE AND FUNCTIONS

The placenta is an important and unique organ that develops in women only during pregnancy. The placenta connects a woman's body to the embryo and then the fetus through the umbilical cord. The cells that make up the placenta, called trophoblasts, function to control the degree of uterine invasion in the mother and the development of a nutrient, gas, and waste transport for the fetus. The fetus receives oxygen and nutrients from the mother and eliminates wastes through the placenta. The placenta is necessary for the development and survival of the fetus during pregnancy, but it must be delivered from the mother's body after the baby's birth. It is then termed the afterbirth.

In addition to its primary goal of transporting nutrients, oxygen, and waste between mother and fetus, the placenta also serves as a major endocrine organ. The placenta synthesizes and secretes sex steroid and protein hormones. One hormone in particular, human chorionic gonadotropin (hCG), is secreted by the placenta about one week after an egg has been fertilized (conception). This hormone stimulates the production of the steroid hormone progesterone, which is needed for survival of the baby. The detection of hCG in a mother's urine is the most common test for pregnancy.

DISORDERS AND DISEASES

In most pregnant women, the placenta forms and grows normally. In some cases, however, the placenta does not grow properly, is poorly positioned in the uterus, or does not function properly. It may be too large or small or connect abnormally. Placental problems are among the most common complications with pregnancy.

Placenta previa is a condition that occurs during pregnancy when the placenta implants in the lower part of the uterus and obstructs the cervical opening to the birth canal. The incidence of placenta previa is approximately one of two hundred births.

Placenta abruptio during pregnancy is a condition in which the placenta separates from the uterus before the fetus is born. This condition occurs in about one of every ninety deliveries. A woman is more likely to develop this condition if she has preeclampsia. The cause is not known, but preeclampsia usually occurs in the second half of pregnancy. Signs include high blood pressure, swelling, and protein in the urine. The risk of preeclampsia is higher in women carrying multiple fetuses, in teenage mothers, and in women older than age forty.

Most women with preeclampsia still deliver healthy babies, but a rare few may develop a condition called eclampsia (seizures caused by toxemia), which is very serious for the mother and the baby. Approximately 8 percent of pregnant women will develop preeclampsia.

When the placenta fails to develop or function properly, the fetus cannot grow and develop normally; this is called placental insufficiency. The earlier in pregnancy that this occurs, the more severe the resulting problems. If placental insufficiency occurs for a long time during pregnancy, then it may lead to intrauterine growth retardation or restriction (IUGR), a condition in which the fetus does not grow as large as it should while in the uterus. These babies are very small for their gestational age. IUGR can be caused by decreased blood flow to the placenta, drug use, smoking, alcoholism, or placental abnormalities. A diagnosis can be made through ultrasound to measure fetal growth and a non-stress test that measures the heart rate and movement of the fetus. Between 3 and 5 percent of all pregnancies are complicated by IUGR caused by placental insufficiency. A baby with severe IUGR is more likely to have health problems in the newborn period, as well as throughout childhood.

PERSPECTIVE AND PROSPECTS

The placenta is a unique organ essential for the birth of a child. The most common problems in pregnancy involve the placenta; fortunately, many are manageable. With preeclampsia, delivery of the baby is the best way to protect both the mother and the baby. This is not always possible, however, because it may be too early for the baby to live outside the womb. In this case, steps can be taken to manage the preeclampsia until the baby can be delivered, including decreasing blood pressure with bed rest or medicine. Fortunately, preeclampsia is usually detected early in women who obtain regular prenatal care, and most problems can be prevented. Most cases of IUGR cannot be prevented, especially if they are the result of genetic causes. Some cases can be prevented by taking the following precautions: abstinence from alcohol, tobacco, and illicit drugs; careful monitoring and early treatment for high blood pressure and diabetes; and a diet high in folate before and during pregnancy to protect against certain birth defects.

—*Thomas L. Brown, Ph.D.*

FOR FURTHER INFORMATION

Benirschke, Kurt, Graham Burton, and Rebecca Baergen. *Pathology of the Human Placenta*. 6th ed. New York: Springer, 2012.

Berven, Eirik, and Andras Freberg. *Human Placenta: Structure and Development, Circulation, and Functions*. New York: Nova Biomedical Books, 2010.

Harding, Richard, and Alan D. Bocking, eds. *Fetal Growth and Development*. New York: Cambridge University Press, 2001.

Kay, Helen H., D. Michael Nelson, and YupingWang. *The Placenta: From Development to Disease*. Chichester, England: Wiley- Blackwell, 2011.

Power, Michael L, and Jay Schulkin. *The Evolution of the Human Placenta*. Baltimore, Md.: Johns Hopkins University Press, 2012.

Plastic surgery

CATEGORY: Procedure

KEY TERMS:

congenital: existing at birth; often used in reference to certain mental or physical malformations and diseases, which may be hereditary or caused by some influence during gestation

cosmetic surgery: the application of plastic surgical techniques to alter one's appearance for purely aesthetic reasons

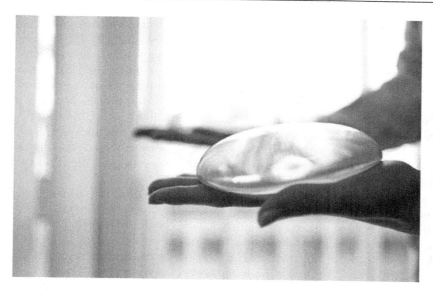

Breast augmentation is a popular plastic surgery procedure. (FDA via Wikimedia Commons)

debridement: the excision of contused and devitalized tissue from a wound surface

dermis: the second layer of skin, immediately below the epidermis; it contains blood and lymphatic vessels, nerves, glands, and (usually) hair follicles

epidermis: the outermost thin layer of skin that encompasses structures superficial to the dermis

granuloma: a nodular, inflammatory lesion that is usually small, firm, and persistent and usually contains proliferated macrophages

plastic surgery: the branch of operative surgery concerning the repair of defects, the replacement of lost tissue, and the treatment of extensive scarring; it accomplishes these ends by direct union of body parts, grafting, or the transfer of tissue from one part of the body to another

reconstructive surgery: the application of plastic surgical techniques to repair damaged tissues

turgor: fullness and firmness; the quality of normal skin in a healthy young person

INDICATIONS AND PROCEDURES

The intent of plastic, reconstructive, and cosmetic surgery is to restore a body part to normal appearance or to enhance or cosmetically alter a body part. The techniques and procedures of all three surgical applications are similar: extremely careful skin preparation, the use of delicate instrumentation and handling techniques, and precise suturing with extremely fine materials to minimize scarring.

Reconstructive surgery. Notable examples of reconstructive surgery involve the reattachment of limbs or extremities that have been traumatically severed. As soon as a part is separated from the body, it loses its blood supply; this leads to ischemia (lack of oxygen) to tissues, which in turn leads to cell death. When an individual cell dies, it cannot be resuscitated and will soon start to decompose. This process can be greatly slowed by lowering the temperature of the severed body part. Packing the part in ice for transport to a hospital is a prudent initial step.

An important consideration in any reconstructive procedure is site preparation. The edges, or margins, of the final wound must be clean and free of contamination. Torn skin is removed through a process called debridement. A sharp scalpel is used gently to cut away tissue that has been crushed or torn. All bacterial contamination must be removed from the site prior to closure to prevent postoperative contamination. Foreign material such as dirt, glass, gunpowder, metals, or chemicals must be completely removed. The margins of the wound must also be sharply defined. Superficially, this is done for aesthetic reasons. Internally, sharply defined margins will reduce the chances for adhesions to form. Adhesions are bands of scar tissue which bind adjacent structures together and restrict normal movement and function. Therefore, both the body site and the margins of the severed part must be debrided and defined. Reconstruction consists of the painstaking reattachment of nerves, tendons, muscles, and skin, which are held in place primarily by sutures although staples, wires, and other materials are occasionally used. Precise alignment of the skin to be closed is accomplished by joining opposing margins. Postoperative procedures include careful handling of the wound site, adequate nutrition, and rest in order to maximize healing. Abnormalities in the healing process can lead to undesirable scarring from the sites of sutures. Such marks can be avoided with careful attention to correct techniques.

Bones are reconstructed in cases of severe fractures. The pieces are set in their proper positions, and the area is immobilized. Where immobilization is not possible, a surface is provided onto which new bone can grow. These temporary surfaces are made of polymeric materials that will dissolve over time.

Congenital anomalies such as a deformed external ear or missing digit can be corrected using reconstructive techniques. In the case of a missing thumb, a finger can be removed, rotated, and attached on the site where the thumb should have been. This allows an affected individual to write, hold objects such as eating utensils, and generally have a more nearly normal life. Similar procedures can be applied to replace a missing or amputated great or big toe. The presence of the great toe contributes significantly to balance and coordination when walking.

Prosthetic materials are implanted in a growing variety of applications. There are two basic types of materials used in prostheses, which are classified according to their surface characteristics. One is totally smooth and inert; an example is Teflon or silicone. The body usually encloses these materials in a membrane, which has the effect of creating a wall or barrier to the surface of the prosthesis. From the body's perspective, the prosthesis has thus been removed. With any prosthesis, the problem most likely to be encountered is infection, which is usually caused by contamination of the operative site or the prosthesis. Infection can also occur at a later, postoperative date because of the migration of bacteria into the cavity formed by the membrane. This is a potentially serious complication. A smooth prosthesis can also be used to create channels into which tissue can later be inserted. In such an application, the prosthesis may be surgically removed at some time in the future. A second type of prosthesis does not have a smooth surface; rather, it has microscopic fibers similar to those found on a towel. This type of surface prevents membranes from forming, contributing to a longer life for the prosthesis by reducing postoperative infections.

An important procedure in reconstructive surgery is skin grafting. A graft consists of skin that is completely removed from a donor site and transferred to another site on the body. The graft is usually taken from the patient's own body because skin taken from another individual will be rejected by the recipient's immune system. (Nevertheless, fetal pig skin is sometimes used successfully.) Skin grafting is useful for covering open wounds, and it is widely used in serious burn cases. When only a portion of the uppermost layer of the skin is removed, the process is called a split thickness graft. When all the upper layers of the skin are removed, the result is a full thickness graft. Whenever possible, the donor site is selected to match the color and texture characteristics of the recipient site.

A skin flap is sometimes created. This differs from a graft in that the skin of a flap is not completely severed from its original site but simply moved to an adjacent location. Some blood vessels remain to support the flap. This procedure is nearly always successful, but it is limited to immediately adjacent skin.

A wide variety of flaps has been developed. A flap may be stretched and sutured to cover both a wound and the donor site. Flaps may be created from skin that is distant to the site where it is needed and then sutured in place over the donor site. Only after the flap has become established at the new site is it cut free from the donor site. Thus, skin from the abdomen or upper chest may be used to cover the back of a burned hand, or skin from one finger may be used to cover a finger on the other hand. This two-stage flap process requires more time than a skin graft, but it also has a greater probability of success.

Plastic surgery. Plastic surgery consists of a variety of techniques and applications, often dealing with skin. Some common procedures that primarily involve skin are undertaken to remove unwanted wrinkles or folds. Folds in skin are caused by a loss of skin turgor and excessive stretching of the skin beyond which it cannot recover. Common contributors to loss of skin turgor in the abdomen are pregnancy or significant weight loss after years of obesity. Both women and men may undergo a procedure known as abdominoplasty (commonly called a "tummy tuck"). The skin that lies over the abdominal muscles is carefully separated from underlying tissue.

Portions of the skin are removed; frequently, some underlying adipose (fat) tissue is also removed or relocated. The remaining skin is sutured to the underlying muscle as well as to adjacent, undisturbed skin. A major problem with this procedure, however, is scar formation because large portions of skin must be removed or relocated. The plastic surgeon must plan the placement of incisions carefully in order to avoid undesirable scars.

Plastic surgery is also used to reduce the prominence of ears, a procedure called otoplasty. In some children, the posterior (back) portion of the external ear develops more than the rest of the ear, pushing the ears outward and making them prominent. By reducing the bulk of cartilage in the posterior ear and suturing the remaining external portion to the base of the ear, the plastic surgeon can create a more normal ear contour. The optimal time to perform this procedure on children is just prior to the time that they enter school, or at about five years of age.

Cosmetic surgery. The most common site for cosmetic surgical procedures is the face. Correction may be desired because of a congenital anomaly that causes unwelcome disfigurement or because of a desire to alter an unwanted aspect of one's body. The cosmetic procedures that have been developed to correct abnormalities of the face include closure of a cleft lip or palate. The correction of a cleft lip is usually done early, ideally in the first three months of life. Closure of a cleft palate (the bone that forms the roof of the mouth) is delayed slightly, until the patient is 12 to 18 months old. These procedures allow affected individuals to acquire normal patterns of speech and language.

Among older individuals, common procedures include blepharoplasty and rhinoplasty. The former refers to the removal of excess skin around the eyelids, while the latter refers to a change, usually a reduction, in the shape of the nose. Both procedures may be included in the more general term of face lift. The effects of aging, excessive solar radiation, and gravity combine to produce fine lines in the face as individuals get older. These fine lines gradually develop into the wrinkles characteristic of older persons. For some, these wrinkles are objectionable. To reduce them—or more correctly to stretch them out—a plastic surgeon removes a section of skin containing the wrinkles or lines and stretches the edges of the remaining epidermis until they are touching. These incisions are placed to coincide with the curved lines that exist in normal skin. Thus, when the edges are sutured together, the resultant scar is minimized. Rhinoplasty often involves the removal of a portion of the bone or cartilage that forms the nose. The bulk of the remaining tissue is also reduced to maintain the desired proportions of the patient's nose. As with any plastic surgical procedure, small sutures are carefully placed to minimize scarring.

A third body area that is commonly subjected to cosmetic procedures is the breast. A woman who is unhappy with the appearance of her breasts may seek to either reduce or augment existing tissue. Breast reduction is accomplished by careful incision and the judicious removal of both skin and underlying breast tissue. Often the nipples must be repositioned to maintain their proper locations. A flap that includes the nipple is created from each breast. After the desired amount of underlying tissue is removed, the nipples are repositioned, and the skin is recontoured around the remaining breast masses.

USES AND COMPLICATIONS

Reconstructive, plastic, and cosmetic surgeries all have their complications, ranging from severe—such as the rejection of transplanted tissue—to minor but unpleasant—such as noticeable scars. In addition, there is an inherent risk in any procedure that requires the patient to undergo general anesthesia. With reconstruction, which involves the repair of damaged tissues and structures, the initial injuries sustained by the patient present further obstacles and dangers. The following examples from each type of surgery illustrate the risks involved. For example, a surgeon who must perform a skin graft can choose between a split and a full thickness graft. A split thickness graft site will heal with relatively normal skin, thus providing opportunities for additional grafting at a later date. It also produces less pronounced scarring. A limitation of this technique, however, is an increased likelihood for the graft to fail. Full thickness grafts are stronger and more likely to be successful, but they lead to more extensive scarring, which is aesthetically undesirable and renders the site unsuitable for later grafts. The surgeon's decision is based on the needs of the patient and the severity of the injury.

The minimization of scarring is a major concern for many patients undergoing plastic surgery. The prevention of noticeable scars involves an understanding of the natural lines of the skin. All areas of the body have lines of significant skin tension and lines of relatively little skin tension. It is along the lines of minimal tension that wrinkles and folds develop over time. These lines are curved and follow body contours. As a rule of thumb, they are generally perpendicular to the fibers of underlying muscle. The plastic surgeon seeks to place incisions along the lines of minimal tension. When scars form after healing, they will blend into the line of minimal tension and become less noticeable. Furthermore, the scar tissue is not likely to become apparent when the underlying muscles or body part is moved. Undesirable scarring is a greater problem in large procedures, such as abdominoplasty, than in procedures confined to a small area, such as rhytidectomy (face lift), because of the difficulty in following lines of minimum tension when making incisions.

One of the most popular cosmetic procedures is breast enlargement. According to the American Society of Plastic Surgeons, 296,203 augmentation mammoplasties were performed in the United States in 2010, and the total number of women with implants in the United States is more than 2 million. Initially, the most commonly used prosthesis, or implant, was made of silicone. In some patients, silicone leaked out, causing the formation of granulomatous tissue. Such complications led to a voluntary suspension of the production of silicone prostheses by manufacturers and of their usage by surgeons. Different materials, such as polyethylene bags filled with saline solution or solid polyurethane implants, were soon substituted. Saline will not cause tissue damage if it leaks, and few adverse reactions to polyurethane have been reported. Silicone implants made a comeback in 2006, when the US Food and Drug Administration began approving them for use in women aged twenty-two years or older.

Alongside possible surgical complications of breast augmentation, women may also have concerns regarding screening methods for breast cancer, and how their surgical history would

affect these methods of assessment. Routine screening with a mammography is done the same way as women without implants, but for women with implants, the mammography would include multiple views of the breasts, as the implants may result in false or misleading results. The implants could also get in

---

In the News:
Wrinkle Treatment with Botox and Artefill

As a person ages, the collagen and elastin proteins in the skin that keep it supple and smooth begin to weaken. The skin begins to thin and lose fat, and gravity causes the skin to sag. Wrinkles and deep facial folds develop. While these changes once seemed inevitable and were reversible only through major plastic surgery, new products and treatments are rejuvenating aging faces. Two such products are Botox and Artefill (sold as Artecoll in countries outside the United States).

Botulinum toxin type A (Botox cosmetic) is a compound produced by the bacterium *Clostridium botulinum* and is the same toxin that causes the potentially lethal food poisoning known as botulism. When used to combat wrinkles, the toxin is highly purified and diluted thousands of times, then injected in very small, safe doses into facial muscles, particularly between the eyebrows and at the sides of the eyes. The toxin blocks the release of a chemical signal called acetylcholine from nerve cells, which normally leads to muscle contraction. Botox paralyzes the muscles to eliminate frowning and to relax the associated furrows and lines around the eyes and between the eyebrows. The effect lasts for three to four months or more, and then the procedure must be repeated to maintain the wrinkle-free appearance.

Botox was first approved for use in treating eye muscle disorders in 1989, and in April, 2002, the Food and Drug Administration (FDA) approved Botox for wrinkles, although it had been used legally to treat wrinkles prior to official approval. In 2001, more than 1.6 million Botox injections were given to an estimated 850,000 patients in the United States. The number of people using Botox is anticipated to increase over the next several years.

As an alternative to Botox treatment for wrinkles, Artefill has the advantage of being a long-term or potentially permanent treatment. Artefill is an injectable implant that contains tiny non-biodegradable polymer microspheres of poly(methyl methacrylate) (PMMA) suspended in a solution containing 75 percent collagen. Artefill is injected into the wrinkle or facial fold, where the microspheres stimulate the body to produce its own collagen, which surrounds and encapsulates the microspheres. Within three to six months, the implant becomes permanently anchored in place by the body, where it plumps up the wrinkle.

Artefill has been used successfully to treat more than 200,000 patients outside the United States. Clinical trials of the implant in the United States were completed in September, 2001. In 2003, an FDA advisory panel recommended approval of Artefill for the treatment of wrinkles.

—*Karen E. Kalumuck, Ph.D.*

the way of getting a clear view of small lesions and make compression of the breast during imaging harder than with women without implants. Mammograms can also show complications related to the implant, including rupture or content leakage. Ultrasound can also be conducted on women with breast implants as a screening tool for breast cancer.

PERSPECTIVE AND PROSPECTS

The origins of plastic, reconstructive, and cosmetic surgery are fundamental to the earliest surgical procedures, which were developed to correct superficial deformities. Without any viable methods of anesthesia, surgical interventions and corrections were limited to the skin. For example, present day nose reconstructions (rhinoplasty) are essentially similar to procedures developed four thousand years ago. Hindu surgeons developed the technique of moving a piece of skin from the adjacent cheek onto the nose to cover a wound. Similar procedures were developed by Italians using skin that was transferred from the arm or forehead to repair lips and ears as well as noses. Ironically, wars have provided opportunities to advance reconstructive techniques. As field hospitals and surgical facilities became more widely available and wounded soldiers could be stabilized during transport, techniques to repair serious wounds evolved.

Skin grafts have been used since Roman times. Celsus described the possibility of skin grafts in conjunction with eye surgery. References were made to skin grafts in the Middle Ages. The evolution of modern techniques can be traced to the early nineteenth century, when Cesare Baronio conducted systematic grafting experiments with animals. The modern guidelines for grafting were formulated in 1870. Instruments for creating split thickness grafts were developed in the 1930s, and applications of this procedure evolved during World War II.

Plastic, reconstructive, and cosmetic procedures have all become important in contemporary surgical practice. Reconstructive surgery allows the repair of serious injuries and contributes greatly to the rehabilitation of affected individuals. Cosmetic surgery can help individuals feel better about themselves and their bodies. Both use techniques developed in the broader field of plastic surgery.

There are both positive and negative aspects of plastic surgery. Positively, many individuals who sustain serious and potentially devastating injuries are able to return to relatively normal lives. Burn victims and those having accidents are more likely to return to normal activities and resume their occupations than at any time in the past. Miniaturization and new materials have extended the range of a plastic surgeon's skills. Negatively, there is growing criticism concerning the number of elective procedures undertaken for the repair of cosmetic defects.

The quest for perfection and physical beauty has prompted some critics to question the correctness of some unnecessary procedures. Although such procedures are not usually covered by insurance policies, their utilization has increased. The continuation of such activities invokes both ethical and personal considerations; there is no clearly defined, logical endpoint. Clearly, while plastic surgical techniques have benefited millions, there are opportunities for abuse. Society must decide if any limitations are to be placed on plastic surgical procedures and what they should be.

In the meantime, advances in materials, instruments, and techniques will benefit plastic, reconstructive, and cosmetic surgery. As but one example, the advent of magnification and miniaturization and the development of tiny instruments and new suture materials have allowed the reconstruction of many injury sites. Blood vessels and nerves are now routinely reattached and a mere nine individual sutures are required to join the severed portions of a blood vessel one millimeter in diameter.

—*L. Fleming Fallon, Jr., M.D., Ph.D., M.P.H.*
Updated by Danielle T. Um

FOR FURTHER INFORMATION

Grazer, Frederick M., and Jerome R. Klingbeil. *Body Image: A Surgical Perspective.* St. Louis, Mo.: Mosby Year Book, 1980.

Loftus, Jean M. *The Smart Woman's Guide to Plastic Surgery.* 2d ed. Dubuque, Iowa: McGraw-Hill, 2008.

MedlinePlus. "Plastic and Cosmetic Surgery." *MedlinePlus,* May 2, 2013.

Narins, Rhoda, and Paul Jarrod Frank. *Turn Back the Clock Without Losing Time: Everything You Need to Know About Simple Cosmetic Procedures.* New York: Three Rivers Press, 2002.

Townsend, Courtney M., Jr., et al., eds. *Sabiston Textbook of Surgery.* 18th ed. Philadelphia: Saunders/Elsevier, 2012.

Venkataraman, Shambhavi, and Priscilla J. Slanetz. "Breast Imaging for Cancer Screening: Mammography and Ultrasonography." *UpToDate*, 26 Nov. 2018, www.uptodate.com/contents/breast-imaging-for-cancer-screening-mammography-and-ultrasonography.

Weatherford, M. Lisa, ed. *Reconstructive and Cosmetic Surgery Sourcebook*. Detroit, Mich.: Omnigraphics, 2001.

Polycystic ovary syndrome

CATEGORY: Disease/Disorder

KEY TERMS:

biguanide: a type of medication to lower blood glucose by increasing sensitivity to insulin and possibly lowering the liver's glucose production

gonadotropin: hormone secreted by the pituitary gland; the primary gonadotropic hormones are luteinizing hormone (LH) and follicle-stimulating hormone (FSH)

hirsutism: excess facial hair

hyperandrogenism: higher-than-normal levels of androgens in the blood

ovarian follicle: a fluid-filled sac that contains an immature egg, or oocyte

CAUSES AND SYMPTOMS

In polycystic ovary syndrome (PCOS), ovaries contain numerous follicles, or small collections of fluid, and may interrupt the releasing of ova. PCOS seems to be caused by a combination of genetics and environmental factors. PCOS is very common as it affects 5-10 percent of women. Researchers are currently using candidate gene research to try to determine which genetic sequences may lead to susceptibility for PCOS. First-degree relatives of someone with PCOS are at higher risk of developing the condition themselves. Exposure to prenatal androgens may play a role, although this exposure may occur anywhere from the prenatal period through puberty. Additionally, in the prenatal period, the androgens appear to be from the fetus and not the mother.

Hyperinsulinemia and obesity both contribute to higher levels of androgens, called hyperandrogenism.

Insulin may directly stimulate the production of androgens from the ovary, or it may indirectly affect androgen levels by inhibiting sex hormone-binding globulins. Obesity is associated with hyperinsulinemia.

The signs and symptoms can be ambiguous. The most common are related to the hyperandrogenism and include hirsutism (excess facial hair), infertility, and menstrual irregularities. Acne and male-pattern baldness may also occur. The 1990 National Institutes of Health classification of PCOS requires disordered ovulation and clinical or biochemical evidence of hyperandrogenism. In 2003, the Rotterdam European Society of Human Reproduction and Embryology/ American Society of Reproductive Medicine consensus workshop included having polycystic ovaries but suggested that two of these three symptoms were enough on which to base a diagnosis. Thus, a woman with PCOS may have disordered ovulation and polycystic ovaries with androgen excess, or androgen excess with polycystic ovaries but no disorder in ovulation. However, other scenarios are possible.

Hyperandrogenism can be evaluated through laboratory tests, including testosterone levels, sex hormone-binding globulins, and other androgen levels. However, these tests have not always reliably reflected PCOS symptoms. Ultrasound is used to detect the presence of polycystic ovaries and may include an assessment of follicle number and ovary size. Criteria for ultrasound evaluation include having twelve or more follicles that are two to nine millimeters in diameter or ovarian volume greater than ten cubic centimeters.

TREATMENT AND THERAPY

The main goal of treatment and therapy is to normalize menstrual cycles and ovulation and, if desired, achieve a successful pregnancy. The least-invasive approach to achieving this goal is weight loss in those who are overweight. Weight loss of 5 to 10 percent has been shown to have a positive impact on symptoms of PCOS—hirsutism, infertility, and menstrual irregularities as well as hyperinsulinemia. This goal can be achieved by a reduction in caloric intake and increased physical activity, although it is difficult to maintain. Although weight loss is helpful, it may not alleviate all symptoms of PCOS in overweight females. In addition, only about half of those with PCOS are estimated to be overweight.

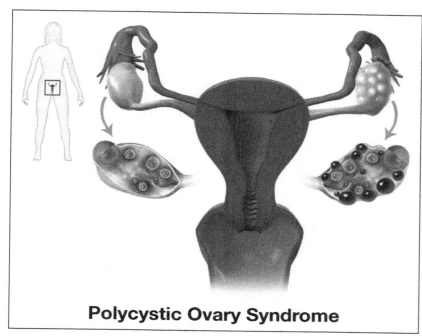

Polycystic Ovary Syndrome

(BruceBlaus via Wikimedia Commons)

Medications may be prescribed to achieve menstrual regularity or normalize blood glucose levels. Birth control medications will help to regulate menses if the woman is not trying to conceive. However, they may also result in weight gain and insulin resistance, which would be a negative effect for the PCOS treatment overall. Clomiphene citrate, a selective estrogen receptor modulator (SERM), may be prescribed to enhance the chances of conception, if this is desired. However, only 35 to 40 percent of women receiving this medication become pregnant. If clomiphene citrate fails to induce conception, then exogenous gonadotropins or laparoscopic ovarian surgery may be tried. However, gonadotropin therapy is associated with multifetus pregnancy, which is not found as often with surgery. However, regimens with low doses of gonadotropins have had some success over traditional doses in achieving single pregnancy. If these options fail to produce pregnancy, then in vitro fertilization is also an option.

For blood glucose normalization, oral hypoglycemic agents such as the biguanide metformin are usually prescribed. Some studies have suggested this medication may also enhance fertility, although other studies have found no such result. Current recommendations are to discontinue metformin when pregnancy is confirmed. Some suggest that metformin may be continued through pregnancy if type 2 diabetes is present. Nonsteroidal antiandrogen medications may help improve the symptoms of androgen excess, although they are not commonly used in adolescents. While several medications may improve hirsutism to some extent, nonpharmacological treatment can also be used, including waxing, electrolysis, bleaching, plucking, and heat or laser therapy.

PERSPECTIVE AND PROSPECTS

First described by Irving F. Stein and Michael L. Leventhal in 1935, PCOS was for a time referred to as the Stein-Leventhal syndrome. At that time, surgical resection of the ovaries was fairly successful treatment, although complications with internal adhesions eventually made other treatments more desirable.

The prevalence of PCOS has been estimated from 2 to 30 percent of premenopausal women. While women of childbearing age were at one time believed to be the primary group afflicted with PCOS, adolescents are now also being diagnosed with the disorder. The diagnosis is somewhat more difficult because menses are often irregular until at least two years past menarche.

Polycystic ovaries by themselves have no long-term negative effects, although women with polycystic ovaries without the symptoms of the syndrome are at higher risk for hyperstimulation syndrome. Those with PCOS are at higher risk of complications associated with diabetes and cardiovascular disease. Depression and a reduced quality of life have been reported in women with PCOS, possibly as a result of difficulties with conception, dissatisfaction with appearance, and issues associated with chronic disease.

—*Karen Chapman-Novakofski, R.D., L.D.N., Ph.D.*

FOR FURTHER INFORMATION

Dunaif, Andrea, et al., eds. *Polycystic Ovary Syndrome: Current Controversies, from the Ovary to the Pancreas.* Totowa, N.J.: Humana Press, 2008.

Franks, Stephen. "Polycystic Ovary Syndrome." *Medicine* 37, no. 9 (September, 2009): 441–444.

Hoeger, Kathleen M. "Role of Lifestyle Modification in the Management of Polycystic Ovary Syndrome." *Best Practice and Research: Clinical Endocrinology and Metabolism* 20, no. 2 (June, 2006): 293–310.

MedlinePlus. "Polycystic Ovary Syndrome." *MedlinePlus*, May 13, 2012.

Norman, Robert J., et al. "Polycystic Ovary Syndrome." *The Lancet* 370, no. 9588 (August 25, 2007): 685–697.

Radosh, Lee. "Drug Treatments for Polycystic Ovary Syndrome." *American Family Physician* 79, no. 671 (April 15, 2009): 671–676.

Polyps

CATEGORY: Disease/Disorder

KEY TERMS:

colonoscopy: an endoscopic procedure used for visualization of the intestine

endometrial curettage: a surgical procedure in which the endometrial lining of the uterus is scraped to remove tissue or growths

endoscopy: procedure with a flexible tube that allows direct viewing inside the body

inherited disorder: a disorder caused by an alteration of a gene and passed through families

hysteroscopy: procedure in which a small lit tube is inserted into the vagina and used to examine the cervix and the inside of the uterus

saline infusion sonography: an ultrasound scan of the uterus while the it is being filled with sterile saline (salt water). This helps outline the uterine wall and cavity

transvaginal ultrasound: an ultrasound scan obtained via a probe inserted into the vagina; it is used to examine female reproductive organs

CAUSES AND SYMPTOMS

Polyps are abnormal tissue growths that can look like small bumps or tiny stalks, and can occur in various places including the nose, the vocal cords, the stomach, the colon, the bladder and the female reproductive tract. The cause of polyps varies with the location of the polyp growth in the body. Symptoms are also site dependent.

Nasal polyps consist of inflamed tissue in the mucous membrane lining of the nose or sinuses. Causes of nasal polyps may be allergies, chronic infection, cystic fibrosis, and asthma. They usually develop around the ethmoid sinuses (inside the top of the nose) and may block the airway, resulting in difficulty breathing or shortness of breath because of obstruction. Cold-like symptoms such as breathing through the mouth, loss of the sense of smell, and a runny nose are also common symptoms.

Vocal cord polyps are typically caused by mechanical injury such as shouting and can occur either on one or on both vocal cords. One type of vocal cord polyp called polypoid corditis is thought to be due to smoking. Symptoms include a hoarse and raspy voice that develops over days or weeks. Vocal cord polyps are not to be confused with nodules, which are similar to calluses and are generally caused by chronic overuse of the voice such as singing.

Stomach polyps are rare and are usually discovered incidentally— for example, during an upper gastrointestinal endoscopy (a viewing of the interior of the stomach). Causes include *Helicobacter pylori* (*H. pylori*) bacteria or chronic gastritis (inflammation of the stomach) caused by an autoimmune response. Stomach polyps usually do not cause symptoms, but if symptoms do occur they may include nausea, vomiting, abdominal pain, bleeding, or a feeling of fullness after eating even small amounts.

Colorectal polyps grow on the lining (mucous membrane) of the colon (also known as the large intestine) or rectum and may be caused by abnormal cell growth, heredity (family history or inherited disorder), or inflammatory diseases such as ulcerative colitis or Crohn's disease. Small polyps do not usually cause symptoms. If symptoms do occur, then they may include change in bowel habits (constipation or diarrhea), blood in a bowel movement, rectal bleeding, fatigue due to anemia from loss of blood, and pain.

Polyps of the female reproductive tract most commonly occur in the uterus (endometrial polyps) and cervix (cervical polyps). They most commonly present in perimenopausal and multigravida women between the ages of 30 and 50 years. Polyps are most commonly asymptomatic and are usually an incidental finding during a routine gynecologic pelvic examination. Symptoms may include bleeding, heavy or irregular menstrual periods, leukorrhea (a white or yellow

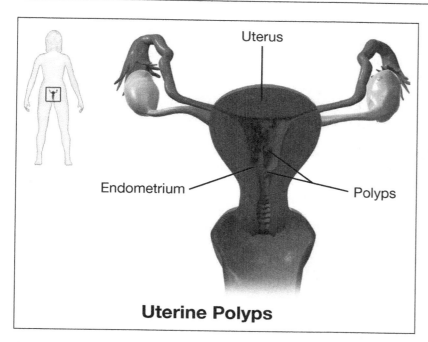

Uterine Polyps

(BruceBlaus via Wikimedia Commons)

discharge of mucus), and possibly infertility. The exact cause of endometrial polyps and cervical polyps is unknown, but may be related to estrogen hormone level, chronic inflammation, or genetics. The risk associated with polyps increases with a woman's age. Younger women have little risk associated with cervical polyps while women in their perimenopausal to postmenopausal years have a slightly higher likelihood of a malignancy associated with cervical polyps. The risk is greatest in postmenopausal women with abnormal uterine bleeding. Literature exists suggesting that polyps may contribute to subfertility and pregnancy loss, though this is an area that is not well understood. It may be related to mechanical interference with sperm transport or embryo implantation. However, many women with polyps have successful pregnancies. The diagnostic modalities that are commonly used to evaluate endometrial polyps include a two- or three-dimensional transvaginal ultrasound, saline infusion sonography and hysteroscopy.

PREVENTION, TREATMENT AND THERAPY

It is possible to prevent some polyps. Controlling allergies and managing chronic sinusitis may prevent nasal polyps. Vocal cord polyps are directly related to injury from yelling such as at a sporting event, so less abuse may lessen the potential for development. Stomach polyps caused by *H. pylori* may be controlled by treating the underlying bacteria and controlling gastritis may diminish the occurrence. Vocal cord polyps usually require surgical removal to restore the normal speaking voice. Voice therapy with a speech pathologist may be needed to prevent future occurrences.

The goal of treatment for nasal polyps is to reduce the size of the polyp or to remove it. Because nasal polyps may occur in response to allergies or chronic sinusitis, medications that treat allergies or chronic sinusitis such as corticosteroids (a drug that reduces inflammation), antihistamines, and antibiotics may be effective in shrinking the size of the polyp. If the polyp is in the sinus cavity, then endoscopic surgery using a small camera and tube inserted into the sinus allows the physician to remove the polyp.

Stomach polyps require biopsy and, if there is concern, surgical removal. Medications to treat gastritis, including antibiotics, may be used. Routine colonoscopy and flexible sigmoidoscopy are recommended for routine cancer screening, and if a colorectal polyp is seen during the procedure, it is removed. If colorectal polyps are causing symptoms, then surgical removal either through colonoscopy or removal of a portion of the intestine may be needed.

Uterine polyps may be watched, medications may be used to shrink them, or surgery may be used to remove them; if the polyps are cancerous, then a hysterectomy (removal of the uterus) is usually necessary. In asymptomatic young women with small polyps smaller than 10 mm in size, conservative management can be safely followed by monitoring the polyp growth. In cases where polyps are affecting fertility, mechanical hysteroscopic resection is advisable. If the infertility was caused by a polyp, the patient often becomes spontaneously pregnant shortly after removal. Endometrial curettage may be recommended to rule out sub clinical endometrial hyperplasia or cancer.

PERSPECTIVE AND PROSPECTS

Polyps are usually benign (not cancerous), but they can become malignant (cancerous) over time or in certain areas. Risk factors include age, obesity, family history, poor overall health (including allergies and chronic infections), stomach ulcers, infections, and inherited disorders such as familial adenomatous polyposis. Prevention and screening, routine visits to the physician for health maintenance, and good health behaviors are important to prevent, recognize, or manage polyps. Prompt treatment is indicated if polyps cause symptoms or if a biopsy demonstrates malignant cells. Research is continuing on the causes of polyps and factors that transform polyps from benign to malignant.

—*Patricia Stanfill Edens, Ph.D., R.N., FACHE*
Updated by Shiliang Alice Cao, B.A.

FOR FURTHER INFORMATION

Bremmer, H., et al. "Colorectal Cancers Occurring after Colonoscopy with Polyp Detection: Sites of Polyps and Sites of Cancers." *International Journal of Cancer* 133, no. 7 (October, 2013): 1672–1679.

Ghoubara, A., Sundar, S. and Ewies, A. A. A. (2018) Predictors of malignancy in endometrial polyps: study of 421 women with postmenopausal bleeding, Climacteric, 21:1, 82-87

Lev, R., et al. *Adenomatous Polyps of the Colon: Pathobiological and Clinical Features.* New York: Springer-Verlag, 2012.

Maydeo, A., and Dhir, V. "The Gallbladder Polyp Conundrum: A Riddler on the Wall." *Gastrointestinal Endoscopy* 78, no. 3 (September, 2013): 494–495.

Schnatz, P. F., et al. "Cervical Polyps in Postmenopausal Women." *Menopause*, vol. 16, no. 3, 2009, pp. 524–528., doi:10.1097/gme.0b013e3181927286.

Tanos, V, Berry, K.E., Seikkula, J., Raad, A.E., Stavroulis, A., Sleiman, Z., Campo, R. and Gordts, S.: The management of polyps in female reproductive organs. Int J Surg. 43:7–16. 2017.

Thakkar, K., Sihman, and Gilger, M. A. "Colorectal Polyps in Childhood." *Current Opinion in Pediatrics* 24, no. 5 (October, 2012): 632–637.

Wethington, S. L., et al. "Risk and Predictors of Malignancy in Women with Endometrial Polyps." *Annals of Surgical Oncology*, vol. 18, no. 13, 2011, pp. 3819–3823., doi:10.1245/s10434-011-1815-z.

Postpartum depression

CATEGORY: Disease/Disorder

KEY TERMS:

baby blues: depression affecting a woman after giving birth; symptoms usually lessen without medical intervention

major depressive disorder: a pattern of major depressive episodes that form an identified psychiatric disorder

major depressive episode: a syndrome of symptoms characterized by depressed mood; required for the diagnosis of some mood disorders

postpartum: following childbirth or the birth of young

CAUSES AND SYMPTOMS

For most women, the symptoms of depression are fairly common in the first week after childbirth. According to *Healthy Children* magazine, approximately 70 to 80 percent of women who have given birth experience what are often called the "baby blues" or the "fourth-day blues." These symptoms often disappear or lessen without medical intervention within one- or two-weeks following birth. In contrast, postpartum depression (PPD) is more severe and longer lasting. It occurs in about one in every ten women who have given birth. Additionally, an important distinction between baby blues and PPD is that the blues typically do not interfere with the mother's ability to care for a baby, whereas PPD can affect the ability of the mother to care for her child and herself.

PPD symptoms often include sadness, restlessness, guilt, unexplained weight changes, insomnia, frequent crying, irrational fears, irritability, decreased energy and motivation, and even lessened feelings of self-worth. Doctors also look for the presence of a depressed mood or a significantly diminished interest or pleasure in nearly all activities. Postpartum depression also commonly interferes with a mother's ability to care for the baby.

A personal or family history of depression, bipolar disorders, or other mental illnesses puts one at higher risk for PPD. Other factors that seem to play a role are an unwanted pregnancy, a complicated or difficult labor, a fetal anomaly, a lack of social support, and a temporary upheaval, such as a recent move, death of a loved one, or job change. Women who have previously suffered from depression following the birth of a child have an increased risk of becoming depressed following a subsequent delivery. In women with a history of PPD, the risk of recurrence is about one in three to one in four.

PPD is best understood as resulting from several causes. One factor is that the sudden change in body hormones caused by childbirth can affect the mother's mood. There is also a psychological sense of anticlimax after an event that has been anticipated for many months. Many new mothers are very tired, and some are a little apprehensive and lacking confidence about the challenges of motherhood. Another factor is the sudden change that may occur in lifestyle and an associated feeling of shrunken horizons, especially if the mother had been working before the birth. Additionally, environmental, social, and sexual difficulties can predispose some women to develop PPD.

PPD may be accompanied by a rare but very severe symptom known as postpartum psychosis. Symptoms may include dramatic mood swings, delusional thoughts about the baby, hallucinations, and severe sleep disturbances. Often a danger with this condition is that the mother contemplates or fears that she will kill her child. When such symptoms develop, immediate care is vital, as it will protect both the mother and the child. Additionally, immediate care will help to reduce the distress of the mother, which will in turn help her to regain her health more quickly and return to healthy mothering after treatment.

TREATMENT AND THERAPY

It is important for all new mothers to be aware of the baby blues and the more serious problem of PPD. Awareness of the possibility of PPD may encourage expectant mothers to better care for themselves psychologically and to prepare in advance for what may be a psychologically and physically challenging first few weeks of motherhood. In terms of prevention, it is important for new mothers to avoid becoming too tired and to obtain assistance in baby and household care as much as possible. The loving support of a husband or significant other, relatives, and close friends is extremely helpful. The baby's father can take turns caring for the baby when the baby is unsettled or distressed. During the day, friends or family can help with shopping or looking after the baby while the mother rests.

If the depression develops and persists, a physician should be consulted for an evaluation of PPD.

Antidepressant medication, such as sertraline hydrochloride (Zoloft), is usually effective if administered in the early stages of depression. Counseling is also beneficial to PPD sufferers. In severe cases, in which postpartum psychosis develops or the level of depression becomes life-threatening, admission to a psychiatric hospital for treatment may be necessary. Finally, it is important to note that anyone receiving medications, especially antidepressants, should be in regular contact with their physicians. Side effects, such as increased thoughts of suicide, may be an associated risk.

—Alvin K. Benson, Ph.D.;
Updated by Nancy A. Piotrowski, Ph.D.

FOR FURTHER INFORMATION

Bennett, Shoshana S., and Pec Indman. *Beyond the Blues: A Guide to Understanding and Treating Prenatal and Postpartum Depression.* Rev. ed. San Jose, Calif.: Moodswings Press, 2006.

Kleiman, Karen R., and Valerie D. Raskin. *This Isn't What I Expected: Overcoming Postpartum Depression.* Boston, Mass.: Da Capo, 2013.

Lundberg-Love, Paula K., Kevin L. Nadal, and Michele Antoinette Paludi. *Women and Mental Disorders.* Santa Barbara, Calif.: Praeger, 2012.

Nason, Juliana K., Patricia Spach, and Anna Gruen. *Beyond the Birth: A Family's Guide to Postpartum Mood Disorders.* Seattle: Postpartum Support International of Washington, 2012.

Nicholson, Paula. *Postnatal Depression: Facing the Paradox of Loss, Happiness, and Motherhood.* New York: Wiley, 2001. O'Hara, Michael W. *Postpartum Depression: Causes and Consequences.* New York: Springer, 1995.

Postpartum Support International. http://www.postpartum.net. Sebastian, Linda. *Overcoming Postpartum Depression and Anxiety.* Omaha, Nebr.: Addicus Books, 2006.

Postpartum depression in female veterans

CATEGORY: Disease/Disorder

DESCRIPTION

Postpartum depression (PPD) is defined as clinical depression that has lasted for at least 2 weeks and has an onset within 4 weeks of giving birth. It can take up to a year to develop these depressive symptoms to still be diagnosed as PDD.

PPD is the most common complication of pregnancy and childbirth, with 10 percent of new mothers in the United States experiencing it. Postpartum "baby blues" are experienced by up to 80 percent of new mothers; the symptoms are less severe than those of PPD and are transitory, not extending beyond 2 weeks postpartum. Symptoms of PPD include sadness, tearfulness, decreased motivation, decreased interest in food and self-care, withdrawal from family, poor self-esteem regarding ability to parent, anxiety, mental confusion, feelings of shame and guilt, and/or loss of interest in the baby.

There has been limited research on postpartum depression among women in the military, but some studies report that between 11 percent and 24 percent of new mothers in the military experience PDD. Approximately 15 percent of active-duty members of the military are females. The Navy and Marines have recently extended maternity leave from 6 weeks to 18 weeks. The Air Force and Army, however, still allow only 6 weeks of maternity leave. The Air Force recently changed its policy on postpartum deployment: whereas before women had a 6-month deferment after giving birth, they now have a 12-month deferment.

Researchers in a study of servicewomen who gave birth while on active-duty status found that 11 percent had met criteria for PPD. The highest prevalence (16.6 percent) was among women who had been deployed before childbirth and reported combat-related exposure and trauma symptoms. It is unclear whether the increased risk for PPD among women who had been deployed in combat zones was attributable to combat exposure, experiencing childbirth, leaving another young child for deployment, or a combination of any of these factors.

Another study found that the prevalence of PPD among active-duty servicewomen was 9.9 percent. The highest incidence was found in the Army, 12.0 percent, and the lowest in the Air Force, 7.3 percent. Among servicewomen it was found that the youngest age group, 18- to 20-year-olds, was about 40 percent higher than that in the oldest age group, women over 40, to experience PPD. It was also found that the risk of suicide was higher for servicewomen with PPD compared to those without PPD.

RISK FACTORS

There are several risk factors for postpartum depression, including the following:

- A prior history of depression or bipolar disorder diagnosis.
- A prior history of postpartum depression.
- Lack of social support, especially if missing from the father of the baby or the mother's partner (if the mother is a single parent or is unsupported in her relationship).
- Deployment can increase this lack of support from the father of the baby.
- A previous or current deployment.
- Personal, familial, and professional stressors common to military life, such as frequent moves, prolonged deployment in combat, and being away from extended family.
- A history of severe premenstrual syndrome.
- A family history of depression
- Lower socioeconomic status and/or financial stressors.
- An infant in poor health or one with a difficult temperament.
- Young age.

Women in the military may be hesitant to disclose mental health concerns for fear that this may have a negative effect on their military careers; because of this, symptoms of PPD in this population may go unidentified and untreated.

ASSESSMENT AND SCREENING TOOLS

There are screening tools available to both medical and mental health personnel to screen for postpartum depression or risk for postpartum depression if the woman is still pregnant. These are meant for screening only; they are not used to diagnose.

The Postpartum Depression Screening Scale (PDSS) is a 35-item self-reporting measure; higher scores indicate a higher degree of depressive symptoms present.

The Edinburgh Postnatal Depression Scale (EPDS) is a 10-item self-report measure in which items on the scale correspond to symptoms of clinical depression (suicidal ideation, anhedonia, sleep disturbances).

The Patient Health Questionnaire 2-item (PHQ-2) is another preferred screening tool of the U.S. Department of Veterans Affairs (VA).

The VA/Department of Defense recommends that women be screened for depression at both prenatal and postnatal appointments; use of the EPDS or PHQ-2 is preferred by the VA.

INTERVENTIONS

The interventions that typically are used for depression have been shown to be effective for PPD. These include mental health therapy including cognitive behavioral therapy (CBT), antidepressant medications, and medication combined with mental health therapy. Support group therapy that incorporates mental health support and educational elements.

Other supports found to help reduce risk of PDD include social support services, recreational opportunities, financial assistance, and hospital-sponsored support programs. The MIST (Maternal Infant Support Team) program at Camp Pendleton in San Diego hosts group meetings with case managers, social workers, medical officers, lactation consultants, pediatric nurses, professionals from military relief groups, community Women, Infants, and Children (WIC) staff, community program representatives, and community visiting nurses. The program also includes mental health counseling and a 10-week program, Moms in Transition, which offers education and support to active-duty women and civilian wives of military spouses who have recently given birth.

—*Jessica Therivel, LMSW-IPR*

FOR FURTHER INFORMATION

Appolonio, Kathryn Kanzler, and Randy Fingerhut. "Postpartum Depression in a Military Sample." *Military Medicine*, vol. 173, no. 11, Nov. 2008, pp. 1085–1091., doi:10.7205/milmed.173.11.1085.

Do, Tan, et al. "Depression and Suicidality during the Postpartum Period after First Time Deliveries, Active Component Service Women and Dependent Spouses, U.S. Armed Forces." *Medical Surveillance Medical Report*, vol. 20, no. 9, Sept. 2013, pp. 2–7.

Nguyen, Stacie, et al. "Is Military Deployment a Risk Factor for Maternal Depression?" *Journal of Women's Health*, vol. 22, no. 1, 10 Jan. 2013, pp. 9–18., doi:10.1089/jwh.2012.3606.

Shivakumar, Geetha, et al. "Managing Posttraumatic Stress Disorder and Major Depression in Women Veterans During the Perinatal Period." *Journal of Women's Health*, vol. 24, no. 1, 21 Jan. 2015, pp. 18–22., doi:10.1089/jwh.2013.4664.

Spooner, Shawn, et al. "Maternal Depression Screening During Prenatal and Postpartum Care at a Navy and Marine Corps Military Treatment Facility." *Military Medicine*, vol. 177, no. 10, 1 Oct. 2012, pp. 1208–1211., doi:10.7205/milmed-d-12-00159.

Tan, Michelle. "Army Reviewing Rules for Maternity, Paternity Leave." *Army Times*, 7 Aug. 2015, www.armytimes.com/story/military/careers/army/2015/08/07/army-reviewing-rules-maternity-paternity-leave/31285283/.

Postpartum depression treatment: Psychosocial support

CATEGORY: Disease/Disorder Social issue

DESCRIPTION

Postpartum depression (PPD) is defined as clinical depression that has lasted for at least two weeks and has an onset within four weeks of giving birth. Symptoms of PPD include sadness, tearfulness, decreased motivation, decreased interest in food and self-care, difficulty concentrating, poor self-esteem regarding ability to parent, anxiety, mental confusion, feelings of shame and guilt, and/or loss of interest in the baby.

A significant risk factor for PPD is either thinking about or actually experiencing decreased levels of psychosocial support. Psychosocial support is looking at the impact of relational interactions on the mother's mental health. A new mother may be missing support in various areas of her life causing her to be at risk for PPD.

RISK FACTORS

The woman's family and friends may be absent, critical, or intrusive. The woman also may be experiencing emotional or physical abuse. The practices of a woman's culture can serve as a protective factor or a risk factor depending on how that culture supports and assists new mothers.

The woman may be experiencing stress related to work (including the absence from work, the decision regarding whether to return to work, loss of career), money, and other potential losses.

Stress and how it relates to the parenting role has been consistently linked to PPD. This stress may be episodic stress or chronic stress. Episodic stressors are stressful life events, daily hassles, or catastrophic events. Chronic stress includes perceived stress, chronic strain, and parenting stress. Perceived stress is when a mother feels overwhelmed and unable to cope with her current situation. Chronic strain may come from low socioeconomic status, work demands, insufficient food, and the like.

Parenting stress can be measured and evaluated using three domains. These are parental distress, difficult child stress, and parent–child dysfunctional interaction (PCDI), Parental distress involves the mother's feelings of incompetence in parenting and the responsibilities that go along with parenting. Difficult child stress is related to the mother's perception of how challenging the child is. PCDI measures how the mother feels about her interactions with the child. This stressor can be affected by partner support, and if the mother is working outside the home, reduced interaction occurs naturally.

In 2014, the Centers for Disease Control and Prevention (CDC) published information from 2009 reporting that in the United States, 11.9 percent of women between the ages of 18 and 44 who gave birth experienced symptoms of depression.

Women with PPD may feel tearful, anxious, hopeless, and inadequate at caring for the baby; may have difficulty sleeping and experience loss of appetite; may experience inability to experience pleasure and memory problems; and may develop suicidal thinking.

Parenthood, whether through childbirth or adoption, can be a time of crisis for new parents due to drastic change in someone's identity. It causes transitions in roles, relationships, and patterns of interpersonal functioning. Emotions are more difficult to regulate. Social expectations that new mothers will experience joyful bonding with their infants may serve to minimize the stress and discomfort that may also be present.

Because it is assumed that adoption is a desired, positive experience, adoptive parents can feel as though they are unable to seek help or express negative emotions even though they may encounter the same issues of loss of identity, independence, career, and so on that biological parents experience.

SUPPORT

Instrumental support includes actual physical assistance such as meals preparation, laundry, or house cleaning.

Informational support consists of advice or suggestions.

Emotional support produces expressions of love, caring, and compassionate support.

Relationship quality between parents, rather than marital status, provides the protective social support.

Single mothers did not show a higher rate of PPD when relationship quality was taken out of the equation.

Another aspect that can reduce the risk of developing PDD includes validating or supportive statements (called appraisal support) such as "I trust your judgment" or "You are doing a good job."

Today, new mothers can find these kinds of supports through online education, social media, message boards, forums, and support groups.

Adolescent mothers are at a higher risk for PPD because they often lack these supports.

Often women need less actual support than believed; however, they seem to benefit from awareness that the support exists if needed.

Parental self-efficacy refers to the beliefs held by a parent about his or her abilities, powers, and capabilities to complete the needed tasks to care for a child. High self-efficacy in a new mother has shown to reduce the risk of PDD.

Psychosocial support (referrals to education, support groups, and assistance with home/childcare) offered by the social worker will only be useful if the woman feels this support meets needs that she has identified and if it is acknowledged that she may be experiencing PPD.

Often women may not seek treatment for PPD until symptoms are severe or family and/or friends ask them to get help.

Women may be ashamed to recognize a need for help and may not know how or where to find help.

Women may intellectually understand PPD but not recognize the symptoms in themselves.

Commonly, new mothers will minimize their symptoms and may deny the severity of their depression.

Partner and/or family support can be the most beneficial even when support is coming from other sources.

Cultural considerations may affect whether women seek treatment, and PPD is more likely to go undetected and untreated in minority groups.

Social hierarchy and cultural disadvantages can increase risk for PPD.

Women in minority groups may feel shame related to PPD, perceive stigma, or be coping with cultural beliefs that minimize depression by seeing mental health issues as a sign of weakness or with a cultural bias against disclosing any negative feelings to family or friends. This is a common experience, as minority groups overall seek less mental health treatment. For example, some black mothers reported a community belief that "strong" mothers do not "catch" PPD.

Research showed that the most beneficial interventions used to reduce risk of PDD were interpersonal psychotherapy, home visits conducted by a postpartum nurse or midwife, postpartum peer-based phone support, and flexible postpartum care by midwives.

Assessment

There are screening tools that measure social supports for women. The Maternal Support Scale is an index of emotional, informational, childcare, financial, respite, household, and other supports that may or may not be available from the baby's father, mother's parents, in-laws, and extended family. The Postpartum Social Support Questionnaire (PSSQ) is a 50-item questionnaire that measures emotional and instrumental social support from spouse/partner, parents, in-laws, other family members, and friends.

The stress and coping model for PPD theorizes that it is the psychosocial stressors listed above that are a main risk factor for PPD. The model proposes that positive actual supports or perceived supports will help the woman to have improved self-confidence, general satisfaction, and positive self-evaluation.

Treatment

Any counseling interventions for PPD will be more likely to have positive outcomes if they work to build up the new mother's ability to cope with stress and enhance her support system through advocacy and finding resources.

Organizations exist that provide community-based psychosocial support for women experiencing PPD by linking them with volunteers who have survived PPD and with healthcare workers/clinicians who are specialists in the treatment of PPD.

Support groups such as Postpartum Education and Support and Postpartum Support International were created to help women with PPD and their families. Support is provided through outreach, education, and local referrals for treatment, services, and volunteer contacts. These groups project a common message of validation that the woman is are not alone, reassurance that it is not her fault, and hope that she will be able to overcome PDD.

It is important for women experiencing PDD to reach out for support. They should do their own research to find the resources and supports for PDD in their community.

For Further Information

Banker, J. E., & LaCoursiere, D. Y. (2014). Postpartum depression: Risks, protective factors, and the couple's relationship. *Issues in Mental Health Nursing, 35*(7),503-508.doi:10.3109/01612840.2014.888603

Dagher, R. K., McGovern, P. M., Alexander, B. H., Dowd, B. E., Ukestad, L. K., & McCaffrey, D. J. (2009). The psychosocial work environment and maternal postpartum depression. *International Journal of Behavioral Medicine, 16*(4), 339-346. doi: 10.1007/s12529-008-9014-4

Dennis, C. L., & Dowswell, T. (2014). Psychosocial and psychological interventions for preventing postpartum depression. *Cochrane Database of Systematic Reviews*, 2. Art. No.: CD001134.

Leahy-Warren, P., McCarthy, G., & Corcoran, P. (2012). First-time mothers: Social support, maternal parental self-efficacy, and postnatal depression. *Journal of Clinical Nursing, 21*(3-4), 388-397. doi: 10.1111/j.1365-2702.2011.03701.x

Thomason, E., Volling, B. L., Flynn, H. A., McDonough, S. C., Marcus, S. M., Lopez, J. F., & Vazquez, D. (2014). Parenting stress and depressive symptoms in postpartum mothers: Bidirectional or unidirectional effects?. *Infant Behav Dev, 37*(3), 406-415.

Yim, I. S., Stapleton, L. R. T., Guardino, C. M., Hahn-Holbrook, J., & Schetter, C. D. (2015). Biological and psychosocial predictors of postpartum depression: Systematic review and call for integration. *Annual Review of Clinical Psychology, 11*, 99-137.

Postpartum psychosis

CATEGORY: Disease/Disorder

DESCRIPTION

Psychosis refers to specific symptoms such as hallucinations, delusions, grossly disorganized thought, abnormal motor behaviors,, and looks at their severity, and their duration. (For more information on psychosis, see *T709378*.) Experiencing these symptoms does not automatically lead to a psychotic diagnosis. Currently postpartum psychosis (PPP) is not a distinct diagnosis in the *DSM-5*. The classifications "with peripartum onset" or "with postpartum onset" can be applied to a variety of mood disorders as an impacting element. Despite its absence from the *DSM-5* there is consensus on which elements of psychosis combine in the syndrome called PPP. There is also consensus that PPP is the most extreme manifestation of postpartum psychological occurrences, which range from so-called baby blues through postpartum depression to PPP.

Briefly, baby blues are transient disturbances or problems of adjustment that usually appear within the first few days after giving birth and that do not significantly impair function. Between 50 percent and 70 percent of postpartum women experience baby blues, which may include tearfulness, headaches, low self-esteem, emotional lability, fatigue, and ambivalent feelings toward the new infant. Postpartum depression includes the same symptoms as major depressive disorder; it impacts functioning and affects 10 percent to 20 percent of women who have recently given birth, usually within 12 weeks of delivery with an onset up to a year postpartum. Since the mother's functioning is impacted by mood disturbances such as depressed mood loss of interest in normal activities, and possibly intrusive thoughts about harming the newborn or guilt about not being a good mother it is extremely important to seek professional assessment and treatment as soon as possible. In more severe cases where the mother's level of functioning is significantly impacted and the health and development of the newborn may be compromised it may be necessary to have involvement of agencies such as Child Protective Services (CPS).

Due to the severity of the symptoms, PPP is a medical emergency that requires immediate intervention. Early intervention is necessary to address the increased risk of suicide and harm to the baby and to decrease the impact of the current episode. Onset is sudden and rapid, usually from 2 days to 4 weeks after delivery, and most often starts with mania (hyperactivity or elevated mood) or other mood symptoms and progresses rapidly to symptoms that may include delusions (frequently centered on the new baby), mood lability, hallucinations, bizarre behavior, mania, severe depression, confusion, and obsessions (frequently centered on the new baby). Although PPP frequently occurs in women with a history of mental health diagnoses, the symptoms of PPP appear suddenly. PPP has a profound negative impact on functioning, although if mania is present the mother's vastly increased activity level may mask the impairment. It was found that 73 percent of women who developed PPP recalled symptoms appearing within 3 days of giving birth and that the most common symptoms were feeling excited, elated, or "high" (52 percent); not needing sleep or not being able to sleep (48 percent); feeling active or energetic (37 percent); and being very talkative (31 percent). Symptoms of PPP may appear similar to those of a primary psychotic disorder (e.g., schizophrenia) or a mood disorder (e.g., bipolar disorder). Aside from the obvious factor of recently having given birth, other factors associated with the onset of PPP are a history of mental health disorder(s), including previous PPP, family history of psychotic illness, recent stressful events beyond the immediate impact of giving birth, absence of a family or social support system, delivering one's first child, emergency caesarean section or otherwise complicated birth, and perinatal death.

Numerous causes for postpartum psychological distress have been investigated, including increased levels of emotional stress caused by pregnancy and the responsibilities of child rearing, sudden endorphin decrease with labor, abrupt hormone level changes after delivery, low serum levels of free tryptophan (which is an essential amino acid associated with the development of major depression), thyroid gland dysfunction, a prior mental health diagnosis, a family history of mental health disorder(s), occurrence of unexpected adverse life events, lack of social or family support, genetic factors, and maternal age $\geq$ 35 years. One approach (Spinelli, 2009) views PPP as the manifestation of a lifetime vulnerability to mood disorders that is precipitated by childbirth. The outcome varies with speed of diagnosis and treatment. Most women recover within 12 weeks, but up to 15 percent continue to experience depressive symptoms for more than 24 weeks. Approximately 40 percent have the same symptoms again after a subsequent pregnancy. Treatment may include voluntary or involuntary hospitalization, medications, and psychoeducational therapy for the affected individual and the family.

FACTS AND FIGURES

Heron (2008) and Spinelli (2009) report that PPP occurs in 1–2 mothers per 1, 000 deliveries. Spinelli reports that approximately 4 percent of women with PPP commit infanticide. Sadock (2015) reports that 50 to 60 percent of PPP episodes occur after the birth of a first child, that 50 percent of cases involve women with a family history of mood disorders, and that 50 percent of cases involve deliveries that had complications of a non-psychiatric nature.

RISK FACTORS

Risk factors include a personal or family history of a mental health disorder(s), particularly a mood or psychotic disorder; a prior episode of PPP; recent stressful events; lack of social or family support; first delivery; emergency caesarean section or other delivery complications, including perinatal death; and lack of sleep.

SIGNS AND SYMPTOMS

Signs and clinical presentation include recent childbirth, sudden and rapid onset of symptoms, hallucinations, delusions (frequently centered on the infant), withdrawal and disconnection, disorganized thinking and behavior, mood lability, obsessions (frequently involving birth or the new infant), and sleep deprivation. Mania (hyperactive or elevated mood) frequently is present and may be mistaken for better than average adjustment to the presence of a new baby.

ASSESSMENT

Shame about not being able to care for a newborn infant may prevent or delay seeking treatment. A brief assessment for postpartum depression and PPP should be conducted at every contact with women who have recently delivered a baby. If the brief assessment indicates there is a need, an in-depth assessment using relevant diagnostic and assessment tools should be conducted.

When assessing for PPP consider the following:

1. Complete a standard bio-psycho-social-spiritual history;
2. Thoroughly assess personal and family mental health history, including prior mental health diagnoses and medication;
3. Assess for suicidal thinking or thoughts of harming the baby and otherwise harming self or others; and
4. Assess family support and care system for the newborn.

ASSESSMENTS AND SCREENING TOOLS

A. Postpartum Bonding Questionnaire (PBQ)
B. Edinburgh Postnatal Depression Scale (EPDS)
C. Postpartum Depression Screening Scale (PDSS)
D. Mood Disorder Questionnaire (MDQ)

TREATMENT

Treatment of PPP should start with preventive measures throughout the pregnancy, including assessment of prior PPP or other mental health disorders, family history of mental health disorders, education about possible postpartum mood lability ranging from baby blues to PPP, involvement of family and support network with the pregnancy, and brief assessments of mood at every visit.

When PPP does occur treatment should first include considerations of the safety, health, and well-being of the newborn. Appropriate referrals should be made immediately for assessment and intervention if needed to care for the newborn. Child Protective Services or analogous agencies may need to be involved. There may be times when the best interests of the mother and those of the child are in conflict.

It is important to be aware of cultural values, beliefs, and biases when working with different people. Treatment should include knowledge about the histories, traditions, and values of the people with whom you are working.

APPLICABLE LAWS AND REGULATIONS

Each jurisdiction (e.g., nation, state, province) has its own standards, procedures, and laws for involuntary restraint and detention of persons who may be a danger to themselves or others. The lack of a formal *DSM-5* diagnosis for PPP may complicate legal and detention issues. It is important to understand protocols in your jurisdiction to best help support mothers struggling with PPP.

As mandated reporters all medical and mental health professionals must report any suspicion of neglect or abuse of a child to Child Protective Services or local agency.

Since 1922 the laws of England have recognized the biological and psychiatric circumstances that may surround infanticide, and probation and psychiatric treatment are mandated when appropriate. Twenty-nine other countries have made similar adjustments to their laws; however, the U.S. judicial system continues to punish rather than treat mothers with postpartum mental disorders who kill their children.

Each country has its own standards for cultural competency and diversity in social work practice. Social workers must be aware of the standards of practice set forth by their governing body (e.g., National Association of Social Workers in the United States, British Association of Social Workers in England), and practice accordingly.

SERVICES AND RESOURCES

- Brain & Behavior Research Foundation (formerly NARSAD), http://bbrfoundation.org/
- National Alliance on Mental Illness (NAMI), http://www.nami.org/
- U.S. National Institutes of Health (NIH), http://www.nih.gov/
- U.S. National Institute of Mental Health (NIMH), http://www.nimh.nih.gov/index.shtml
- National Association of Social Workers (NASW), http://www.socialworkers.org/
- Royal College of Psychiatrists (RCP), http://rcpsych.ac.uk

FOOD FOR THOUGHT

The case of Andrea Yates, the Texas woman who drowned her five children in June 2001, encapsulates many issues surrounding PPP and infanticide, including the failure of family, society, and failure of the mental health and legal communities to intervene appropriately. Yates had been pregnant or breastfeeding for 7 years, cared for her bedridden father, home-schooled her older children, taught evening Bible study, baked cookies, designed crafts, made costumes— in short, she was a "super mom." However, she also had a history of psychiatric illness, with the first reported psychotic episode after the birth of her first child, two suicide attempts that were attributed to efforts to resist satanic voices commanding her to kill her fourth child soon after birth, numerous other hospitalizations and disrupted medication regimens, plus an immediate family history of bipolar disorder and major depressive disorder. At her first trial the jury acknowledged the tragedy of the situation and their own conflicted feelings by returning a guilty verdict after 3 and one half hours of deliberations and by taking only 35 minutes to deny the prosecutor's request for the death penalty. The incident was treated as a legal question rather than a mental health issue when Yates was sentenced to life in prison rather than to intensive treatment. A second trial overturned the first verdict on a technicality and she is now in a state mental hospital. This case highlights the fact that PPP is an extremely serious mental health crisis where immediate intervention is necessary.

RED FLAGS

Assess for suicidal, infanticidal, or homicidal ideation.

Monitor changing medication regimens, or non-adherence to regimen, particularly if breastfeeding.

Evaluate mother-child attachment, as it may be adversely impacted by PPP. Social workers are mandated reporters for abuse and neglect of children and must report any suspicions that abuse or neglect is happening to CPS or the appropriate local agency.

—*Chris Bates, MA, MSW*

FOR FURTHER INFORMATION

American Psychiatric Association. (2013). Diagnostic and Statistical Manual of Mental Disorders. Fifth edition. DSM-5. In (5th ed., pp. 45-47). Washington, DC: American Psychiatric Publishing.

Doucet, S., Dennis, C. L., Letourneau, N., & Blackmore, E. R. (2009). Differentiation and clinical implications of postpartum depression and postpartum psychosis. *Journal of Obstetric, Gynecologic & Neonatal Nursing, 38*(13), 269-279.

Hall, S. D., & Bean, R. A. (2008). Family therapy and childhood-onset schizophrenia: Pursuing clinical and bio/psycho/social competence. *Contemporary Family Therapy, 30*(2), 61-74.

Heron, J., McGuinness, M., Blackmore, E. R., Craddock, N., & Jones, I. (2008). Early postpartum symptoms in puerperal psychosis. *BJOG: An International Journal of Obstetrics & Gynaecology, 115*(3), 348-353.

Monzon, C., di Scalea, T. L., & Pearlstein, T. (2014). Postpartum psychosis: Updates and clinical issues. *Psychiatric Times, 31*(1), 1-6.

Posmontier, B. (2010). The role of midwives in facilitating recovery in postpartum psychosis. *Journal of Midwifery and Women's Health, 55*(5), 430-437.

Sadock, R. J., Sadock, V. A., & Ruiz, P. (2015). Kaplan & Sadock's synopsis of psychiatry: behavioral sciences/clinical psychiatry. In (pp. 831-840). Philadephia, PA: Wolters Kluwer.

Spinelli, M. G. (2009). Postpartum psychosis: Detection of risk and management. *American Journal of Psychiatry, 166*(4), 405-408.

Posttraumatic stress disorder

CATEGORY: Disease/Disorder

KEY TERMS:

avoidance: a conscious or unconscious defense mechanism by which a person tries to escape from unpleasant situations or feelings, such as anxiety and pain

eye movement desensitization and reprocessing (EMDR): a structured therapy that encourages the patient to briefly focus on the trauma memory while simultaneously experiencing bilateral stimulation (typically eye movements), which is associated with a reduction in the vividness and emotion associated with the trauma memories

personal trauma narrative: the story of a traumatic experience will be told repeatedly through verbal, written, or artistic means; sharing and expanding upon a trauma narrative allows the individual to organize their memories, making them more manageable, and diminishing the painful emotions they carry

CAUSES AND SYMPTOMS

Post-traumatic stress disorder (PTSD) is said to occur when a person experiences symptoms such as intense fear, helplessness, or horror following exposure to a traumatic event (an event outside the range of normal human experiences). The traumatic event may involve threatened death, serious injury, or other threat to physical integrity; witnessing the death of or threat to another person; or learning about the death of or threat to a family member or close friend. Events such as natural disasters (earthquakes, mudslides, fires, floods, tsunamis, tornados), war, domestic violence, crime, accidents, and medical procedures may trigger the development of PTSD.

PTSD is the only disorder in the *Diagnostic and Statistical Manual of Mental Disorders* (DSM) with a cited etiology. PTSD involves reexperiencing the trauma, avoidance of things that remind the person of the trauma, and an uncomfortable state of arousal usually connected to readiness to avoid re-experiencing a trauma. Re-experiencing includes recurrent and intrusive thoughts, recurrent distressing dreams, feeling as if the event is happening again, intense psychological distress at exposure to any reminders (internal or external) of the event, or intense physical reactivity to any reminders of the event. Persistent avoidance includes anything associated with the event, as well as a numbing of general responsiveness.

Such numbing may be indicated by several of the following: avoiding thoughts, feelings, or conversations associated with the event; avoiding activities, places, or people that remind one of the event; forgetting an important aspect of the event; experiencing markedly diminished interest or participation in significant activities; feeling detached or estranged from others; having a restricted range of feelings, such as not being able to love; or feeling that the future is foreshortened. Increased arousal includes at least two of the following: difficulty with sleep; irritability or outbursts of anger; difficulty concentrating; hypervigilance; or exaggerated startle response.

The re-experiencing, avoidance, and arousal start after the traumatic event, last more than one month, and cause clinically significant distress or impairment in social, occupational, or other important areas of functioning. The course of the disorder varies, with some individuals not experiencing symptoms until years later, but most individuals experience symptoms within three months of the initial trauma. If the trauma occurs early in life, it may have profound effects on stress response throughout the individual's lifetime.

Persons with PTSD may describe painful guilt feelings about surviving when others did not, or about what they had to do to survive. Their phobic avoidance of situations or activities that resemble or symbolize the original trauma may interfere with interpersonal relationships and lead to marital conflict, divorce, or job loss.

The likelihood of developing PTSD increases as intensity and physical proximity to the event increase. Recent immigrants from countries where there is considerable social unrest and civil conflict may have elevated rates of PTSD. The disorder may occur at any age. Women are more likely to develop PTSD than men; this gender difference is thought to exist in part because some traumatic events that women experience occur directly to their persons.

Not everyone who experiences a significant trauma will develop PTSD. Individual differences in terms of immediate stress response, physical health, and other biological factors may explain a lack of occurrence in some individuals.

TREATMENT AND THERAPY

Treatments for PTSD include individual therapy, group therapy, antianxiety and antidepressant drugs, and eye movement desensitization and reprocessing (EMDR). Combinations of therapies can also be effective. In general, the sooner the victim of PTSD receives treatment, the greater are the chances of complete recovery. It is important to note, however, that complex techniques such as trauma debriefing and critical incident debriefing should be attempted only by well-trained persons. Discussing traumatic events in a way that is not sensitive to the experience of the victim may retraumatize them, so caution is advised. For untrained persons, the best way to help someone affected by a trauma is to help them get to a qualified treatment professional as quickly as possible. This is especially important because research has suggested that treatment delivered soon after the trauma may reduce the overall negative impacts of the trauma.

Psychotherapy can help the person come to grips with the traumatic event. Different approaches are used, including exposure (or imaginal) therapy, anxiety management/relaxation training, cognitive therapy, and supportive psychotherapy. Also, hypnosis, journaling (such as thought diaries and grief letters), creative arts, and a critical-incident stress debriefing may be used in treating PTSD, either alone or in conjunction with psychotherapy.

Group therapy, in which victims of PTSD can share their experiences and gain support from others, is especially helpful. Groups are typically small (six to eight persons) and are often composed of individuals who have undergone similar experiences. Also, marital and family therapy or parent training may be used in treating PTSD.

In general, the goals of psychotherapy include facilitating "victims" emotional engagement with the trauma memory, helping them organize a personal trauma narrative, assisting them in correcting dysfunctional cognitions that often follow trauma, helping them develop increased trust in others, and decreasing their emotional and social isolation. The therapist typically provides empathy, validation, safety, consistency, and sensitivity to cultural and ethnic identity issues.

Antianxiety and antidepressant drugs can relieve the physiological symptoms of PTSD. The major pharmacological agents include benzodiazepines, serotonin receptor partial agonists, tricyclic antidepressants, MAO inhibitors, and selective serotonin reuptake inhibitors. Because of the many biological abnormalities presumed to be associated with PTSD, and because of the overlap between symptoms of PTSD and other comorbid disorders, almost every class of psychotropic agent has been administered to PTSD patients. Whether it includes individual or group therapy, drugs, or some combination of these three, the treatment approach must be tailored to the individual PTSD sufferer and his or her unique situation. EMDR is a newer therapy for PTSD. It combines many aspects of the other therapies described and works to facilitate reprocessing of traumatic information and experience.

Guided discussion and therapeutic work may involve specific eye movements while remembering different aspects of the traumatic event. It is suggested that this type of activity creates an orienting response that facilitates trauma processing. The technique requires a high level of skill and sophistication and should be used only by appropriately trained professionals. EMDR is very highly recommended for trauma and remains a topic of great research interest.

It is important to remember that PTSD, like many other mental health disorders, may not occur in isolation. Comorbidity, or the presence of more than one disorder, is the rule rather than the exception with PTSD. Depressive disorders, substance use disorders, and other anxiety disorders are the disorders most likely to occur with PTSD. Treatment must address the comorbid conditions when they are present. PTSD can be reliably assessed through semi-structured interview and self-report measures. Treatment typically occurs on an outpatient basis, but it also may occur on an inpatient basis if the symptoms are severe.

PERSPECTIVE AND PROSPECTS

PTSD was observed in World War I, when some soldiers had intense anxiety reactions to the horrors they were experiencing. At that time, it was called combat neurosis, shell shock, or battle fatigue. It was formally diagnosed as an anxiety-based personality disorder in the 1960s among Vietnam War veterans, but it is no longer considered a personality disorder and is instead seen as an anxiety disorder. It is also now known that traumatic events may include not only war but also violent personal assault, kidnapping, terrorist attacks, torture, natural or human-made disasters, severe automobile accidents, or different aspects of life-threatening illness. For children, sexually traumatic events may include sexual experiences that were developmentally inappropriate, even if no threatened or actual violence occurred. PTSD may be especially severe when the trauma is of human origin (for example, torture) and directly related to damage to one's person.

Promising research identifying change to the stress response system in younger persons following trauma, as well as gender differences in trauma response, are expected to fuel greater understanding of the mechanisms of trauma response. Such knowledge will in turn be useful for developing new drug, biological, and interpersonal therapies for children and adults and for both women and men.

IMPACT ON WOMEN

PTSD has long been thought of as something that primarily impacts men based on the belief that it only results from combat and war experiences. We now know that PTSD impacts both men and women, and women at an even higher rate than men. This may be due to the increased traumatic experiences women are subject to, including the sexual violence of rape and sexual assault. Women fall victim to sexual violence and domestic violence more often than men due and therefore have more likelihood of experiencing lasting

trauma symptoms. Unfortunately, PTSD in women is still overlooked and underdiagnosed. This may be due to the different expressions of PTSD in women compared to how professionals are used to seeing it in men. Women may show signs of depression, anxiety, hypervigilance, and fear, while their male counterparts may show more symptoms of anger, rage and hostility. Since we also know sexual violence is highly underreported, women may not come forward with their struggles.

Trauma experienced in childbirth is another common source of PTSD developments. Since childbirth is seen as a natural occurrence, despite how challenging, painful or scary it is, the traumatic experience the woman has is often discussed as normal. This results in women again not seeing support for their emotional struggles, due to invalidation of their experience by friends, family, and medical professionals around them. Women who fear for the lives of their babies during pregnancy, childbirth or if their baby is brought to the NICU may have increased risk of developing PTSD. Loss of pregnancy, such as miscarriage or stillbirth may also result in the woman experiencing trauma symptoms.

Medical professionals should always look for PTSD symptoms in women when they are presenting with other symptoms such as depression, anxiety, fear, chronic pain, headaches, eating or sleeping issues and other fear or anxiety-based symptoms. Treating women should include validation of their experiences and their feelings of victimization and unsafety in the world. Along with the empirically supported treatment methodologies, it is important for women to feel heard and understood about their experiences. Support groups can be particularly helpful for women experiencing PTSD, due to the peer support aspect, and community building.

—*Lillian M. Range, Ph.D.*
Updated by Nancy A. Piotrowski, Ph.D.
and Kimberly Ortiz-Hartman, Psy.D., LMFT

FOR FURTHER INFORMATION

American Psychiatric Association. *Diagnostic and Statistical Manual of Mental Disorders:DSM-5.* 5th ed. Arlington, Va.: Author, 2013.

Bremner, Douglas J. *Does Stress Damage the Brain? Understanding Trauma-Related Disorders from a Neurological Perspective.* New York: W. W. Norton, 2002.

EMDR Institute, 2011.

Foa, Edna B., Terence M. Keane, and Matthew J. Friedman, editors. *Effective Treatments for PTSD: Practice Guidelines from the Society for Traumatic Stress Studies*. 2d ed. New York: Guilford, 2009.

McNally, Richard J. *Remembering Trauma*. Rev. ed. Cambridge, Mass.: Harvard University Press, 2005.

National Center for Posttraumatic Stress Disorder. US Department of Veterans Affairs, May 21, 2013.

"Post-Traumatic Stress Disorder." *MedlinePlus*, May 14, 2013.

"————". *National Institute of Mental Health*, Dec. 3, 2012.

Riley, Julie Smith, and Brian Randall. "Post-Traumatic Stress Disorder." *Health Library*, Mar. 15, 2013.

Schiraldi, Glenn R. *Post-traumatic Stress Disorder Sourcebook*. 2d ed. New York: McGraw-Hill, 2009.

Sidran Institute—Traumatic Stress Education and Advocacy, 2013.

Posttraumatic stress disorder in military service personnel

CATEGORY: Disease/Disorder

DESCRIPTION

Posttraumatic stress disorder (PTSD), as defined by the *Diagnostic and Statistical Manual of Mental Disorders, Fifth Edition* (*DSM-5*), can occur when an individual has experienced or witnessed a traumatic event, learned of a traumatic event happening to a close family member or friend, or experiences repeated or extreme exposure to the details of the event. The event needs to involve actual or threatened death or serious injury or involve a perceived threat to the physical safety of the affected individual or others.

Women now make up close to 15 percent of active-duty forces in the U.S. military. Female service members and veterans who have experienced combat often encounter physically and psychologically traumatic situations and as a result are at risk for developing PTSD. In addition to combat-related trauma, female military personnel are at significant risk for military sexual trauma (MST). MST is a term that is defined by the U.S. Department of Veterans Affairs (VA) as "sexual harassment that is threatening in character or physical assault of a sexual nature that occurred while the victim was in the military, regardless of geographic location of the trauma, gender of the victim, or the relationship to the perpetrator." MST encompasses both the harassment/assault as well as the trauma associated with the assault. Exacerbating such experiences is the fact that a female in the military cannot always easily transfer to another duty station or quit, so she may be subject to repeated interactions or casual contact with the perpetrator.

Female military service personnel and veterans have a higher rate of premilitary stressors and traumatic life experiences than nonmilitary women. Females in the military have very high rates of nonmilitary service–related trauma, including sexual assault, childhood abuse, adult abuse, and intimate partner violence (IPV). Researchers have found that many women join the military to escape violent or traumatic home situations. This nonmilitary service–related trauma can lead to an increased risk for PTSD. In addition, because females are underrepresented in the military, the unit cohesion that is present as a social support for male soldiers may be absent.

FACTS AND FIGURES

Demand by veterans for treatment for PTSD has greatly increased in the last 10 years. Veterans Affairs records indicate that 155,704 veterans were treated for PTSD in 1998; by 2008 this number had grown to 438,248. Prevalence estimates of PTSD in veterans of current foreign wars range from 12 to 24 percent. Individuals with PTSD frequently also abuse alcohol and other substances: it is estimated that 35 to 50 percent of those in whom a substance use disorder has been diagnosed also have a diagnosis of PTSD. These individuals also often have more severe drug use and worse outcomes than patients without PTSD. Many more veterans receive a diagnosis of PTSD than receive treatment: VA and Department of Defense (DOD) data show that only about half of veterans in whom the disorder is diagnosed receive treatment. Female veterans also contend with a lower diagnosis rate than male veterans. Results from a study indicate that 59 percent of males received a diagnosis whereas 62.7 percent met the criteria for diagnosis of PTSD; female veterans had a 19.8 percent diagnosis rate whereas 40.1 percent met the criteria.

Studies have reported conflicting findings with respect to differences in risk for PTSD between males and females. A systematic review identified seven

Information on Post-traumatic Stress Disorder

Causes: Exposure to traumatic event

Symptoms: May include recurrent and intrusive thoughts; reliving of traumatic event; intense psychological distress with exposure to reminders of event; recurrent disturbing dreams; difficulty sleeping; irritability or outbursts of anger; detachment; difficulty concentrating; hypervigilance; exaggerated startle response

Duration: Often chronic with acute episodes

Treatments: Individual therapy, group therapy, anti-anxiety medications, antidepressants

studies that found servicewomen post-deployment at a higher risk for PTSD than servicemen, four studies with servicewomen at a decreased risk, and seven studies in which no gender difference was determined. A study of veterans found that female veterans were more likely to have internalizing symptoms related to concentration and distress from reminders of the traumatic events. Male veterans were more likely to have externalizing symptoms including nightmares, hypervigilance, and emotional numbing. Researchers in a study found that women veterans who had been exposed to combat reported higher levels of PTSD, depression, and alcohol misuse than women veterans who had not been exposed to combat.

RISK FACTORS

Factors that may increase the risk for PTSD in female military personnel and veterans include combat experience; long deployments; multiple deployments; having been wounded; having witnessed death; service on graves registration duty; being tortured or captured by the enemy; exposure to stress that is unpredictable and uncontrollable; poor social support; poor family support; MST; previous lifetime traumas history of physical or sexual abuse in childhood or adulthood); mild traumatic brain injury (TBI); and alcohol dependence and/ or substance use. Meta-analysis has shown that lack of social support may be the primary risk factor for developing PTSD. The symptoms of PTSD have a negative effect on relationships, which serves to reduce the social support that is needed to combat the PTSD. Female

servicemembers who have been sexually assaulted in the military have a 9 times greater chance of developing PTSD. Being a member of a particular racial or ethnic group has not been determined to increase one's vulnerability to developing PTSD; although rates of PTSD differ across racial and ethnic groups, it is not clear whether these differences stem from greater exposure to traumatic stress, from sociodemographic factors, or from true ethnic vulnerability. This finding was supported in a study of female veterans that found more similarities than differences with respect to rates of PTSD between Caucasian, Hispanic, and African American subjects.

SIGNS AND SYMPTOMS

Psychological symptoms include anxiety, depression, anger, emotional detachment, numbing, hallucinations, dissociative episodes, and restricted range of affect.

Behavioral problems include sleep disturbances (trouble falling asleep, trouble staying asleep, nightmares), alcohol or substance use, excessive smoking, not exercising, aggression, overeating, decreased appetite and dietary intake, avoidance behaviors, physical abuse of partner or children, diminished interest in activities that were normally of interest, and increased risk-taking behaviors.

Sexual symptoms include decreased interest in sexual activity or increased interest in sexual activity.

Physical problems involve increased risk of diabetes, obesity, and heart disease; exaggerated startle reflex; trouble concentrating; elevated heart rate; elevated blood pressure; and elevated risk for premature mortality possibly due to medical conditions connected to poor health behaviors (smoking, drinking, obesity) but also from chronic stress.

Social problems may include marital or relationship distress, difficulty parenting, and isolation and withdrawal from family and friends.

ASSESSMENT

Professionals who are helping those with PTSD may perform any or all of the following assessments: perform a complete bio-psycho-social-spiritual history to explore all potential symptoms or manifestations of PTSD, assess risk factors for PTSD, and/or assess and explore social and family functioning and measure available supports.

Professionals may also use screening tools such as Combat Exposure Scale (CES) (determines exposure to combative situations and enemy contact from light to heavy, which can provide information regarding risk for PTSD), PTSD Checklist—Military (PCL-M), Clinician-Administered PTSD Scale (CAPS), Beck Depression Inventory (BDI), Dissociative Experiences Scale (DES), Impact of Event Scale (IES), Traumatic Life Event Questionnaire (TLEQ), The State-Trait Anger Expression Inventory-2 (STAXI-2), The PTSD Symptom Scale Interview (PSS- 1), The Mississippi Scale for Combat-Related PTSD, and/or The Inventory of Psychosocial Functioning (IPF) (specific to active-duty military personnel and veterans).

Professionals may also perform laboratory testing for alcohol and illegal drug use or an MRI or CT scan to determine if a TBI is a comorbidity that may be indicated depending on symptom clusters.

TREATMENT

Accurate assessment of PTSD is important to correctly guide treatment. Having an accurate assessment will improve treatment planning and also help with determination of disability. Treatment for PTSD will most likely involve counseling and/or medication. The most common therapeutic intervention for the treatment of PTSD is one of the variations of cognitive behavioral therapy (CBT), specifically cognitive processing therapy (CPT), prolonged exposure therapy (PE), or imagery rehearsal (IR), which can be provided to individuals or groups. In group-based work, participants work towards a common goal, which is an experience familiar to them from military culture. Some clinicians who specialize in trauma work and have the appropriate training may also use an intervention called eye movement desensitization and reprocessing (EMDR). All of the therapeutic interventions are goal-oriented, active, engaging, and skill-based. The most commonly prescribed medications for treatment are the selective serotonin reuptake inhibitors (SSRIs).

CPT can work for people who are feeling stuck in memories or recurrent thoughts related to the trauma. CPT focuses on learning about symptoms, becoming aware of thoughts and feelings, learning skills to challenge these thoughts and feelings (cognitive restructuring), and understanding how trauma typically affects one's beliefs.

PE therapy helps to address the avoidance symptoms and behaviors that the person may be utilizing. Repeating exposure to the thoughts, situations, and emotions that the person has been avoiding can help them learn that these reminders do not have to be avoided. PE has four main parts: (1) education on symptoms and how treatment can provide symptom relief, (2) breathing retraining to assist with relaxation and decrease distress, (3) real-world rehearsals (in vivo exposure) in a safe environment to reduce emotional distress in avoidance situations, and (4) imaginal exposure (talking through the trauma) to regain control over emotions and cognitions.

In IR, the person takes an image or nightmare related to the trauma and actively works on changing the image or nightmare, so it is less upsetting and then mentally rehearses the changed image or nightmare. Elements of psychoeducation and muscle relaxation are included as well.

EMDR has the person focus on hand movements or tapping motions while she relays information about the traumatic memories. The rapid eye movements have been found to help the brain process the memories. Over time, the person will change her reaction to the memories and learn relaxation strategies. EMDR has four main parts: (1) identifying a specific targeted memory, belief, or image related to the trauma, (2) desensitizing and reprocessing, which is the process of the eye movements, (3) learning how to replace negative images with positive images and thoughts, and (4) learning how to complete a body scan: she will look for areas of tension or unusual sensations to identify any additional areas that need to be addressed.

Yoga has emerged as a potential treatment for symptoms of hyperarousal (anger, sleep problems). In a study in which participants attended yoga sessions researchers found a significant decrease in hyperarousal symptoms. Results from a similar study of veterans with PTSD who had participated in yoga and meditation sessions for 8 to 12 weeks indicated statistically significant reduction of stress, anxiety, and depression as well as improvements in quality of sleep, social functioning, and spiritual well-being.

Many veterans with PTSD do not receive the treatment they need because of barriers such as stigma related to going to a mental health treatment facility, time constraints, and lack of transportation. To reduce barriers for veterans with PTSD, the VA is implementing a telephone-based collaborative care model, which utilizes care teams consisting of nurse care managers, pharmacists, psychologists, and psychiatrists who provide care by phone or videoconference. The nurses manage care, the pharmacists review medication histories, the psychologists deliver CPT via interactive video, and the psychiatrists supervise the team and provide consultations. Initial results from studies of this new model indicate that it is effective in reducing PTSD symptoms and in providing care for veterans who would not otherwise have sought treatment.

Professionals who work with female military service personnel or veterans need to understand the unique features of military culture for female veterans in order to appropriately refer for any follow-up care. They may also need to educate the person and families about PTSD, including the need for good self-care to reduce symptoms and negative side effects, refer to specialized PTSD programs and clinicians as appropriate, encourage person to join a PTSD support group (preferably a military-supported group), encourage evaluation by physician and/or psychiatrist to address physical symptoms (sleep disturbances, shortness of breath, tension), advocate as needed with the VA or Social Security Administration for benefits or services, and safeguard confidentiality and privacy and maintain awareness of what impact releasing records can have on the woman's military service record and military career.

APPLICABLE LAWS AND REGULATIONS

PTSD has been used in the criminal justice system as an insanity defense and stress from exposure to combat has been allowed in consideration for sentencing.

The U.S. Supreme Court has officially recognized the need for defendants' military service including mental health issues to be taken under consideration in capital cases.

Since 2008, many states have established veterans' treatment courts to serve criminal defendants who are veterans and have mental health and/or substance use issues. These dockets usually involve a combination of biweekly court appearances, random drug/alcohol testing, and mandatory treatment/counseling sessions. State legislation is required to establish these courts; many state legislators have

specifically named PTSD as the rationale for the veterans-only docket and treatment model.

The VA and the DOD have set forth clinical practice guidelines for psychosocial rehabilitation of veterans (job training, social skills training, self-care, education, employment, psychoeducation, peer counseling, and intensive case management). These include the following:

1. The safety of the veteran is paramount.
2. The veteran should have a discharge plan that includes a plan for safe, stable housing.
3. The veteran should have an option of work or another productive activity.
4. The veteran and family should be educated about his or her disorders and provided with resources, including referral to support groups.
5. The veteran should be assigned a case manager if needed.
6. The veteran should receive job skills training.
7. The veteran must be assigned to a primary care team in either a medical or mental health setting.
8. The veteran must have access to psychiatrists, psychologists, social workers, and/or nurses as needed.

Professionals need to be aware of military regulations regarding confidentiality when providing mental health services to active-duty personnel and recognize that these limits may be a barrier to disclosure of traumatic events. Before President Clinton's executive order in 1999, there was no patient-therapist confidentiality protection in the military setting. Military Rules of Evidence, Rule 513 (MRE 513), does not protect rights as strongly as federal laws for civilians do, however. If the professional is court-ordered to reveal information, he or she may ask the judge to include a protective order to admit only portions of the records, not the records in their entirety, and to seal the record of the hearing in order to safeguard privacy. Under MRE 513, there are several exceptions to confidentiality: Deceased patient; evidence of spousal abuse or child abuse; mandatory reporting under federal, state, or military law; danger to any person, including the patient; fraud committed by the patient; a constitutional requirement (the accused's right to due process may be weighed against the accuser's right to privacy); or the need to ensure the safety and security of military personnel, military dependents, military property, classified information, or the accomplishment of a military mission. This military mission inclusion is considered a grey area: it gives the military great leeway in requesting records.

SERVICES AND RESOURCES

The VA maintains the National Center for PTSD, which is a vast source of information for patients and professionals, http://www.ptsd.va.gov

The VA also has a veterans' crisis hotline: 1-800-273-8255. This hotline connects veterans in crisis or their loved ones with a qualified responder through the Department of Veteran Affairs.

The VA has PTSD-specific treatment programs that include outpatient programs and intensive programs that may be inpatient or residential. PTSD specialists are available at VA medical centers.

Every VA medical center also has on staff a women veterans program manager to serve as an advocate and referral source.

Female-specific programs and treatments include women's stress disorder treatment teams; outpatient mental health programs with a primary focus on PTSD and other issues related to experienced trauma; specialized inpatient and residential programs for female veterans who require more intensive support; and women's comprehensive health centers, which are female-specific VA health centers located in some VAs that often provide outpatient mental health services.

The National Alliance on Mental Illness (NAMI) has a veterans resource center with resources on PTSD, treatments, programs, news and media reports, and online discussion forums, http://www. nami. org/template.cfm?section=ptsd

FOOD FOR THOUGHT

In 2009, a jury in Oregon found a defendant who had killed an unarmed man guilty but legally insane due

Problem	Goal	Intervention
Person is exhibiting signs and symptoms of PTSD.	Person will have relief from PTSD symptoms and return to baseline functioning.	Review assessments and tools to learn where symptoms are clustering and in what areas the person is experiencing the most distress. Evaluate for drug or alcohol use that may be exacerbating symptoms. Evaluate available supports and enlist as appropriate. Begin therapeutic intervention (CPT, PE, EMDR) or refer to outside mental health resource. Refer for group support if appropriate and if the person is receptive.
Person is experiencing high levels of anger and increased potential to be violent.	Decrease anger and violent impulses. Improve safety for person and family and social supports.	Screen for IPV risk or perpetration. Address any physical aggression and what the triggers are. Work on behavioral interventions and breathing exercises to help reduce anger and violent impulses. Show how repeated stress due to violence will destabilize the family. Establish a safety plan.
Person has disclosed that she experienced sexual trauma in the military and is now exhibiting signs and symptoms of PTSD.	Person will have a reduction in symptoms and feel empowered and more in control of her personal safety.	Utilize CBT to work on symptom reduction. Access a self-defense or personal safety empowerment intervention that will reduce feelings of fear and help her feel she is in control of her personal safety and will not suffer a sexual trauma again.
Person's family is experiencing negative symptoms such as stress, family discord, anxiety, and depression as a result of the patient's PTSD.	Reduce negative symptoms and improve family coping and family support.	Address numbing and avoidance behaviors that create the most conflict with relationships and family functioning. Encourage the woman to be more expressive and regain emotional intimacy with her partner and/or family. Reduce self-isolation from family members and friends by breaking cycle of avoidance and withdrawal. If the woman has been away for a long period, educate on the age-appropriate needs of and discipline for her children. Encourage positive parent-child interactions.

to PTSD. The defendant was being treated for service-connected PTSD; he faced a 25-year prison sentence but instead was committed to a psychiatric hospital.

Some police departments are training their crisis response teams in management of suspects who have PTSD (hostage situations in which the hostage-taker is a veteran with PTSD).

Veterans with PTSD and mild traumatic brain injuries (TBI) have an increased risk for suicide only if the PTSD symptoms are severe. Having a mild TBI and mild PTSD symptoms does not increase risk for suicide.

Accidental motor vehicle death rates may be higher among veterans because of an increase in high-risk behaviors (not using seatbelts, driving while intoxicated).

A new area of research is using personal safety training or self-defense training to empower female veterans who have been traumatized sexually and who have PTSD. This is in effect a behavior therapy technique that shows promise but needs further testing and evaluation.

Women serving in Iraq or Afghanistan are more likely to be unmarried and poorer than their male counterparts. The combination of less social support and increased financial stress can increase the risk of PTSD.

Seeking Safety is a CBT-based group intervention for women with PTSD and a co-occurring substance use disorder that has had successful outcomes.

Partners and family members living with veterans with PTSD can experience emotional strain, intimacy problems (for partners), and low satisfaction with life. It is important to include partners and family members in PTSD treatment if they are willing and able to address the social support relationships.

RED FLAGS

Suicide is the third leading cause of death among members of the military currently serving in combat zones, with suicide rates among active-duty personnel at record highs.

In one study, veterans with PTSD were found to have a higher incidence of IPV perpetration than veterans who do not have PTSD. Fifty-three percent of the veterans in the study identified at least one physically aggressive act they had perpetrated in the previous 4 months. Sixty percent of veterans who had current or recent partners reported mild-to-moderate IPV perpetration some time in the past 6 months.

If a person is in crisis (suicidal ideation, ongoing trauma), the crisis problems need to be resolved before beginning any type of CBT treatment.

—*Jessica Therivel, LMSW-IPR, and Melissa Rosales Neff, MSW*

FOR FURTHER INFORMATION

Crum-Cianflone, N. F., & Jacobson, I. (2014). Gender differences of postdeployment post-traumatic stress disorder among service members and veterans of the Iraq and Afghanistan conflicts. *Epidemiologic Reviews, 36*(1), 5-18. doi:10.1093/epirev/mxt005

Fiore, R., Nelson, R., & Tosti, E. (2014). The use of yoga, meditation, mantram, and mindfulness to enhance coping in veterans with PTSD. *Therapeutic Recreation Journal, 48*(4), 337-340.

Hoerster, K., Jakupcak, M., Stephenson, K., Fickel, J., Simons, C., Hedeen, A.,... Felker, B. (2015). A pilot trial of telephone-based collaborative care management for PTSD among Iraq/Afghanistan war veterans. *Telemedicine Journal and E-Health, 21*(1), 42-47. doi:10.1089/tmj.2013.0337

Middleton, K., & Craig, C. D. (2012). A systematic literature review of PTSD among female veterans from 1990 to 2010. *Social Work in Mental Health, 10*(3), 233-352. doi:10.1080/15332985.2011.639929

Ready, D. J., Sylvers, P., Worley, V., Butt, J., Mascaro, N., & Bradley, B. (2012). The impact of group-based exposure therapy on the PTSD and depression of 30 combat veterans. *Psychological Trauma: Theory, Research, Practice, & Policy, 4*(1), 84-93.

Suris, A., Lind, L., Kashner, T. M., Borman, P. D., & Petty, F. (2004). Sexual assault in women veterans: An examination of PTSD risk, health care utilization, and cost of care. *Psychosomatic Medicine, 66*(5).

Precocious puberty

CATEGORY: Disease/Disorder

Also known as: Sexual precocity, gonadotropin puberty, pubertas praecox

KEY TERMS:

gonads: ovaries in girls

hormones: chemicals produced by glands such as the thyroid, pituitary, or adrenals that stimulate bodily changes or growth and that regulate body functions

hypothalamic hamartomas: tumors in the hypothalamic region of the brain, which are usually benign

hypothalamus: the region of the brain that stimulates glands to secrete hormones

idiopathic: having an unidentified cause

puberty: secondary sexual development that involves the maturation of the reproductive system and is typified by significant physical growth

CAUSES AND SYMPTOMS

Secondary sexual development is commonly known as puberty. It is typically characterized by growth of pubic and underarm hair, acne, and rapid physical development until about age eighteen. During puberty, a girl develops breasts and begins to menstruate and ovulate.

Puberty is the result of hormonal changes triggered by the hypothalamus region of the brain. The brain releases luteinizing hormone-releasing hormone (LHRH) in periodic bursts, which causes the pituitary gland to secrete gonadotropin- releasing hormone (GnRH). Gonadotropins stimulate the ovaries in girls to secrete sex hormones. These hormones—estrogen and progesterone in girls start the sexual maturation process and stimulate rapid physical growth.

Onset of puberty, especially in girls, appears to be occurring earlier than previously reported. Current data approximates puberty beginning around age ten in girls and age eleven in boys. Different factors have been proposed for this trend including changes in dietary habits, increasing incidence of childhood obesity, and greater inclusion of different population groups in the normative sample (e.g., African-American females who typically initiate puberty at an earlier age than their caucasian peers). Approximately one in every ten thousand children begins puberty abnormally early, between infancy and approximately age eight in girlsThis condition, known as precocious puberty, affects both sexes but is two- to five-times more common among girls than boys. Early onset of puberty is also more likely to occur in overweight children.

In addition to prematurely developing secondary sexual characteristics, children with precocious puberty are initially tall for their ages. Left untreated, however, they rarely reach their full adult height potential because the same sex hormones that trigger early growth also end it prematurely. Many females final height is under 5 feet and males often grow no taller than 5 foot 2 inches. Precocious puberty frequently results in adolescent behaviors such as moodiness, irritability, and aggressiveness, as well as the early development of a sex drive. Children with precocious puberty reach sexual maturity at varying rates, and some characteristics may even begin to regress to their normal state.

When an underlying cause for precocious puberty cannot be determined, the condition is known as idiopathic precocious puberty. About 80 percent of cases in females and 40 percent of male cases are idiopathic. Common causes for precocious puberty that can be identified include genetic disorders or tumors in the hypothalamic region of the brain. Such tumors, known as hypothalamic hamartomas, are usually benign.

Between 5 and 10 percent of boys with precocious puberty genetically inherit the condition from their fathers or indirectly from their maternal grandfathers. This genetic transmittal of precocious puberty only occurs in about 1 percent of girls with the condition. Less common causes of precocious puberty include other kinds of brain tumors, ovarian tumors or cysts, and adrenal gland disorders such as adrenogenital hyperplasia or congenital adrenal hyperplasia. Precocious puberty can also be caused by pituitary lesions, hydrocephalus, radiation therapy, nervous system disorders such as neurofibromatosis, thyroid disorders (specifically severe hypothyroidism), and a rare condition called McCune-Albright syndrome.

Children with precocious puberty are often self-conscious about their early physical and sexual development, since they appear older than their ages. Mental development is not affected by the condition, however, so children with precocious puberty are usually not as emotionally mature as they appear. Early pubertal girls are especially at risk of being confronted with social or sexual pressures (e.g., involving early exposure to drugs and alcohol or sexual advances from older adolescents) for which they are emotionally unprepared. Associated distress may result in withdrawal or acting out, which can be serious enough to warrant therapeutic intervention. There is some evidence of greater behavioral problems in girls with precocious puberty in comparison to peers, which

Information on Precocious Puberty

Causes: Hormonal imbalance; possibly linked to genetic disorders, tumors in hypothalamus, adrenal gland disorders, hydrocephalus, radiation therapy, nervous system disorders, McCune-Albright syndrome

Symptoms: Premature development of secondary sexual characteristics; above-average height until adulthood but failure to reach full growth potential, moodiness, irritability, aggressiveness, early development of sex drive

Duration: Chronic

Treatments: Hormonal therapy

also points to the need for education and communication with patients and parents regarding psychosocial development, coping skills, and healthy body image.

TREATMENT AND THERAPY

Underlying causes of precocious puberty, if known, are often difficult or impossible to treat. Surgical removal of noncancerous hypothalamic hamartomas and other brain tumors, for example, may not be feasible and rarely halts sexual development. Other causes such as neurofibromatosis are incurable, and treatments for conditions such as adrenal disorders may not stop the effects of precocious puberty.

Therefore, many forms of precocious puberty are treated by changing patients' hormonal balance. Synthetic hormones called LHRH analogs and gonadotropin-releasing hormone agonists (GnRHa) block the body's production of sex hormones and thus slow down or stop pubertal symptoms. The synthetic hormone histrelin acetate, also known by its brand name Supprelin, has been shown to be effective in reducing early sexual changes in both sexes and to slow bone growth. Leuprolide acetate, sold under the brand name Lupron-Depot PED, is another successful treatment for this condition. Daily injections of these drugs are stopped when the patient reaches the appropriate age for onset of puberty. Synthetic versions of GnRH or LHRH interrupt the chain of hormonal events that result in sexual maturation. Some research, however, suggests a link between these therapies and bone mineral density loss. Treatments are administered in daily or monthly injections.

Girls with precocious puberty caused by congenital adrenal hyperplasia can be treated by suppressing the hormone known as ACTH with a glucocorticoid. Precocious puberty associated with McCune-Albright syndrome can be treated with testolactone, which blocks the production of estrogens. Some forms of precocious puberty involving the gonadotropins can be treated with the hormone suppressant nafarelin acetate. Genetic counseling is recommended for families of patients with inherited precocious puberty. Psychological counseling may also benefit patients, since they may not fit in with peers because of the physical ramifications of the condition.

PERSPECTIVE AND PROSPECTS

Previous treatments for precocious puberty included the use of synthetic progesterone, an artificial version of a sex hormone secreted by the ovaries. Synthetic progesterone frequently stops menstruation and reduces breast size in girls, but it has little or no effect on boys. Unfortunately, it fails to stop rapid growth in either sex. Synthetic progesterone can also result in several serious side effects. Experimental treatments for idiopathic precocious puberty include a combination of spironolactone and testolactone for male patients, as well as another drug called deslorelin or Somagard for either sex. Puberty is a time of many changes for children. Emotional changes and challenges may occur. Children may struggle in relationships that they previously were successful in. Additional support for adolescents, including peer support and connectedness. If emotional struggles become significant, mental health therapy may be indicated.

—*Cheryl Pawlowski, Ph.D.;*
Updated by Lenela Glass-Godwin, M.W.S.
and Paul F. Bell, Ph.D.

FOR FURTHER INFORMATION

Garibaldi, Luigi and Chematailly, Wassim. Disorders of pubertal development, In (eds.) Kliegman, Robert, Stanton, Bonita, Schor, Nina, St. Geme, Joseph, and Behrman, Richard. *Nelson Textbook of Pediatrics*. 20th Edition, Vol. 2: 2656-2662. Philadelphia: Elsevier. 2016.

Huffman, Grace Brooke. "Reassessing the Age Limit of Precocious Puberty in Girls." *American Family Physician* 61, no. 6 (March 15, 2000): 1850.

Kar, Sujita and Choudhury, Ananya. Understanding normal development of adolescent sexuality: A bumpy ride. *Journal of Reproductive Sciences*, 8, no. 2 (April-June, 2015): 70-74.

Kim, Eun and Lee, Moon. "Psychosocial aspects in girls with idiopathic precocious puberty." *Psychiatry Investigation*, no. 9(1) (March, 2012): 25-28.

National Institutes of Health. "Puberty and Precocious Puberty: Overview." *NIH: Eunice Kennedy Shriver National Institute of Child Health and Human Development*, April 3, 2013.

Preeclampsia and eclampsia

CATEGORY: Disease/Disorder

KEY TERMS:

gestational hypertension: blood pressure of at least 140/90 mm Hg at or after 20 weeks' gestation

hemolysis: the rupture of red blood cells and release of hemoglobin into the blood, which can cause anemia

ischemia: restriction of blood supply that causes a shortage of oxygen in tissues

perinatal mortality: number of stillbirths and deaths in the first week of life per 1,000 total births

proteinuria: the presence of protein (typically albumin) in the urine

tonic-clonic seizures: also known as grand mal seizures. These produce bilateral, convulsive muscle contractions

CAUSES AND SYMPTOMS

Preeclampsia, formerly known as toxemia, is a serious disease that develops in 2% to 8% of pregnant women and remains a leading cause of maternal and perinatal morbidity and mortality. It is characterized by gestational hypertension and significant proteinuria at or after 20 weeks' gestation. Mild preeclampsia is defined as a blood pressure of 140/90 mmHg or higher with proteinuria of 0.3-3g/day. Severe preeclampsia includes an additional adverse feature such as blood pressure between 160-170/100-110 mm Hg, proteinuria of 3-5g/day, and/or headache. Other symptoms may include progressive lower extremity or abdominal swelling, changes in vision, abdominal

pain, nausea or vomiting, impaired liver function, and shortness of breath. Typically, early-onset preeclampsia (<34 weeks of gestation) is associated with worse maternal and neonatal outcomes compared to late-onset preeclampsia (>34 weeks of gestation). Intrauterine growth restriction (IUGR) in the developing fetus is a potential complication of preeclampsia and can lead to low birth weight and predisposes the fetus to various adult diseases such as diabetes and coronary artery disease.

An estimated 15% of women with preeclampsia develop HELLP syndrome, which is characterized by hemolysis, elevated liver enzymes, and a low platelet count. HELLP syndrome usually occurs in the last trimester, with women complaining of nausea, vomiting, and upper abdominal pain. In severe cases, the syndrome leads to intravascular blood clotting, kidney failure, liver failure, respiratory failure, systemic failure, and death. Eclampsia is a complication that occurs in 1-2% of severe preeclampsia cases and is characterized by new onset of tonic-clonic seizures or coma that cannot be attributed to other causes in addition to the symptoms of preeclampsia. Most cases of eclampsia occur within 24 hours of delivery. Organ damage, especially injury to the kidneys, liver, brain, and placenta, may occur.

The cause of preeclampsia and eclampsia remains largely unknown. The leading hypotheses involve placental dysfunction in early pregnancy. Placental ischemia leads to the release of factors into the maternal blood circulation that contribute to vessel damage and inflammation, both of which increase the risk of developing preeclampsia. However, placental impairment alone is not sufficient to trigger preeclampsia. Predisposing cardiovascular and metabolic disorders may result in late-onset preeclampsia. Interactions between genetics and environmental factors are thought to be important as well. The incidence of preeclampsia is rising in the United States, which may be related to higher prevalence of predisposing disorders and a general trend of delayed childbearing. The risk of preeclampsia is higher in women with personal or family histories of preeclampsia; women who already have chronic hypertension; women younger than 18 or older than 40; women experiencing their first pregnancy or their first pregnancy with a new partner; women who are obese (BMI > 30); women with inadequate prenatal care; and women with other conditions such as diabetes, kidney disease, and

Information on Preeclampsia and Eclampsia

Causes: Unknown; risk factors include first pregnancy, personal or family history of disorder, age younger than eighteen or older than forty, more than one fetus, obesity, and certain diseases (polycystic ovarian syndrome, diabetes, kidney disease, hypertension, autoimmune disorders)

Symptoms: For preeclampsia, high blood pressure, proteinuria, headaches, abdominal pain, vision problems; for eclampsia, convulsive seizures, organ damage, sometimes coma or death

Duration: Chronic during pregnancy

Treatments: Strict bed rest, balanced salt solution, sedatives, blood pressure medications, magnesium sulfate, diazepam, diuretics, delivery of baby as soon as possible

autoimmune disorders. Black women are more likely to die from preeclampsia or eclampsia than white women, though this disparity may be confounded by a higher prevalence of chronic hypertension in black women and disproportionate levels of care. Interestingly, smoking is associated with a reduced risk of preeclampsia in low-risk pregnancies.

DIFFERENTIAL DIAGNOSIS

Preeclampsia shares clinical symptoms with many other diseases, including chronic hypertension, thrombotic thrombocytopenic purpura (TTP), antiphospholipid syndrome, HELLP syndrome, pheochromocytoma, systemic lupus erythematosus (SLE), and acute fatty liver of pregnancy (AFLP).

TREATMENT AND THERAPY

Preconception counseling and assessment is recommended for women at high-risk of preeclampsia. Some research has demonstrated efficacy of antiplatelet agents, low-dose aspirin, and calcium supplementation in preventing preeclampsia. Severity of the disease and maturity of the baby are primary considerations for treatment. The only definitive cure for preeclampsia is delivery, which means treatment of preeclampsia for women who are remote from term (<34 weeks' gestation) is largely symptomatic. Patients who are experiencing severe symptoms and whom are close to term may undergo induction of labor or c-section. Management of hypertension during pregnancy is essential and can be accomplished with antihypertensive agents including nifedipine (*Procardia*), hydralazine (*Apresoline*), and labetalol (*Normodyne*). First-line treatment and prevention of eclampsia is magnesium sulfate (Epsom salt), which is neuroprotective and reduces the incidence of seizures. Women treated for preeclampsia and eclampsia should also be monitored for other symptoms, including headaches, blurred vision, abdominal pain, vaginal bleeding, and loss of fetal heart sounds.

PERSPECTIVE AND PROSPECTS

The first known description of preeclampsia was by Hippocrates in the 5th century B.C. Recent research has focused on the underlying mechanisms of preeclampsia and the role of gene-gene and gene-environment interactions. Some research has postulated that epigenetic changes – modifications to gene expression – to the gametes, placenta, and fetus are implicated. Concurrent research has identified excessive or atypical maternal immune responses as another potential cause of preeclampsia. Additional pharmacological studies are needed to develop treatments that target placental dysfunction and subsequent consequences. These insights could help improve preventive and therapeutic measures, particularly for high-risk patients.

—*David M. Lawrence;*
Updated by Robin Kamienny Montvilo, R.N., Ph.D.,
and Derrick Cheng, BSc, BA, and Carol Shi, BA

FOR FURTHER INFORMATION

Duley, L. "The global impact of pre-eclampsia and eclampsia." *Seminars in Perinatology*, 33, no. 3, 2009, 130-137.

Haram, K., et al. "The HELLP syndrome: clinical issues and management. A Review." *BMC Pregnancy and Childbirth*, 9, no., 2009, 8.

Jeyabalan, A. "Epidemiology of preeclampsia: impact of obesity." *Nutrition Reviews*, 71, 2013, S18-S25.

Phipps, E., et al. "Preeclampsia: updates in pathogenesis, definitions, and guidelines." *Clinical Journal of the American Society of Nephrology*, 11, no. 6, 2016, 1102-1113.

Sibai, B. M. "Etiology and management of postpartum hypertension-preeclampsia." *American Journal of Obstetrics and Gynecology*, 206, no. 6, 2012, 470-475.

Steegers, E. A., et al. "Pre-eclampsia." *The Lancet*, 376, no. 9741, 2010, 631-644.

Von Dadelszen, P., et al. "Subclassification of pre-eclampsia." *Hypertension in Pregnancy*, 22, no. 2, 2003, 143-148.

Pregnancy and gestation

CATEGORY: Biology

KEY TERMS:

amniotic sac: the sac that surrounds the fetus in the uterus and is filled with amniotic fluid

blastocyst: the fertilized egg after it has divided several times to form a hollow ball of cells in one of the earliest stages of development

cervix: the constricted lower end of the uterus

chorion: the membrane in the embryo that further differentiates into the placenta and umbilical cord

chromosomes: rod-like structures inside cells that carry the genetic material

embryo: the unborn child from the second through the eighth week of development

endometrium: the lining of the uterus

Fallopian tube: the structure that leads from the internal cavity of the uterus to the ovary

fetus: the unborn child from the eighth week after fertilization until birth

placenta: the organ that connects the mother to the embryo or fetus through the umbilical cord and is necessary for the child's nourishment

trimester: a division of pregnancy into three equal time periods of about thirteen weeks

PROCESS AND EFFECTS

Pregnancy begins conception or fertilization with the fusion of an egg and sperm within a woman's body and continues until childbirth, typically thirty-eight weeks later. This gestational time is divided into three approximately equal periods called trimesters, each associated with specific physical and biochemical hallmarks.

Prior to conception, a mature egg, or ovum, ruptures from a fluid-filled follicle within the ovary and is swept into the Fallopian tube by large fringes on the tube that caress the ovary's surface. The empty follicle is transformed into a structure called the corpus luteum which secretes hormones that help to prepare the woman's body for pregnancy. If the ovum is fertilized within twenty-four hours, pregnancy will occur. If it is not fertilized, the uterine lining will be shed during menstruation.

Sperm ejaculated into a woman's vagina travel through the cervix and uterus and into the Fallopian tubes. Only about 200 of the original 500 million sperm delivered to the woman may reach the vicinity of the ovum. Enzymes in the sperm heads dissolve protective outer layers of the egg. When one sperm finally breaks through the plasma membrane, the innermost covering of the ovum, chemical changes on the surface of the ovum prevent additional sperm from entering. The genetic material contained in the sperm and ovum fuse. If the fertilizing sperm is a gynosperm, which carries an X chromosome, then the baby will be female; if it is an androsperm, which carries a Y chromosome, then the baby will be male.

About twelve hours after fusion of the genetic material, the first cell division occurs. Divisions continue at intervals of twelve to fifteen hours, doubling the number of cells each time, and the fertilized ovum is now called a blastocyst. The blastocyst is gently guided through the Fallopian tube to the uterus by the beating of the millions of tiny hairs, called cilia, that line the inner surfaces of the Fallopian tubes. This journey to the uterus takes about three days.

Upon arriving in the uterus, the blastocyst "explores" the endometrium, the uterine lining, for an appropriate site to settle. Prior to this implantation in the endometrium, the blastocyst ruptures from the clear protective sheath that helps to prevent it from settling in the Fallopian tube. By ten to fourteen days after fertilization, the blastocyst implants securely within the endometrium and the embryonic stage begins.

At this point, it consists of several hundred cells and is about the size of the head of a pin. After implantation, chemical signals produced by the blastocyst prevent the mother's immune system from recognizing the blastocyst as a foreign invader and destroying it. Other chemical signals cause the endometrium to thicken and extend blood vessels to the blastocyst for nourishment from the mother. The uterine wall softens and thickens, and the cervical opening is sealed with a mucus plug.

At this point, the cells of the blastocyst divide into two distinct clusters: One part will form the

Stages of Fetal Development

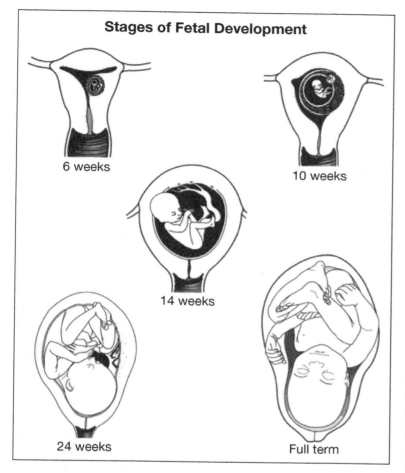

6 weeks

10 weeks

14 weeks

24 weeks

Full term

© EBSCO

embryo itself, and the other part will join with the woman's tissue to form the placenta, the structure that will provide nourishment from the mother to the growing embryo. These early placental cells produce the hormone human chorionic gonadotropin (hCG). This hormone signals the ovary to cease ovulation and stimulates it to produce the hormone progesterone, which prevents menstruation and causes the endometrium to grow even thicker.

During the second week after fertilization, a cavity surrounding the embryo begins to form. This is destined to become the amniotic sac, which will contain the shock-absorbing amniotic fluid in which the fetus floats during development. At this time, the hCG being produced by the blastocyst and ovaries can be detected by pregnancy tests.

Three weeks after conception, the size of the embryo is about 2 millimeters (0.08 inch). The embryonic cells have divided into germ layers, distinct groupings of cells that are destined to produce specific body parts. The rudimentary brain appears at the end of a long tube. The heart is forming and will be beating within a week. At this point, the mother has missed her menstrual period and may be experiencing symptoms of pregnancy, such as nausea, heartburn, and tender breasts.

During the fifth through seventh weeks of embryonic development, massive physical changes occur. The crown-to-rump length of the embryo increases to around 1.25 centimeters (0.5 inch). The embryo's face, trunk, and limbs grow, and by the end of this period distinct fingers and toes are formed. The backbone is in place, and ribs begin to develop, as do skin, eyes, and all of the organ systems and the circulatory system. At this point, the placenta is connected to the embryo by the umbilical cord, and placental cells penetrate the blood vessels of the endometrium to provide transit of nutrients from the mother's bloodstream to the embryo. The placenta also filters out some potentially dangerous substances from the mother's bloodstream and aids in disposing of embryonic waste products.

By the eighth week of development, the embryo is about 4 centimeters (1.5 inches) long, weighs about 14 grams (0.5 ounce), and is composed of millions of cells. All organs are formed, and the embryo is officially called a fetus. The woman's uterus has increased in size, and her waistline may begin to enlarge. At this point, hormonal shifts stabilize, which frequently relieves morning sickness and other discomforts of early pregnancy.

Growth and organ system interconnection continue during the third month of fetal life, and the cells of the immune system are formed. During the fourth month, facial features develop, and the fetus may begin to respond to sound. Hair on the head and the eyebrows coarsens and develops pigment. The distinction between male and female fetuses becomes apparent with a visible vagina or penis. Sixteen to eighteen weeks after fertilization, the mother may feel the first fetal movements. She has gained several pounds, and changes in her body shape are readily visible. Frequently, this second trimester is associated with feelings of joy and minimal discomfort.

The third trimester is largely a period of growth for the fetus. Its weight increases rapidly. The fetus becomes very active within the amniotic fluid and responds to sound from both within and outside the mother. The weight gain may put incredible stress on the mother's body, and pressure on internal organs may cause frequent urination, heartburn, and difficulty breathing and sleeping.

Normal pregnancies vary from thirty-eight to forty-two weeks long. The lungs are the final organs to mature, and by the end of the eighth month all organ systems are established and functional. The fetus continues to gain weight until the end of pregnancy. At this time, the fetus will weigh around 3 kilograms (7 pounds) and have a crown to rump length of approximately 37 centimeters (14.4 inches). The end of pregnancy is heralded by the beginning of uterine contractions, and frequently by the rupture of the amniotic sac and expulsion of its fluid. Labor leads to the birth of a unique individual created from the developmental programs contained in the genetic material inherited from each parent.

COMPLICATIONS AND DISORDERS

Since the developing embryo or fetus is dependent on the placental connection to the mother for nourishment, its health is directly tied to the diet and lifestyle of the mother. Any environmental substance that may cause a developmental defect is known as a teratogen. Women must take care to avoid teratogens such as drugs or nicotine during pregnancy. Pregnant women must ingest adequate levels of protein, vitamins, and iron to remain healthy and have a healthy baby. Smoking during pregnancy has been linked to heart defects, and it decreases the amount of oxygen available to the fetus, which causes poor growth. Consumption of alcohol is associated with a host of defects collectively called fetal alcohol syndrome. Whether any level of alcohol consumption is safe during pregnancy is not yet known. The use of drugs such as heroin and cocaine during pregnancy increases the likelihood of stillbirths and unhealthy babies.

The loss of a fetus before the twentieth week of pregnancy is called a miscarriage. The most common cause of miscarriage during the first trimester is a major genetic defect in which the embryo has missing or extra chromosomes and therefore cannot develop normally. Other common causes are physical abnormalities in the embryo, a malformed uterus in the mother, an "incompetent" cervix that opens as the fetus enlarges, scarring of the uterus, and hormonal deficiencies. Increasing age of the mother, smoking, and alcohol and drug consumption are also correlated with miscarriage. To prevent future miscarriages of a nongenetic cause, hormone therapy, medications, and surgery are options.

Ectopic pregnancies occur when the fertilized egg implants in the wall of the Fallopian tube instead of in the uterus. The growing embryo may rupture the tube, endangering the mother's life and necessitating emergency surgery and possible loss of that Fallopian tube. Unruptured ectopic pregnancies can be treated with medication or laparoscopic surgery. Scarring of the Fallopian tube from an infection can narrow this passage and cause ectopic pregnancy, as can early "hatching" of the blastocyst from its protective covering.

Neural tube defects result from a problem in the ectodermal layer of the embryo resulting in improper closure of the brain and spinal cord in early embryonic development. The outcomes of this defect are anencephaly (absence of a complete brain and part of the skull), a lethal condition, or spina bifida (portions of the spinal cord protruding from the spine), which can vary from mild to severe. These disorders seem to occur in families with a history of neural tube defects in pregnancy. Folic acid, an important component of prenatal vitamins, can reduce the risk of neural tube defects.

Neural tube defects can be detected prenatally by ultrasound, in which high-frequency sound waves are bounced off the contents of the uterus. The echoes are converted to an image, or sonogram, on a screen. Another test for neural tube defects is the alpha fetoprotein test, which measures levels of a fetal protein in the mother's blood; high levels indicate a neural tube defect.

Down syndrome, which results from the presence of one extra chromosome number 21, is the leading cause of mental retardation in the United States and occurs in about 1 in every 800 live births. Many other genetic disorders are caused by missing or extra chromosomes. Some inherited diseases are attributable to errors in small pieces of chromosomes. Examples of these sorts of disorders include cystic fibrosis, hemophilia, Tay-Sachs disease, and sickle cell disease. Many

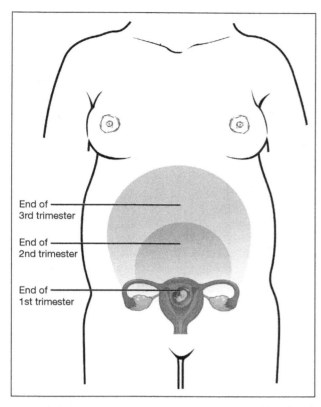

The abdomen stretches and grows during pregnancy to accommodate the fetus. (OpenStax via Wikimedia Commons)

of these genetic diseases can be detected by prenatal tests.

Amniocentesis is performed between the fifteenth and seventeenth weeks of pregnancy. A needle is inserted through the mother's abdomen, and a sample of the amniotic fluid is removed. Fetal cells present in the fluid are cultured for two to three weeks. The fetal cells are then analyzed for chromosome complement or tested for small genetic changes that can result in specific genetic diseases. Occasionally amniocentesis is done in the third trimester to determine fetal lung maturity when delivery of a premature infant is expected. Chorionic villus sampling provides a similar means to examine the genetic material of the fetus. This test is performed as early as the eighth week of pregnancy when a small piece of the chorionic villus, a tissue of embryonic origin that surrounds the early placenta, is removed and genetic analysis is immediately performed. Prenatal diagnosis of a chromosome abnormality or genetic

disease allows the parents to terminate the pregnancy or to prepare for the birth of an affected child.

Infections acquired by a pregnant woman may be only inconveniences for her, but they may have severe consequences for an unborn child. Rubella, or German measles, can cause fetal death or severe impairment during the first trimester and permanent hearing loss during the second trimester. Vaccination prevents contraction of rubella but cannot be given during pregnancy. Cytomegalovirus (CMV) can cause physical and mental retardation, blindness, and deafness to the fetus if the mother first contracts CMV during pregnancy.

Toxoplasmosis is an infection that can cause serious fetal consequences including miscarriage, stillbirth, and neonatal death if contracted in pregnancy. Avoidance of gardening where cats defecate and avoiding any contact with cat litter are measures counseled to pregnant women to reduce risk. Transmission of the sexually transmitted diseases syphilis and gonorrhea to the fetus can be prevented with antibiotic therapy. Human immunodeficiency virus (HIV), the virus that causes acquired immunodeficiency syndrome (AIDS), can be transmitted from mother to fetus through the placenta. Newborns with AIDS have a host of disorders and usually die within one or two years.

Rh factor is a substance on the surface of red blood cells. Individuals with and without this substance are Rh positive and Rh negative, respectively. If a woman is Rh negative and has an Rh-positive fetus, during delivery some of the baby's blood cells will enter the woman, and her body will manufacture antibodies to destroy the foreign cells. If with a subsequent pregnancy the fetus is Rh positive, these antibodies could attack and destroy the fetus. This problem is avoided by blood-typing of mother and fetus during the first pregnancy and by administering Rho(D) immune globulin (human), which destroys the fetal red blood cells entering the mother before her body can produce antibodies. Hence, future pregnancies are not at risk for Rh incompatibility.

A host of medical problems in the mother can develop during pregnancy that could jeopardize both her health and the health of her fetus. Blood pressure problems develop in about 7 percent of pregnant women as a result of the enormous changes in blood volume and pressure. The largest danger is that the fetus will not receive enough oxygen, which may lead to growth problems or sudden death during the final months of pregnancy. Preeclampsia is a cluster of symptoms related to high blood pressure, including edema (swelling caused by water retention) and kidney malfunction. Eclampsia (convulsions and coma) is life-threatening and needs emergency treatment. Bed rest, diet modification, close monitoring by a physician, or hospitalization may be prescribed for mild to severe cases of high blood pressure during pregnancy.

The effect of the hormones induced by pregnancy on the production of insulin, which regulates sugar levels in the body, is not well understood. In some pregnancies, insulin levels are not regulated properly, which results in gestational diabetes. Untreated, this can result in loss of the fetus late in pregnancy, the birth of a baby with high body fat content and an immature pancreas, or maternal convulsions and coma. Proper medical intervention and monitoring can correct or ease the effects of gestational diabetes on both mother and fetus.

Up to half of pregnant women develop anemia, a deficiency in red blood cells, because of a lack of iron or folic acid. The demand for the production of red blood cells in both mother and fetus leads to this disorder, which can cause poor growth in the fetus and increased susceptibility to infection, fatigue, and severe bleeding during childbirth for the mother. Proper diet and dietary supplements can alleviate anemia.

PERSPECTIVE AND PROSPECTS

Until the mid-twentieth century, what was known about fetal development was derived mainly from the study of miscarriages. The development and use of ultrasound techniques in the 1960s allowed a more accurate picture of developmental progression of normal, active fetuses, and such techniques subsequently became indispensable for the detection of some developmental abnormalities.

While physicians had been able to sample the amniotic fluid surrounding a fetus since the late nineteenth century, it was not until 1970 that they discovered that the fluid contained fetal cells which could be analyzed for chromosomal composition. At this time, amniocentesis became a tool for prenatal genetic analysis and sex determination and a routine test for pregnant women over the age of thirty-five, who are at a higher risk of carrying a fetus with a genetic abnormality.

The liberalization of abortion laws in the United States in the 1960s gave parents of abnormal fetuses the option of pregnancy termination. In the early 1980s, chorionic villus sampling allowed much earlier detection of genetic defects and facilitated decision making for the expectant parents. In the 1980s, some physicians began performing surgery on fetuses within the mother's uterus to correct problems threatening the life of the fetus, such as kidney disorders. Advanced monitoring and intervention techniques have vastly decreased maternal deaths during pregnancy and childbirth.

Increased knowledge about infectious and toxic agents and about the ill effects of certain lifestyle habits upon a developing fetus has led to better education and prenatal care for both mother and fetus. Because of career and personal considerations, older women frequently wish to begin families. Medical advances have made it not uncommon for women past the age of forty to conceive for the first time and give birth to healthy infants.

Much research has been focused on the initial stages of pregnancy and infertility. Techniques have been developed to circumvent damaged Fallopian tubes. In the procedure called in vitro fertilization, a woman is given hormones to induce ovulation. Several mature eggs are removed from her ovaries and fertilized in a glass dish. The resulting blastocysts are then implanted into the woman's uterus. In some cases in which a woman is unable to carry the fetus herself, a surrogate mother has been used as an "incubator" for the embryo. Unused embryos fertilized in vitro are stored in a deep freeze and may be thawed for future use. Early embryos have been separated into individual cells, which then develop into genetically identical blastocysts, each with the potential to become an infant. These technological advances have raised a host of ethical questions concerning disposal of the embryos and their genetic manipulation.

Human reproductive research is focused on the reversal or circumvention of infertility, the alleviation of maternal and fetal distress, and the prenatal detection and treatment of genetic disease. The knowledge gained about reproduction serves to enhance a sense of awe and wonder at the beauty and complexity of the gestational process. Pregnancy and gestation are impacted by many factors such age, socioeconomic status and location of the woman. Medical prenatal care is highly recommended for all that have access to it. Trained midwives or doctors are utilized by women around the world to assist in the process and ensure the highest chance of safety for the mom and baby. Since the prenatal process brings about many vast changes for women, it is important for them to also seek emotional support when needed. The knowledge and information of wise women around the mother-to-be can be immensely helpful in this transition. When further physical or emotional struggles arise, it can also be important to seek outside help, such as a prenatal support group or individual counseling. Postpartum medical care and pediatric care for the infant are recommended to follow.

—*Karen E. Kalumuck, Ph.D.;*
Updated by Robin Kamienny Montvilo, R.N., Ph.D.
and Kimberly Ortiz-Hartman, Psy.D., LMFT

For Further Information

Cunningham, F. Gary, et al., editors. *Williams Obstetrics.* 23d ed. New York: McGraw-Hill, 2010.

Curtis, Glade B., and Judith Schuler. *Your Pregnancy Week-by-Week.* 6th ed. Cambridge, Mass.: Da Capo Press, 2008.

Eisenberg, Arlene, Heidi E. Murkoff, and Sandee E. Hathaway. *What to Expect When You're Expecting.* 4th ed. New York: Workman, 2009.

Moore, Keith L., and T. V. N. Persaud. *The Developing Human.* 8th ed. Philadelphia: Saunders/Elsevier, 2008.

Simkin, Penny. April Bolding. Ann Keppler. Janelle Durham. *Pregnancy, Childbirth, and the Newborn: The Complete Guide.* Hopkins, Minnesota: Meadowbrook Press, 2010.

Tsiaras, Alexander, and Barry Werth. *From Conception to Birth: A Life Unfolds.* New York: Doubleday, 2002.

Pregnancy and human immunodeficiency virus (HIV)

Category: Disease/Disorder

Key Terms:

boosting: the combination of an anti-HIV drug (usually a protease inhibitor) with another agent (e.g., ritonavir) that inhibits the liver enzymes that metabolizes that anti-HIV drug, which increases the serum concentration of the anti-HIV drug and its efficacy

dendritic cell: an antigen-presenting cell that acts as a key regulator of the adaptive immune response that is capable of activating naïve T cells and stimulating the growth and differentiation of B cells

integrase: an enzyme associated with the HIV virion that can insert the retroviral dsDNA and insert it into the genome (i.e. the chromosomes) of the host cell

macrophages: professional phagocytic cells that detect, phagocytose, and destroy bacteria and other harmful invading organisms, and regulate the immune response by presenting antigens to T cells and initiating inflammation by releasing signaling molecules known as cytokines that activate other cells

monocytes: a type of large white blood cell that can differentiate into macrophages, or dendritic cells

helper T cells: a type of lymphocyte that recognizes foreign antigens and secretes signaling molecules called cytokines to regulate the immune response; there are two different subtypes of helper T cells, one of which (Th1) activates cell-mediated immune responses for defending against intracellular viral and bacterial pathogens, and the other (Th2) of which drives B cells to produce antibodies against antigens in the humoral response

reverse transcriptase: an enzyme associated with the HIV virion that copies or replicates the viral single-stranded RNA molecule into a double-stranded DNA copy of it

Description

The human immunodeficiency virus (HIV) targets the human immune system. As HIV infects and destroys specific immune cells, the function of immune system begins to wane, resulting in immunodeficiency. When the patient's immune system fails, opportunistic infections begin to overwhelm her. At this point she is suffering from acquired immune deficiency syndrome (AIDS).

There are two forms of HIV: HIV-1 and HIV-2. HIV-1 is the cause of AIDS in the United States and worldwide. HIV-2 is rare and is found mainly in Western Africa and Southern Asia. Therefore, our descriptions of AIDS will exclusively cover those caused by HIV-1.

HIV infects CD4-positive cells, which includes dendritic cells, helper T cells, monocytes, and macrophages. The CD4 protein is a cell surface protein that helps the cells of the immune system communicate with one another. The HIV surface protein gp120 binds to CD4 but requires the presence of a co-receptor, which is either CXCR4 or CCR5. CXCR4 tends to be specific to helper T cells, CCR5 is found in the surfaces of T cells, macrophages, monocytes, and dendritic cells. Furthermore, different strains of HIV vary in their propensity or specificity for either CXCR4 or CCR5. The co-receptor, however, is essential for HIV infection since some people with mutations in the gene that encodes CCR5 are resistant to HIV infection.

HIV is a single-stranded RNA virus that is a member of a larger group of viruses known as the retroviruses. Upon exposure to bodily fluids that contain the virus, HIV-contaminated blood products, or HIV-contaminated needles, the virus typically infects dendritic cells found in peripheral tissues. The infected dendritic cell then carries the virus to a local lymph node where the virus spreads widely among the host of CD4 positive cells within the lymph node. Within the infected cells, HIV uses an enzyme called "reverse transcriptase" to reverse transcribe its single-stranded RNA into a double-stranded DNA copy. HIV then uses another enzyme called an "integrase" to integrates the viral DNA into the genome of the host cell. Now whenever the host cell divides, each daughter cell will receive a copy of the viral DNA. Also, whenever the immune cell transcribes those genes required to help it fight infections, the viral genes will be transcribed as well.

After the initial infection, the number of T cells in the patient's blood will plummet for about the first twelve weeks while the number of HIV virus particles rapidly rise. During this time the patient will experience flu-like symptoms that may mimic the symptoms of infectious mononucleosis. However, the patient's immune system will respond against the virus and the number of virus particles will decrease to a low but easily detectable number. The patient has now entered the chronic phase of the disease. The chronic phase may last anywhere from 2 to 10 years.

The HIV reverse transcriptase is error-prone and can make many mistakes when it is reverse transcribing the viral RNA into DNA. Consequently, the virus is subject to remarkable levels of variation within each patient. Some of his variation may affect the gene that encodes gp120 which will result in viruses that may tend to infect specific cell types or resist certain antiretroviral drugs. Whatever the case may be, the waning immune system is left trying to fight an intruder that varies every time the immune system starts to gain the upper hand against the virus.

During the chronic phase of HIV infection, the virus slowly chips away at the numbers of T cells as the number virus particles in the blood slowly rises. The patient may lose 1 to 2 billion T cells a day. When T-cell counts remain above 500 cells / mm3, the patient will usually have enough of an immune response to fight off most infections. However, other infections, such as tuberculosis, may become more common in severe cases. If the resident virus inside the host undergoes mutations that cause its gp120 preferentially bind the CXCR4 co-receptor, then the virus will become far more T-cell specific. Such a virus can now lay low in lymphoid tissue while destroying T cells. Since 90 percent of all T cells are in lymphoid tissue, such an event can rapidly deplete the patient's pool of T cells. Without helper T cells, the B lymphocytes cannot receive the proper signals to make antibodies and cell-mediated immunity against virus-infected cells is abrogated.

When the patient's T-cell counts fall to between 200 to 500 cells per cubic millimeter of blood, the patient will usually experience swollen lymph nodes, harry leukoplakia, and oral candidiasis. When T-cell counts fall below 200 cells / mm3 of blood, opportunistic infections that people with normal immune systems can easily keep it may will begin to infect the patient again and again. These infections include recurrent bacterial pneumonias, pneumocystis pneumonia, esophageal candidiasis, and tumors, such as Kaposi sarcoma, and primary lymphoma. At this point the patient is in full-blown AIDS.

HIV is transmitted from one person to another in blood, semen, vaginal secretions, and breast milk. To cause infection, the virus must pass through the skin or mucous membranes and enter the body's tissues. This can occur during sexual intercourse, breastfeeding, or through penetration of the skin by a contaminated hypodermic needle, among other circumstances. It is estimated that one third to one half of perinatal transmission occurs during breastfeeding. Epidemiological studies have shown that women are now the fastest-growing population of individuals with

HIV infections and AIDS. Male-to-male sexual transmission is the most common mode of transmission in the United States. Male-to-female sexual transmission is the most common mode of transmission in resource limited countries. Female-to-male sexual transmission is less common but possible since HIV is present in cervical and vaginal fluid. Sexual intercourse account for 75 percent of all HIV transmission. This underscores the importance of educating young women about the dangers of unprotected sex. Other modes of transmission include intravenous drug abuse, mother-to-child transmission by means of the placenta at birth or through breast milk, accidental needle sticks, or, rarely, the administration of contaminated blood products.

Although pregnancy does not appear to significantly expedite the progression of HIV infection, HIV-infected women who are pregnant are at greater risk for its complications, which include malnutrition, preterm labor, preeclampsia, and having an infant of low birthweight. Therefore, intervention and treatment are essential for a woman with HIV infection and measures to prevent infection are necessary for her fetus.

To prevent mother-to-child transmission (MTCT) of HIV, the mother is prescribed highly active antiretroviral therapy (HAART), which consists of a combination of drugs designed to reduce the replication of HIV in the body and decrease the number of virus particles in the blood. The mother must continue to take these medications beyond childbirth as lifelong therapy. Additionally, antiretroviral therapy is commonly given to the newborn infants of HIV-infected women within 6 to 12 hours after their delivery and is generally continued for the first 4 to 6 weeks of life.

The consistent use of combination antiretroviral therapy (ART) and abstention from breastfeeding reduces the risk of MTCT of HIV, also known as *perinatal transmission* of the virus, to less than 1 percent. Additionally, pregnant women who are infected with HIV should avoid any unnecessary medical procedures (amniocentesis, episiotomy) during pregnancy and delivery, to minimize the risk of contact of their fetus or infant with HIV. Fetal scalp electrode and scalp pH sampling should be avoided during delivery because these procedures may increase the risk of HIV transmission. Preconception counseling of HIV-infected pregnant women about the risks of HIV infection to themselves and their fetuses is crucial.

Pregnant women with HIV may also benefit from individual and family/couples therapy and participation in support groups.

HIV diagnosis includes antibody tests, which detect antibodies against the virus in the blood, antibody\antigen tests, which detect both antibodies against the virus and viral antigens in the blood, and RNA/DNA tests that detect HIV RNA or DNA. Antibody\antigen tests are the recommended tests and if the tests are positive, they should be confirmed with RNA/DNA tests and antibody tests.

FACTS AND FIGURES

In the United States, women constitute 19 percent of the nearly 40,000 new HIV diagnoses and 24 percent of the approximately 18,000 AIDS diagnoses in 2016. Among those newly infected women, who received a diagnosis of HIV in 2016, minorities were disproportionally affected: 61 percent were African American, 19 percent were white, and 16 percent were Hispanic/Latina. Fortunately, these numbers represent a decline in HIV among women in the past several years, since HIV diagnoses decreased by 20 percent among African-American women, by 14 percent among Hispanic/Latina women, and remained stable among white women.

Unfortunately, HIV acquisition through injection drug is on the rise. Worldwide, there was a 33 percent increase in the number of cases of HIV infection through injection drug use from 2011 to 2015. However, in the United States, from 2012 to 2016, HIV diagnoses decreased 18% among women who inject drugs. In 2017, people who inject drugs accounted for 6% of HIV diagnoses, and women who inject drugs accounted for 3% (1,016) of HIV diagnoses.

By the end of 2017, there were 38,739 new HIV diagnoses in the United States and dependent areas. An estimated 1,122,900 people had HIV, and 6 of 7 knew that they had the virus. Approximately half of all persons with HIV infection and/or AIDS are females, and these are the leading causes of death for women of reproductive age. The U.S. Centers for Disease Control and Prevention (CDC) recommends that all pregnant women be screened for HIV infection as early as possible. Based on estimates from 2006, which is the year from which the most recent data is available, approximately 8,500 women living with HIV gave birth each year. There were an estimated 21,956 cases of perinatally-acquired HIV prevented between 1994 and 2010. Of the estimated 174 children in whom HIV infection was diagnosed in 2014, 73 percent were infected perinatally, and 88 percent of the estimated 104 children in whom AIDS was diagnosed in 2014 got HIV through perinatal transmission. In 2016, 99 children under the age of 13 received a diagnosis of perinatally-acquired HIV. At the end of 2015, 1,872 children were living with HIV infections that they have acquired perinatally and 9,728 adults and adolescents (aged 13 and older) were diagnoses with HIV that had been acquired through perinatal transmission.

RISK FACTORS

Risk factors for the acquisition of HIV infection among women are multiple sex partners, intravenous drug use, unprotected anal or vaginal intercourse, blood transfusion before 1985, the presence of opportunistic infections (which may be misdiagnosed as other conditions), tattooing and body piercing with contaminated needles, sexually transmitted diseases (STDs), and lack of education and resources. A pregnant woman with HIV/AIDS is at risk of transmitting the disease to her fetus if she is unaware that she is infected; has had no prenatal care or HIV testing; experiences preterm labor; has a low number of CD4 T-lymphocytes as a measure of how HIV has affected the immune system; has a high viral load as a measure of how much HIV is in the blood; lacks access to antiretroviral drug therapy; is malnourished; or delivers her infant vaginally.

SIGNS AND SYMPTOMS

Psychologically, effects of HIV infection and/or AIDS in a pregnant woman can include feelings of loneliness, guilt, anxiety, anger, denial, fear, or depression, the last of which affects an estimated 30 percent of HIV-infected pregnant women. Behavioral manifestations of these conditions can include substance abuse, withdrawal from social relationships because of the stigma attached to HIV infection and AIDS, and weight loss.

Physical effects of HIV infection and/or AIDS during pregnancy include changes in general appearance, malnourishment, severe diarrhea and other influenza like symptoms, respiratory problems, and symptoms of opportunistic infections. Fewer than 40 percent of HIV-infected newborns show signs of infection by the virus at birth; however, by 4 months of age, almost all HIV-infected children have detectable HIV in their blood.

TREATMENT

All pregnant women, especially those who are members of high-risk groups, should be tested for HIV infection. Pregnant women who are HIV infected, or who present with active AIDS, or women with either condition who have given birth should undergo a complete biological, psychological, physical, and social assessment. Such assessments should include ascertaining the onset, duration, and presenting symptoms of her HIV infection or AIDS; a history of recurrent infections and of her prenatal care; and assessments for substance abuse and for past and present mental health, stress management skills, and coping mechanisms. Tests for HIV infection of the woman may be needed if her status is unknown, and if she has a newborn infant, it should be tested for HIV within 24 hours after its birth. The woman should also be asked for permission to obtain additional relevant information from her family members.

Early treatment for HIV infection and/or AIDS in pregnancy reduces the risk of MTCT of HIV. The recommended treatment regimens for pregnant women include two nucleoside reverse transcriptase inhibitors (NRTIs) and a third drug that is either a protease inhibitor or an integrase inhibitor.

NRTIs target the HIV reverse transcriptase. Upon entering cells, NRTIs are phosphorylated to form active metabolites that compete for incorporation into viral DNA. The phosphorylated NRTIs inhibit the HIV reverse transcriptase enzyme competitively and terminate synthesis of DNA chains. Thus, NRTIs prevent viral replication within cells, and are effective medications when combined with other antiretroviral drugs. The two-drug NRTI combinations recommended for pregnant women are tenofovir disoproxil fumarate and emtricitabine (TDF-FTC), tenofovir disoproxil fumarate and lamivudine, or abacavir and lamivudine. TDF-FTC is an important component of the antiretroviral treatment (ART) cocktail if the patient is also infected with hepatitis B, because it is active against hepatitis B. The third drug in this ART cocktail is either a boosted HIV protease inhibitor or an integrase inhibitor. Protease inhibitors (PIs) inhibit the HIV protease required for the proteolytic cleavage of viral polyprotein precursors into individual functional proteins. PIs prevent the formation of function HIV polypeptides and arrest productive infection of cells. Integrase inhibitors target the HIV integrase and prevent HIV DNA from being integrated into the host cell DNA.

For women presenting in the first trimester, a boosted protease inhibitor is the first choice (either atazanavir/ritonavir or darunavir/ritonavir). Ritonavir is the boosting agent in this case. For women presenting after the first trimester, then the integrase inhibitor dolutegravir is the third drug of choice, as it is better tolerated than the protease inhibitors. The integrase inhibitor raltegravir is an acceptable alternative, but since this drug must be administered twice a day, it is not as convenient. Alternative agents include:

1. NRTIs zidovudine plus lamivudine – not first-line because it causes headaches and anemia and requires twice-a-day dosing;
2. ritonavir-boosted lopinavir (PI) – also second-line because it can exacerbate the nausea of pregnancy;
3. The non-nucleoside reverse transcriptase inhibitor (NNRTI) efavirenz – second-line because it can aggravate mental health disorders and has significant drug-drug interactions with methadone;
4. NNRTI rilpivirine – has the advantage of being formulated in a single pill in combination with tenofovir and emtricitabine, but there is less data on the use of this drug during pregnancy.

If the woman is already on an antiretroviral treatment when she discovers that she is pregnant, she must see her primary healthcare provider immediately, because some anti-HIV drugs are not safe for pregnant women and their fetuses. For example, antiretroviral regimens that contain the drugs, stavudine, didanosine, full-dose ritonavir, or nelfinavir, should be discontinued immediately once the woman discovers she is pregnant.

In order to decrease the risk of HIV infection, all infants born to HIV-infected mothers should receive antiretroviral prophylaxis soon after birth. If the mother has good suppression of HIV infection (≤1000 copies / mL), then her baby should be treated with 4-6 weeks of zidovudine. If the mother

has not experienced good viral suppression (≥1000 copies/mL), then combination antiretroviral prophylaxis is warranted. Such treatments include zidovudine for six weeks, plus three doses of nevirapine given 48 hours after birth, 48 hours after the first dose, and 96 hours after the second dose. An alternative combination antiretroviral prophylactic treatment is zidovudine, lamivudine, and nevirapine for six weeks. If the infant cannot tolerate this drug regimen, then the lamivudine and nevirapine are discontinued after two weeks if the nucleic acid amplification tests at birth was negative for HIV-specific nucleic acids. Women with concurrent sexually transmitted infection, genital ulcers, or other health concerns that increase the risk of excess bleeding have increased risk of MTCT of HIV, and combination antiretroviral prophylactic treatments may be warranted regardless of their viral load.

It is essential that HIV-positive pregnant women understand the importance of adhering to medication schedules and dosages, both for themselves and for their newborn infants, and to the possible consequences of failing to do so. In addition to HAART and the treatment of any opportunistic infections, pregnant women with HIV infection and/or AIDS may benefit from individual and family/couples therapy, participation in support groups, nutritional evaluations, and case management services. The American Academy of Pediatrics Committee on Pediatric AIDS recommends that pregnant women with HIV infection avoid breastfeeding because of the risk of MTCT of the virus to their infants in breast milk. Mothers with HIV infections and/or AIDS can prevent the spread of HIV infection through safe sex and routine gynecological care (pelvic examinations every 6 months). Health care providers and social workers can offer or provide referrals to support services and follow-up counseling.

Many expectant mothers may not know that they are infected. For this reason, the CDC recommends that all women be tested for HIV as part of routine prenatal care. Research conducted by the CDC has established that pregnant women agree to the HIV test if the "opt-out approach" is used. The opt-out approach involves telling a pregnant woman that she will be given an HIV test as part of her routine prenatal care unless she opts out or chooses not to have the test. Also, HIV diagnoses are not evenly distributed throughout the United States. In 2017, the population rates (per 100,000 people) of people who received an HIV diagnosis were highest in the South (16.1), followed by the US 6 dependent areas (12.3), the Northeast (10.6), the West (9.4), and the Midwest (7.4). If the mother-to-be is from a part of the country where HIV among women is more common, then the CDC recommends a second test during the third trimester of pregnancy.

In 2016, the American Medical Association (AMA) created a new Common Procedural Terminology (CPT) code that includes HIV testing in the Obstetric Panel. This allows prenatal care providers to order just one panel that includes many standard serologic tests for pregnant women, including HIV.

Also, women who live with HIV may not realize that they are pregnant, or they might be unaware how to plan a pregnancy, or how to reduce the risk of transmitting HIV to their baby. For women who live with HIV, it is important that they visit their primary care health provider regularly. Second, they should take any and all HIV medications as directed, regularly, and throughout their pregnancy, labor, and delivery. Third, they should make sure that their baby received HIV medicine after delivery. Fourth, as painful as it might be, they should avoid breastfeeding, since the HIV is effectively transmitted to infants through infected breastmilk. Finally, they should avoid the practice of pre-chewing food for their baby or for anyone else's baby.

Social and economic factors affect access to health care. Poverty in particular, can be a major barrier to people living with HIV properly receiving the care that they and their unborn children desperately need. Pregnant women living with HIV may face additional obstacles to accessing proper medical care if they also use injection drugs or other substances; or are homeless, incarcerated, mentally ill, or uninsured.

APPLICABLE LAWS AND REGULATIONS

The United States Rehabilitation Act of 1973 Section 504 protects individuals against discrimination because of disability, and the United States Health Insurance Portability and Accountability Act of 1996 (HIPAA) protects individuals by ensuring the privacy of their health information and their right to review and make corrections to their medical records. Additionally, each state of the United States has its own laws regarding testing for HIV, criminal exposure to

HIV, and laboratory reporting. State specific information about these laws can be found at http:// www. cdc.gov/hiv/policies/law/states/index.html

—*Noelle Ainslie, MSW,*
and Jessica Therivel, LMSW-IPR
Updated David Hernandez

FURTHER READING

Robert Casanova, et al., editors. *Beckmann and Ling's Obstetrics and Gynecology*, 8th ed. Wolters Kluwers, Philadelphia, PA, 2018.

Becquet, R., et al. "Children who acquire HIV infection perinatally are at a higher risk of early death than those acquiring infection through breastmilk: A meta-analysis." *PloS One*, vol. 7, no. 2, 2012, e28510. doi:10.1371/ journal.pone.0028510

Centers for Disease Control and Prevention. "HIV among pregnant women, infants, and children." Published March 2018. https://www.cdc.gov/ hiv/pdf/group/gender/pregnantwomen/cdc-hiv-pregnant-women.pdf.

Money, D., et al. "Guidelines for the care of pregnant women living with HIV and interventions to reduce perinatal transmission: Executive summary." *Journal of Obstetrics and Gynaecology Canada: JOGC*, vol. 36, no. 8, 2014, 721.

Senise, J., Castelo, A., & Martinez, M. "Current treatment strategies, complications and considerations for the use of HIV antiretroviral therapy during pregnancy." *AIDS Review*, vol. 13, no. 4, 2011, 198-213.

Pregnancy and smoking cessation

CATEGORY: Disease/Disorder

WHAT WE KNOW

Smoking during pregnancy is associated with significant health risks for both the mother and fetus, including increased risk for low birth weight, intrauterine growth retardation, sudden infant death syndrome (SIDS), ectopic pregnancy, premature birth, and miscarriage. Smoking during pregnancy is associated with development of major health problems in infants and children, including asthma, bronchitis, and impaired development.

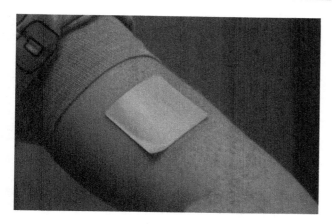

A nicotine patch is a small, self-adhesive patch that releases a slow, steady amount of nicotine into the body through the skin. (Wikimedia Commons)

Smoking during pregnancy exposes the fetus to toxic chemicals, including nicotine, carbon monoxide, and lead. When a pregnant woman smokes, the fetus is exposed to nicotine concentrations that are approximately equal to those in the mother's body, reducing the amount of nutrients and oxygen that are able to reach the fetus.

There is a relationship between how much a pregnant woman smokes and how much her baby will weigh at birth. Light smoking and heavy smoking are associated with an increase in the risk of low birth weight of 53 percent and 130 percent, respectively.

If all pregnant women quit smoking during pregnancy and maintained nonsmoking status for the duration of their pregnancies, there would be an 11 percent reduction in stillbirths and a 5 percent reduction in neonatal deaths. Most pregnant women know that smoking is bad for their baby. Historically, pregnant women underreport any current smoking, although some physicians may have in-office saliva testing for more accurate results.

Smoking cessation interventions for pregnant women can reduce the rate of maternal smoking and consequently reduce smoking-related morbidity and mortality. For example, infants of women who quit smoking during the first trimester tend to have weight and body measurements comparable to those of infants born to nonsmokers. Prenatal smoking cessation programs have decreased the incidence of intrauterine growth retardation and preterm births.

Women who quit smoking early in pregnancy (for example, during the first trimester) produce significant healthcare cost savings by decreasing the number of low birth weight babies. Although quitting smoking early in pregnancy offers the greatest benefit to both mother and fetus, significant benefits can still be achieved when mothers quit later in pregnancy.

Despite high rates of women who go back to smoking after their baby is born, supporting smoking reduction and cessation in pregnant women remains worthwhile and effective. Informal smoking cessation interventions during pregnancy are effective, but more intensive interventions are even more effective. The exception to this is group-based intensive interventions. Group interventions tend to be poorly attended and are less effective than individual intervention strategies

Smoking cessation interventions include cognitive behavioral therapy, motivational programs that offer incentives (such as financial rewards, either cash or gift cards, tied to specified behavior such as attending cessation meetings or testing nicotine-free), motivational interviewing, nicotine replacement therapy (NRT), and giving pregnant women the opportunity to experience real-time ultrasound feedback of fetal health status. According to researchers, providing incentives is the most effective intervention.

Teenage pregnant smokers had an increased interest in cessation and in getting help with cessation after utilizing an online tool that was specific to adolescent pregnant smokers. The participants stated that the tool increased their awareness of the dangers associated with smoking while pregnant and increased their motivation to quit.

Smoking with a partner or with family or friends can be a social interaction. Partner or family member participation in cessation attempts is critical for the long-term success of smoking cessation interventions in pregnant women. It is important to provide an opportunity for the partner to learn about smoking cessation if he or she is a smoker.

Although NRT increases the likelihood of successful smoking cessation by 50–70 percent, research results differ on the effectiveness of NRT in pregnancy. Results of clinical studies suggest that the use of NRT by pregnant women increases the risk of preterm and low birth weight births. It is unclear whether these findings are related to NRT being prescribed to heavier smokers, who may already have been at risk for fetal health concerns, or if NRT itself adversely affects the developing fetus.

Researchers who analyzed a trial of NRT in pregnancy to determine factors associated with cessation found that women who are better educated and have lower pretreatment cotinine (the predominant metabolite in nicotine) concentrations were more likely to stop smoking with the NRT treatment.

60 percent of pregnant smokers continue to smoke past their first prenatal visit. For these women, interventions that are not pharmacologically based have smoking cessation rates that usually are less than 20 percent. These interventions have almost no impact on heavier smokers, who tend to be poor and undereducated and whose social networks are filled with smokers.

Women who smoke are 30 percent less likely than nonsmokers to breastfeed their infants. Researchers who studied women who smoked during the postpartum period but had previously quit smoking found that the longer a women quit smoking during pregnancy, the more likely she was to at least begin breastfeeding her baby.

Vouchers with monetary value and a free breast pump are likely the most effective incentives for women to quit smoking while pregnant and to breastfeed after their child is born (and continue to not smoke). Other effective parts of cessation programs are support through having a "quitting pal" as well as initial daily text/telephone support.

Although 20–40 percent of female smokers stop smoking during pregnancy, they are vulnerable to relapse. Up to 60 percent of mothers who quit smoking during pregnancy resume smoking within 6 months of giving birth, and 80–90 percent do so within 12 months. Risk factors for smoking relapse after delivery include intending to quit smoking only for the duration of the pregnancy, not breastfeeding, using smoking as a way to cope with stress, lack of social support, and living with smokers. Researchers have found that a low-intensity smoking cessation program combined with relapse prevention can improve the quit rates in pregnant women and lead to smoking abstinence of up to one year postpartum.

—*Jessica Therivel, LMSW-IPR, and Chris Bates, MA, MSW*

FOR FURTHER INFORMATION

Association of Women's Health, Obstetric & Neonatal Nursing. (2010). AWHONN position statement. Smoking and women's health. *JOGNN: Journal of Obstetric, Gynecologic & Neonatal Nursing, 39*(5), 611-613. doi:10.1111/j.1552-6909.2010.01178.x

Crossland, N., Thomson, G., Morgan, H., Dumbrowski, S., & Hoddinott, P. (2015). Incentives for breastfeeding and for smoking cessation in pregnancy: an exploration of types and meanings. *Social Science & Medicine, 128,* 10-17. doi:10.1016/j.socscimed.2014.12.019

Dias-Dame, J., & Cesar, J. (2015). Disparities in prevalence of smoking and smoking cessation during pregnancy: a population-based study. *BioMed Research International, 345430.* doi:10.1155/2015/345430

Morgan, H., Hoddinott, P., Thomson, G., Crossland, N., Farra, S., Yi, D., & Campbell, M. (2015). Benefits of Incentives for Breastfeeding and smoking cessation in pregnancy (BIBS): A mixed-methods study to inform trial design. *Healthy Technology Assessment, 19*(30), 1-300. doi:10.3310/hta19300

Phelan, S. (2014). Smoking cessation in pregnancy. *Obstetrics & Gynecology Clinics of North America, 41*(2), 255-266. doi:10.1016/j.ogc.2014.02.007

Pregnancy and substance misuse

CATEGORY: Disease/Disorder

DESCRIPTION

Misuse of substances, including alcohol, illicit drugs, and prescription drugs taken for non-medical reasons, during pregnancy has serious implications for both the mother and fetus. In 2013 the fifth edition of the *Diagnostic and Statistical Manual of Mental Disorders* (*DSM-5*) was published, replacing the *DSM-IV*. The DSM-IV chapter on "Substance-Related Disorders" included substance dependence, substance misuse, substance intoxication, and substance withdrawal, and then discussed specific substances (e.g., alcohol, amphetamines). The *DSM-5* instead separates these disorders into two categories: substance use disorders and substance-induced disorders (intoxication, withdrawal, and other substance/medication-induced mental disorders). Thus, it removes the distinction between abuse and dependence and instead divides each disorder into mild, moderate, and severe subtypes. Drug craving was added as a criterion for substance use disorder, whereas "recurrent legal problems" was removed. Substance use disorders refer to a pattern of continued use of a substance (e.g., alcohol, cannabis, opioids, sedatives) that causes cognitive, physiological, and behavioral symptoms, resulting in problems in various areas of functioning. The substance may be illegal (e.g., cannabis, cocaine, heroin), legal (e.g., alcohol), or prescription medications used for purposes (i.e., recreational use) other than for which they were prescribed. The pattern of use is pathological. The individual may experience impaired self-control and may continue to use even when risks are present. There also may be tolerance and withdrawal.

Abuse of substances during pregnancy has effects on the mother; effects on the course of pregnancy, including delivery; and effects on the fetus, newborn, and/or developing child. Substances abused during pregnancy cross the placenta and can affect the fetus directly or indirectly, as when abuse during pregnancy leads to poor maternal nutrition and sleep deprivation. Alcohol is a teratogen (i.e., a substance that can cause birth defects); the use of alcohol during pregnancy, particularly heavy or binge drinking, has been identified as the leading preventable cause of intellectual disability and is associated with an array of physical, cognitive, and behavioral issues that fall under the umbrella term fetal alcohol spectrum disorder (FASD). (For more information about the effects of alcohol abuse during pregnancy, see *Quick Lesson About …Alcohol Abuse and Pregnancy*). The use of stimulants (e.g., nicotine, cocaine, methamphetamine)and/or repeated episodes of withdrawal can reduce blood supply to the fetus, causing fetal growth restriction, spontaneous termination, neurological abnormalities, premature birth and its associated morbidity, and low birth weight. Chronic opiate use during pregnancy has been linked with smaller head circumference. Substance misuse in pregnancy can continue to cause problems for the neonate after birth as well. Neonatal abstinence syndrome (NAS), a condition in which babies develop physical dependence on narcotic drugs in utero and experience withdrawal symptoms after delivery, may cause irritability, feeding issues, tremors, increased muscle tension (i.e., hypertonia), vomiting, diarrhea, seizures, and respiratory problems. Most infants with NAS require care in a neonatal intensive care unit (NICU), which is

expensive and frequently is stressful for parents. Prenatal substance exposure is associated with a heightened risk of long-term cognitive, language, and behavioral issues, although lasting effects may be subtle and difficult to differentiate from psychosocial issues that often accompany maternal substance misuse (e.g., poverty, unstable living situations, inadequate nutrition and care, maternal mental illness).

Treatment barriers for pregnant women who are abusing substances can be categorized into four types: accessibility, acceptability, availability, and affordability. Accessibility may include issues with transportation, employment, child care, family responsibilities, social support, and incarceration. Acceptability refers to fears of stigmatization, self-denial, and fear of loss of custody. Availability refers to whether the client qualifies for treatment, if the program accepts women or pregnant women, and whether there is a waiting list. Affordability refers to financial and insurance issues that may prevent treatment.

In some cases, pregnancy provides an opportunity to motivate women who abuse substances to begin treatment. Pregnant women already in treatment should be encouraged to pursue good prenatal care. A multidisciplinary approach that includes medical support for the mother as well as addiction treatment and supportive counseling may be the most effective. Women who are coping with substance misuse in pregnancy often feel stigmatized by society and by the healthcare professionals they may be seeing for prenatal care. Treatment must be approached nonjudgmentally and supportively. Treatment may include psychiatric or psychological counseling (cognitive-behavioral therapy, psychodynamic therapy), pharmacotherapy (e.g., methadone, buprenorphine), residential treatment, and/or support groups.

FACTS AND FIGURES

Substance misuse is more common in adolescents and younger adults; younger pregnant women report higher rates of substance misuse than older pregnant women. Alcohol is the most commonly used substance during pregnancy: 9.4 percent of pregnant women between ages 15 and 44 report alcohol use. Maternal binge drinking may cause preterm birth and low birth weight: a study found that women ages 40 to 44 had the highest binge-drinking rates and the highest rate of preterm births. In the United States, prevalence rates for substance-affected live births decreased for cocaine from 1999 to 2008 but increased for narcotics and hallucinogens.

The increase in narcotic use during pregnancy is believed largely to be due to non-medical use of prescription opioids. Marijuana is the most commonly used illicit drug during pregnancy. One United States study found that although the rate of women being admitted to substance misuse treatment during pregnancy remained fairly stable from 1992 to 2012, at approximately 4 percent of all female admissions, there has been a significant increase in women who report marijuana use upon admission (from 29 percent to 43 percent) and who report that marijuana is their primary substance (from 6 percent to 20 percent). Approximately 15 percent of pregnant women between ages 15 and 17 use illicit drugs, with this number decreasing to 9 percent of pregnant women ages 18 to 25 and to 3 percent of pregnant women ages 26 to 44. An estimated 6 percent of pregnant women reported using an opioid analgesic at some point during pregnancy, of which only 20 percent had a current or lifetime medical condition that might require treatment with opioids.

In 2009 NAS was diagnosed in 3.39 per 1,000 U.S. births. These newborns were more likely to have breathing issues, low birth weight, feeding problems, and seizures. Pregnant women in detoxification programs who live in rural areas have been found to have higher rates of illicit drug use than pregnant women in detoxification programs who are from urban areas. In one study of rural women who were pregnant and abusing substances, researchers found that 83 percent of the respondents had experienced a barrier to treatment, with respondents reporting two barriers each on average. Higher rates of family discord, often including violence, were associated with greater drug use in a study of pregnant women entering substance use treatment.

RISK FACTORS

Substance misuse in pregnancy occurs across all races, ethnicities, and socioeconomic statuses, but the highest risk is found among women who are extremely poor; have high levels of stress; have poor self-esteem and coping skills; have comorbid mental health issues, including depression; have histories of physical, sexual, or interpersonal violence; have lower levels of education; and have inadequate access to healthcare and social services. Youth increases the risk for substance misuse during pregnancy, as stated above. A past history before pregnancy of using substances increases risk for substance misuse during pregnancy.

SIGNS AND SYMPTOMS

Signs and symptoms will vary depending on the specific substance being used or consumed. Psychological: mood swings, feelings of sadness and hopelessness, worry, irritability, memory problems, anxiety, paranoia, euphoria, anger, guilt, loneliness.

Behavioral: panic attacks, disorientation, suicidal ideation or suicide attempts, sedation, inebriation, frequent falls, problems at school or work, driving while impaired, periods of violence.

Physical: dilated pupils, rapid eye movement, tremors, track marks or infected injection sites, inflamed nasal passages, increased pulse rate and blood pressure, hair loss, gum disease, skin conditions, weight loss, frequent hospitalizations.

Social: withdrawal from family, friends, and other social supports, self-isolation.

TREATMENT

For any pregnant client who is using alcohol or illicit substances, a reduction in use is imperative, with abstinence preferred in most situations if possible. Pregnant clients should be informed about the risks of substance use during pregnancy; the process of asking detailed questions about substance use may itself raise the client's awareness of risks and prompt her to reduce or cease use. Screening all clients for substance misuse is recommended but universal urine testing is not. Social workers often employ the transtheoretical stages of change model when approaching clients who are abusing substances. In this model there are five stages involved in making changes in behavior: precontemplation, contemplation, preparation, action, and maintenance. If a client is in the precontemplation stage, in which she is unaware that a problem exists and has no plans to change her behavior, the social worker will approach counseling differently from counseling the client who is actively taking action to change. In the contemplation stage the individual is beginning to recognize that a problem exists and is starting to think about making changes. In the preparation stage the client is starting to make small steps, whereas the action stage involves more overt modifications. The maintenance stage is also referred to as relapse prevention.

From a health perspective abstinence is the preferred approach for pregnant clients. For clients who cannot be successfully abstinent, a harm reduction approach can be appropriate. Social workers employing harm reduction look for underlying issues, encourage the client to keep track of substance use, try to reduce frequency of use and amount used, encourage avoidance of substance-using peers, and help the client plan for the future.

Treatment approaches vary widely in intensity; care should be individualized based on comprehensive assessment of the pregnant client. Twelve-step approaches conceptualize substance misuse as a disease and focus on abstinence, socialization, and enhancing self-efficacy. Motivational interviewing focuses positively on why an individual changes behavior, not why he or she does not. This approach uses collaboration and empathy to engage the client in change, and often is used in combination with other treatment approaches. Psychodynamic therapy techniques examine underlying trauma and conflicts, stress and negative emotions resulting from which the client copes with through substance misuse. Cognitive-behavioral therapy helps individuals identify and change the dysfunctional thoughts and behaviors that are leading to substance misuse in order to gain control and make changes. More intensive treatment (e.g., day treatment, residential treatment, inpatient treatment) may be indicated for women who have severe substance misuse and/or mental health issues and/or an unsupportive living situation. Pregnant women have complex treatment needs and are most successful in programs that are comprehensive (e.g., include child care and offer assistance with employment, education, and housing), designed for women, and culturally sensitive. Opioid maintenance treatment often is recommended for pregnant women who are dependent on opioids; medical support may be required for initial detoxification and stabilization depending on the substance(s) involved (e.g., benzodiazepines, alcohol).

LAWS AND REGULATIONS

In the United States there has been a trend to criminalize substance misuse during pregnancy, with 18 states classifying substance misuse during pregnancy as child abuse under their child-welfare statutes and 3 states allowing for involuntary commitment of pregnant women to mental health or substance misuse

facilities. One state, Tennessee, recently enacted a law that makes women who use certain substances while pregnant eligible to be charged with assault. This trend has raised concerns that incarceration or the threat of incarceration is not an effective method of reducing substance misuse and may instead lead to women avoiding prenatal care if they are worried about incarceration, involuntary commitment, custody loss, or housing loss. Criminalization treats substance misuse as a moral failing rather than as a sign of the biological and behavioral disorder of addiction. Social workers need to become knowledgeable regarding the rules and legislation of their state and nation to ensure that they can safeguard their clients' rights without breaking the law.

In 2001 the U.S. Supreme Court heard the case *Ferguson et al. v. City of Charleston*, which arose from the practice of nurses testing pregnant women for cocaine use without consent and sending positive results to the Charleston police for those women to be prosecuted. The Supreme Court ruled that women could not be tested by a hospital without a warrant or their expressed consent.

SERVICES AND RESOURCES

Alcoholics Anonymous, www.aa.org

Narcotics Anonymous, www.na.org

Harm Reduction Coalition, www.harmreduction.org

World Health Organization (WHO), http://www.who.int/topics/substance_abuse/en/

National Institute on Alcohol Abuse and Alcoholism (NIAAA), www.niaaa.nih.gov

National Institute on Drug Abuse, www.drugabuse.gov

Substance misuse and Mental Health Services Administration (SAMHSA), www.samhsa.gov

Canadian Centre on Substance misuse, http:// www.ccsa.ca/

FOOD FOR THOUGHT

Universal screening of all women for risk of substance use and dependence is recommended in healthcare settings beginning in adolescence, ideally before conception.

Many controversies surround the testing of pregnant women for substance use. There are concerns about biased selection of women to be tested versus the expense of testing all pregnant women, about the limitations of testing in terms of contributing

Problem	Goal	Intervention
Pregnant client is exhibiting signs and symptoms of substance misuse	Client will reduce or discontinue substance use while pregnant	Educate client on the risks and consequences of substance misuse during pregnancy. Evaluate client's support system and try to build up deficient areas. Provide counseling interventions or refer client to an addictions specialist to aid in recovery. Provide a safe, supportive, non-judgmental environment for client
Client who is pregnant and abusing substances is encountering barriers preventing her from receiving treatment	Barriers will be removed, and client will be able to access treatment	Have client share what barriers she is facing (e.g., accessibility, availability, acceptability, affordability). Advocate for client and try to broker appropriate services. Provide a non-judgmental environment to reduce feelings of stigma. Assist client in finding child care or other supports that are needed for her to receive treatment
Client has limited access to services	Increase services and program availability for pregnant women with substance misuse issues	Advocate for an increase in pregnancy-specific treatment programs. Advocate with the state legislature and/or the agency/facility for policies and laws regarding substance misuse in pregnancy that decriminalize substance misuse and encourage treatment versus punishment. Educate the local physician communities on how to avoid judgment in practice to foster trust and decrease stigma

meaningful information to the care of the child and concerns that possible legal consequences will prevent women from seeking care during pregnancy.

Members of impoverished and ethnic and racial minority populations are screened more often for drug and alcohol use in pregnancy than members of other populations.

Very few addiction treatment programs are equipped to specifically manage substance misuse and pregnancy. Only 19 U.S. states have substance misuse treatment programs specifically for pregnant women. Often the drug treatment facilities that do accept pregnant women are expensive and unable to help with childcare arrangements, which precludes them as an option for some clients.

In one study the fathers and fathers-to-be in couples in which both partners were abusing substances (binge drinking, using marijuana) did not significantly reduce use during their partner's pregnancy and the mothers returned quickly to the same behaviors of drinking and marijuana use after giving birth.

A study found that the majority of women who were pregnant and using drugs or who had recently delivered after using drugs during pregnancy felt that health and social care professionals were critical, unsupportive, or adversarial. These women often felt that because of their drug use history they were not afforded choices during pregnancy or delivery.

Preconception counseling (i.e., providing medical knowledge to women of childbearing age with a chronic disorder) is recommended for women of childbearing age who are attending addiction treatment centers.

RED FLAGS

Many of the substance misuse screening tools are validated on adults, so if the social worker is working with pregnant adolescents who are abusing substances he or she needs to be aware of possible effects on validity and reliability due to age differences.

Women who deliver babies exposed to drugs in utero frequently have histories of physical and sexual abuse. Researchers in one study found that 80 percent reported having experienced physical violence, 63 percent reported having experienced forced sexual activity, and 48 percent reported having experienced sexual abuse in childhood.

The social worker needs to be aware of his or her country's/state's statutes regarding mandatory reporting of prenatal substance misuse or substance exposure in newborns, as well as any mandatory reporting regulations at the facility or agency that employs him or her.

Universal screening is recommended, but even when this is in place clients may not be honest in their reporting of substance use. In a study, investigators found that 4.6 percent of the study population reported using illicit drugs during pregnancy yet 20 percent of the study population had positive urine drug screens.

Postpartum pain management needs to be considered for clients with a past or present substance use history. One option may be for the physician to order opioids immediately postpartum while the patient is in the hospital but not to discharge the patient with an opioid prescription.

—*Jessica Therivel, LMSW-IPR*

For Further Information

American College of Obstetricians and Gynecologists. (2011, January). Substance misuse reporting and pregnancy: The role of the obstetrician-gynecologist. *Committee on Health Care for Underserved Women: Committee Opinion, 473*, 200-201.

Bandstra, E. S., & Accornero, V. H. (2011). Infants of substance-abusing mothers. In R. J. Martin, A. A. Fanaroff, & M. C. Walsh (Eds.), *Fanaroff and Martin's neonatal-perinatal medicine: Diseases of the fetus and infant* (9th ed., pp. 735-757). St. Louis, MO: Elsevier Mosby.

Brandon, A. R. (2014). Psychosocial interventions for substance use during pregnancy. *Journal of Perinatal & Neonatal Nursing, 28*(3), 169-177. doi:10.1097/JPN.0000000000000041

Gopman, S. (2014). Prenatal and postpartum care of women with substance use disorders. *Obstetrics and Gynecology Clinics of North America, 41*(2), 213-228. doi:10.1016/j.ogc.2014.02.004

Narkowicz, S., Plotka, J., Polkowska, Z., Biziuk, M., & Namiesnik, J. (2013). Prenatal exposure to substance of abuse: a worldwide problem. *Environment International, 54*, 141-163. doi:10.1016/j.envint.2013.01.011

National Institute on Drug Abuse (NIDA). (2011, May). Prenatal exposure to drugs of abuse: A research update from the National Institute on Drug Abuse. *Topics in Brief: NIDA*. Retrieved July 18, 2015, from http://www.drugabuse.gov/sites/default/files/prenatal.pdf

Smith, M., Costello, D., & Yonkers, K. (2015). Clinical correlates of prescription opioid analgesic use in pregnancy. *Maternal & Child Health Journal, 19*(3), 548-556. doi:10.1007/s10995-014-1536-6

Visconti, K. C., Hennessy, K. C., Towers, C. V., & Howard, B. C. (2015). Chronic opiate use in pregnancy and newborn head circumference. *American Journal of Perinatology, 32*(1), 27-31. doi:10.1055/s-0034-1374817

Pregnancy test

Category: Procedure

Key Terms:

false negative: a test result which incorrectly indicates that the individual is not pregnant

false positive: a test result which incorrectly indicates that the individual is pregnant

human chorionic gonadotropin (hCG): a glycoprotein hormone similar in structure to luteinizing hormone that is secreted by the placenta during early pregnancy to maintain corpus luteum function and is commonly tested for as an indicator of pregnancy

Indications and Procedures

Pregnancy tests are a rapid, inexpensive, and accurate way to assess whether or not a woman is pregnant. Pregnancy occurs when a sperm fertilizes an egg after sexual intercourse. The newly fertilized egg implants in the wall of the uterus about 6-12 days after fertilization. This implantation causes a hormone called human chorionic gonadotropin (hCG) to be released. After implantation, hCG continues to be released by the placenta triggering other physiological changes that occur throughout pregnancy. It can be detected in the blood and urine of a pregnant woman. It is not present in males or non-pregnant females, which makes the test very reliable.

HCG is the basis for pregnancy tests available over the counter in most drugstores and in medical settings. Pregnancy tests can reliably detect the presence of hCG 1-2 weeks after the first missed period. It is possible to detect the presence of hCG sooner, but the test results may be less accurate with higher false

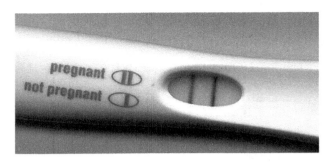

A positive pregnancy test. (Klaus Hoffmeier via Wikimedia Commons)

negative rates. For women without regular menstrual cycles, pregnancy tests may detect hCG about 3 weeks after sexual intercourse.

Pregnancy tests usually come in the form of a stick, strip, or cassette. There are also electronic forms available. The test is usually performed by urinating on the stick/strip or dropping urine into a reservoir on the cassette. Each of these methods contains antibodies designed specifically to target hCG. In the presence of hCG, these antibodies bind the hormone and undergo a chemical reaction to turn blue. If hCG is detected, this means the test is positive for pregnancy.

While the majority of pregnancy tests detect hCG in urine, hCG can also be detected in blood. HCG can be detected in blood about 1 week after ovulation, which is sooner than in urine. The blood test is also less convenient as it requires getting blood drawn in a medical center, and it usually takes longer to obtain these results. Usually, the urine hCG test is preferred in medical settings unless there are other indications for a blood test to verify the results.

USES AND COMPLICATIONS

There are several ways to perform a pregnancy test depending on the brand of the test. Some of the common ways to perform pregnancy tests are: urinating directly onto a stick or strip, dipping the strip into a cup of urine, or using a dropper to drop urine onto a cassette. Usually after applying the urine, it takes a few minutes for the reaction to complete and display the results. In most tests, if hCG is present the antibodies will bind and turn blue, which can be visualized in the form of a line or a cross. Electronic pregnancy tests may also display words like "pregnant" or "not pregnant." The readings may vary depending on the brand of the test so be sure to read and follow the directions provided.

HCG pregnancy tests are most accurate starting 1 week after a missed period. They may detect pregnancy earlier, but the results may be less accurate. There will be a higher false negative rate because it takes time for hCG levels to build up to a detectable range after its initial release. There is evidence to suggest that digital pregnancy tests may be both easier to use and more accurate for early home pregnancy tests than strips or cassettes.

While pregnancy tests are generally reported to be 99% accurate, it is possible to obtain false positive or false negative results. False positive results may be due to loss of a pregnancy soon after implantation in the uterine lining, medications that contain hCG (e.g. fertility drugs), or medical problems with the ovaries. False negatives as mentioned above may be due to taking the test too soon after fertilization. HCG levels increase over time so if an initial pregnancy test is negative, rechecking in 1-2 weeks may improve the accuracy of results. Checking the strip too early before the antibody reaction can fully develop or using dilute urine may also cause false negative results. Urine is most concentrated in the morning, so tests taken first thing in the morning may be slightly more accurate. If you have mixed positive and negative results, you may need to follow up with a health care provider to obtain a blood test or an ultrasound to verify pregnancy.

—*Kathleen Chung, B. A.*

FOR FURTHER INFORMATION

ELISA for Home Pregnancy Test. (n.d.). Retrieved October 27, 2017, from http://www.elisa-antibody. com/ELISA-applications/home-pregnancy-test

Parenthood, P. (n.d.). When to Take a Pregnancy Test | Options, Cost and Accuracy. Retrieved October 27, 2017, from https://www.plannedparenthood. org/learn/pregnancy/pregnancy-test

Tomlinson, C., Marshall, J., & Ellis, J. E. (2008). Comparison of accuracy and certainty of results of six home pregnancy tests available over-the-counter. Current Medical Research and Opinion, 24(6), 1645-1649. doi:10.1185/03007990802120572

Knowing if you are pregnant. (2017, February 01). Retrieved October 27, 2017, from https://www. womenshealth.gov/pregnancy/you-get-pregnant/ knowing-if-you-are-pregnant

Premature (Preterm) birth

CATEGORY: Disease/Disorder

KEY TERMS:

antenatal steroids: medications given to pregnant women expecting preterm delivery; they have been shown to reduce the morbidity and mortality of hyaline membrane disease

cervical cerclage: the process of encircling a cervix with sutures or synthetic tape that is abnormally liable to dilate (an incompetent cervix) with a ring or loop to prevent a miscarriage

cone biopsy: a biopsy to remove abnormal tissues high in the cervical canal; called a cope biopsy because a cone-shaped wedge of tissue is removed for examination

fetal fibronectin: a protein produced by fetal cells; found at the interface of the the fetal sac and the uterine lining; it can be thought of as an adhesive or "biological glue" that binds the fetal sac to the uterine lining; when it starts "leaking" into the vagina it indicates a possible preterm delivery

necrotizing enterocolitis: the death of tissue in the intestine; occurs most often in premature or sick babies

prostaglandins: cyclic fatty acids with varying hormone-like effects, notably the promotion of uterine contractions

transvaginal ultrasound (TVUS): a test used to look at a woman's uterus, ovaries, tubes, cervix and pelvic area; the ultrasound probe is placed inside the vagina

CAUSES AND INDICATIONS

Labor is defined as cervical change with contractions. Premature or preterm birth is defined as delivery before 37 weeks of gestation, though the vast majority of premature babies are born between 34 and 37 weeks. In the US, about 10% of all pregnancies are preterm, with the number reaching as high as 14% among African American women. The rate has increased in recent years, and this may be due to the increasing number of multiple births—the risk of prematurity increases with multiple babies vying for space and resources during the same gestation.

Preterm birth does not have a single, identifiable cause but rather multiple potential causes, and some of them are not very well understood. The risk factors discussed below put a mother at higher risk of preterm birth but do not guarantee that a baby will not have a term gestation (37-40 weeks). Term pregnancy is important for a baby's outcome—it allows for important organs to fully develop and prevents serious complications from occurring. Many times, preterm birth can be out of the hands of the mother and physician; some genetic mutations lead to conditions that naturally lead to premature birth or are incompatible with life. Prenatal care is very important in trying to identify potential risk factors and optimizing a baby's early development. Establishing care early on can also lead to genetic counseling if abnormalities are found.

If frequent contractions happen between 24-34 weeks and the cervical change is minimal (<3 cm) or cervical length is between 20-30mm on transvaginal ultrasound (TVUS), a physician may opt to do a fetal fibronectin test (fFN). This test has an excellent negative predictive value—if it is negative, then there is a 99% chance of no delivery for 1 week. Other important parts of a workup include taking a detailed history (identifying risk factors), doing a complete physical exam, ordering appropriate labs looking for blood/electrolyte abnormalities and sexually transmitted infections, and determining the baby's condition at presentation.

RISK FACTORS AND COMPLICATIONS

Common risk factors include previous preterm delivery, low socioeconomic status, smoking during pregnancy, uterine anomaly, history of cervical procedures (e.g. cone biopsy), sexually transmitted infections (STIs), and preterm premature rupture of membranes (membranes rupturing before the onset of labor before 37 weeks). Chorioamnionitis is a clinical condition that can increase the risk of preterm labor. It is an intrauterine infection that leads to an inflammatory reaction by the mother's body. The inflammation then initiates a cascade that increases the amount of prostaglandins circulating the blood. Prostaglandins are known for stimulating uterine contractions, while another product of the inflammatory cascade, metalloproteases, can ripen the cervix leading to membrane rupture. As previously mentioned, each additional baby in a multiple gestation increases the risk of prematurity, and the incidence of multiple gestations is increasing due to the popularity of assisted reproductive techniques (ART) and increasing maternal age (associated with higher rates of multiple gestations).

Problems arise when babies aren't given enough time to fully develop. Therefore, conditions associated with preterm birth like respiratory distress syndrome (RDS), intraventricular hemorrhage (IVH), and retinopathy of immaturity (ROP) occur when the lungs, brain, or eyes, respectively, are immature and could have benefited from a couple of more weeks of development. Cerebral palsy is another neurologic condition closely tied with premature birth, especially if the baby is born before 32 weeks. Necrotizing enterocolitis can happen in any neonate but this condition is commonly associated with prematurity due to an underdeveloped immune system and reduced oxygen and blood flow. It is not surprising that premature birth is the leading cause of death worldwide for children under 5 years old—these complications increases a neonate's morbidity significantly and can have permanent consequences.

PROGNOSIS

The long-term outlook partly depends on how early the baby is born. Late-preterm, born between 34 and 37 weeks, babies have the highest survival rate among preterm births but still have a higher risk of developing the complications above compared to a term baby. Birth weights in the late-preterm cohort are comparable to term pregnancy weight (about 8 pounds), differing by two pounds or less. A baby is considered to have low birth weight if it weighs less than 5 pounds 8 ounces, and this can happen if a baby is born very premature (before 34 weeks) or there has been some restriction in its growth (e.g. placental insufficiency). This is an important consideration given that low birth weight means a baby will have a harder time keeping warm due to less body fat and can sometimes have problems gaining weight and eating. Their immune system immaturity also puts them at risk of infection, and oxygenation is a concern if they have RDS due to small underdeveloped lungs.

Prognosis is also affected by the outcomes of the complications a premature baby deals with after birth. If the child suffers from intraventricular hemorrhage, most of the time the complication will resolve with minimal impact, but there are cases where the

bleeding can lead to irreversible brain damage. Ninety percent of babies with ROP fall in the "mild" category and do not require treatment, but those with the more severe types can develop blindness or serious vision problems later in life, such as myopia, strabismus, glaucoma, and retinal detachment. If a premature baby develops bronchopulmonary dysplasia (BPD) after having RDS for an extended period, the child can see long-term decrease in pulmonary function compared to a term baby. BPD can lead to a chronic cough and increased air trapping, leading to problems with air flow and oxygenation. This airway obstruction can limit a child's level of physical activity.

PREVENTION

Administering antenatal steroids is one of the most important interventions that can be done for a premature baby—it improves survival rates by decreasing the risk of several complications. Studies have found that before 28 weeks of gestation, steroids can help reduce the rate of the IVH, and after 28 weeks, it can help rapidly mature a baby's lungs, giving it a better shot at reducing pulmonary distress. It also dramatically decreases the rate of NEC. If there are indications of imminent preterm labor before 34 weeks, a physician may consider giving a tocolytic agent, or a drug to delay labor, to give the steroids at least 48 hours to continue maturation of the lungs before delivery.

Antibiotics (e.g. penicillin) are also important for preventing transmission of neonatal group B streptococcus (GBS), a common bacterium that can lead to meningitis and sepsis in a neonate. Magnesium sulfate is given before 32 weeks for potential fetal neuroprotection against cerebral palsy. If there have been prior preterm births or a prior second trimester loss, the use of progesterone can be considered from 16-36 weeks to prevent contractions and promote the pregnancy. If there is cervical insufficiency, sometimes from prior cervical procedures, a cervical cerclage may be placed early in pregnancy, around 12 to 14 weeks, to try to prevent miscarriage and delay delivery to 37 weeks.

CONCLUSION

Premature birth is complex to say the least. At the end of the day, each gestation is unique, and studies and statistics can only tell a mother and her medical team what to look for and implement optimization strategies that aren't foolproof. Controlling for smoking and diabetes, monitoring maternal and fetal vital signs, and curing STIs can reduce risk factors for premature birth but not guarantee that it will not occur. That is why establishing prenatal care and developing a close relationship with a medical provider is so important: to help troubleshoot problems along the way and to assist with parent education. There is a natural psychological toll on parents who have premature babies, and it will be important to not only look after the neonate but also check in with parents who may experience stages of grief if they are informed of their child's prematurity. Parent education early on in gestation is key so that parents can prepare for the unexpected and talk about different scenarios should they happen. The more knowledge acquired, the better parents can deal with difficult situations and execute treatment plans to help their baby grow. Mothers of premature babies may be more susceptible to experiencing birthing trauma, and perinatal mood or anxiety disorders. Due to the increased stress of having a premature baby these mothers may need additional mental health support and should be assessed frequently by medical and mental health professionals.

—*Brian A. Campos, BA*

FOR FURTHER INFORMATION

Keelan, Jeff A, and John P Newnham. "Recent Advances in the Prevention of Preterm Birth." *F1000Research*, vol. 6, 18 July 2017, p. 1139., doi:10.12688/f1000research.11385.1.

Mayo Clinic Staff. "Premature Birth." *Mayo Clinic*, Mayo Foundation for Medical Education and Research, 21 Dec. 2017, www.mayoclinic.org/diseases-conditions/premature-birth/symptoms-causes/syc-20376730.

"Premature Babies." *MedlinePlus*, U.S. National Library of Medicine, 26 May 2015, medlineplus.gov/prematurebabies.html.

"Preterm Birth." *CDC*, Centers for Disease Control and Prevention, 24 Apr. 2018, www.cdc.gov/reproductivehealth/maternalinfanthealth/pretermbirth.htm.

Sen, Cihat. "Preterm Labor and Preterm Birth." *Journal of Perinatal Medicine*, vol. 45, no. 8, 21 Oct. 2017, doi:10.1515/jpm-2017-0298.

Premenstrual syndrome (PMS)

CATEGORY: Disease/Disorder

Also known as: Menstrually related mood disorder (MRMD), premenstrual tension, late luteal phase disorder (LLPD), premenstrual dysphoric disorder (PMDD)

KEY TERMS:

endorphins: hormones, found mainly in the brain, that bind to opiate receptors, reducing the sensation of pain and affecting emotions

luteal phase: the second half of the menstrual cycle after ovulation; during this phase, the corpus luteum secretes progesterone

menses: the monthly flow of blood and cellular debris from the uterus that begins at puberty in women

premenstrual dysphoric disorder (PMDD): a severe form of premenstrual syndrome characterized by affective symptoms causing significant disturbances in relationships or social adaptation

progesterone: a hormone produced in the ovary that prepares and maintains the uterus for pregnancy

serotonin: a neurotransmitter involved in sleep, depression, and memory

CAUSES AND SYMPTOMS

Several causes of premenstrual syndrome (PMS) have been proposed. Changes in hormone levels during the luteal phase of the menstrual cycle, when the ovaries are making progesterone, may deplete neurotransmitters such as enkephalins and endorphins, which are responsible for a sense of well-being; gamma-aminobutyric acid (GABA), which aids in relaxation; and serotonin, which stimulates the central nervous system. The disorder may be more likely to occur in women who have enhanced sensitivity to progesterone, a disposition related to serotonin deficiency. PMS may be related to excess prostaglandin, a hormone-like substance that may affect blood pressure and metabolism and smooth muscle activity. Some evidence suggests that women with PMS have lower blood levels of allopregnanolone, a by-product of progesterone that plays a role in mood.

Up to 85 percent of women experience mild to moderate forms of PMS. Another 5 percent of women have symptoms so severe that they interfere with daily activity and may be diagnosed with premenstrual dysphoric disorder (PMDD). In some women, symptoms of PMS increase with age, perhaps because serotonin levels are altered with changes in estrogen levels.

PMS symptoms can be subdivided into physical, behavioral, and psychological. Physical symptoms include fatigue; headache; breast tenderness and swelling; back and abdominal pain; acne; heart palpitations; bloating; weight gain; nausea; muscle and joint pain; water retention; swelling of ankles, feet, and hands; and decreased tolerance to noise or light. Behavioral symptoms include fatigue, insomnia, dizziness, changes in sex drive, cravings for salty or sweet food, and increased appetite. Psychological symptoms include irritability, anger, depressed mood, crying, anxiety, tension, mood swings, and lack of concentration, confusion, forgetfulness, restlessness, loneliness, decreased self-esteem, and tension. The symptoms of depression, anxiety disorders, perimenopause, and thyroid dysfunction are similar to PMS.

A distinguishing feature of PMS is its cyclic occurrence. Researchers at the University of California, San Diego suggests the following criteria for diagnosing premenstrual syndrome: At least one psychological (affective) and physical (somatic) symptom occurs during the five to seven days before menses in each of the previous three cycles, and symptoms are relieved during days four through thirteen of the menstrual cycle. The National Institute of Mental Health and the American Psychiatric Association give similar diagnostic criteria. Blood tests are not necessary for the diagnosis of PMS. Laboratory studies such as a blood count or thyroid function tests may be recommended to screen for other medical conditions that cause fatigue, such as anemia and thyroid disease.

TREATMENT AND THERAPY

Treatment for premenstrual syndrome can be divided into three categories: non-pharmacologic therapy, dietary supplementation, and pharmacologic therapy.

Non-pharmacologic therapies include patient education, supportive therapy, and behavioral interventions. Women who receive educational materials about PMS may gain an increased sense of control and relief of symptoms. Supportive therapies include relaxation and cognitive-behavioral therapy. A therapist may also be able to teach coping methods. Behavioral interventions include keeping a daily symptom

---

Information on Premenstrual Syndrome (PMS)

Causes: Unknown; possibly depletion of neurotransmitters resulting from hormonal changes and sensitivities

Symptoms: Physical (fatigue, headache, breast tenderness and swelling, back and abdominal pain, muscle and joint pain, weight gain, water retention, acne, nausea, palpitations); behavioral (insomnia, dizziness, changes in sex drive, cravings for salty or sweet food, increased appetite); psychological (irritability, anger, depression, anxiety, mood swings, lack of concentration, confusion, forgetfulness, restlessness, decreased self-esteem)

Duration: Often chronic with acute episodes

Treatments: Patient education; exercise; adequate sleep; stress avoidance; dietary changes (increased complex carbohydrates, decreased sodium and caffeine); vitamin E supplements; calcium carbonate supplements; diuretics (spironolactone); antianxiety medications (benzodiazepines); selective serotonin reuptake inhibitors; hormonal therapy (Gonadotropin-releasing hormone agonists, oral contraceptives); Non-steroidal anti-inflammatory drugs (NSAIDs)

---

diary. Each day for three months, a woman records in a diary and ranks any health complaints on a scale of "none at all" to "extreme." The PMS pattern is an increase in symptoms during the fourteen days before menstruation and then a decrease in symptoms within one hour to a few days after bleeding begins.

In addition to keeping the diary, exercising thirty minutes a day (to stimulate the release of enkephalins and endorphins and to reduce swelling through sweat), sleeping six to eight hours every night, avoiding stress, and making dietary changes may help symptoms. Increasing the intake of complex carbohydrates (fruits, vegetables, and whole grains) may relieve mood-related symptoms by boosting the level of tryptophan, a precursor of serotonin. Lowering sodium intake can reduce bloating, fluid retention, and swelling. Restricting caffeine consumption may reduce irritability and insomnia. Vitamin E supplements may reduce breast pain. Vitamin E as a dietary supplement is also a potentially beneficial antioxidant and poses minimal risk. Calcium carbonate supplementation may also improve PMS symptoms.

Nonprescription drugs, such as diuretics for bloating and analgesics for pain, may diminish the symptoms of PMS. Prescription treatments for PMS include anti-anxiety medication such as the benzodi-azepines, which mimic the effects of GABA to relieve irritability; selective serotonin reuptake inhibitors (SSRIs), which increase serotonin levels; hormone treatments such as gonadotropin-releasing hormone (GnRH) agonists and birth control pills that stop the production of estrogen and progesterone; spi-ronolactone, a diuretic that relieves breast tenderness and fluid retention; and non-steroidal anti-inflamma-tory drugs (NSAIDs), or prostaglandin inhibitors, for pain such as headache.

Some treatments that have no proven benefit in relieving the symptoms of PMS include: Progesterone, antidepressant drugs such as Tricyclic Antidepres-sants (TCA), Monoamine Oxidase Inhibitors (MAOI), lithium, and popular dietary supplements such as evening primrose oil, essential free fatty acids, and ginkgo biloba.

PERSPECTIVE AND PROSPECTS

Hysteria (literally, "wandering womb") was described in Egypt in about 1900 BCE as an abnormality of the uterus caused by its "migration" to different parts of the body, resulting in various symptoms, such as head-ache and swollen feet. The term "premenstrual ten-sion" was first used by mental health professionals in the 1930s.

Research on PMS gained momentum in the 1980s. Whereas only one article on PMS appeared in 1964, 425 articles were published on the topic between 1988 and 1989. What had once been considered a pseudocondition, with PMS as a catchall phrase for up to 150 symptoms occurring before menstruation, was recognized as a medical disorder. Research has focused on biomedical and psychosocial causes and treatments.

—*Elizabeth Marie McGhee Nelson, Ph.D.;*
Updated by Uzma Shahzad, M.D., and Christi N.
Gandham, D.O.

FOR FURTHER INFORMATION

Dickerson, Lori M., J. Mazyck, and Melissa H. Hunter. "Premenstrual Syndrome." *American Family Physi-cian* 67, no. 8 (April, 2003): 1743-1752.

Taylor, Diana, and Stacey Colino. *Taking Back the Month: A Personalized Solution for Managing PMS and Enhancing Your Health.* New York: Perigee, 2002.

Vliet, Elizabeth Lee. *Screaming to Be Heard: Hormonal ConnectionsWomen Suspect and Doctors Still Ignore.* New York: M. Evans, 2001.

Yonkers, Kimberly A., and Robert F. Casper. "Clinical Manifestations and Diagnosis of Premenstrual Syndrome and Premenstrual Dysphoric Disorder." *UpToDate*, edited by Robert L. Barbieri, William F. Crowley, Jr., and Kathryn A. Martin.

Prenatal care healthcare costs

CATEGORY: Treatment

WHAT WE KNOW

Prenatal care (PNC) is an important part of main-taining a healthy pregnancy. The typical schedule for PNC in the United States includes visiting a medical professional (such as an OBGYN or Midwife) about once each month during the first 6 months of preg-nancy, every 2 weeks during the 7th and 8th months of pregnancy, and weekly in the last month of preg-nancy, for a total of about 14 visits. PNC should begin as soon as a woman suspects she is pregnant.

In 2013, an analysis was conducted of PNC costs in the United States. Investigators found that in 2010, average total charges for a vaginal birth were $29,800 for Medicaid and $32,093 for commercial insurance. For cesarean births, charges were $50,373 for Medicaid and $51,125 for commercial insurance.

PNC includes a medical history, establishing a due date to assist in monitoring fetal growth, a physical exam, a pelvic exam, diagnostic tests (e.g., blood type and Rh factor; rubella titer; screenings for syphilis and hepatitis B; urinalysis), discussion of lifestyle issues (e.g., nutrition, prenatal vitamins, exercise), and fetal ultrasound.

Costs for diagnostic tests during pregnancy typi-cally were about $1,000 in 2004; costs may increase if the pregnancy is high-risk (requiring more tests) or if a woman chooses to undergo additional, optional tests (e.g., genetic testing).

Costs vary by site of care. In 2007, for instance, Kaiser Permanente, a self-insured provider, reported that PNC and hospital delivery cost on average about $10,000 per pregnancy in 2004.

The costs incurred during the inpatient stay related to birth account for the majority of the total cost related to pregnancy.

In 2014, researchers in California found that charges for delivery varied widely depending on hospital. In studying uncomplicated births in 2011, the researchers found that for a vaginal delivery, charges ranged from $3,296 to $37,227; for a cesarean delivery, they ranged from $8,312 to $70,908. Market-level (i.e., location) and institution-level differences (i.e., different hospitals charging different amounts for same services) accounted for only about 35 percent of the variation between hospitals, leaving approximately two thirds of the variation unexplained.

From 2004 to 2010 the average amount paid by commercial insurance plans for maternal care increased substantially: payments for cesarean births increased 41 percent and those for vaginal birth increased 49 percent. Out-of-pocket costs for mothers increased almost 4-fold in this same time period.

In 2007, about 75 percent of pregnancy-related prescription drug expenses were for prenatal vitamins and other nutritional supplements.

When complications develop during pregnancy, they are responsible for a significant increase in healthcare costs. Complications during pregnancy often are associated with high-risk pregnancy, which can increase the length of hospital stay and costs associated with care.

Pre-pregnancy factors that may make a pregnancy high-risk include younger or older maternal age, being overweight or underweight, having complications in previous pregnancies (e.g., pregnancy-induced hypertension, preterm labor), and certain medical conditions, such as high blood pressure, diabetes, and HIV infection.

Conditions occurring during pregnancy that make a pregnancy high-risk include preeclampsia and eclampsia, gestational diabetes, HIV infection/AIDS, multiple births, and preterm labor.

In the last 30 years, the percentage of women over age 40 having twins or higher multiples has increased 200 percent. The Affordable Care Act (ACA) identified PNC as an essential health benefit, but prior to the act, in 2011, 62 percent of individuals and families

who purchased their own health insurance did not have maternity coverage.

Because all plans purchased through the health insurance exchanges created by the ACA cover pregnancy and childbirth, it was anticipated that in 2014, 8.7 million Americans would be able to obtain maternity coverage.

Prenatal healthcare programs may be able to reduce costs overall.

Home visits by clinicians during a high-risk pregnancy may reduce overall pregnancy-related healthcare costs.

Prenatal care provided in a group setting (e.g., the Centering Pregnancy model) improves birth outcomes and is cost-effective.

Centering Pregnancy brings together pregnant women with similar due dates for a series of clinician-facilitated educational discussions and health evaluation activities that provide a social setting in which the women can receive care and build a support network.

—*Amy E. Beddoe, RN, PhD, and Jessica Therivel, LMSW-IPR*

FOR FURTHER INFORMATION

Akkerman, D., Cleland, L., Croft, G., Eskuchen, K., Heim, C., Levine, A.,... Westby, E. (2012). Health care guideline. Routine prenatal care. Retrieved March 29, 2016, from http://www.icsi.org/_asset/13n9y4/Prenatal.pdf

Anastas, J. W., & Clark, E. J. (2013). NASW standards for social work case management. Retrieved April 5, 2016, from http://www.socialworkers.org/practice/naswstandards/CaseManagementStandards2013.pdf

Briery, C. M., & Morrison, J. (2013, May). Overview of High-Risk Pregnancy. Retrieved March 29, 2016, from http://www.merckmanuals.com/home/womens_health_issues/pregnancy_at_high-risk/definition_of_high-risk_pregnancy.html

Hsia, R. Y., Antwi, Y. A., & Weber, E. (2014). Analysis of variation in charges and prices paid for vaginal and caesarean section births: A cross-sectional study. *BMJ Open*, *4*(1), e004017. doi:10.1136/bmjopen-2013-004017

Martin, J. A., Hamilton, B. E., & Osterman, M. J. K. (2012). Three decades of twin births in the United States, 1980-2009. *NCHS Data Brief, No. 80*, 1-8.

National Association of Social Workers. (2015). *Standards for cultural competence in social work practice*. Retrieved March 26, 2016, from http://www.socialworkers.org/practice/standards/PRA-BRO-253150-CC-Standards.pdf

---

Prenatal substance exposure

Category: Disease/Disorder

What we Know

The use of illicit drugs, alcohol, tobacco, and prescription drugs other than as prescribed during pregnancy has negative ramifications for both mothers and their unborn children and is a significant public health concern.

The *Diagnostic and Statistical Manual of Mental Disorders*, 5th edition (*DSM-5*), replaced the terminology used in the *DSM-IV* (i.e., substance dependence and substance abuse) with substance use disorder (SUD), the severity of which (i.e., mild, moderate, or severe) is determined by the number of criteria that are endorsed. In research, and clinical and treatment settings, the language used to describe problematic consumption of substances changes over time and varies greatly. Many terms have no specific definition, or may have different meanings in different settings (e.g., addiction in a medical setting might refer to the potential for physical withdrawal, whereas in a 12-step meeting addiction would have a unique meaning for each person in the meeting).

The 2013 National Survey on Drug Use and Health found that among pregnant women in the United States ages 15-44, 9.4 percent reported current alcohol use, 5.4 percent reported current use of illicit drugs, and 15.4 percent reported tobacco use within the past month. Although substantial, these rates are lower than those of non-pregnant females in the same age range, of whom 55.4 percent reported current alcohol use, 11.4 percent reported current use of illicit drugs, and 24.0 percent reported tobacco use within the past month.

Polysubstance abuse is common among women who use substances during pregnancy, including concurrent use of legal substances such as alcohol and tobacco that are potentially the most harmful to the developing fetus.

Data from the Infant Development, Environment, and Lifestyle Study (IDEAL), a longitudinal study of infants whose mothers used methamphetamine during pregnancy, have shown that:

Among women who used methamphetamine during pregnancy, the highest number (84.3 percent) reported using during the first trimester compared to 56.0 percent reporting use during the second trimester and 42.4 percent during the third trimester. 25.7 percent of women used at low to moderate levels throughout the pregnancy, 29.3 percent maintained consistently high levels of use, 35.6 percent reduced usage over the course of the pregnancy, and 9.4 percent showed an increase in use.

Almost 75 percent of women who used methamphetamine while pregnant met criteria for substance dependence, now identified in the fifth edition of the *DSM* as substance use disorder.

Ninety percent of the women reported using from one to five substances in addition to methamphetamine.

Women who continue using substances during pregnancy have been found to have higher levels of depression, anxiety, and novelty-seeking than those who stop using.

Women who abuse substances are widely recognized as having an array of psychosocial issues and often have more complex treatment needs than men who abuse substances.

Although substance use patterns among women vary globally, studies from several countries have found that women seeking treatment tend to have lower levels of education, employment, and income and more health, family, and social problems than men seeking treatment and are more likely than men to have substance-using partners, family histories of substance abuse, and personal histories of physical and sexual abuse. The majority also have co-occurring, untreated mental health issues.

Substance abuse among women is also associated with intimate partner violence, incarceration, homelessness, sexually transmitted diseases, and unplanned pregnancies.

Social disadvantage, including low levels of education and employment and not living with a spouse or partner, is associated with higher levels of psychosocial stress, substance use, and medical issues during pregnancy, such as low birth weight and early births.

Detrimental effects of prenatal substance exposure have been documented during fetal development, at birth, and in infancy; however, outcomes vary widely among individual children depending in part on the type and amount of substance(s) used, the stage(s) of pregnancy during which use occurred, and other factors related to substance use such as exposure to violence and inadequate maternal nutrition and prenatal care.

Prenatal substance exposure is associated with increased risk of medical complications such as placental abruption; intrauterine growth restriction, prematurity, and low birth weight; and increased risk of both maternal and child mortality.

Some drugs, in particular alcohol, may cause birth defects during the embryonic and fetal stages.

Substance-exposed newborns may have difficulty with orientation (e.g., difficulty responding to auditory and visual stimuli) and autonomic regulation (e.g., heart rate, breathing); and may have abnormal muscle tone (e.g., rigid or limp), poor alertness, increased startle response, tremors, and irritability.

Neonatal abstinence syndrome, in which babies are born dependent on drugs and withdrawal must be medically managed, is noted in the majority of infants who have been exposed to opiates and benzodiazepines.

Infants with signs of neonatal abstinence syndrome require special care including minimizing light, noise, and handling; swaddling; and small, frequent feedings.

Extended hospitalization may interfere with bonding between mother and child.

Fetal alcohol spectrum disorders (FASD) encompass a group of conditions resulting from prenatal alcohol exposure.

The use of alcohol during pregnancy has been identified as the leading preventable cause of mental retardation.

Although individual outcomes among infants vary and are influenced by an array of factors, maternal binge drinking (i.e., over 3 drinks at a time) is associated with particularly high risk.

Fetal alcohol syndrome (FAS) is diagnosed when three conditions are present in conjunction with a history of prenatal alcohol exposure: growth deficiency (i.e., at or below 10th percentile), characteristic facial abnormalities (e.g., smaller eye openings, smooth philtrum [the surface between the nose and the upper lip], thin upper lip), and central nervous system dysfunction (e.g., seizures, deficits in cognition, communication, memory, adaptive behavior, social skills, attention, academic achievement).

Prenatal substance exposure is associated with a heightened risk of long-term cognitive, language, and behavioral issues, school difficulties, and substance abuse among exposed children, although lasting effects may be subtle and difficult to differentiate from associated psychosocial issues.

Higher rates of prenatal cocaine exposure were associated with higher rates of attention-deficit/hyperactivity disorder in a sample of 5-year-old children, but no association was found with oppositional defiant disorder or separation anxiety disorder.

Prenatal substance exposure was associated with rates of behavior problems that were slightly higher than those among non-exposed youth in the California Long-Range Adoption Study, but this difference did not increase with age.

A review of 27 studies examining the effects of prenatal cocaine exposure on adolescents showed that the majority demonstrated small to medium effects on multiple areas of development that persisted from childhood but did not increase in adolescence.

A large, matched cohort study of children under the age of 3 years found associations between prenatal cocaine exposure and deficits in mental development and between opiate exposure and deficits in psychomotor development, but these differences were not significant once birth weight and other risk factors were controlled for.

Environmental risk factors associated with prenatal substance exposure such as poverty, low educational level, unemployment, homelessness or transient living situations, inadequate nutrition and healthcare, poor parenting, intimate partner violence, parental incarceration, and child maltreatment contribute to negative outcomes among children with a history of prenatal substance exposure.

Variability in the effects of prenatal substance exposure is strongly associated with the level of care the child receives following birth. The quality of the home environment plays a pivotal role in achieving positive developmental outcomes for children with a history of substance exposure.

A study of children with a history of prenatal cocaine exposure found that developmental outcomes at age 2 were predicted by the children's living situation and not prenatal exposure to cocaine. Those children in non-parental, non-kin care had more favorable outcomes and their homes scored higher on measures of caregiving environment.

The combination of traumatic stress combined with prenatal alcohol exposure has been found to have a significant impact on children's development, intelligence scores, and behavior.

Genetic factors may also play a role in that parents with substance use disorders also have higher rates of mental health disorders (e.g., attention-deficit/hyperactivity disorder, bipolar disorder, major depression, anxiety disorders), which are heritable and may affect children's functioning.

The United States Keeping Children and Families Safe Act of 2003 amended the Child Abuse Prevention & Treatment Act to require states to implement requirements that medical staff report children identified with prenatal exposure to substances to child protective services (CPS) and that plans be developed to ensure their safety.

Social workers should be aware of their state's statutes regarding mandatory reporting of newborns with prenatal substance exposure. Many, but not all, states have enacted laws that address substance use during pregnancy. Seventeen states include prenatal substance abuse in child welfare statutes and fifteen states mandate that suspected prenatal exposure be reported to child protective services.

Prenatal substance exposure alone does not determine the disposition of a CPS report, but the child welfare agency is mandated to complete a comprehensive assessment of the family's situation and implement safety planning as needed to ensure the child's safety.

As many as 21-50 percent of prenatal cocaine-exposed children are in nonparental care by the age of 2 years.

Substance use during pregnancy may be identified through screening and maternal self-report or through biological drug testing (i.e., urine, hair, or meconium), but under-identification is common with either approach.

Many controversies surround the testing of pregnant women for drug use. There are concerns about biased selection of women to be tested versus the expense of testing all pregnant women, about the limitations of testing in terms of contributing

information meaningful to the care of the child and concerns that possible legal consequences will prevent women from seeking care during pregnancy.

Universal screening of all women for risk of substance use and abuse is recommended in healthcare settings beginning in adolescence, before women become pregnant.

The Screening, Brief Intervention, and Referral for Treatment (SBIRT) protocol developed by the U.S. Substance Abuse and Mental Health Services Administration (SAMHSA) is used in many primary healthcare settings in the United States.

Several brief questionnaires have shown potential as screening tools, including T-ACE, T-ACER3, AUDIT-C, and TWEAK. T-ACE is noted as highly sensitive with all races, whereas TWEAK is less sensitive with races other than white.

Pregnancy can be a critical period for engaging women in treatment, building on motivating factors such as concern for the developing fetus and social pressures experienced as women become visibly pregnant.

Brief interventions such as motivational interviewing may be useful to assist women to resolve ambivalence about abstinence and to engage in treatment

Motivational interviewing, a directive counseling approach that seeks to facilitate behavioral change by exploring and resolving ambivalence about substance use and building on the individual's intrinsic motivation and commitment, has demonstrated effectiveness both as a freestanding intervention and in conjunction with other treatment.

Comprehensive, women-specific, culturally sensitive outpatient or residential treatment programs are recommended in order to address the complex service needs of pregnant and/or parenting women.

Programs should incorporate screening and treatment for issues commonly associated with substance abuse, including mental health conditions and intimate partner violence.

A survey of women entering substance abuse treatment within a year of pregnancy reported high rates of mental health disorders (78 percent), past-year victimization (66 percent), and criminal justice system involvement (64 percent).

Medical support may be required for initial detoxification and stabilization when physical dependency on a substance is involved.

Treatment may not include total abstinence. Current practice for women who are dependent on opioids (e.g., heroin, oxycodone, morphine) is a maintenance program using carefully monitored levels of methadone or buprenorphine accompanied by counseling.

Potential clinical issues include shame and guilt regarding substance use during pregnancy and potential effects on the child; self-efficacy; and relationship issues, including the positive or negative impact of the woman's partner, rebuilding family relationships, and building a network of non-using supports.

Children's developmental and behavioral needs should be monitored on an ongoing basis. Children with prenatal substance exposure may need early intervention and other supportive services to address treatment of withdrawal, self-regulation, secure attachment, and attainment of developmentally appropriate motor, cognitive, speech, and language skills.

—*Jennifer Teska, MSW*

FOR FURTHER INFORMATION

Brocato, C. L. (2015). Managing opioid addiction in pregnancy. *The Clinical Advisor, 18*(10), 28-35.

Burns, E., Gray, R., & Smith, L. A. (2010). Brief screening questionnaires to identify problem drinking during pregnancy: A systematic review. *Addiction, 105*, 601-614. doi:10.1111/j.1360-0443.2009.02842.x

State policies in brief: Substance use during pregnancy. (2014). *Guttmacher Institute.* Retrieved November 8, 2015, from http://www.guttmacher.org/statecenter/spibs/spib_SADR.pdf

Hamilton, G. (2012). Neonatal abstinence syndrome as a consequence of prescription opioid use during pregnancy. *International Journal of Childbirth Education, 27*(3), 69-72.

Jones, T. B., Bailey, B. A., & Sokol, R. J. (2013). Alcohol use in pregnancy: Insights in screening and intervention for the clinician. *Clinical Obstetrics and Gynecology, 56*(1), 114-123. doi:10.1097/GRF.0b013e31827957c0

Massey, S. H., Lieberman, D. Z., Reiss, D., Leve, L. D., Shaw, D. S., & Neiderhiser, J. M. (2010). Association of clinical characteristics and cessation of tobacco, alcohol, and illicit drug use during pregnancy. *The American Journal on Addictions, 20*(2), 143-150. doi:10.1111/j.1521-0391.2010.00110.x

Mittal, L. (2014). Buprenorphine for the treatment of opioid dependence in pregnancy. *Journal of Perinatal & Neonatal Nursing, 28*(3), 178-184.

Sun, A. (2004). Principles for practice with substance-abusing pregnant women: A framework based on the five social work intervention roles. *Social Work, 49*(3), 383-394.

Prostitution

CATEGORY: Social issue

DESCRIPTION

Prostitution is the delivery of sexual services to an individual who is not a spouse, partner, or friend in exchange for money, housing, food, or drugs. The individuals who engage in prostitution usually are women or girls; men or boys can prostitute themselves as well. Prostitution is illegal in 49 U.S. states; in some counties in Nevada prostitution is legal if provided in a licensed brothel. Prostitution may be off-street, in which services are provided by an escort or call-girl service with prearrangement of time and place or provided in a brothel setting. Prostitution also commonly is provided at the street level, meaning the prostitute is found by the customer on the street and not in a prearranged meeting. The street-level prostitute and client might then go to a motel, apartment, car. Globally, some countries have legalized prostitution by adult prostitutes or decriminalized elements of prostitution by legalizing the sale but not the purchase of sexual services.

Social, economic, and cultural factors create marked differences in the societal perception of prostitution. One view sees prostitution as a crime involving high degrees of violence, discrimination, and human rights violations. The opposite viewpoint regards prostitution as an acceptable occupational choice. Juvenile prostitution is understood and responded to very differently from adult prostitution. Because juveniles are not of legal age to consent to sex, the assumption is made that any engagement in prostitution by a juvenile is coerced. Juveniles should thus be considered victims of prostitution, not criminal offenders, although this is not always how they are treated. Juvenile prostitution is a significant problem both in the United States and internationally.

Professionals come into contact with those who are currently prostituting themselves or have in the past in a variety of practice areas, including in the areas of criminal justice, substance use, mental health, trauma, and child welfare. Such settings can be courts, hospitals, public health clinics, substance abuse treatment programs, homeless shelters, domestic and sexual violence centers, child protective services, and counseling centers/private practice. Professionals need to recognize this population as being very vulnerable and disenfranchised. Even though technically both the client and the adult prostitute are guilty of breaking the law, the customers of prostitutes are much less likely to be arrested than the prostitute. Many individuals engaged in street prostitution have very poor physical health; it is estimated that HIV rates among prostitutes are high, with hepatitis B and C, gonorrhea, herpes, syphilis, and human papillomavirus (HPV) also common. Prostitutes are also at risk for violence, substance abuse, exploitation, and coercion, as well as isolation from social support.

To address the individual and economic costs of prostitution, some communities are instituting diversion programs for arrested prostitutes to try to stop the cycle of arrest, jail, and release.

FACTS AND FIGURES

An accurate estimate of prostitution is hard to obtain because most data derive only from those prostitutes who are arrested and do not include the prostitutes who are not arrested. Professionals can encounter prostitutes in practice knowingly or unknowingly depending on the population with which they work. Prostitution will often result in risky behavior choices due to risk of violence and substance use. Street prostitution is a violent experience for those who provide it. In the United States, rates of physical and sexual abuse of prostitutes range from 60 to 93.5 percent. British researchers found that 92 percent of prostitutes expressed having experienced violence in their lifetime; 72 percent had experienced abuse as children. A Portland, Oregon, program that assists prostitutes to leave prostitution found a history of childhood sexual abuse in 85 percent of the program participants. Many studies also have found links between prostitution and high rates of post-traumatic stress disorder (PTSD) symptoms. Prostitutes who report abuse or assaults to authorities are not always given the proper attention; the criminal

justice system sometimes is reluctant to investigate or prosecute claims of violent victimization made by prostitutes. In the United States almost 3 percent of female homicide victims are women working as prostitutes; women involved in prostitution have a risk of death 12 times greater than that of similarly aged women.

There is also a strong association between substance use and prostitution. There is disagreement in the research community over whether drug use precedes prostitution or prostitution leads to substance abuse. At one health clinic, 86 percent of women engaged in prostitution were using illegal drugs compared to 23 percent of the total female clinic population. In a study of current and former prostitutes in the United Kingdom, researchers found that 83 percent were either currently addicted or had been addicted to drugs or alcohol when they were working as prostitutes. Researchers interviewing providers of drug and alcohol services in the United Kingdom found that approximately 25 percent of service users were women who were exchanging sex for money and/or drugs. The researchers also found that only 34.7 percent of providers offered information on prostitution and only 23.9 percent had harm reduction programs on prostitution. In contrast, 87.5 percent of programs designed for helping individuals exit prostitution had counseling and information on substance use, and 93.7 percent had harm reduction programs.

RISK FACTORS

Incidents of child abuse and family dysfunction in childhood have been reported in the background history of many of the individuals involved in prostitution.

School truancy can be a risk factor for juvenile prostitution.

Young people who run away from home can turn to prostitution as "survival sex," in which they exchange sex for resources.

In the United States, African Americans have the highest rate of juvenile entry into prostitution.

Individuals who entered prostitution as juveniles are also at a higher risk of suicide.

Many prostitutes abuse substances; individuals might prostitute themselves to pay for their drug habits and they might use substances as a means of coping with prostituting themselves.

Problem	Goal	Intervention
Person is actively prostituting self, putting self at risk.	Successfully exiting prostitution if the person wants to exit and receiving necessary formal support services to avoid reentry. Enhanced safety and self-care through harm-reduction strategies for the person who wants to continue to be a sex worker.	Prioritize and address active problems that are linked to prostitution (substance abuse, depression, PTSD). Design treatment plan to address active problems and minimize risk of reentry into prostitution. Provide individual and/or group therapy to address underlying issues. Establish safety plan if there is risk of violence from a pimp who has threatened person working as street prostitute.
Person is prostituting self to support substance addiction.	Person will be drug and alcohol free and will not need to prostitute self to support addiction.	Detoxification if medically necessary. Assist in accessing appropriate drug treatment program to address addiction and provide the means to be sober or pursue a harm-reduction model of recovery if appropriate. Provide supportive environment for sobriety. Assist in finding appropriate housing/ social support to maintain sobriety or harm reduction. Counsel and support to improve low self-esteem and reduce negative emotions that are being experienced.

SIGNS AND SYMPTOMS

There are no obvious physical or emotional signs and symptoms that will indicate that a person is or has been a prostitute. A professional needs to complete a thorough bio-psycho-social-spiritual assessment while providing a nonjudgmental setting for the person to feel comfortable to disclose.

ASSESSMENT

A professional should perform a comprehensive bio-psycho-social-spiritual assessment that includes the person's past prostitution history, relevant family history, family relationships, substance use history, any childhood abuse, and other traumatic events.

A detailed interview and history with a self-reporting questionnaire should be the primary screening tool to help determine whether a person has been involved in prostitution, which can have a major impact on need for services. Other screening tools can identify whether a person has risk factors that can lead to prostitution. These screening tools may include the Child Trauma Questionnaire—Short Form (assesses childhood physical and sexual abuse using a Likert scale), the Davidson Trauma Scale or the Trauma Symptom Checklist (assesses the frequency and severity of PTSD symptoms), and the Impact of Event Scale—Revised (determines the impact of traumatic events on the client's life experiences). If indicated by history, the Addiction Severity Index can be used to evaluate the behaviors and problems associated with substance use.

Depending on the setting, a blood alcohol screening or drug test may either be required or medically ordered, and testing for sexually transmitted diseases (STDs) may be appropriate, including HIV and hepatitis.

TREATMENT

The Eaves study in the United Kingdom resulted in a five-stage model for exiting prostitution that professionals may utilize. This model is not linear or rigid but can serve as a guideline. The stages are readiness/engagement, treatment/support, transition/stabilization, reconstruction/rebuilding, and new roles/identities. Women who are involved in prostitution and are seeking counseling support may also benefit from a person-centered approach with elements of psychodynamic work and attachment theory.

APPLICABLE LAWS AND REGULATIONS

Prostitution is illegal in 49 U.S. states. Nevada is the only state that allows some legal prostitution, with eight counties having active brothels.

Some U.S. cities and counties have formal diversion programs in which arrested prostitutes are directed to specific programs to treat underlying issues (drug use) rather than being sentenced to jail or prison.

Human trafficking laws may help minors engaged in prostitution in the United States. As of 2018, twenty-two states (Alabama, California, Connecticut, Florida, Illinois, Indiana, Kentucky, Michigan, Minnesota, Mississippi, Montana, Nebraska, New Hampshire, North Carolina, North Dakota, Rhode Island, South Carolina, South Dakota, Texas, Tennessee, Vermont, West Virginia) plus Washington D.C. have laws that provide immunity from prosecution for all minors who engage in prostitution, under the assumption that because minors cannot give consent, they are victims of human trafficking. Under so-called safe harbor laws, 19 states allow the minor who is under 18 and arrested for prostitution to enter an affirmative defense that his or her prostitution was due to trafficking. Michigan and South Dakota's safe harbor law applies only to minors who are age 16 or younger. Texas's safe harbor laws apply only to minors under the age of 14.

Seventeen states (Alaska, Arizona, Arkansas, Georgia, Hawaii, Iowa, Kansas, Louisiana, Maryland, Massachusetts, Nevada, New York, Oklahoma, Utah, Washington, Wisconsin, Wyoming) have significant protection for Commercially Sexually Exploited Children (CSEC), but do not consider all prostituted minors to be trafficked, so minors can still be criminalized for prostitution.

Eleven states (Colorado, Delaware, Idaho, Maine, Missouri, New Jersey, New Mexico, Ohio, Oregon, Pennsylvania, Virginia) have no significant safe harbor laws protecting minors from being arrested for prostitution.

SERVICES AND RESOURCES

Many individuals who are prostitutes may qualify for benefits or programs to address physical or mental health needs, but because of stigma or fear of arrest they will not or cannot access the services. Many need help with housing, employment, medical care, drug treatment, and mental health services, but low self-esteem, depression, resistance by providers to helping them, and the structure of the criminal justice system can all be barriers to access. The stigmatization of prostitutes often is internalized by the individual, who then feels he or she is not worthy of being helped.

Sex Industry Survivors Anonymous is a peer-support group for men or women who are either trying to escape prostitution or need support and recovery after leaving prostitution, http://www.sexindustry-survivors.com/

Arizona, California, Washington, D.C., Hawaii, Illinois, Maryland, Minnesota, Missouri, Nebraska, Nevada, New York, Ohio, Oregon, Washington, and Wisconsin have programs and resources for individuals trying to leave prostitution.

FOOD FOR THOUGHT

In a study, researchers found that in the United States, trafficked U.S. women who were engaging in prostitution received less empathy from study subjects than foreign trafficked women. There was a tendency by study subjects to believe that women should have known better and a tendency to blame those who participate in prostitution.

Research indicates that secure housing is a major need that must be met for individuals to be able to leave prostitution.

The illegal status of prostitution compounded by strong moral judgments make prostitutes a difficult population to study.

A formal support process improves the success rate of programs designed to assist individuals in exiting prostitution. In the absence of formal programs, many prostitutes try to exit while utilizing substance abuse treatment or domestic violence shelters but have less success.

Participants in Ohio's CATCH (Changing Actions to Change Habits) court program, for women who have been arrested multiple times for solicitation, have lower rates of re-arrest for prostitution. Women who meet the program criteria are able to enter a two-year treatment program that addresses the physical, mental health, social, and community consequences of prostitution.

Engaging in prostitution leaves individuals vulnerable to loss of social services, removal of children and termination of parental rights, and expulsion from family or church social support. The stigma attached to prostitution makes it difficult for individuals to return to legitimate employment.

RED FLAGS

Providers working with this population need to be alert to signs of secondary or vicarious traumatization. While counseling with or working with this population, hearing about the traumas experienced can result in traumatic stress for the provider.

—*Jessica Therivel, LMSW-IPR*

FOR FURTHER INFORMATION

Begun, Audrey L., and Gretchen Clark Hammond. "CATCH Court: A Novel Approach to 'Treatment as Alternative to Incarceration' for Women Engaged in Prostitution and Substance Abuse." *Journal of Social Work Practice in the Addictions*, vol. 12, no. 3, 4 Sept. 2012, pp. 328–331., doi:10.1080/1533256x.2012.703920.

Holly, Jennifer, and Gemma Lousley. "The Challenge of Change – Improving Services for Women Involved in Prostitution and Substance Use." *Advances in Dual Diagnosis*, vol. 7, no. 2, 2014, pp. 80–89., doi:10.1108/add-02-2014-0005.

Roe-Sepowitz, Dominique E., et al. "The Impact of Abuse History and Trauma Symptoms on Successful Completion of a Prostitution-Exiting Program." *Journal of Human Behavior in the Social Environment*, vol. 22, no. 1, 24 Jan. 2012, pp. 65–77., doi:10.1080/10911359.2011.598830.

———— "Adult Prostitution Recidivism: Risk Factors and Impact of a Diversion Program. *Journal of Offender Rehabilitation*, vol. 50 no. 5, July 2011, pp. 272-285. do i:10.1080/10509674.2011.574205

Wiechelt, Shelly A., and Corey S. Shdaimah. "Trauma and Substance Abuse Among Women in Prostitution: Implications for a Specialized Diversion Program." *Journal of Forensic Social Work*, vol. 1, no. 2, 20 Sept. 2011, pp. 159–184., doi:10.1080/1936928x.2011.598843.

Psoriasis

CATEGORY **Disease/Disorder**

KEY TERMS:

dermatologist: a physician who treats the skin and its structures, functions, and diseases

dermis: the layer of skin directly beneath the epidermis, consisting of dense connective tissue and numerous blood vessels

epidermis: the outermost part of the skin, composed of four or five different layers called strata

methotrexate: a powerful drug, originally developed to treat cancer, that is used to treat patients with severe cases of psoriasis

psoralens: chemicals found in plants that make the skin more sensitive to light

PUVA: a treatment for psoriasis in which the patient is exposed to ultraviolet A (UVA) light after receiving one of the psoralens

stratum corneum: the outermost layer of the epidermis; its cells are normally dead, hard, and removed by normal bathing

ultraviolet light: invisible light composed of waves that are shorter than the ordinary light waves able to be seen by humans

CAUSES AND SYMPTOMS

Psoriasis is a common skin problem that afflicts approximately two of every hundred people, affecting males and females with relatively equal frequency. Although it affects all races, it is most prevalent among northern Europeans. This stubborn, chronic, and as yet incurable disease most commonly appears in one's teens or twenties, although it can appear in early childhood. While 70% of those who develop psoriasis do so by the age of twenty, there is another common danger period in the fifties and sixties, with a large number of patients developing their first symptoms at that time. Psoriasis often accompanies other diseases such as psoriatic arthritis, diabetes, cardiovascular disease, inflammatory bowel disease, and many others. There are certain triggers that have been associated with the development of psoriasis. Some of which include: obesity, infections, certain medications, sunlight, pregnancy, stress, alcohol, and smoking. Previously thought to be a result of a dysfunction of the barrier of the skin, many studies have found that the development may be a result of a dysfunction of the immune system.

There are several different types of psoriasis, making diagnosis difficult. By far the most widespread is the plaque type; because it accounts for 95% of all cases, this type is also called common psoriasis. Plaque-type psoriasis gets its name from the appearance of the patches of affected skin. Each patch resembles a plaque or small disk stuck to the body's surface. These dull, wine-colored patches of abnormal skin are often rounded or oval; they may be very irregular in shape when several nearby patches join together.

The surface of each thickened patch is rough and scaly, with the scales ranging in color from red to white to the most typical silvery gray. These psoriatic plaques can be small (the size of coins) or become palm-sized and larger. Whatever their final size, they generally begin as purple or reddened areas the size of a pinhead. The original areas expand in size, usually for a few weeks, until they reach a stable phase and stop expanding. The average size of a plaque in the stable phase is between two and three inches. A patch of stable psoriasis may eventually grow pale, become less scaly, and disappear completely, or it may begin to enlarge for no apparent reason. Even those plaques that have disappeared may be reactivated and reappear in the same place at some later time.

Certain parts of the body seem most prone to psoriatic lesions, namely the elbows, the knees, the scalp, and the lower back. The patches may appear elsewhere, including the genitals and the buttocks, but the face, hands, and feet are rarely affected. Severe cases may cover the entire chest or back. In a few cases, psoriasis is symmetrical, appearing in the same area on the left and right sides of the body simultaneously.

The patches are, however, more likely to develop in a random, scattered manner. Almost 50% of patients with psoriasis have lesions on their scalps. When these plaques are very large and widespread, they are difficult to treat and very difficult to hide. Although very uncomfortable, scalp psoriasis does not affect the growth of hair or cause baldness. It can cause a temporary thinning of the hair, but the hair grows normally again once the disease is controlled by medication. About one-third of psoriasis patients have affected fingernails and toenails. The diseased nails show pits or pinpoint indentations, loosening, thickening, and a yellowish discoloration. Surprisingly, in some people the condition remains on the nails alone, never developing elsewhere.

In addition to psoriasis of the nails, there are several rare and unusual types of psoriasis that are quite different from the common or plaque type. These include flexural or inverse, guttate, pustular, and erythrodermic psoriasis. Flexural psoriasis appears in folds and creases on the body and is often found on people who are particularly overweight and who are in their mid-forties or older. The patches tend to be very moist rather than scaly and are particularly sore and uncomfortable. Guttable psoriasis consists of an enormous number of highly scattered but minute plaques. It is extremely rare and occurs between the ages of eight and sixteen. Although the spots usually clear up in a few weeks, they sometimes recur or change into the large lesions of common psoriasis. Pustular psoriasis is the only form of the disease that occurs on the palms of the hands or the soles of the feet. It was named for the yellow or white pus-filled spots that form on the skin and eventually drop off. These spots form when enormous numbers of white blood cells invade the skin even though there is no infection present and, therefore, no need for these infection-killing cells.

Erythrodermic psoriasis literally means "red skin." This very rare condition is so named because the entire body is covered by flaming red patches that do not turn scaly. Since the extensive nature of this condition makes internal temperature control very difficult and dehydration inevitable, it can be very dangerous and may require hospitalization.

Common psoriasis, by comparison, is not dangerous or life-threatening. It is usually not painful and does not even cause itching in most patients. It is, however, very annoying because of its unsightly appearance and its tendency to flare up repeatedly. Once the disease has appeared, it stays with the person for life, improving or worsening periodically. After periods of relative quiet, during which the skin may appear quite normal, patients with psoriasis experience new eruptions and scaling for no apparent reason. Plaques continue to form for an unpredictable amount of time, until the condition spontaneously quiets down again.

The source of the plaques is a failure in the mechanism by which normal skin renews itself. Ordinarily, the cells at the base of the epidermis reproduce themselves at a slow and steady rate. They then move upward in about twenty-eight days, changing chemically, dying, and detaching from the surface, the stratum corneum. In psoriatic skin, however, there is a huge increase in the number of basal cells in the epidermis, which reproduce so rapidly that they push upward to the surface in only four days, forming thick disks of sticky, abnormal cells. Below the epidermis, the dermis of a patient with psoriasis is also abnormal. Its normally fine blood vessels are wide and extremely twisted, which results in the red appearance of the plaques and causes bleeding to occur easily when the skin is bumped or scratched. An unusually high number of the white blood cells called neutrophils and T lymphocytes are also present. They move up into the epidermis, creating inflammation and swelling within the plaques.

Long before modern dermatology discovered these facts about the structure and the functioning of psoriatic skin, it was noted that the disease does seem to run in families. If one parent has the problem, there is a one-in three chance that a child will eventually be afflicted; if both parents have the disease, the risk for their offspring is one in two. With nonidentical twins, there is a 70% chance that if one has psoriasis, they both will; with identical twins, the figure can be as high as 90%, according to some studies. Investigators suspect that psoriasis is not handed down by a simple pattern, such as with eye color inheritance. It seems more likely that the condition results from a combination of several genetic factors from each parent, much like the manner in which height and intelligence are inherited.

TREATMENT AND THERAPY

More than 90% of psoriasis patients can be cleared significantly of their lesions or even made lesion-free by the medicines and methods developed by modern technology. For minor outbreaks, limited to a small area of the body, the first choice for treatment is a corticosteroid cream or ointment applied directly to the plaques. Corticosteroids are hormones, produced by the adrenal glands, that are able to reduce inflammation. Corticosteroids are produced in the laboratory and combined with other chemicals to reduce inflammation even more effectively by decreasing blood flow to the psoriatic lesions. Dermatologists have a large variety of such preparations ranging from mild to extremely potent. They must find one that is strong enough to suppress the inflammation but not so strong that it causes unwanted side effects.

There are two major undesirable side effects of corticosteroid therapy. Psoriatic skin absorbs all substances more easily than normal skin; the excess hormones enter the bloodstream and can change the output of hormones by the pituitary and adrenal glands, dangerously altering the body's chemical balance. The other danger is to the skin itself, which becomes abnormally thin, easily damaged, and prone to infections. Another drawback to the use of corticosteroids is the tendency for the psoriatic plaques to reappear soon after the creams or ointments are discontinued.

Many patients find relief from a completely different class of medications, those which contain tar.

This thick, black, oily liquid is produced from coal. It contains thousands of chemical substances, and biochemists do not know which of those substances actually help to heal the skin. Tar-containing ointments, creams, gels, shampoos, and bath additives are useful for removing the scales without worrisome side effects. A major drawback, however, is their tendency to stain clothing, bedding, bathroom tiles, and bathtubs. Some staining can be avoided by covering the treated skin area with bandages, cotton underwear, or a shower cap. In addition to the staining, many patients find the tar odor quite unpleasant; pharmaceutical companies are constantly trying to improve this aspect of these quite effective products.

A third type of preparation is particularly effective for removing very thick scales. These medications contain a compound called salicylic acid. Like the corticosteroids, salicylic acid ointments and gels are most effective when they are in contact with the plaques for a long period of time. After treatment, it is often recommended that patients cover their lesions with plastic gloves, plastic bags (for the feet), or taped-down plastic wrap for four to eight hours. Patients with psoriasis have noted for years that exposure to the sun is very helpful in clearing their lesions.

Daily sunlight exposure is effective for as many as 80% of patients. This treatment is relatively accessible for at least part of the year and inexpensive compared to the various medications available. Given the increased risk of skin cancer, it is strongly recommended that patients have repeated but brief sun exposures and avoid sunburn by using creams and lotions. Although sun exposure is helpful to most patients with common psoriasis, it rarely helps and can even worsen the pustulate and erythrodermic types. Since too much exposure to sunlight will damage rather than help any skin, even plaque-type patients are advised to stop their sun exposure once the psoriasis has improved.

For patients in many climates, sunbathing is possible for only a few months of the year. The development of sunlamps for use at home or in a dermatologist's office, hospital, psoriasis care center, or tanning parlor has made this therapy possible all year round. Because of the danger of severe sunburns, sunlamp treatments remain controversial. To reduce their danger, a dermatologist must carefully

Information on Psoriasis

Causes: Failure inmechanism bywhich normal skin renews itself; often hereditary

Symptoms: Red, scaly patches; thick, silvery-gray scales; physical discomfort; loose, thick, and yellowish fingernails and toenails; thinning hair

Duration: Chronic with acute episodes

Treatments: Corticosteroids, tar-containing agents, sun exposure, methotrexate

determine the amount of time of each treatment, the precise distance from the lamp, and the appropriate frequency of treatments for each individual patient to achieve maximal and safe results.

The curative effect of sunlight depends on the presence of the very short wavelength part of the light, called ultraviolet. It is ultraviolet B (UVB) waves that help heal psoriasis, possibly by slowing down the high growth rate of cells in the epidermis. Both natural sunlight and sunlamps contain UVB and, therefore, have the potential to help psoriasis. They also have the potential, however, to burn the skin. Patients with severe psoriasis may require the use of ultraviolet A (UVA) waves from a special kind of sunlamp.

The patient is given a dose of a psoralen, a substance that makes the skin more light-sensitive, and is then exposed to UVA inside a full-body light cabinet. Thirty treatments may be required to completely clear the skin. The psoralen is often given in tablet form, although some patients suffer fewer side effects if it is painted onto the skin or if they bathe in it. The early side effects of PUVA (psoralen plus UVA) treatment include nausea, itching, colored blotches on the skin, and occasional worsening of the psoriasis. More worrisome are the possible later side effects: skin cancer and the development of cataracts in the eyes. The danger of developing cataracts also exists from natural sunlight and UVB sunlamps; patients using any light therapy must use excellent sunglasses that block out all rays harmful to the eyes.

For the patient with widespread psoriasis who is not responsive to corticosteroids, tar preparations, or the various light therapies, the drug methotrexate is effective in more than 80% of patients. This powerful drug was originally developed to treat various kinds of cancer because it slows down the process of cell multiplication. Thus the psoriatic epidermal cells are prevented from reproducing and forming the scaly plaques. Often methotrexate must be taken for six months or a year, in pill form or by injection, to have a significant impact on an extensive case. Such a dosage poses a risk of numerous and serious side effects, including persistent feelings of sickness, indigestion, and diarrhea.

Frequent tests are necessary to monitor the condition of the blood, since methotrexate can interfere with the bone marrow's production of normal blood cells. Most important, periodic liver biopsies, the removal of sample liver cells by means of a special needle, are necessary because methotrexate can cause irreversible damage to this crucial organ. It is very important that a pregnant woman never take methotrexate or that a woman never become pregnant while taking it. The drug's ability to interfere with cell growth can cause many abnormalities in a developing embryo or fetus. Similar fetal abnormalities can be caused by the drugs called retinoids.

For patients with pustular and erythrodermic psoriasis, the retinoids etretinate and acitretin can be very useful, if side effects are carefully monitored. Some dermatologists have been especially successful combining PUVA and etretinate therapies; the improvement in the psoriasis is greater than with either alone, while the lower dosage of each minimizes risk and side effects.

Another medication effective in treating severe psoriasis is cyclosporine. It has brought dramatic improvement to patients with lifelong disabling symptoms. Many people, however, can tolerate the drug only for short periods. Because of its potential to cause high blood pressure and kidney damage, as well as an increased risk of cancer, this medicine is prescribed only with extreme caution.

People with moderate or severe psoriasis may benefit from a relatively new type of treatment used called biologics. Biologics are proteins produced with or from a living organism and they have the ability to target the immune system with high specificity. Biologics include a variety of classes such as monoclonal antibodies and kinase inhibitors. An example of a monoclonal antibody is called Adalimumab or Humira®. Previously approved for psoriatic arthritis, Adalimumab was approved in 2017 to treat fingernail psoriasis.

All the many therapies described can bring partial or total clearing of lesions and even result in the remission of the disease for a period of time. Until the cause of psoriasis is completely understood, however, it is likely that no permanent cure will be developed.

PERSPECTIVE AND PROSPECTS

Descriptions of psoriasis are found in the records of the earliest known civilizations. The term "psora" comes from the ancient Greek language. Psoriasis was considered a form of leprosy in biblical times. Despite this ancient history and extensive modern research, however, the exact cause of psoriasis is still unknown. Unlike many human diseases, psoriasis does not afflict any animals; therefore, it cannot be studied through controlled laboratory testing.

Early work on psoriasis by dermatologists centered on differential diagnosis. This is the ability to distinguish psoriasis from various rashes caused by fungi, such as ringworm, and from the many forms of eczema or dermatitis caused by allergies. Skin biopsies developed by oncologists can now determine that the condition is not a cancer; the portion of skin removed, when placed under a microscope, will clearly show the dermal and epidermal appearance characteristic of psoriatic skin.

While skin scientists have proven that psoriasis is not contagious, it has been known since the 1930s that many cases develop soon after strep throat and other upper respiratory infections. The bacteria involved are not the cause of the psoriasis, however, but rather a trigger for the development of a condition for which the patient is genetically predisposed. Another trigger, excessive scratching or rubbing of the skin, can precipitate outbreaks in susceptible people; this is named the Koebner phenomenon, for its discoverer. With the help of neurologists and psychologists, it has been proven that the disease is not caused by "nerves," yet stress of all kinds is definitely able to make its symptoms worse, and patients must be helped to lower their stress levels if they are to keep the disease under control.

Nutritionists have searched for ways to use diet to help psoriatics, but to no avail. Although no particular foods either help or hinder the course of the disease, most dermatologists now recognize that drinking alcohol can both precipitate and aggravate the disfiguring plaques.

Immunologists have been very involved in the study of psoriasis even though it is not an allergic reaction to any substance in one's environment. In the late twentieth century, they pursued many possible connections between the streptococci bacteria that cause strep throat, the white blood cells called T lymphocytes that seek to destroy them, and the development of psoriasis. They believe that, in predisposed people, chemicals from the bacteria cause the T lymphocytes to give off substances that trigger the skin's uncontrolled and excessive production of epidermal cells.

Geneticists have been searching diligently for the source of the predisposition to psoriasis. Among the genes children receive from their parents are those that build particular proteins on their white blood cells called human leukocyte antigens (HLAs). Out of the hundreds of different HLAsthat one can possibly inherit, those who develop psoriasis always seem to possess similar combinations. The identification of the genes responsible for HLAs and the role of those genes in precipitating psoriasis may bring about major improvements in the treatment and possibly a cure for this disease afflicting millions of people throughout the world.

—*Grace D. Matzen*
Updated by Brittany Polizzi, RN

FOR FURTHER INFORMATION

"An Overview of Psoriasis and Psoriatic Arthritis." *National Psoriasis Foundation*, Feb. 2011.

"About Psoriasis." *National Psoriasis Foundation*, 2013.

Camisa, Charles. *Handbook of Psoriasis*. 2d ed. Hoboken, N.J.: John Wiley & Sons, 2004.

Leikin, J. B. (2019). Biologics for the primary care physician: Review and treatment of psoriasis. Disease-a-Month, 65(3), 50. doi:10.1016/j.disamonth.2018.06.002

Shuman, Jill, and Purvee S. Shah. "Psoriasis." *Health Library*, Feb. 25, 2013.

Turkington, Carol, and Jeffrey S. Dover. *The Encyclopedia of Skin and Skin Disorders*. 3d ed. New York: Facts On File, 2007. Weedon, David. *Skin Pathology*. 3d ed. NewYork: Churchill Livingstone/ Elsevier, 2010.

"What Is Psoriasis?" *National Institute of Arthritis and Musculoskeletal and Skin Diseases*, Sept. 2009.

Psychiatric disorders

Category: Disease/Disorder

Key Terms:

biomedical model: a way of viewing and understanding psychiatric disorders which emphasizes customary medical practice in identifying and treating a particular disorder from which a person suffers

diagnostic codes: the method used in the *Diagnostic and Statistical*

Manual of Mental Disorders (DSM) to record psychiatric diagnoses for statistical and administrative purposes

multiaxial classification: the classification system used in the DSM to account for several factors when making psychiatric diagnoses, including present condition, developmental/ personality disorders, physical disorders, life stresses, and overall functioning

neuroscience: the scientific specialization that seeks to understand mental processes, occurrences, and disturbances in terms of underlying mechanisms in the brain and the nervous system

psychodynamic model: a way of viewing and understanding psychiatric disorders which emphasizes the recognition and treatment of underlying psychological and developmental traumas

psychopharmacology: the use of drugs to study effects on brain chemistry; drugs are used to treat mental disorders, study brain chemistry, and promote new disease classifications

psychosocial treatment: a significant specialization in treating people with psychiatric disorders through employing principles of psychology, human behavior, family and group dynamics, and social and occupational learning

somatic treatment: the treatment of people with psychiatric disorders using specialized drugs and electroconvulsive therapy; some major drug groups used are antidepressants, antipsychotics, mood stabilizers, anxiolytics, and psychostimulants

Causes and Symptoms

Many centuries ago, physicians began to understand that psychiatric disorders such as depression arose from abnormalities in brain structure or chemistry. As the field of psychiatry developed, medicine has had a profound influence in establishing the biomedical model to define and treat mental disorders. Sigmund Freud and other influential psychiatrists working in the late nineteenth century broadened the understanding of how emotional pain and trauma experienced during a person's childhood can contribute profoundly to the occurrence and course of mental disorders. The medical influence on the field of psychiatry was deepened and broadened by the contribution of neuroscience. Scientists who began studying the brain more intensively, beginning in the early twentieth century, proved the relationship of brain function to speech, learning, comprehension, memory, emotional regulation, and other important human abilities. Technologies developed in the late twentieth century, such as functional magnetic resonance imaging (fMRI) and genetic testing, have furthered psychiatrists' understanding of the biological, genetic, and neurological basis of a number of mental disorders.

Despite long and exacting efforts to understand mental illness, much remains to be explored. While psychiatrists would prefer to base their diagnoses on knowing the causes and the biological or neurological mechanisms of mental disorders, this knowledge has proved to be elusive. Therefore, most psychiatric diagnoses are based on the psychiatrist recognizing a pattern of symptoms and a typical course of disease. During World War II, psychiatrists realized that their colleagues differed widely in how they recognized and described various mental illnesses. Bureaucratic and professional forces coalesced in a drive to make the diagnosis of psychiatric disorders more systematic.

In 1952, the American Psychiatric Association issued a manual that sought to clarify the diagnostic process. Unfortunately, the early manuals proved to be impractical and were largely ignored by psychiatrists. This changed when a more rigorous effort culminated in the publication of the third edition of the *Diagnostic and Statistical Manual of Mental Disorders* (DSM-III) in 1980. This text became widely accepted as the standard reference for psychiatrists to use when diagnosing psychiatric disorders. The manual has been strengthened and revised several times; a fifth edition, known as DSM-5, was published in 2013. Scientists and clinicians continue their work on the manual to correct flaws, incorporate research findings, and explore new areas. However, shortly before the publication of the DSM-5 in May 2013, the US

National Institute of Mental Health issued a statement condemning the DMS-5's "lack of validity," noting that "DSM diagnoses are based on a consensus about clusters of clinical symptoms, not any objective laboratory measure."

While psychiatrists agree that standard definitions of psychiatric disorders are needed to clarify their thinking, permit easier communication, improve treatment planning, and stimulate further research, a growing number of psychologists recognize the need for more accurate diagnostic criteria that are based on genetic, neurophysiological, and biological measures. While psychiatrists agree that a more accurate diagnostic system based on biomarkers is needed, the technology and research to establish such diagnostic criteria are not yet available. Therefore, the symptom-based diagnostic criteria put forth in the DSM-5 remain the most widely used in the field of psychiatry. When using the DSM-5, psychiatrists must find that the person exhibits specific signs and symptoms and has maintained this clinical picture for a sufficient length of time to warrant being diagnosed with a psychiatric disorder.

The DSM-5 assigns a specific code for each psychiatric diagnosis, which facilitates administrative and statistical work. The diagnostic codes in the DSM-5 are compatible with the coding system used in the International Classification of Diseases (ICD-10-CM), published by the World Health Organization as update to the previous edition in 2015. The ICD-10-CM coding system uses a combination of letters and numbers in its codes, and the DSM-5 contains both the previous ICD-9-CM and the ICD-10-CM coding systems to facilitate the transition to the ICD-10-CM coding system.

Furthermore, the DSM-5 combined the first three axes of the multiaxial diagnostic system used in the fourth edition of the DSM (DSM-IV-TR) into one list that includes all disorders. The DSM-IV-TR had listed clinical disorders on five separate axes, with Axis I referring to the principal disorder, Axis II indicating any additional personality disorder that might affect the Axis I disorder, Axis III indicating any medical problems that might affect the presentation or treatment of the principal disorder; Axis IV noting any psychosocial or contextual factors, and Axis V noting any disability. The DSM-5 introduced a nonaxial diagnostic system, combining Axes I, II, and III into one list, with an expanded set of ICD-10-CM codes to note any psychosocial or environmental factors and disability (formerly Axes IV and V).

Several major diagnostic categories of psychiatric disorders are shown in the DSM-5. These include neurodevelopmental disorders; schizophrenia spectrum and other psychotic disorders; bipolar and related disorders; depressive disorders; anxiety disorders; obsessive-compulsive and related disorders; trauma- and stressor-related disorders; dissociative disorders; somatic symptom and related disorders; feeding and eating disorders; sleep-wake disorders; sexual dysfunctions; gender dysphoria; disruptive, impulse-control, and conduct disorders; substance-related and addictive disorders; neurocognitive disorders; and paraphilic disorders. This listing demonstrates the breadth of problems that are seen and treated by psychiatrists and other mental health practitioners.

Research shows that, as of 2016, 18.3 percent of adults in the United States will experience any mental illness, with the prevalence being higher in women (21.7%) compared to men (14.5%). Globally, approximately 10 percent of the adult population will have a psychiatric disorder, although psychologists believe the actual rates of mental illness are underreported in many developing countries. The most common disorders are anxiety disorders and mood disorders, such as depression.

Researchers learned that people who experience their first symptoms later in life generally have a better chance of recovering, but almost all people who suffer from a psychiatric disorder will experience distressing symptoms for several years. According to researchers, the differences in prevalence among the races may be more reflective of survey methods than of ethnic origins. Higher rates of mental illness are found among people who are poor and who fail to complete high school. People who suffer from one psychiatric disorder were found by researchers to be at a high risk (60 percent) for having another mental health disorder at some time during their lives.

TREATMENT AND THERAPY

Making an accurate diagnosis of psychiatric disorders is essential to treating problems properly, since many can be improved through the application of psychosocial, somatic, drug, and adjunctive therapies. For example, it is said that most people who suffer from major depression can be treated successfully with brief psychotherapy, a course of medication, or a combination of both. The somatic technique of exposing a person each day to a bank of bright lights (light therapy) has been used successfully to treat seasonal affective disorder (depression associated with a specific season, especially winter). Many depressed people and their families have been helped by the adjunctive therapy of participating in a support group.

The use of laboratory tests to clarify psychiatric diagnosis is growing in importance. Only a few disorders can be revealed by laboratory tests, but research is being conducted to validate such testing and to increase its scope and usefulness. Some tests are done routinely to rule out medical problems that may be causing the psychiatric problems the person is experiencing or to ensure that the patient can take needed medication.

Drugs have been used in the United States to treat psychiatric disorders since the early 1950s, and new medications are introduced frequently. The distressing thought disturbances experienced by people suffering from schizophrenia have been treated with antipsychotic drugs. Antipsychotics also are used to treat psychotic symptoms such as the hallucinations and delusions experienced by some people who are suffering from depression or other mood disorders. Several classes of antipsychotics have been developed. Mood stabilizing medication, such as lithium and valproic acid, as well as antipsychotics are the drugs most commonly used to treat people suffering from bipolar disorders, in which patients experience swings in mood from the highs of mania to the lows of depression.

Various classes of antidepressants such as selective serotonin reuptake inhibitors (SSRIs), serotonin-norepinephrine reuptake inhibitors (SNRIs), tricyclics and monoamine oxidase inhibitors (MAOIs) are used to treat people suffering from depression. Many people experiencing symptoms associated with anxiety disorders have been helped through the use of benzodiazepines and other anxiolytics. Central nervous system stimulants (psychostimulants) are used to treat narcolepsy, a disorder in which people have trouble staying awake. Psychostimulants also are used to treat attention-deficit hyperactivity disorder (ADHD), because the stimulants have the paradoxical effect of reducing the behaviors that disrupt classroom work and life at home. The drugs decrease excessive physical activity and have been shown to improve an individual's attention to adult

---

Information on Psychiatric Disorders

Causes: Genetic and environmental factors, medications, substance abuse

Symptoms: Wide ranging; may include emotional distress, mental impairment, abrupt changes in mood or personality, anxiety, depression, manic behavior, substance abuse, difficulty sleeping

Duration: Acute to chronic

Treatments: Depends on type and severity; may include drug, psychosocial, somatic, and adjunctive therapies

---

guidance, increase attention span and memory, and lessen Zthe individual's tendency to be distracted from tasks and to act impulsively. The person with ADHD also is helped with behavior management techniques and careful control of the environment to reduce sources of external stimulation.

Unfortunately, the use of drugs in treating psychiatric disorders is not problem-free. Almost all psychopharmaceuticals have side effects that can be serious enough to prevent their use in treatment. A growing number of psychiatrists have expressed their concern over what they believe to be widespread overdiagnosis and overtreatment for psychiatric disorders in the United States; many patients respond well to simple lifestyle changes, such as increased physical activity or brief therapeutic interventions, so psychiatrists should prescribe psychopharmaceutical medications judiciously. Some people must take other prescription drugs that preclude the use of the drug needed to treat the psychiatric disorder. The possibility of overdose by people who have thoughts of taking their lives can limit the use of possibly toxic drugs. Some people are not helped by drug therapy, are reluctant to take drugs, or fail to take drugs properly.

For such people, it is fortunate that other forms of treatment can be used. Many people who suffer from psychiatric illness have been helped by trained psychotherapists, such as psychiatrists, psychologists, social workers, counselors, and members of the clergy. Many forms of psychotherapy are practiced. The aims of psychotherapy can be to help the person deal well with life's stresses and crises, confront and resolve psychological conflict, avoid interpersonal problems, and find more satisfaction and fulfillment in life.

Psychotherapy is delivered to individuals, couples, families, and other groups. More emphasis is being placed on conducting psychotherapy only for a limited time, because this approach is preferred by most patients and their insurance companies and because research results support its effectiveness.

Behavioral therapy can be used to help the person to change specific behaviors that cause problems. Behavioral therapy has been used to treat several psychiatric disorders, including alcohol and drug dependence, anxiety, phobias, autism spectrum disorders, and eating disorders. Systematic desensitization has been used to help people who have irrational fears, or phobias. The patient is gradually introduced to the situation that elicits the fearful response and is taught to use relaxation techniques to reduce anxiety and to bring fears under personal control. In behavior modification programs, unwanted behavior is defined, targeted, reduced, and eliminated. At the same time, the person is rewarded for behaving properly.

Electroconvulsive therapy (ECT), formerly called shock therapy, is used generally to treat people with severe depression who have not responded to less intrusive treatment methods. In ECT, the patient is exposed to an electric current that is passed through electrodes taped to the scalp. The current causes the person to experience a brief seizure, usually for less than a minute. This treatment method has been used for many years, and several improvements have been made to make the procedure safer and less damaging to the person's memory.

Treatment of psychiatric disorders is usually delivered in the community where the affected person lives. In the United States, legislation in the 1960s caused federal funds to be used to build and staff community mental health centers. Many health insurance providers will pay part of the fees charged by private therapists, which allows some people to afford their services. Alcohol and drug treatment programs generally offer people either short-term residential or outpatient services. Many people are served in institutional settings, such as mental hospitals and nursing homes. Some use services provided by governmental funding.

Many people who have suffered psychiatric disorders recover completely; investigators find a 38 percent remission rate. The researchers were surprised to learn that people are most likely to recover from alcohol and drug abuse, generalized anxiety, and antisocial personality. Complete freedom from distressing symptoms and episodes is less likely for those who suffer from mania, obsessive-compulsive disorder (in which the person performs repetitive rituals to allay anxiety caused by disturbing thoughts or fears), and schizophrenia (a disorder typified by thought disturbances such as hallucinations and delusions, mood changes, communication problems, and unusual behaviors). However, with a combination of pharmacological and psychosocial treatments and interventions, 70 to 90 percent of patients with psychiatric disorders experience a reduction of symptoms and improved quality of life, even without achieving full remission. A large number of people who suffer mental illness have never been treated. In 2016, about 44.7 million individuals suffered from mental illness, but only about 19 million received treatment, which is only 43%. However, women were more likely to seek out treatment (48.8% vs 33.9%). Researchers estimate the economic cost of untreated psychiatric disorders in the United States to be more than $100 billion each year.

PERSPECTIVE AND PROSPECTS

Early medical documents show that mental illness has always been an area of significant concern. Symptoms of mental illness were described in the Bible, and they were studied and treated in classical times. Interest in understanding mental disorders waned during the medieval period, when it was thought that sufferers were possessed by demons or were being punished by God. Mentally ill people were often maltreated and incarcerated. Finally, the foundation was laid in the late sixteenth century for a more complete understanding of psychiatric disorders: In 1586, Timothy Bright, a physician, published the first English-language text on mental illness, entitled *Treatise of Melancholie.*

In late eighteenth-century France, Philippe Pinel took over the management of a hospital for insane men and not only advocated more humane treatment of mentally ill people but also took steps to free them from the chains and other punishing devices that they were forced to endure. Pinel instituted the scientific study of mental illness. He tracked the prevalence of mental disorders, conducted studies to learn the natural course of mental illness, and established a treatment model followed by the more progressive psychiatric facilities.

The brain was studied even more intensely in the nineteenth century. During this era, scientists made important contributions to the understanding of how certain parts of the brain are responsible for specialized functions. They learned that particular brain regions are related to speech and language, movement, sensations, learning, understanding, and emotions. Emil Kraepelin correlated information about the age of onset, natural course, and length of time of particular mental disorders. He used the information that he organized to develop the first classification system of psychiatric disorders. Among the maladies he named were dementia praecox (now called schizophrenia), dementia in the elderly (now called Alzheimer's disease), and manic-depressive illness (bipolar disorder).

While neuroscientists were making significant contributions to the understanding of the brain, psychiatrist Sigmund Freud was advancing his study of hysteria and its connection with childhood trauma. He used hypnosis and free association to release and resolve underlying misconceptions and fears and to give the patient relief from debilitating trauma and its associated symptoms. He also produced theories on psychological function and structure and on psychotherapy. During the twentieth century, psychiatrists drew on a broad array of disciplines to improve the diagnosis and treatment of psychiatric disorders, including the study of brain chemistry, biology, structure, and functioning. Advances in neuroimaging techniques allowed scientists to study and sometimes diagnose brain dysfunction. Specialized drugs were developed to be used in the treatment of specific mental disorders. Since 1952, the American Psychiatric Association has published a series of diagnostic and statistical manuals designed to bring order to the study, diagnosis, and treatment of psychiatric disorders. Psychiatrists continue to work toward developing more accurate diagnostic criteria and more effective treatments for psychiatric disorders.

—*Russell Williams, M.S.W.*
Updated by Nancy A. Piotrowski, Ph.D.
and Oi-Lee Tiffany Wong, RN, MS

FOR FURTHER INFORMATION

Ahrnsbrak R, Bose J, Hedden SL, Lipari RN, Park-Lee E. "Key Substance Use and Mental Health Indictors in the United States: Results from the 2016 National Survey on Drug Use and Health. Substance Abuse and Mental Health Services Administration." *Substance Abuse and Mental Health Services Administration* (SAMHSA), September, 2017, https://www.samhsa.gov/data/sites/default/files/NSDUH-FFR1-2016/NSDUH-FFR1-2016.htm.

American Medical Association. *The ICD-10-CM 2019: The Complete Official Codebook, First Edition.* USA: American Medical Association Press, 2018.

Insel, Thomas. "Transforming Diagnosis." *National Institute of Mental Health,* April 29, 2013.

Kring, Ann M., et al. *Abnormal Psychology.* 11th ed. Hoboken, N.J.: John Wiley & Sons, 2010.

Oltmanns, Thomas F., et al. *Case Studies in Abnormal Psychology.* 9th ed. Hoboken, N.J.: John Wiley & Sons, 2012.

Sadock, Benjamin J., Virginia A. Sadock, and Pedro Ruiz, eds. *Kaplan and Sadock's Comprehensive Textbook of Psychiatry.* 9th ed. Philadelphia: Lippincott Williams & Wilkins, 2009.

Psychiatric disorders and aging

CATEGORY: Specialty

KEY TERMS:

acute confusion syndrome: a transient condition caused by the action of various biological stressors on vulnerable older persons, who may experience inattention, disorganized thinking, other cognitive impairments, and emotional problems

anxiety: a condition characterized by nervousness or agitation; in older people, it is often caused by the existence of a psychiatric disorder such as depression, a general medical condition such as hypothyroidism, or a side effect of medication

depression: a condition characterized by a persistent mood of sadness, weight loss, greatly decreased interest in life, and sometimes psychotic episodes; biological factors, family history of depression, underlying medical problems, and medication side effects all can contribute to these symptoms

hypochondriasis: a condition in which the patients believe strongly that they are suffering from one or more serious illnesses, even when this belief is unsupported by medical evidence

insomnia: disturbed sleep, which occurs in older people more often than in any other age group;

insomnia in older people can be caused by many factors, such as dysfunctional sleep cycles, breathing problems, leg jerking, underlying medical and psychiatric disorders, and the side effects of medication

memory loss syndrome: a condition in which a person gradually but progressively loses capacity in many cognitive areas, but especially in the ability to remember; Alzheimer's disease is considered the most common factor causing serious memory loss in older people

suspiciousness: a range of symptoms from increasing distrust of others to paranoid delusions of conspiracies; changes related to aging are thought to be major factors causing increased suspiciousness in older people

SCIENCE AND PROFESSION

Growing numbers of old and very old people and the increased complexity of diagnosis and treatment of this age group have driven the growth of geriatric psychiatry. Psychiatrists who specialize in working with the geriatric population note that the psychiatric problems experienced by older people often fit poorly in the diagnostic categories set down in the *Diagnostic and Statistical Manual of Mental Disorders: DSM-IV-TR* (4th ed., 2000). The interplay among declining physical health, decreasing mental functioning, social withdrawal and isolation, and vulnerability to stress makes proper diagnosis and appropriate treatment more difficult. In response to this complexity, practitioners of geriatric psychiatry tend to take a broader approach to diagnosis and to use an interdisciplinary model in developing a treatment plan. The profession of geriatric psychiatry has developed most in Great Britain and Canada but is attracting growing numbers of practitioners in the United States and other Western countries.

DIAGNOSTIC AND TREATMENT TECHNIQUES

Geriatric psychiatrists tend to follow the lead of specialists in geriatric medicine, who have found that taking a syndromal approach to diagnosis appears to work better with older patients.

Among the psychiatric syndromes used by geriatric psychiatrists are acute confusion, anxiety, depression, hypochondriasis, insomnia, memory loss, and suspiciousness. Special attention must be given by geriatric psychiatrists to the older person's overall ability to function, general health status, social support system, family history, and preexisting conditions. Geriatric psychiatrists are forced to acknowledge the role played by changes in the brain as it ages and to separate changes that are relatively benign from those that pose real threats to the patient. Hospitalization and significant medical intervention tend to occur more often in the later stages of a person's life, and geriatric psychiatrists are aware that these events can have a great impact on the patient's mental well-being.

When they can, geriatric psychiatrists draw readily upon the help of other health-care providers in treating elderly persons, including the use of specially qualified clinical psychologists, social workers, nurses, occupational therapists, speech pathologists, dietitians, and physical therapists. Improving the understanding of family members and providing them with supportive advice and services can be an important part of the overall treatment plan.

With the aging baby boomer population, the number of older women in the United States will continue to increase significantly. Older women with mood disorders and schizophrenia that began in their early adulthood will continue to require psychiatric treatment, although these treatments may need to be modified with age. Late-onset depression is more common among older women than older men for a variety of reasons: illness, widowhood, loss of support structures, financial stress, and the like. Late-onset schizophrenia and bipolar disorders are less common in aging women, but they affect older women more often than older men; studies indicate that women experience late-onset schizophrenia at nearly double the rate of men and perhaps as much as twenty-two times the rate of men. Psychiatric issues related to Alzheimer's disease and care giving also affect the psychological well-being of older women. Anxiety disorders, including general anxiety disorder, are more common among older women than among older men. Clinicians will remain alert to the need to prescribe lower doses of psychiatric medications to aging women to reduce side effects. These medications might worsen physical conditions, including metabolic syndromes, Parkinson's disease, low blood pressure, and fracture.

PERSPECTIVE AND PROSPECTS

In the United States, federal funding has expanded for qualified providers, such as clinical psychologists and social workers, to render mental health services to older people, especially those who live in long-term care facilities. Funds have increased for the proper training of those who provide mental health services to older people. Examinations have been established to show evidence of "added qualifications" in geriatric medicine and psychiatry. More textbooks and specialty journals devoted to geriatric mental health are now in circulation. The federal government has sponsored important national conferences on various aspects of geriatric mental health. With the costs of hospital and long-term care continuing to rise, more emphasis has been given to preventive services and day-care services.

Furthermore, some hospitals have established specialized geropsychiatric units to improve diagnosis and treatment and to decrease the time that older people spend in the hospital. Services are expected to increase for adult children who care for older parents with mental illnesses. Research efforts have increased concerning the causes and appropriate treatment of psychiatric problems in older people. Older people are becoming healthier as they learn more about how mental health and physical health are affected by the way in which one lives. They are advised to stop smoking, eat a better diet, exercise more, and continue to take an active part in family and community life. All these trends are expected to continue in the future.

—*Russell Williams, M.S.W.*
Updated by Michael J. O'Neal

FOR FURTHER INFORMATION

Andreasen, Nancy C., and Donald W. Black. *Introductory Textbook of Psychiatry.* 5th ed. Washington, D.C.: American Psychiatric Press, 2011.

Bee, Helen L., and Barbara L. Bjorklund. *The Journey of Adulthood.* 7th ed. Upper Saddle River, N.J.: Prentice Hall, 2011.

Birren, James E., and K. Warner Schaie, editors. *Handbook of the Psychology of Aging.* 7th ed. Boston: Academic Press/Elsevier, 2011.

Blazer, Dan G., Dan G. Blazers, and David C., Steffens, editors. *Essentials of Geriatric Psychiatry.* Washington, D.C.: American Psychiatric Publishing, 2012.

Lavretsky, Helen, Martha Sajatovic, and Charles F. Reynolds, eds. *Late-Life Mood Disorders.* New York: Oxford University Press, 2013.

Lehmann, S. W. "Psychiatric Disorders in Older Women." *International Review of Psychiatry* 15, no. 3 (August 2003): 269–79.

Miller, Mark D., and Lalith Kumar K Solai, editors. *Geriatric Psychiatry.* New York: Oxford University Press, 2013.

Sadock, Benjamin J., and Virginia A. Sadock, eds. *Kaplan and Sadock's Comprehensive Textbook of Psychiatry.* 9th ed. Philadelphia: Lippincott Williams & Wilkins, 2009.

Puberty and adolescence

CATEGORY: Biology

KEY TERMS:

contrasexual pubertal development: development of male characteristics in pubescent girls

estrogen: the chemical compound produced by the female ovaries that is involved in the regulation of menstrual periods and in the development of female sexual traits

gonadotropins: chemical compounds produced by the pituitary gland of the brain that cause the growth and maturation of the gonads

gonads: the reproductive organs; the ovaries in females and the testes (testicles) in males

hormones: chemical messengers produced in one part of the body that greatly influence activity in another part; examples include the gonadotropins estrogen and testosterone

ovaries: the female reproductive organs, which contain the ova (eggs); the ovaries are almond-shaped and are found in the lower pelvic area

pituitary gland: a small structure located near the base of the brain that produces the gonadotropins

premature adrenarch: the appearance of public hair without any other signs of puberty

premature menarch: the onset of periods without other signs of puberty

premature thelarche: development of breasts without any other sign of puberty

testes: the male reproductive organs and the site of sperm production; also known as the testicles *testosterone:* the male sex hormone produced by the testes and responsible for the male sexual traits; a small amount is also produced by the adrenal glands in females and is responsible for the growth of hair during adolescence in both sexes

CAUSES AND SYMPTOMS

The development period known as adolescence encompasses a host of biochemical, physical, and psychological changes in an individual that result in maturation as an adult capable of sexual reproduction. Collectively, the biochemical changes that lead to sexual maturity are called puberty. The process occurs over several years, and its time of onset is difficult to detect because the initial physical changes are quite subtle. For boys and girls in the United States and Western Europe during the last half of the twentieth century, the average age at which the onset of puberty occurred was between eight and thirteen years in girls, and nine and fourteen years in boys. Medical researchers are noting an earlier onset of puberty for many children around the world, but the reasons for this shift are not yet well understood.

One of the most dramatic physical changes that occurs in puberty is a tremendous growth spurt. The rate of height increases per year doubles as compared with height gain prior to puberty. On the average, girls gain approximately 3 inches of height during this period, and boys grow by about 8 inches.

The bulk of this growth is accounted for by an elongation of the thigh bones, followed by growth in the trunk. During this time, the thighs become wider, and shoulder width also increases. Both sexes accumulate fat during early puberty. Boys frequently appear rather chubby early in adolescence, but they generally lose this excess fat during their growth spurt. Most of this accumulated fat in girls is redistributed on their bodies and results in the typically curved silhouette. The average girl gains approximately 25 pounds during the adolescent period, while boys gain about 40 pounds, most of which is in the form of muscle.

Additional physical changes that occur during adolescence include changes in the facial bones, especially an elongation of the jawbone. Muscle size and strength increase during puberty, with a boy's development in this area extending years past the end of muscle strength increase in the typical girl. Prior to puberty, muscular strength is equivalent in both sexes, but the increase stops at the time of the first menstrual period in girls. Each of the major organs of the body, including the digestive tract, liver, kidneys, and heart, increases in size for both sexes during puberty. The size and activity of various glands adjust to reflect their increasing or decreasing role in the maturing individual.

Both girls and boys experience a characteristic increase in the distribution of hair on their bodies. Axillary (armpit) hair and pubic hair increase in density and coarseness, finally achieving the characteristic adult pattern.

Major alterations in the reproductive systems of boys and girls occur during puberty. In girls, the vagina enlarges and undergoes changes in chemical composition and cellular structure, and it begins producing typical adult secretions. Menarche, the first menstrual period, takes place even though ovulation (the maturation and release of an egg by the ovaries) may not occur for many months. The ovaries increase in size, and chemical changes prepare them to ovulate on a monthly basis. Breasts evolve from the pre-adolescent form to that of adult women. Boys undergo enlargement of the testicles, which are experiencing biochemical changes that prepare them for the continuous process of sperm production, as well as enlargement of the penis.

Because of the complexity of the many physical changes that occur during puberty, as well as the wide variation in the normal age of onset of this period, physicians have adopted a "sex maturity rating" scale to aid in their assessment of normal adolescent development. For both sexes, a rating of 1 (least mature) to 5 (most mature) is used to rank information collected by the visual observation of secondary sexual characteristics. For girls, breast and pubic hair development are the physical traits assessed. Boys are ranked based on the appearance of their genitals (penis and testicles) and the amount and distribution of their pubic hair.

All these physical changes are the direct result of global biochemical changes occurring in the adolescent's body. Just prior to puberty, a hormone called luteinizing hormone-releasing factor (LHRF) is produced by a portion of the brain called the hypothalamus. The LHRF travels to another structure in the brain, the pituitary gland. Upon receiving this hormonal signal, the pituitary gland produces two additional hormones called gonadotropins. The gonadotropins stimulate the development and enlargement of the ovaries in girls and the testicles in boys. As a result of the stimulation of the gonadotropins, the gonads produce sex hormones; the ovaries produce estrogen, and the testes produce testosterone. Females also produce a small amount of testosterone in the adrenal glands, which are located above the kidneys. These sex hormones enter the bloodstream and signal the start of the physical changes associated with puberty.

Examples of the effects of these hormones include the development of axillary hair in both boys and girls, which is initiated and maintained by testosterone. Breast development in girls is triggered by the estrogen produced by the ovaries. Maturation of the larynx in boys is accomplished by the action of testosterone. The other physical changes noted above are the result of sex hormones working alone or in concert with each other and of hormonal action on the genetic information of the individual.

The psychological changes that take place during puberty, although normal, may be dramatic. Thinking and cognitive skills mature during this period, accompanied by a tendency to analyze the rules and values of families, friends, and society. Frequently, this is a period of rebellion against parents and other authority figures. The confusion frequently associated with the rapid changes in adolescents' bodies and minds and their changing perceptions of their role in the world, coupled with the beginnings of adult responsibility, can lead to problems with self-esteem, anxiety, and depression. Critical and unreasonable self-assessment of appearance and abilities may lead to psychological illness. Socialization and self-identity come into prominence in the adolescent's life and can result in additional confusion, feelings of rejection, and experimentation with alcohol and drugs.

Sexual feelings are awakened in the adolescent and can be particularly challenging to understand and channel in an appropriate and responsible manner. Discovery of a sexual orientation contrary to heterosexual interests can create severe psychological problems for the adolescent because of fear of rejection by family and society. The possibilities of pregnancy or fatherhood or the contraction of a sexually transmitted disease may add gravity to early sexual explorations. Many groups argue that adolescents should have access to accurate and nonjudgmental information on contraception and disease prevention.

COMPLICATIONS AND DISORDERS

A number of medical disorders can result from abnormalities in the biochemical processes that mediate puberty. Other, less serious varieties of physical afflictions are natural and temporary side effects of the normal changes that accompany adolescence. Psychological disturbances may be associated with the extensive upheaval in the physical, mental, and social aspects of an adolescent's life, and in most cases they do not reach severe proportions. In some instances, however, professional intervention is indicated.

If the onset of puberty is not evident by age thirteen in girls or age fourteen in boys, or if puberty is initiated but little progression is observed for six to twelve months, detailed medical evaluation of the situation is recommended. Oral histories and a complete physical examination are conducted, and the individual's sex maturity rating is determined. The level of the gonadotropic hormones will first be assessed in order to determine if the delay of puberty is caused by a lack of the gonad-stimulating hormones produced by the brain or if the sex hormone production by the gonads is deficient.

A permanent deficiency in the amount of gonadotropic hormones produced by the pituitary gland prevents the sex organs from maturing and producing the sex hormones estrogen (in girls) and testosterone (in boys). This syndrome is referred to as hypogonadotropic hypogonadism and can be caused by a variety of central nervous system abnormalities.

Congenital defects (abnormalities present at birth) in the pituitary gland can inhibit the production of gonadotropins. Likewise, tumors at certain positions in the brain, including the pituitary gland, may block hormone production. Deficiency in another hormone, human growth hormone, results in short stature and delayed puberty. Other conditions, such as genetic abnormalities, chronic disease, pathologies of the thyroid gland or its functions, malnutrition, and excessive exercise, can also be the root cause of delayed puberty.

Delayed puberty can also be caused by failure of the ovaries or testes to mature despite normal levels of gonadotropins produced by the brain. In the vast majority of cases, the root cause of this syndrome, hypogonadotropic hypogonadism, is linked to defects in the normal chromosomal complement of the individual; that is, it is a genetic defect. Usually, it is caused by the presence of abnormal sex chromosomes and is diagnosed by examination of the chromosomes by a procedure called karyotyping.

A third category of delayed puberty is termed "constitutional delay in puberty." At the latest extreme of what is classified as the "average" age of onset of puberty, the individual's stature may be short, menarche may be delayed in girls, and the sex maturity ranking for both sexes would be low. In reality, these individuals are merely slightly beyond the age of onset considered "normal" and will, without medical intervention, proceed through normal puberty and develop into fully mature adults of normal height. Patience and close observation of changes are the best course of action in cases of constitutional delay in puberty.

True cases of precocious puberty-that is, puberty with an extremely early onset because of physical or biochemical abnormalities- are extremely rare, occurring in about one in every ten thousand children. In these cases, there is usually a defect in one or more of the glands producing the hormones that initiate puberty. Skilled medical diagnosis is indicated in these cases. When puberty begins much earlier than expected, the physician will check for a number of potentially serious problems such as adrenal gland disorders, reproductive system cysts, nervous system disorders, and thyroid abnormalities. Early pubertal onset is considered to be prior to eight and one-half years in girls or nine and one-half years in boys.

Acne, or pimples and blackheads on the skin of the face and upper back, commonly appears during adolescence. This skin disorder is a by-product of the hormones produced at puberty, which also stimulate the production of oil in the glands of the face and back. Acne may be treated with over-the-counter remedies and frequent washing of the skin, and it usually disappears as the individual approaches adulthood. In some severe cases, however, in which infection and scarring are distinct possibilities, medical intervention is recommended.

Preoccupation with personal appearance, difficulties with self-esteem, and a host of other psychological factors connected with the upheavals experienced during adolescence can lead to eating disorders.

Anorexia nervosa, which will affect about 0.9 percent of women during their lifetime, is a syndrome characterized by extremely low food intake, preoccupation with losing weight, maintaining a weight that is more than 15 percent below a normal level for age and height, disturbed perception of personal weight (seeing oneself as obese when one is pathologically thin), and (in girls) skipping three or more sequential menstrual periods. This is a serious disorder and is fatal for approximately 5 percent of affected individuals. Death is related to the extremely poor nutritional state of these patients; it may occur from heart failure or kidney failure, among other causes, and is associated with diseases afflicting the entire body. A physician's supervision, psychological counseling, and behavioral modification are very successful in the improvement of patients with this disorder.

Bulimia nervosa is characterized by "binge-purge" cycles of rapid, uncontrolled eating followed by self-induced vomiting, the use of laxatives, and extreme dieting. For a diagnosis of bulimia, which will affect about 1.5 percent of women during their lifetime, these episodes must occur at least twice a week for three months. In contrast to anorectics, bulimics are of normal to slightly above normal weight, so are not as often suspected of having an eating disorder. Bingeing and purging usually occur in private. Severe medical consequences of the behavior include cardiac arrest, rupture of the esophagus (the tube that runs from the mouth to the stomach), eroding of tooth enamel, and severe dehydration. As with anorexia, medical intervention and psychological counseling are necessary to control and defeat this harmful behavioral pattern.

There are other common physical complaints for adolescents during this period. "Growing pains" are a very real phenomenon during the rapid growth period of puberty. Sharp pains, especially in the legs, may sometimes awaken the sleeping adolescent. This discomfort is best treated with massage or a mild over-the-counter pain reliever. Pain associated with menstrual periods is common in adolescent, as well as adult, females. In most cases, over-the-counter medications provide relief, but in severe cases, or when pain is associated with heavy menstrual flow, a physician's intervention is recommended.

Depression, a feeling of gloom and hopelessness about the present and the future, is a disorder that may afflict the adolescent. Many factors can provoke or heighten depression, including rejection by peers and/or parents, chronic illness, economic turmoil, severe family problems, and stress associated with school. Frequently, the situation quickly resolves itself, but if depression occurs for an extended period (for days or weeks, depending on the teenager), medical intervention and psychological counseling are recommended. Untreated depression can lead to eating and sleeping disorders, a desire to escape problems through the abuse of drugs or alcohol, severe behavioral problems, or psychosomatic disorders such as headaches, chest pains, stomach problems, and fatigue.

Anxiety, unfocused fear that sometimes leads to extreme situations including panic attacks, is another psychological disorder sometimes associated with puberty. The most severe outcome of depression and/or anxiety is suicide. Any indication that a teenager is considering suicide, no matter how seemingly inconsequential, must be taken seriously; medical and psychological intervention must be obtained at once.

PUBERTY IN GIRLS

Researchers and clinicians identify a number of causes for puberty disorders in girls. Among them are heredity, hormonal disorders (including polycystic ovary syndrome, a set of symptoms associated with elevated androgen levels), genetic disorders, pituitary or thyroid problems that interfere with secretion of hormones needed for body growth and development, chromosomal disorders, eating disorders, excessive exercise, tumors, infections, and chemotherapy. Among girls, symptoms may include lack of breast development by age thirteen, lack of public hair by age fourteen, and more than five years between breast development and menarche. Clinicians will also be alert to girls whose periods have not started by age sixteen and those who show breast growth, pubic hair, and other signs of puberty before age seven or eight. Types of puberty disorders that affect girls include delayed puberty (i.e., puberty has not started by age thirteen), precocious puberty (i.e., puberty begins before age seven or eight), contrasexual pubertal development (i.e., development of male characteristics in girls), premature thelarche (i.e., development of breasts without any other sign of puberty), premature menarche (i.e., periods start without other signs of puberty, and premature adrenarche (that is, the appearance of public hair without any other signs of puberty).

It is worth noting that the leading causes of death and disability among adolescent girls are injuries sustained in motor vehicle accidents and interpersonal violence.

PERSPECTIVE AND PROSPECTS

Extensive historical evidence dating back as far as the time of Aristotle (384-322 BCE) suggests that the onset of puberty in modern times occurs much earlier than at most other periods of recorded history. Nevertheless, there are many exceptions to this trend. During times of severe stress-for example, in Western Europe during World War II-the age of onset of puberty was several years later than in calmer political times.

Many factors are responsible for the earlier onset of adolescence in Western societies, including improved nutrition and elevated economic status. Improved public health, in terms of immunizations to prevent and treatment to cure childhood diseases, likewise contributes to the improved health of the individual and onset of puberty at an earlier age. Modern society, however, creates stresses that in some cases delay the age of pubertal onset. These factors include poverty, the divorce and remarriage of parents, separation from siblings, and increasing responsibilities assigned to children whose parents are unavailable to the child for much of the day.

In cases of delayed puberty attributable to deficiencies in gonadotropin production or a failure of the gonads to mature despite adequate levels of gonadotropins, medical intervention can compensate for the resulting physical immaturity. Boys can be given increasing doses of testosterone over a period of time, which will lead to the development of the external physical traits characteristic of puberty. Girls initially may be given oral doses of estrogen and then be given a combination of estrogen and another sex hormone, progesterone, as therapy progresses. These hormones lead to normal external pubertal development in most cases.

Some individuals with delayed puberty are deficient in human growth hormone and also experience greatly shortened stature as compared with the normal range of heights for other individuals in their age group. Until the 1980s, human growth hormone was isolated from cadavers, and its cost was prohibitively high for most people. With the revolution in recombinant DNA technology, human growth hormone is synthesized quite cheaply and is available to individuals who need it. Unfortunately, the accessibility of this drug creates the possibility of its abuse by parents who want their normal children to be exceptionally large and strong.

In the latter third of the twentieth century, psychologists and other health professionals began to recognize an increase in the rate of disturbed behavior exhibited by adolescents. These behavioral anomalies included alcohol and drug abuse, promiscuity (with the accompanying risk of infection with sexually transmitted diseases and/or pregnancy), depression, and suicide. Educators, health professionals, and concerned adults recognize these syndromes and address them through counseling, medication when indicated, outreach programs, and peer counseling programs, among other efforts. As the medical and psychological communities gain further understanding of the physical, psychological, and social consequences of puberty, additional interventions will be developed to smooth out this turbulent period of human development.

—Karen E. Kalumuck, Ph.D.;
Updated by Lenela Glass-Godwin, M.W.S.
and Michael J. O'Neal

FOR FURTHER INFORMATION

Garrod, Andrew, et al. *Adolescent Portraits: Identity, Relationships, and Challenges.* 6th ed. Boston: Pearson/Allyn & Bacon, 2008.

Kroger, Jane. *Identity Development: Adolescence Through Adulthood.* 2d ed. Thousand Oaks, Calif.: Sage, 2007.

Santrock, John W. *Adolescence.* 13th ed. Boston: McGraw-Hill, 2010.

Pulmonary diseases

CATEGORY: Disease/Disorder

KEY TERMS:

alveoli: the many tiny air sacs at the ends of the terminal bronchioles, where oxygen and carbon dioxide are exchanged

asthma: a condition in which spasms of the bronchial smooth muscle cause narrowing and constriction of the airways

bronchi: the branching airways from the single large trachea to the multiple terminal bronchioles

bronchoscopy: a procedure that uses a flexible or rigid fiberoptic telescope to visualize the bronchial tree directly; it also permits samples of tissue to be removed for analysis

cancer: a tumor (or growth) of abnormal, genetically transformed cells that invade and destroy normal tissue; also referred to as a malignancy

emphysema: progressive destruction of the alveolar walls, leading to highly inflated and stiffened lungs

interstitial pulmonary fibrosis (IPF): the scarring and thickening (fibrosis) of the lung tissue, which causes breathing difficulty, chest pain, coughing, and shortness of breath; the lungs become increasingly stiffer until heart failure ensues

pathology: the study of the nature and consequences of disease

pleurisy: the inflammation and swelling of the pleurae, the membranes that enclose the lungs and line the chest cavity; a complication of several pulmonary diseases

pneumonia: an inflammation of the lung tissue in which the alveolar sacs fill with fluid

pulmonary: the Latin word for lung, used to describe both the lung tissue and the bronchial tree

respiration: a process that includes both air conduction (the act of breathing) and gas exchange (oxygen and carbon dioxide transfer between the air and blood)

CAUSES AND SYMPTOMS

Disorders of the pulmonary system are among the most common diseases. Because it acts as an interface between the external and internal environments, the pulmonary system is subject to continual attacks on its health and integrity. A wide variety of disease-causing agents reach the lung with each breath. Infectious organisms (such as bacteria, viruses, and molds), environmental toxins (such as tobacco smoke and air pollutants), and various airborne allergens are the primary causes of lung disease.

The pulmonary system consists of an intricate bronchial tree terminating in very delicate, thin-walled sacs known as alveoli, each of which is surrounded by blood vessels. The entire network is contained within the supporting tissue of the lungs. These individual parts are perfectly suited to efficiently carry out their two life-sustaining functions: air conduction and the gas exchange between oxygen in the air and carbon dioxide (a waste product) in the bloodstream. Disruption of either function renders a person vulnerable to potentially fatal consequences.

All pulmonary diseases can be categorized in two ways. The first is based on the cause, such as a virus, asbestos, or cigarette smoke; the second is based on the result, the specific loss of a structure and its function. Infectious diseases are the most common causes of respiratory problems. Infection usually occurs through inhalation, although it can come from another source within the body as well. A vast number of microorganisms are trapped by the hairs, mucus, and immune system cells that line the respiratory tract. Those that are not repelled generally infect the upper tract, namely the nose and throat, but it is the few that reach the bronchi and lungs that cause the most serious illnesses—bronchitis, pneumonia, and tuberculosis.

Bronchitis, an inflammation of the bronchial tree, is the result of viruses or bacteria that invade the airways and infect the bronchial cells. In a counterattack, the body responds by sending large numbers of immune system cells (white blood cells), which destroy the invaders both by direct contact and by releasing chemical substances. The inflamed bronchi begin to leak significant amounts of fluids, producing the most obvious symptom of bronchitis: a frequent cough that yields initially clear white and later yellow or green phlegm. Rarely does bronchitis progress to serious disability; more often it resolves, although recurrence is common.

Unlike bronchitis, pneumonia is extremely serious. It can develop from bronchitis or can occur as a primary infection. Pneumonia is an infection that goes beyond the airways into the alveoli and supporting lung tissue. While the process of the disease is the same as that of bronchitis, fluid accumulates not only in the bronchi but also in the alveolar sacs, which cannot be efficiently cleared by coughing. The normally air-filled sacs, now fill with fluid, and cannot perform their vital function of gas exchange. If the fluid continues to accumulate, larger and larger areas

of lung become unable to function, and the person literally drowns.

In the case of tuberculosis (TB), one specific bacterium (*Mycobacterium tuberculosis*) is inhaled, generally from the spray of coughs or sneezes of infected persons. The bacterium settles in the bronchus, where it begins to invade and multiply. Unlike the organisms that cause bronchitis and pneumonia, it passes through the airways into the substance of the lung. Again, the body reacts in an attempt to confine the organisms" spread by forming walled-off circular areas (cavities) around the destruction. Up to this point, the person may have been only minimally ill. However, while the cavities are successful at containing the spread, some bacteria within them may not have been killed and remain dormant for many years. Later, when the person's immune system is weakened by disease, alcoholism, drug abuse, or another disorder, the bacteria reawaken and invade the lung, producing massive destruction and the loss of both structure and function. If it is left untreated, the result is death.

Though men are more affected by TB, women can experience particularly severe consequences, especially during pregnancy. An expecting mother with TB is six times as likely to lose her baby and two times as likely to birth a child prematurely or with low birth weight. Pregnant women who have both HIV and TB are 400% more at risk of both maternal and infant mortality.

In ways different from infectious diseases, toxic substances such as tobacco smoke cause severe disability and death either through permanent structural damage (emphysema) or by transforming respiratory cells into abnormal ones (lung cancer). Many toxic chemicals are released when tobacco is burned, and these substances affect the entire lining of the respiratory tract both in the short term and in the long term. In the immediate period, the small hairs that line the upper tract no longer function to filter the air, and large amounts of fluid enter the airways because they are constantly inflamed, producing the familiar smokers' cough. As the irritation continues for years, permanent damage ensues.

Emphysema, which is present in nearly all smokers to some degree, is characterized by widespread destruction of the walls of individual alveolar sacs. As adjacent walls break, the alveoli coalesce into very large, balloon-like structures. The supporting lung tissue, which is normally soft and spongy, becomes stiff and hard, making breathing very difficult. Although the lungs become overinflated, the air is stale as it is unable to move in and out with each breath. The picture of a patient with severe emphysema is dramatic: the patient labors forcefully with an open mouth, trying unsuccessfully to draw air in and out. Both air conduction and gas exchange are seriously affected. If lung function falls below a critical minimum, death occurs.

A combination of chronic bronchitis and emphysema results in chronic obstructive pulmonary disease (COPD), which is now the third leading cause of death in the U.S. The disease often presents few symptoms until it is well-developed in the lungs, usually detected when an individual is over fifty years old. COPD results in a chronic cough and shortness of breath that progressively limits tolerance to physical activity. These symptoms are exacerbated over time and further progression of COPD may affect the heart if the lungs can no longer supply adequate amounts of oxygen to the body. Traditionally, COPD affected more men than women, but the prevalence and mortality rate of the disease has risen more dramatically for women than men. Women made up 53% of COPD deaths in 2009. These changing trends may be due to changing smoking habits and women taking on more traditionally "male" occupations in factories and industrial plants. Individuals who identify as "never-smokers" and develop COPD are 1.5 times more likely to be women.

Lung cancer is a major health problem, claiming tens of thousands of lives each year in the United States alone, more than any other cancer. The mechanism by which toxic substances transform normal cells into cancer cells is complex, involving damage to the cells' genetic material. Many factors interact to allow cancer cells to grow into tumors, including the failure of the immune system to destroy these abnormal cells. Tumors may form in either the bronchial tree or the substance of the lung itself. In either case, the end result is the same: the tumor destroys normal structure by compression and invasion, replacing large areas of lung. Cancer cells also enter the bloodstream and travel to distant sites in the body, where they can grow into equally destructive tumors.

Although lung cancer is often associated with smoking cigarettes, and indeed 85% of individuals with the disease have a history of cigarette use, only 20% of smokers develop lung cancer. This suggests that other factors, including genetics, gender, diet, previous pulmonary diseases and occupational exposure may predispose an individual toward the development of lung cancer. As in COPD, women with lung cancer are 2 to 3 times as likely as men to have never smoked. Possible reasons for this increased susceptibility in women include biological differences including nicotine metabolism, hormonal effects, and an individual's ability to repair damaged DNA. Women seem to survive lung cancer better than men: five-year survival rates for women were 37%, compared to 19% in men.

A pulmonary disease that affects nearly 40 million adults as well as children is asthma. The trachea and bronchial tree of an asthmatic are highly sensitive to a variety of stimuli as diverse as cold air, dust, exercise, and emotional stress. The bronchial muscles respond to the agent by spasm, producing narrow, constricted airways. Thick secretions are released that plug the bronchial tree and add to the serious decline in air conduction. An asthma attack may range from mild bronchial contractions to life-threatening closure. Many asthmatic patients have multiple allergies to foods, animal dander, plant pollen, dust, and so on, implying that their respiratory systems respond abnormally to otherwise harmless substances. Asthma is usually a lifelong problem, and while most attacks subside, death can occur.

Young boys are more likely to have asthma than young girls, but around puberty that statistic shifts and may be related to changing and increasing sex hormones. Asthma tends to become more prevalent, with more severe symptoms, in female patients as they age, while the inverse is true for males. Women with premenstrual asthma require more corticosteroid therapy and are at a higher risk for emergency room visits and hospitalization. As men and women age, another shift occurs. Men over 45 are more at risk of developing severe asthma than women and between 50 to 65 asthma severity drops for women, suggesting that menopause may be a protective factor in asthma cases.

Some respiratory conditions seem to affect women almost exclusively, including pulmonary hypertension (high blood pressure in the lungs' arteries), catamenial pneumothorax (collapsed lung occurring

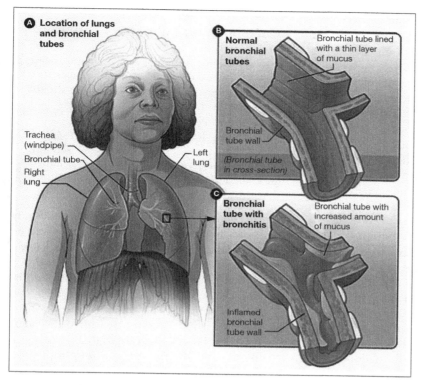

A Location of lungs and bronchial tubes

Trachea (windpipe)
Bronchial tube
Right lung
Left lung

B Normal bronchial tubes
Bronchial tube lined with a thin layer of mucus
Bronchial tube wall
(Bronchial tube in cross-section)

C Bronchial tube with bronchitis
Bronchial tube with increased amount of mucus
Inflamed bronchial tube wall

Figure A shows the location of the lungs and bronchial tubes in the body. Figure B is an enlarged, detailed view of a normal bronchial tube. Figure C is an enlarged, detailed view of a bronchial tube with bronchitis. The tube is inflamed and contains more mucus than usual. (National Heart Lung and Blood Institute via Wikimedia Commons)

within 72 hours before or after menstruation), and pregnancy-related asthma exacerbation.

TREATMENT AND THERAPY

The most common symptoms associated with pulmonary disease are coughing, chest pain, and shortness of breath. Because each of these symptoms is present in such a wide variety of pulmonary diseases, it often is necessary to use other tools to determine the specific illness present. The most important of these diagnostic tools is the chest x-ray, in which nonspecific symptoms can be correlated with structural and functional abnormalities. A critical advancement in the use of x-rays is the computed tomography (CT) scan. Using a computer, a large number of detailed x-rays are combined to create a very detailed picture, allowing an ambiguous abnormality on a chest x-ray to be visualized with much greater accuracy. If further information is needed in order to determine the

exact nature of an abnormality revealed by the chest x-ray and the CT scan, a sample of lung tissue must be obtained.

The bronchoscope, a flexible or rigid fiber-optic tube, is passed through the mouth into the bronchial tree, allowing direct inspection of the pulmonary system. Performed using anesthesia in the hospital operating room, bronchoscopy can be used to remove a small amount of tissue for biopsy. While the procedure has a higher risk than either the chest x-ray or the CT scan, it also has a high yield of information.

Once a specific diagnosis is made, treatment is begun that addresses the particular cause or resulting dysfunction. Infectious agents such as those causing bronchitis, pneumonia, and tuberculosis have the most direct treatment, antibiotics. These drugs, first discovered in the early part of the twentieth century, revolutionized modern medicine. Penicillin, sulfa drugs, erythromycin, and tetracycline are among the most useful antibiotics for pulmonary infections. The particular microorganisms that are destroyed are specific to each drug, although significant overlap exists. Diseases that once claimed millions of lives can now be successfully cured.

Patients with asthma, lung cancer, and emphysema are not as fortunate. All these conditions are progressive pulmonary diseases: asthma can remain stable for years but causes significant disability, emphysema slowly worsens, and lung cancer is sometimes curable but is frequently fatal. No cure exists for asthma; treatment is directed at alleviating the symptoms. The drugs that are used fall into three categories: those that reverse the bronchial constriction and open the airways (epinephrine, methylxanthines), those that reduce the inflammation and hence the thick mucus secretions (steroids), and those that attempt to stabilize respiratory cells, decreasing their abnormal response to stimuli (cromolyn sodium).

During an asthma attack, epinephrine and similar acting compounds are administered through inhalation or as injections in order to relieve the spasms that dangerously narrow bronchial airways. Between attacks, patients may use nasal sprays that contain mild doses of epinephrine-like drugs, as well as steroids that reduce the inflammation associated with asthma. Two other commonly used medications are caffeinelike drugs known as methylxanthines, which also serve to open narrowed airways, and cromolyn sodium, an interesting substance that appears to stabilize the bronchial cells and prevent their hypersensitive reactions to various allergens. The reality of all these drugs is that although they reduce the severity of attacks, they do not prevent their occurrence.

Emphysema is more difficult than asthma to treat. The enlarged alveoli and stiffened surrounding lung tissue are permanent structural changes. Progression of the disease can be significantly reduced if, in the early stages, environmental insults, particularly smoking, cease. Patients with emphysema have frequent serious pulmonary infections because the defense mechanisms of the bronchial tree are severely impaired as well. Such repeated infections hasten the decline in respiratory function. Both air conduction and gas exchange are affected. Supplementing oxygen is the mainstay of treatment, both during sudden deterioration and in later stages. Eventually, when the lungs of the emphysema patient no longer function, mechanical ventilators (artificial respirators) are needed. Need for this technology generally heralds a fatal outcome. Lung cancer has the most dismal prospects of all the pulmonary diseases. Treatment has met with limited success because lung cancer becomes symptomatic relatively late in its course and because it is such an aggressive disease, spreading to other parts of the body. Three main modalities exist in attempting to cure lung cancer: surgical removal of the tumor and surrounding lung tissue, radiation therapy, and chemotherapy.

Surgery and radiation are localized treatments, while chemotherapy is systemic, reaching the whole body via the bloodstream. Very often, the latter two are used to alleviate symptoms when attempts at a cure fail. When lung cancer is discovered early, all three procedures may be used. Bronchoscopy allows a sample of the tumor to be analyzed, and based on various other findings, a treatment plan may be instituted that begins with surgically removing the mass. Radiation is then used in very controlled ways to destroy any remaining cancer cells in the surrounding

---

Information on Pulmonary Diseases

Causes: May include infection, environmental toxins (especially tobacco smoke), allergies, cancer

Symptoms: Frequent coughing, chest pain, wheezing, shortness of breath

Duration: Acute to chronic

Treatments: May include antibiotics, epinephrine, methylxanthines, steroids, cromolyn sodium, mechanical ventilators, surgery, radiation therapy, chemotherapy

---

lung tissue. If it is found that cancer cells have already spread to other regions— such as the bone, brain, or liver—then chemotherapy consisting of highly toxic drugs is given directly into the bloodstream in order to reach migrating cancer cells. Unfortunately, because lung cancer is an extremely destructive disease extending beyond its local site of inception to distant, unrelated organ systems, treatment has been disappointing and fatality rates are high.

A treatment modality that plays a very important role for many pulmonary diseases, and indeed has supported countless lives, is the respirator. This mechanical device, essentially an artificial lung, delivers a preset volume of air rich in oxygen into the lungs through a conducting tube that lies in the trachea, the largest airway, from which the right and left main bronchi divide. Although fraught with ethical issues about unnecessary prolongation of death and suffering, the artificial respirator is clearly indicated when the person will most likely fully recover from a sudden illness. In these cases, mechanical breathing can provide adequate oxygenation to the body as it repairs itself.

Death has long been defined as the cessation of respiration. Artificial respirators have forced a rethinking of that definition, which now requires cessation of brain activity. Many pulmonary diseases in their final stages lead to dependence on these mechanical ventilators. Many of these same diseases, and those of other systems that affect the lungs, can also cause sudden respiratory failure. Cardiopulmonary resuscitation (CPR) is a highly effective emergency procedure that essentially substitutes a rescuer for a machine. Through delivering exhaled air into the unconscious person and simultaneously compressing the chest, the critical functions of breathing and circulation are maintained. CPR is a simple procedure to learn, and one that has saved innumerable victims.

PERSPECTIVE AND PROSPECTS

Pulmonary diseases have caused an extraordinary number of deaths throughout human history. Whereas lung cancer claims the most lives today, infectious diseases, especially pneumonia, claimed many more lives in the thousands of years before the introduction of antibiotics in the early twentieth century. Many potentially fatal illnesses, particularly those that are viral in origin, are transmitted through the respiratory route. Because of the ease with which they can be spread—person to person, through coughs and sneezes—epidemics often occur. Rubella, measles, chickenpox, smallpox, mumps, diphtheria, and pertussis (whooping cough) are among such illnesses. Many of these viral diseases kill by secondary pneumonias that overwhelm the body's defense mechanisms.

The well-known rashes that occur in several of these illnesses are simply manifestations of viremia, the passage of viruses through the lungs into the bloodstream. Most of the victims of these diseases were children; indeed, these illnesses were among the principal reasons for the high child mortality rates. While antibiotics are ineffective in treating viral diseases (as opposed to bacterial or fungal diseases), vaccinations have proven very successful, reducing or even eliminating them. Two epidemic diseases that have killed millions of people throughout recorded history have been the pneumonic plague and influenza. Both have been somewhat controlled by improved sanitation (in the case of the plague) and improved vaccine programs (as with influenza). General sophistication in caring for the victims of these diseases has minimized mortality in those cases that do occur.

The plague has been feared since ancient times, and at least three major epidemics are known in which large portions of populations were destroyed. The first of these was recorded in Europe and Asia Minor during the sixth century, the second (known as the Black Death) was in the fourteenth century, and the last began in China in 1894, an epidemic that eventually spread to all continents, including North America, by 1900. The plague is an infectious disease caused by a bacterium that lives in the bodies of rodent fleas. It is transmitted to humans through bites of rat fleas in particular and enters the bloodstream. High fever, very enlarged and painful lymph glands, and severe weakness characterize the illness, which occurs a few days after the flea bite. In this stage of the disease, known as bubonic plague, the fatality rate ranged from 50 to 90 percent, but the disease was not contagious. As the infection spread from the bloodstream to lung tissue, a highly contagious pneumonia resulted that allowed person-to-person transmission through infectious droplets expelled by coughing. This form of the disease, pneumonic plague, was almost invariably fatal, with nearly 100 percent mortality within a few days of infection. Approximately one-half of the population of Europe died during the Black Death. Improved sanitation methods that separated the rat population from human habitations have played the most important role in stemming the outbreak of new epidemics. Such problems continue to exist in much of the developing world, however, and plagues still occur sporadically.

While influenza was not recorded well historically, the disastrous epidemic of 1918 proved just as deadly as the plague, killing 35 million people worldwide in a few short months. Because of immigration, the disease spread rapidly throughout Europe and North America within a few months. Influenza is caused by a virus and spread solely by the respiratory route, through inhalation. High fever, muscle and joint pain, coughing, chest pain, and weakness are common symptoms. The pneumonia that may develop within a few days of the onset of the illness can rapidly progress to death. Early twentieth- century medicine was completely overwhelmed by the number of cases and the severe pneumonia that followed. Vaccinations with killed virus particles have become routine preventive medicine for those most at risk: the elderly, the sick, and infants. The mortality associated with influenza in the past has been reduced but definitely not eliminated.

—Connie Rizzo, MD, PhD
Updated by Maria Haslip, PhD, RN

FOR FURTHER INFORMATION

American Lung Association. http://www.lungusa. org.

"Catamenial Pneumothorax." Genetic and Rare Diseases Information Center, U.S. Department of

Health and Human Services, 13 Oct. 2015, www.rarediseases.info.nih.gov/diseases/9858/catamenial-pneumothorax.

Hedrick, Hannah L., and Austin K. Kutscher, eds. *The Quiet Killer: Emphysema, Chronic Obstructive Pulmonary Disease.* Lanham, Md.: Scarecrow Press, 2002.

Olak, Jemi, and Yolanda Colson. "Gender Differences in Lung Cancer: Have We Really Come a Long Way, Baby?" *The Journal of Thoracic and Cardiovascular Surgery,* vol. 128, no. 3, 2004, 346–351.

Pinkerton, Kent E., et al. "Women and Lung Disease. Sex Differences and Global Health Disparities." *American Journal of Respiratory and Critical Care Medicine,* 192, no. 1, 2015, 11-6.

World Health Organization. *Tuberculosis in Women Fact Sheet.* World Health Organization, 25 Sept. 2018, www.who.int/tb/areas-of-work/population-groups/gender/en/.

Zein, Joe G and Serpil C Erzurum. "Asthma is Different in Women" *Current Allergy and Asthma Reports,* vol. 15, no. 6, 2015, 28.

R

Rape and sexual assault

CATEGORY: Social issue

KEY TERMS:

date rape: a forced sexual act during a date

deoxyribonucleic acid (DNA): genetic material contained in cells, which can definitively identify an individual

incest: a sexual act between close relatives such as father-daughter or brother-sister

perpetrator: an individual who commits a crime *sexual harassment:* physical behavior of a sexual nature that is aimed at a particular person or group of people, especially in the workplace or school

statutory rape: a sexual act with a child below the legal age of consent, even if the act is consensual

NATIONAL SEXUAL ASSAULT HOTLINE
1-800-656-4673

CAUSES AND SYMPTOMS

Rape is an act of violence; it is an expression of aggression and anger rather than a sexual motivated act. A power imbalance usually exists, with the stronger of two individuals committing the assault. The typical victim of rape is a sixteen- to twenty-four-year-old woman; however, any male, female, or child can be raped. Sexual assault has a broader definition than rape. In addition to vaginal, anal, or oral penetration, sexual assault includes inappropriate touching as well as any physical contact, speech, or presentation of images that an individual does not desire to consent to. Many types of rape and sexual assault exist, including spousal, incest, child, elder, date, acquaintance, coworker, stranger, and same-gender. Cases of women raping women or men also exist.

In the United States, the estimated lifetime prevalence of sexual assault is approximately 18 percent in females and 3 percent in males. The typical rapist is a twenty-five- to forty-four- year-old man who plans the attack and often may select a woman of the same race.

More than half of the time, the victim knows the rapist through work, friends, family, or by living in the perpetrator's neighborhood. More than 50 percent of rapes occur in the victim's home. The rapist may break in or gain entry through a ruse, such as posing as a salesman.

Compared with other men, rapists drink more heavily, begin having sexual experiences earlier, and are more likely to have been physically or sexually abused as children. Individuals who have been sexually assaulted as children are also more likely to be assaulted as adults. Many studies note that more than 50 percent of all physical and sexual assaults involve a perpetrator who was reported to have been drinking. Often, rape victims have also consumed alcohol before the incident (estimates run as high as 60 to 70 percent). Illegal drug use may also be a factor in rapes. The perpetrator may be under the influence of drugs or administer them to the victim. Date rape occurs when a sexual assault occurs during a date. The rapist often gives the victim drugs or alcohol; the most common date rape drug is alcohol. Regardless of the circumstances, victims of sexual abuse are not at fault and should never be blamed. For example, even if the victim is flirting on her date, this never gives another person the permission to make unwanted advances or acts. Most rapes are not reported to the police (80 to 90 percent by most estimates).

Immediately after a rape, the victim may exhibit the following symptoms: erratic behavior, confusion, crying, fear, nervousness, hostility, inappropriate laughter, sleep disturbances, anorexia, physical pain, and/or social withdrawal. Physical symptoms of rape include vaginal and rectal lacerations as well as injuries to other body parts. The presence of semen in the vagina or rectum, which can be subjected to DNA analysis for identification of the perpetrator, confirms the diagnosis of intercourse but not rape. Rape victims may suffer from posttraumatic stress syndrome, which may persist for years and have a marked impact on the victim's life. Following a rape, some victims abuse alcohol and/ or drugs; some become suicidal. More than 50 percent of rape victims develop difficulties with interpersonal relationships (such as with a husband or other partner).

TREATMENT AND THERAPY

Following a rape, the victim should proceed directly to a hospital without changing clothes, showering, douching, or urinating, as these activities may destroy evidence. Often, rape victims are referred to specialized centers that provide focused care and make certain that proper procedures are followed, including preserving the "chain of evidence." Chain of evidence refers to the proper handling of evidence (semen, hair samples, and skin samples) from the time of collection throughout the legal process. Specimens collected for forensic evaluation include mucosal swabs, skin swabs, fingernail clippings, hair samples, blood samples, saliva samples, the victim's clothes, and semen samples, if available. Sperm may be detected up to 72 hours after an assault in vaginal swabs, up to 24 hours in anal swabs, and are rarely detected in oral swabs. A complete evaluation of the victim may take up to six hours. In female victims, areas that should be carefully evaluated include the breasts, perineum, vagina, anus, and rectum.

Non-genital trauma is commonly seen on the victim's extremities, face, and/or neck, which may consist of bruising, abrasions, lacerations, and/or erythema. These are more likely to be present when the victim is examined within 72 hours of the assault, or if the perpetrator is a stranger. Colposcopy may be used to detect milder genital trauma and an ultraviolet (UV) light (ex: Wood's lamp) may assist in detecting semen on the skin. It is important to keep in mind that through this traumatic event, victims often do not know the exact right steps to take due to the emotional difficulty they are experiencing. Since many women do not report rapes at all, there are also times a woman may decide later on to pursue justice, when any physical evidence is gone.

Immediate care includes medical and surgical treatment of injuries, which may be significant. The victim-and, if possible, the rapist-should be tested for sexually transmitted diseases (STDs). Minimal screening consists of testing for gonorrhea, chlamydia, trichomonas, bacterial vaginosis, and candidiasis. Necessity to screen for human immunodeficiency virus (HIV) hepatitis, and syphilis should be

---

Information on Rape and Sexual Assault

Causes: For perpetrators, impulsive and antisocial tendencies, alcohol, illegal drug use, history of sexual abuse as child

Symptoms: For victims, vaginal and rectal tears, bruises, injury to other body parts

Duration: For rapists, many are repeat offenders, who will attempt rape for decades

Treatments: For perpetrators, psychological counseling, drug and alcohol rehabilitation, medication; for victims, medical, surgical, and psychiatric

---

determined on an individual basis. Victims may opt out of testing for STDs if he/she consents to prophylactic treatment. Prophylactic treatment for STDs is recommended due to the poor follow-up visit rates. Postexposure Hepatitis B vaccination is considered adequate protection against Hepatitis B, unless the perpetrator is known to have Hepatitis B. Prophylactic antiviral medications are controversial after a sexual assault.

The risk of HIV transmission after a single consensual episode of vaginal or anal intercourse is estimated to be 0.1-2 percent. Transmission after an assault is presumed to be higher, secondary to the trauma and bleeding. Risk and benefits should be discussed with the patient.

Pregnancy tests should be performed on any female of child-bearing age. If the possibility of exposure to pregnancy exists, then hormonal treatment can be administered to prevent that eventuality. Drug screening may also be performed to detect levels of alcohol, benzodiazepines (for example, the date rape drug, *Rohypnol*), gamma-hydroxy butyrate (GHB), or other common drugs of abuse.

In addition to treatment of the immediate physical and emotional trauma, follow-up care should be arranged. The victim may need long-term counseling, psychiatric care, and psychiatric medication. Posttraumatic stress disorder (PTSD), depression, and anxiety are commonly seen in victims. Victims may avoid any future pelvic exams, which then puts them at higher risk for cervical cancer.

Child molesters, serial rapists, and violent rapists are often given long-term prison sentences. While in prison, they are offered treatment; however, treatment cannot be enforced. An evaluation of sex offenders incarcerated at Atascadero State Hospital in California reported that 80 percent of sex offenders never participated in any treatment. Occasionally, some child molesters and repeat offenders are given suspended sentences or paroled after a short prison sentence.

Some of these offenders have committed further violent attacks, including murder of the rape victim. Sex offenders are required to register with local authorities so that their whereabouts can be made available to the public. Some states define a sexually violent predator as someone who commits a sexually violent crime and who has a mental abnormality or personality disorder. A number of researchers report a high level of success for rapists who undergo a treatment program. A standard premise for counseling and psychiatric care is that the rapist must admit that he or she has a problem for therapy to be successful.

PERSPECTIVE AND PROSPECTS

From the days of ancient Greece through the American colonial period, rape was deemed to be a capital offense. Rapists were subjected to a wide range of punishments, including beatings, castration, and execution. However, in colonial America, the rape of Native American women was not deemed to be a crime because the women were "Pagan and not Christian." Two centuries ago, rape was often not viewed as a type of physical assault; rather, it was deemed to be a serious property crime against the man to whom the woman belonged (her father or husband). The loss of virginity was a particularly serious matter. Under biblical law, if the father agreed, the rapist was required to marry his victim instead of receiving the civil penalty.

Anecdotal reports of rape during warfare have been described since antiquity-Greek, Roman, Persian, and Israelite armies reportedly engaged in rape. During the 1937 Nanking Massacre, it was reported that Japanese soldiers raped as many as 80,000 Chinese women over a six-week period. Anecdotally, by the end of World War II, Red Army soldiers were estimated to have raped approximately 2,000,000 German women and girls. During the 1994 Rwandan genocide, an estimated 500,000 women were raped. One study found that during

Liberia's thirteen-year-long civil war, 92 percent of the women interviewed had experienced sexual assault. Even today, rape is being used as a weapon of war in the Democratic Republic of Congo (DRC) to humiliate, dominate, and instill fear in the civilians of a community.

The medical literature contains numerous analyses of rape and sexual assault. In August 2009, researchers at St. Paul's Hospital in Vancouver, British Columbia, published a study that evaluated the sexual assault of prostitutes. They found an "alarming rate" of violence against these women. They recommended that the following steps were crucial to stem violence against prostitutes: socio-legal policy reforms, improved access to housing and drug treatment, and scaled-up violence prevention efforts, including police-prostitute partnerships.

Although young adult women are the most frequent targets of sexual assault, physical abuse of older women has risen rapidly during the last decade. In October 2009, researchers with the Michigan State University Program in Emergency Medicine published a study comparing a group of postmenopausal victims of sexual assault with younger adult women (eighteen to thirty-nine years old). During the five-year study period, 1,917 adult sexual assault victims qualified for inclusion in the study; 84 percent of the victims were eighteen to thirty-nine years old, and 4 percent were postmenopausal women who were at least fifty years old. The 72 postmenopausal victims were more likely to be assaulted by a single perpetrator, usually a stranger (56 percent versus 32 percent); to be assaulted in their own home (74 percent versus 46 percent); and to have experienced more physical coercion (72 percent versus 36 percent). The younger women were more likely to have used alcohol or illicit drugs before the assault (53 percent versus 18 percent) and to have a history of sexual assault (51 percent versus 15 percent).

Postmenopausal victims had a higher number of non-genital (2.3 percent versus 1.2 percent) as well as anal injuries (2.5 percent versus 1.8 percent). The authors concluded that postmenopausal women are not immune from sexual assault and that the epidemiology of sexual trauma in this age group is different from that of younger women.

Sexual harassment and assault are not uncommon at the workplace. A study published in August 2009, by the University of Southern Maine evaluated the frequency and impact of workplace sexual harassment on the health, work, and school outcomes on high school girls. They noted that sexual harassment has a significant impact on high school girls' connections to work and school; it not only taints their attitudes toward work but also threatens to undermine their commitment to school. They added that as a consequence of sexual harassment experienced at work, teenagers may have their career development or career potential impeded or threatened because of school absence and poor academic performance. In addition, they noted, the physical safety of working students may be at risk under these circumstances, which would create a need for teenagers to receive training to deal with sexual assault and other types of workplace violence.

As it is in adults, alcohol is a frequent component of adolescent peer-on-peer sexual aggression. A study published in September 2009 by the Institute for Research on Women and Gender, University of Michigan, examined the characteristics of adolescents involved in alcohol-related and nonalcohol-related sexual assault of peers. The researchers conducted a Web-based survey of 1,220 students (grades seven through twelve) and found that adolescents who reported alcohol-related and nonalcohol-related sexual aggression had higher levels of impulsivity and more extensive histories of dating, early sexual activity, and alcohol consumption than adolescents who did not assault. Furthermore, perpetrators of alcohol-related assault had higher levels of alcohol use in the past thirty days as well as more alcohol- or drug-related problems than perpetrators of nonalcohol-related assault.

A particularly heinous form of sexual assault is one on a child. In October 2009, investigators at the Crimes Against Children Research Center, University of New Hampshire, Durham, published a study that strove to obtain national estimates of exposure to the full spectrum of childhood violence, abuse, and crime. The researchers conducted a cross-sectional national telephone survey that involved 4,549 children up to age seventeen. The authors found that a clear majority (60.6 percent) of the children had either experienced or witnessed victimization in the previous year. Almost half (46.3 percent) had experienced a physical assault in the study year, almost 25 percent had experienced a property offense, about 10 percent had experienced a form of child maltreatment, 6.1 percent had experienced a sexual victimization, and about 25 percent had been a witness to violence or experienced another form of indirect victimization in the year (including 9.8 percent who had witnessed an intrafamily assault). About 10 percent had experienced a victimization-related injury. More than one-third (38.7 percent) had been exposed to two or more direct victimizations (10.9 percent had five or more, and 2.4 percent had 10 or more) during the study year.

A 2010-2011 survey of adolescents, between the ages of fourteen and twenty-one, revealed that 1 out of 10 adolescents had been the perpetrator of a sexual assault. An association was found with perpetrators and a higher exposure to violent X-rated media. Up to the age of seventeen, the majority of the perpetrators were male. Among those older than seventeen, females and males had an equal representation as perpetrators.

IMPACT ON WOMEN

The vast majority of rape and sexual assault victims are female. This has had a historical impact on women and their experiences in the world. From the time women were seen as male property to the use of rape as a weapon of war and domination, women have been continuously oppressed with sexual violence. Although in modern time women have made strides in equality, the sexual violence against women continues on at an alarming rate. Rape continues to be underreported, based on the burden of proof placed on the victim, re-traumatization of the legal systems approach and continued invalidation of women's experiences. It is essential to continue to emphasize the facts that victims are never to blame, rape and sexual assault are never okay, and women should be protected against sexual violence and supported through the healing process. Lasting emotional symptoms associated with Posttraumatic Stress Disorder are common for these victims. Healing can take a few months or can be a lifelong battle. Immediate care, support and therapy are indicators on how long and challenging the healing process will be. It is also important to be aware that victims of sexual violence may experience a relapse of triggers and symptoms at different times in their lives, therefore treatment may be indicated again.

— *K. Thomas Finley, Ph.D.*
Updated by Kimberly Ortiz-Hartman, Psy.D., LMFT

FOR FURTHER INFORMATION

American College of Obstetricians and Gynecologists. http:// www.acog.org.

Matsakis, Aphrodite. *The Rape Recovery Handbook: Step-by-Step Help for Survivors of Sexual Assault.* Oakland, CA: New Harbinger, 2003.

National Sex Offender Registry. http://www.family watchdog.us.

Reddington, Frances P., and Betsy Wright Kreisel, editors. *Sexual Assault: The Victims, the Perpetrators, and the Criminal Justice System.* Durham, NC: Carolina Academic Press, 2005.

Summerfeld, Leila Rae. *Beyond Our Control: Restructuring Your Life after Sexual Assault.* Grand Rapids, MI: Kregel, 2009.

United Nations Human Rights: Rape: Weapon of War. http:// www.ohchr.org/en/newsevents/pages/rapeweaponwar.aspx.

Violence Against Women: State Resources. http:// www.womens health.gov/violence/state.

World Health Organization (WHO). http://www.who.int/en.

Reproductive system

CATEGORY: Anatomy

KEY TERMS:

bladder: the pouch in the abdominal cavity that collects urine until it can be eliminated from the body; while not a part of the reproductive system, it is located adjacent to the reproductive organs and is an important landmark

fertilization: the process in which the sperm head penetrates the ovum, resulting in the formation of an embryo

gametes: the reproductive cells in the ova

hormone: a chemical signal that is carried in the blood from its site of production to the area where it has an effect

labia majora: relatively large, fleshy folds of tissue that enclose and protect the other external genital organs

labia minora: a pair of thin cutaneous folds that form part of the vulva, or external female genitalia

menstrual cycle: the cycle of ovum development, hormone production, and menstruation in female primates; in humans, the average duration is about twenty-nine days

ovulation: the release of an ovum from its follicle in the ovary

ovum: the female gamete; a large spherical cell that carries the female's chromosomes

STRUCTURE AND FUNCTIONS

The reproductive system in each sex includes the organs that produce the gametes, called the gonads, and those that transport the gametes. In addition, the female mammary glands are also considered reproductive organs since they produce milk to nourish the newborn, a critical step in survival of the species.

In the female reproductive system, the outer opening of the vagina is located behind the urethra, which carries only urine and does not have a reproductive role in the female. Bartholin's and Skene's glands are located near the urethral and vaginal openings; these glands supply moisture and mucus to the female external genitals. The vaginal and urethral openings are located between folds of tissue, the labia majora and the labia minora. At the front junction of these folds is the clitoris, a small round structure containing many touch receptors; stimulation of the clitoris during intercourse is important in promoting sexual gratification in the female. The area that includes the labia, the vaginal and urethral openings, and the clitoris is known as the vulva.

Internally, the vagina consists of a recess with elastic walls and a large blood supply, but little sense of feeling since there are only sparse touch receptors. The vagina slants upward and slightly backward from its outer opening. Near its upper end is the cervix, the lowest portion of the uterus. The cervix consists of strong connective tissue and contains glands that secrete mucus. The cervix has a narrow passageway, the cervical canal, that opens into the main part of the uterus.

The uterus is about 7.5 centimeters long and 5.0 centimeters wide in the nonpregnant woman. The wall of the uterus is composed primarily of involuntary muscle controlled by nerves and hormones. The inner part of the uterus is hollow and is lined with a spongy layer of cells, the endometrium; the endometrium has a large blood supply and contains glands that secrete nutrients for the embryo during pregnancy. The endometrium undergoes growth during

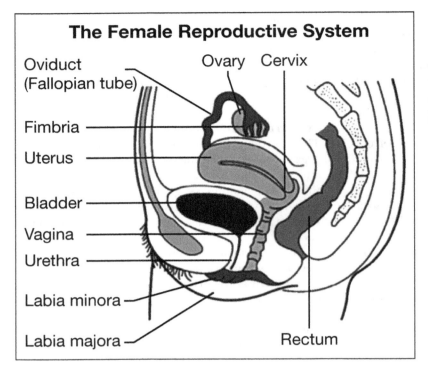

The Female Reproductive System

Oviduct (Fallopian tube)

Ovary   Cervix

Fimbria

Uterus

Bladder

Vagina

Urethra

Labia minora

Labia majora

Rectum

© *EBSCO*

the menstrual cycle and is shed as the menstrual discharge if the woman does not become pregnant.

At either side of the upper end of the uterus are the oviducts, or Fallopian tubes, which are hollow tubes that open into the cavity of the uterus. The oviducts lead upward and sideways away from the uterus toward the ovaries, with their funnel-shaped ends adjacent, but not attached, to the ovaries. The ovaries are the female gonads; they produce ova, the female gametes. Each 3-centimeter-long ovary contains thousands of follicles, spherical structures that each contain one ovum. Hormonal signals cause growth of some of the follicles during the menstrual cycle, and, as they grow, the ova within them mature. The follicles are also sites of production of the hormones estrogen and progesterone. In the middle of the menstrual cycle, one follicle will ovulate, releasing its ovum, which will enter the oviduct to be transported toward the uterus.

During intercourse, after sperm are deposited in the vagina, the sperm will swim in the fluids of the female tract, passing upward through the cervical canal, the uterus, and the oviducts. If an ovum is present in one of the oviducts, it may be fertilized by a sperm. The fertilized ovum will then move downward to the uterus, where it will attach to the endometrium and develop into an embryo. At birth, uterine muscle contractions will cause stretching of the cervical canal and movement of the fetus through the cervix and vagina. Milk production (lactation) in the woman's breasts after childbirth will allow for the nourishment of the newborn. Milk is produced in glands within the breast; ducts carry the milk to openings in the nipple. In between the milk-producing glands are wedges of fat; it is the fat tissue that determines the size of the breast in the non-pregnant woman. Breast size is not related to milk-producing ability.

DISORDERS AND DISEASES

Abnormalities may exist in either the male or the female reproductive tract as a result of deviations during embryonic development, injury, or disease. Anatomical abnormalities in the reproductive system often can be corrected surgically.

In women, problems during embryonic development can lead to malformed reproductive organs. The vagina may be present but may not have an outer opening, or conversely, the outer opening may lead to an abnormally shallow vagina. The uterus may be divided into two separate halves (bicornuate uterus), and the vagina may also show such a division. It is also possible for a normal uterus to have an abnormal placement in the abdomen: It may be tilted backward or bent forward at an atypical angle. Surprisingly, variations in the anatomy of the uterus often have little effect on fertility. Malfunctions in embryonic development of the reproductive organs can lead to intersex conditions, in which an individual has a mixture of male and female reproductive organs. An intersex individual may be either a genetic male or a genetic female. Hormone treatment and surgery can usually assure a fulfilling sex life in adulthood for such individuals.

Stretching of the pelvic area during childbirth sometimes leads to uterine prolapse, a condition in which the uterus sags into the vagina. Other causes of prolapse are developmental abnormalities, lifting heavy objects, and loss of muscle and tissue strength with aging. A prolapsed uterus is associated with pain during intercourse and may cause difficulty in urination. Temporary relief from a uterine prolapse can be achieved with the use of a pessary, a device worn in the vagina to support the uterus. Surgery to restore the supporting tissues in the pelvis may be necessary for long-term relief, but in some cases the uterus cannot be returned to its proper position and so must be removed, a process called hysterectomy.

In endometriosis, patches of endometrial tissue from the uterine lining attach to and grow on other organs in the pelvic cavity, affecting the shape and function of these organs. It is thought that the endometrium escapes into the pelvis through the oviducts during menstruation. The abnormally placed endometrial tissue can cause pain and infertility. Endometriosis can be treated with hormone therapy or with surgery to remove the endometrial patches. In more severe cases and when the woman does not wish to bear children in the future, the removal of the uterus may be required to control the invasion of other organs by the endometrial patches. The ovaries may also be removed in order to eliminate the source of hormones that produce the growth of the endometrium.

In polycystic ovary syndrome, one or both ovaries contain cysts that are formed from follicles that have failed to ovulate. Women with polycystic ovaries either do not menstruate or have irregular patterns of bleeding. Because ovulation does not occur, they are infertile. Another symptom of polycystic ovary syndrome is growth of hair in a male pattern on the face, neck, and chest; the hair growth is caused by certain hormones that are produced in abnormal amounts by the ovaries. Therapy usually involves hormone treatment in an attempt to establish ovulation and to prevent the deleterious effects of abnormal hormone levels on the body.

Both benign (non-spreading) and cancerous tumors may appear in the reproductive organs. Potential sites of tumor growth are the testes and prostate gland in the male and the ovaries, uterus, and breasts in the female. Only rarely do tumors cause pain, but they may be detected during routine self-examination of the testes or breasts or during a doctor's examination. Treatment usually begins with surgery to remove the tumor, and x-ray therapy or chemotherapy prevents further tumor growth. Hormone treatment can also be useful in controlling the growth of some reproductive tumors. The exact factors that cause tumors to form are not well understood, but a family history of such problems, abnormal hormone levels, and exposure to radiation, pollutants, and toxins have all been implicated.

FEMALE CIRCUMCISION

Rituals involving alteration of the reproductive organs have been performed since ancient times. Circumcision of women is practiced in some cultures. Indigenous groups who perform female circumcision are found in the Pacific Islands, Asia, the Middle East, and Africa, and the practice has been carried to the United States by immigrants. The term *female circumcision* refers to three procedures that may be carried out singly or together. In simple circumcision, the flap of tissue covering the clitoris is removed. The entire visible part of the clitoris is removed in clitoridectomy. Infibulation is the sewing together of the labia to cover the vaginal opening, leaving only a small hole for the discharge of urine and menstrual fluid. A woman who has been infibulated cannot have intercourse or give birth; the tissue must be cut open to allow either of these events, after which the area may be sewn closed again.

Female circumcision may take place shortly after a girl's birth or at puberty, and it is performed for a variety of reasons. Infibulation is a means of enforcing female abstinence from sexual activity. A wish to control women's sexual desire is also given as a reason for performing simple circumcision and clitoridectomy. Also involved are the society's views of what the ideal female organs should look like. From a medical standpoint, female circumcision is of concern because of pain and discomfort caused by the development of scar tissue in the vulval area. It is not known how many women die from infection or bleeding following these procedures, which are usually performed by other women under less-than-sanitary conditions.

—*Marcia Watson-Whitmyre, Ph.D.*

FOR FURTHER INFORMATION

Ammer, Christine. *The New A to Z of Women's Health: A Concise Encyclopedia.* 6th ed. New York: Checkmark Books, 2009.

Berek, Jonathan S., ed. *Berek and Novak's Gynecology.* 15th ed. Philadelphia: Lippincott Williams & Wilkins, 2012.

Jones, Richard E., and Kristin H. Lopez. *Human Reproductive Biology*. 4th ed. London: Academic Press, 2013.

Manassiev, Nikolai, and Malcolm I. Whitehead, eds. *Female Reproductive Health*. New York: Parthenon, 2004.

Marieb, Elaine N. *Essentials of Human Anatomy and Physiology*. 10th ed. San Francisco: Pearson/Benjamin Cummings, 2012.

Strauss, Jerome F., III, and Robert L. Barbieri, eds. *Yen and Jaffe's Reproductive Endocrinology: Physiology, Pathophysiology, and Clinical Management*. 6th ed. Philadelphia: Saunders/Elsevier, 2009.

Wade, L. "Learning from Female Genital Mutilation: Lessons from Thirty Years of Academic Discourse." *Ethnicities* 12, no. 1 (February, 2012): 26–49.

Rotator cuff surgery

CATEGORY: Procedure

KEY TERMS:

acromion: the outward end of the spine of the scapula or shoulder blade

arthroscopy: minimally invasive surgical procedure on a joint in which an examination and sometimes treatment of damage is performed using an arthroscope, an endoscope that is inserted into the joint through a small incision

deltoid muscle: the muscle forming the rounded contour of the human shoulder

humeral: relating to the humerus bone, the bone of the upper arm or forelimb, forming joints at the shoulder and the elbow

shoulder impingement: common cause of shoulder pain, often caused by repeated activity of the shoulder; also called "swimmer's shoulder"

rotator cuff: a capsule with fused tendons that supports the arm at the shoulder joint and is often subject to athletic injury

tendonitis: inflammation of a tendon, often caused from overuse

INDICATIONS AND PROCEDURES

The shoulder, considered to be a ball and socket joint, is the most flexible joint in the human body. Because of its structure, a wide range of motion is permitted. This also predisposes the shoulder to a very high risk of injury. To counter this risk, the shoulder is stabilized by a group of four muscles, collectively known as the rotator cuff: the subscapularis, the supraspinatus, the infraspinatus, and the teres minor.

The signs and symptoms of rotator cuff injuries are the same for men and women including point tenderness around the region of the humeral head deep within the deltoid muscle, pain and stiffness within the shoulder region within a day of participating in activities that involve shoulder movements, and difficulty in producing overhead motions involving the upper arm. Pain often occurs at night as a result of sleeping positions that put excess pressure on the joint. Occasionally, a clicking noise can be heard emanating from the joint upon movement or the patient may experience a "sticking point" when shoulder movements are attempted. Injuries to the rotator cuff can mimic other common shoulder region problems, including bursitis (inflammation of a bursa, a soft, fluid-filled sac that helps cushion surfaces that glide over one another) and tendonitis (inflammation of a tendon). Injuries to the rotator cuff include impingement and tears.

Impingement occurs when the rotator cuff tendons are pinched because of a narrowing of the space between the acromion (shoulder blade) process and the rotator cuff. This narrowing commonly occurs with aging, but it can also be traumatically induced. Sports that commonly put excess stress on the rotator cuff include baseball, swimming, and tennis. Besides a traumatic injury, chronic impingement of the rotator cuff tendons can cause partial or complete tears. To evaluate the extent of shoulder dysfunction, the physician will conduct a physical examination to determine range of motion and use diagnostic procedures such as x-rays, an arthrogram (an x-ray after a tracer dye has been injected into the shoulder), magnetic resonance imaging (MRI), and ultrasound. Nonsurgical interventions include rest, ice immediately following an injury or heat twenty-four hours afterward, painkillers, anti-inflammatory medications, and physical therapy.

Rotator cuff surgery is usually recommended when there is little improvement in shoulder function or pain reduction after a course of noninvasive therapies. Surgery to correct rotator cuff tears is more successful if the procedure is performed within three months of the date of injury. If the shoulder is surgically treated later there is a complication of the torn tendons retracting away from each other increasing the difficulty of the surgery and decreasing the chances of a satisfactory outcome. Surgery can be a classic open procedure, requiring a 2- to 3-inch incision in the shoulder, or less traumatic arthroscopy, which requires only a small incision, half an inch or less, just large enough to accommodate the instruments and a video camera apparatus. Occasionally, the surgeon will use a combination of the open procedure and arthroscopy. Either general anesthesia, in which the patient is asleep, or local anesthesia, in which the region is "frozen" but the patient is awake, can be used for the procedure. Often a scalene block is also used which removes all sensation of the extremity that eventually returns shortly after surgery. With local anesthesia, a light sedative may also be used to put the patient at ease, but not asleep. Acromioplasty reduces the impingement of the rotator cuff tendons. In this procedure, a portion of the bone underneath the acromion is shaved in order to give the tendons more room to move and prevent them from becoming pinched. This process is often included in rotator cuff surgical repairs. In rotator cuff repairs, the torn tendons are reattached to the humerus (upper arm bone). The open surgical procedure requires a relatively large incision through the shoulder as well as cutting through the deltoid muscle. Any scar tissue that has formed is removed, and a small ridge is cut into the top of the humerus. Small holes are drilled into the bone, and the tendons are sutured to the bone using these holes as anchors. The surgeon will also correct any other problems encountered, such as removing bone spurs, shaving down the acromion, or freeing up ligaments that may be pressing against the tendons.

During arthroscopic surgery, the majority of these additional procedures are still able to be performed. After the small incision is made into the shoulder, a thin tube is inserted. This tube contains the surgical instruments as well as a video camera that is used to guide the repair procedure. Arthroscopic surgery is becoming more common and is preferred for small to larger tears, as it limits the amount of surgical intervention, reduces surgical risks, and quickens recovery time. If more extensive damage is discovered, then the surgeon may elect to combine the arthroscopic procedure with open surgery. However, arthroscopic tear repair has advanced tremendously,

to the point that tears previously thought to be irreparable or too extensive are now being completed with arthroscopy.

IMPACT ON WOMEN

Currently literature provides limited consistent information on the impact of patients' gender on recovery after rotator cuff repair. One particular study investigated whether gender affects pain and functional recovery in the early postoperative period after rotator cuff repai In the study, eighty patients (40 men and 40 women) were prospectively enrolled. Pain intensity and functional recovery were evaluated, using visual analog scale (VAS) pain score and range of motion on each of the first 5 postoperative days, at 2 and 6 weeks and at 3, 6, and 12 months after surgery. Perioperative medication-related adverse effects and postoperative complications were also assessed.

Results showed the mean VAS pain score was significantly higher for women than men at 2 weeks after surgery ($p = 0.035$). For all other periods, there was no significant difference between men and women in VAS pain scores, although women had higher scores than men. Mean forward flexion in women was significantly lower than men at 6 weeks after surgery ($p = 0.033$) and the mean degree of external rotation in women was significantly lower than men at 6 weeks ($p = 0.007$) and at 3 months ($p = 0.017$) after surgery. There was no significant difference in medication-related adverse effects or postoperative complications.

The authors of this study concluded women had more pain and slower recovery of shoulder motion than men during the first 3 months after rotator cuff repair. The findings can serve as guidelines for pain management and rehabilitation after surgery and can help explain postoperative recovery patterns to patients with scheduled rotator cuff repair.

In another study, researchers wanted to determine the overall differences in disability between men and women and to examine the relationship between factors that represent sex (biological factors) and gender (non-biological factors) with disability and satisfaction with surgical outcome 6 months after rotator cuff surgery.

Patients with impingement syndrome and/or rotator cuff tear who underwent rotator cuff surgery completed several standard assessment forms, such as the Quick Disabilities of the Arm, Shoulder and Hand

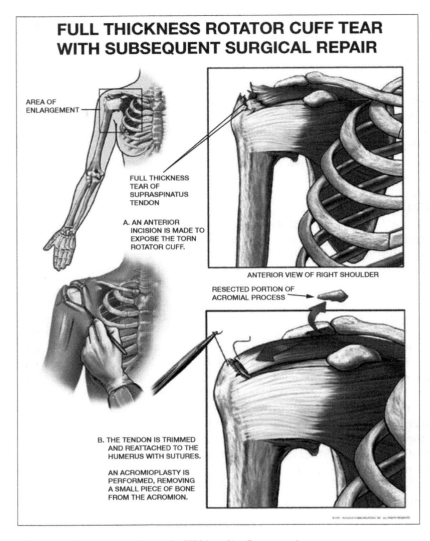

FULL THICKNESS ROTATOR CUFF TEAR WITH SUBSEQUENT SURGICAL REPAIR

AREA OF ENLARGEMENT

FULL THICKNESS TEAR OF SUPRASPINATUS TENDON

A. AN ANTERIOR INCISION IS MADE TO EXPOSE THE TORN ROTATOR CUFF.

ANTERIOR VIEW OF RIGHT SHOULDER

RESECTED PORTION OF ACROMIAL PROCESS

B. THE TENDON IS TRIMMED AND REATTACHED TO THE HUMERUS WITH SUTURES.

AN ACROMIOPLASTY IS PERFORMED, REMOVING A SMALL PIECE OF BONE FROM THE ACROMION.

(Nucleus Communications via Wikimedia Commons)

(QuickDASH) which measures status prior to surgery and 6 months post-operatively. They also rated their satisfaction with surgery at their follow-up appointment. One hundred and seventy patients entered into the study (85 men and 85 women). One hundred and sixty patients (94%) completed the 6-month assessment. Women reported more disability both prior to and after surgery. Disability at 6 months was associated with pain-limited range of motion, participation limitation, age and strength. Satisfaction with surgery was associated with level of reported disability, expectations for improved pain, pain-limited range of motion and strength.

The researchers concluded that this study indicated women with rotator cuff pathology suffer from higher levels of pre- and post-operative disability and sex and gender qualities contribute to these differences. Similar studies in the future regarding differences between men and women prior to and post-op rotator cuff repair will help to promote more effective and tailored care by health professionals.

USES AND COMPLICATIONS

The varying outcomes from rotator cuff surgery range from almost full recovery to no improvement at all. The degree of recovery is dependent upon the extent of damage to the rotator cuff as well as patient compliance with physical therapy after surgery. If the tendon has been torn for a long time, then it may not be reparable.

As with all surgical procedures, the patient may have an adverse reaction to the anesthesia. This risk is greater if the person is obese or has a cardiovascular, pulmonary, or metabolic condition. Surgical incisions always have the risk of infection, but this risk is minimized with the arthroscopic procedure because of the small incision size and the relatively short operative time (one to two hours). In rare instances, there is also the risk of nerve damage resulting in partial paralysis or temporary numbness at the incision area.

After surgery, the recovering arm will be put in a sling with a small shock-absorbing pillow placed behind the elbow. Extreme care should be taken with shoulder movements for the first three months following surgery. Reaching and lifting objects above the head should be avoided during this period. Passive range of motion exercises, in which the arm is moved by the physical therapist, should be started as soon as possible to prevent scar tissue formation and resultant stiffness. Exercises should be done several times a day so that within two to three weeks, the range of motion (flexibility) of the repaired shoulder should be equivalent to that of the uninjured shoulder. After six weeks, more advanced exercises are recommended in order to strengthen the rotator cuff as well as the surrounding shoulder muscles. Full recovery and rehabilitation from rotator cuff surgery can take up to a year.

—Bonita L. Marks, Ph.D.
Updated by Jeffrey P. Larson, PT, ATC

FOR FURTHER INFORMATION

Codsi, Michael Howe, Chris R. Shoulder Conditions: Diagnosis and Treatment Guideline. Phys Med Rehabil Clin N Am. 2015 Aug; 26(3): 467–489. doi: 10.1016/j.pmr.2015.04.007

Pfeiffer, Ronald P., and Brent C. Mangus. *Concepts of Athletic Training.* 6th ed. Sudbury, Mass.: Jones and Bartlett, 2012.

Rotator Cuff Repair. MedlinePlus, a service of the National Library of Medicine National Institutes of Health. http://www.nlm.nih.gov/medlineplus/ency/article/007207.htm.

Rotator Cuff Tears. American Academy of Orthopedic Surgeons. http://orthoinfo.aaos.org/topic.cfm?topic=A00064

Rotator Cuff Tears: Surgery and Exercise. Cleveland Clinic. http://my.clevelandclinic.org/disorders/rotator_cuff/hic_rotator_cuff_tears_surgery_and_exercise.asp....

Shoulder Surgery. American Academy of Orthopedic Surgeons. http://orthoinfo.aaos.org/topic.cfm?topic=a00066.

S

Same-sex adoption

CATEGORY: Social issue

DESCRIPTION

Same-sex families raising and adopting children is not a modern phenomenon but with shifting societal acceptance of sexual minority (lesbian, gay, bisexual, transgender, and queer) communities, same-sex families have become more visible. Recent court cases and federal legal changes within the United States (U.S.) have further allowed for legal acknowledgment of same-sex parental recognition and adoption. With this said, same-sex couples are about four times more likely to adopt than their heterosexual counterparts.

An individual family unit's makeup is unique and diverse, and adoption is no different. Adoption within same-sex couples is often quite similar to heterosexual couples and comes in many diverse forms. Adoption may arise from one spouse adopting the biological child of the other spouse ("2nd-parent adoption"), adopting a child related to them (e.g. a niece or nephew), or adopting an unrelated child (i.e. through an adoption agency). No matter the route though, same-sex partners face many barriers to adopting and raising children, both social and legal.

Lesbian parents' abilities to raise well-adjusted children are well established in scientific literature. Same-sex parents and their children score equally with their heterosexual counterparts on measures of relationship quality, psychological well-being, social adjustment, and parental investment of time and effort. There are no differences in child intelligence or behavioral problems. Further, contrary to popular belief, children of gay and lesbian parents are no more likely to be LGBTQ themselves than if raised by heterosexual parents.

FACTS & STATISTICS

The number of same-sex couples who have adopted children is difficult to determine because this information is not routinely tracked. U.S. adoptions are often only categorized as of married couples, unmarried couples, single women, or single men. Most agencies do not collect data on the sexual orientation of persons who apply to them to become parents. The U.S. census, last performed in 2010, has also not asked about the sexuality of the persons in a household. Further, same-sex marriage in the U.S. was legalized broadly *after* the 2010 census, therefore the census data cannot be truly utilized to extrapolate the number of same-sex families. This said, some estimates indicate that there are roughly 5.2 million to 9.5 million U.S. adults who identify as LGBT, and about 2 million to 3.7 U.S. children being raised by LGBT persons. Of these children, most appear to be raised by single LGBT parents. Of note, same-sex couples are more likely than opposite-sex couples to adopt older children, children with special needs, and children of a different race than their own.

LEGAL CONSIDERATIONS

With the routine shifts of ideological control of state and national governments in the U.S., whether conservative, moderate, or liberal, the ease or the legality of same-sex adoption is constantly shifting. At the U.S. national level in 2019, same-sex marriage is legal and accessible. This was granted with the U.S. court cases of *United States v. Windsor* and *Obergefell v. Hodges,* which legalized same-sex marriage and all the accompanying benefits across the country. Although same-sex marriage is legal in the U.S., there are many legal and policy factors that negatively influence and bar same-sex couples from adopting children.

Although laws continue to open for LGBT families and adoption, discrimination experienced during the adoption process presents a barrier for gay and lesbian prospective parents to adopt. Same-sex couples may be exposed to more scrutiny by adoption agencies than would heterosexual couples. Research suggests that gay and lesbian couples tend to be keenly aware of the multiple layers of stigma present in the adoption process. Since the rules and regulations of same-sex adoption are inconsistent nationwide, checking with local, state, and national laws in your practice areas are critical. "Religious freedom" laws in several states allow for child welfare agencies to refuse services to same-sex couples if it violates their personal beliefs (e.g. Michigan, Oklahoma, Texas, and more). With this said, it is critical to promote and work with adoption agencies that provide LGBT-inclusive adoption services. Yet despite these barriers, adoptions are increasing among same-sex couples. Further, research indicates that the health and well-being of children in families with gay or lesbian parents is improved when the government of the nation in which they live formally acknowledges the relationships of same-sex couples.

Assessment

Health care providers and social workers who are working with gay and lesbian individuals and couples who are prospective adopting parents should be aware of the unique needs, experiences, and discrimination their clients may face during and after the adoption process. When counseling same-sex couples, it may be important to ask and support clients around their coping practices around discrimination and provide additional support mechanisms for coping with homophobia they may face during the adoption process or being adoptive same-sex parents. Further, like all new adoptive parents, counseling around the client's feelings about becoming parents and how they can prepare to transition into parenthood. Further, additional support may be needed for the child, for if, or when, the child experiences prejudice because of their parents' sexual orientation.

Clinicians and social workers should be aware of their own cultural values, beliefs, and biases and develop specialized knowledge about the histories, traditions, and values of the individuals with whom they work. Providers and adoption agency personnel should receive specialized education on heterosexism and homophobia prior to working with LGBT clients.

—*Jan Wagstaff, MA, MSW*
Updated by Michael Anthony Moore, MSN, RN

For Further Information

Family Equality Council. (2019). LGBTQ family building guide: Paths to parenthood for the LGBTQ community [Pamphlet]. https://www.familyequality.org/resources/2019-lgbtq-family-building-guide/

Gates, G. J. (2015). Marriage and family: LGBT individuals and same-sex couples. *The Future of Children*, 67-87.

Gjelten, T. (2017, February). In religious freedom debate, 2 American values clash. National Public Radio website: https://www.npr.org/2017/02/28/517092031/in-religious-freedom-debate-2-american-values-clash

Goldberg, A. E., Allen, K. R., Black, K. A., Frost, R. L., & Manley, M. H. (2018). "There Is No Perfect School": The Complexity of School Decision-Making Among Lesbian and Gay Adoptive Parents. *Journal of Marriage and Family, 80*(3), 684-703.

Harris, C. E. (2016). LGBT parenting. In K. Eckstrand & J. M. Ehrenfeld (Eds.), *Lesbian, gay, bisexual, and transgender healthcare: A clinical guide to preventive, primary, and specialist care* (pp. 115-124). Springer.

Higdon, M. J. (2019). Biological Citizenship and the Children of Same-Sex Marriage. *Geo. Wash. L. Rev., 87*, 124.

Obergefell v. Hodges, No. § 14-556 (2015). Retrieved from https://www.supremecourt.gov/opinions/14pdf/14-556_3204.pdf

United States v. Windsor, No. § 12–307 (2013). Retrieved from https://www.supremecourt.gov/opinions/12pdf/12-307_6j37.pdf

Wald, M. S. (2015, June 26). Obergefell: A victory for children.from https://law.stanford.edu/2015/06/26/obergefell-a-victory-for-children/

Same-sex transracial adoption

Category: Social issue

Description

Gay and lesbian couples are not only four times more likely to adopt than their heterosexual counterparts, but also more likely to adopt older children, children with special needs, and children of a different race than their own (transracial adoption). Gay and lesbian parents' abilities to raise well-adjusted children are well established in the scientific literature, and transracial adoptions are no different. Some studies suggest that gay and lesbian persons are uniquely qualified to adopt transracially because of their own minority status and experiences of oppression. Further, gay and lesbian couples are more likely to be an interracial couple themselves.

Concrete statistical data on the numbers of transracial adoptions by same-sex couples does not exist. As a whole, estimates indicate that there are roughly 5.2 million to 9.5 million U.S. adults who identify as LGBT, and about 2 million to 3.7 U.S. children being raised by LGBT persons. The reason why same-sex couples are more likely to adopt transracially than heterosexual couples is not currently clear. One reason may be that same-sex couples are more likely to be in an interracial relationship than opposite-sex couples.

APPLICABLE LAWS AND REGULATIONS

International adoption may be the most difficult route of adoption to navigate and utilize for same-sex couples. Legality around adopting a child from another country is regulated by not only the laws of the country in which the child lives but of the country in which the adoptive parents live as well. Increased complications may result if the laws of the two countries conflict. This conflict may further escalate if one country has laws barring adoption to same-sex couples. Only a few countries in the world explicitly allow for same-sex international adoption, including Brazil, Columbia, Mexico, and the Philippines. In the United States, many states have "religious freedom" laws, which allow for child welfare agencies to refuse services to same-sex couples if it violates their personal beliefs.

In addition, countries that are party to the international Hague Adoption Convention (1993) may require additional procedures, such as requiring training in the issues surrounding transracial adoption for persons who seek to adopt a child of a race other than their own.

ASSESSMENT

Health care providers and social workers who are working with gay and lesbian individuals and couples who are prospective adopting parents should be aware of the unique needs, experiences, and discrimination their clients may face during and after the adoption process. Social workers should assist gay and lesbian individuals and couples in determining how they will talk to their child about their racial differences and how they will respond to questions or comments from others about the nontraditional makeup of their family. Having a supportive dialogue between family members about how the child experiences race and racism, especially if the child is of color when the parents are white, can be particularly useful.

Health care providers and social workers can support same-sex couples with transracially adopted children by helping the family unit cope with and navigate the intersections of racism, national origin, and homophobia. All parents racially socialize their children. Both unconsciously and explicitly, parents send meaningful messages to their children about race and other social identities. Clinicians can help support parents by helping parents instill a positive sense of racial pride. This can be endorsed, for example, by attending cultural festivals and purposefully choosing a racially diverse school for their children.

Clinicians and social workers should be aware of their own cultural values, beliefs, and biases and develop specialized knowledge about the histories, traditions, and values of the individuals with whom they work. Providers and adoption agency personnel should receive specialized education on heterosexism, homophobia, and racial and cultural diversity prior to working with LGBT clients pursuing transracial adoption.

—*Jan Wagstaff, MA, MSW*
Updated by Michael Anthony Moore, MSN, RN

FOR FURTHER INFORMATION

Battalen, A. W., et al. "Lesbian, gay, and heterosexual adoptive parents' attitudes towards racial socialization practices." *Journal of Evidence-Informed Social Work*, vol 19, 2019, 1-14.

Family Equality Council. "LGBTQ family building guide: Paths to parenthood for the LGBTQ community." January 1, 2019, https://www.family-equality.org/resources/2019-lgbtq-family-building-guide/. Accessed March 16, 2019.

Gates, G. J. "Marriage and family: LGBT individuals and same-sex couples." *The Future of Children*, Vol. 25, No. 2, 2015, 67-87.

HCCH. "Convention and Protection of Children and Cooperation in Respect of Intercountry Adoption." *Hague Convention #33 of 29 May 1993*.

https://assets.hcch.net/docs/77e12f23-d3dc-4851-8f0b-050f71a16947.pdf. Accessed March 16, 2019.

Higdon, M. J. "Biological Citizenship and the Children of Same-Sex Marriage." *Geo. Wash. L. Rev.*, vol. 87, 2019, 124.

Levi, N. "After Obergfell: The next generation of LGBT rights litigation." *UMKC L. Rev*, vol. 84, 2015, 605.

Scoliosis

CATEGORY: Disease/Disorder

KEY TERMS:

adolescent scoliosis: curvature of the spine that is diagnosed in the early stages of puberty

Cobb angle: the commonly used measure of spinal curvature; the angle created by perpendicular lines to the tops of the first and bottom of the last vertebrae in a curve

idiopathic: referring to a medical condition with no known cause

vertebra (pl. *vertebrae*): the individual bones that are stacked upon one another to form the vertebral column, or spine

CAUSES AND SYMPTOMS

Of all the structures that make up the human body, the spine is second only to the closely associated brain in its centrality to human characteristics. The spinal column protects the spinal cord, which carries out critical message-carrying functions in the body. Additionally, it holds the body erect, a distinctly primate feature.

The spine generally consists of thirty-three separate bones named vertebrae, a term derived from the Latin verb "to turn." It also comprises four separate curves, each of which is associated with a distinct set of vertebrae. At the very top of the spine are the cervical vertebrae. In the chest area one finds the thoracic vertebrae, which represent the sites of attachment of the twelve pairs of ribs. The largest of the vertebrae are termed lumbar vertebrae, from the Latin for "loin." Finally, at the very base of the spine are two sets of small vertebrae comprising the sacrum and coccyx.

Abnormal curvature of the skeletal structure of the spinal (or vertebral) column is known as scoliosis. Scoliosis can result from a number of different causes, including birth defects, accidents, and a host of conditions that include poliomyelitis and muscular dystrophy. The cause of this lateral curvature is unknown in the majority of cases, however. It is believed that approximately 80 percent of scoliosis cases have no known cause, and are classified as "idiopathic scoliosis." Within this general subdivision, three separate forms are recognized, based on the age of the patient at the onset of the curvature.

The adolescent form of scoliosis, which is usually recognized between ten and thirteen years of age, is by far the most common form. A brief look, however, at infantile (birth to three years) and juvenile (four to ten years) scoliosis will help to illustrate the difficulty faced by researchers in this field of study. All these age groupings refer to the age at which the deformity is first noted, not the age at which the curvature began.

When the scoliosis is recognized in the youngest range, it is more common in males, with one study citing a 3:2 ratio. While infantile idiopathic scoliosis tends to corrects itself, this natural remission is rarely observed when the diagnosis is made later in life. As with the other variations, there is marked evidence of hereditary influence in the juvenile condition. In this age range, males and females share equal likelihood of diagnosis.

By contrast, in the far more common adolescent condition one finds a striking shift to females, who are three times more likely to be affected. In a recent study of pregnancy-related outcomes, women with adolescent idiopathic scoliosis were slightly more susceptible to symptoms such as back pain and infertility. The psychosocial effects of idiopathic scoliosis on women have been studied at length. There is some evidence to suggest potential impairments to self-esteem and happiness, demonstrating that the condition may compromise quality of life in a variety of ways.

A dozen different types of curves associated with scoliosis have been identified, but four major classes are of greatest frequency and concern. In the chest area, one finds the most common of all curve patterns, the right thoracic curve. It is possible for this condition to progress rapidly. Early treatment is essential. As the curve develops, the ribs on the right side shift and create a deformity which not only is unattractive but also can squeeze the heart and lungs; this so-called rib hump can result in serious cardiopulmonary difficulties.

A similar, but gentler, curve is the thoracolumbar curve. It begins in the same region of the thoracic vertebrae but ends farther down the back, in the lumbar region. The twist may be either right or left and is generally less deforming in its appearance. A lumbar curve is found far down in that region of the back, producing a twist in the hips. In pregnant women and older adults, this twist often causes severe back pain. The current evidence indicates that nearly 13% of postmenopausal women aged 50 years and older have some degree of lumbar scoliosis, highlighting that it is not nearly as rare as one may expect.

The three curves described thus far are single, or C-shaped, curves. The double major curve is an S-shaped curve and is the most common of that type. Curvature begins in the thoracic area and is complemented by a second curve in the opposite direction found in the lumbar region. To some extent, the two curves offset each other and the scoliosis is less deforming. The double major curve can progress and become the source of a rib hump.

These and the other less common curves demand an accurate description beyond their location. John Cobb searched for such an important tool and developed the widely used Cobb angle measurement. His suggestion was to relate the top of the first and the bottom of the last vertebrae of a curve by determining the angle formed by the intersection of lines perpendicular to them. It is not difficult, using an X ray of the spine, to draw lines above and below the vertebrae, construct the required perpendiculars, and measure the angle of their intersection. This technique allows physicians to communicate accurately and have a useful measure with which to note the progression, remission, or stabilization of the patient's scoliosis. In addition to degree of curvature, the complex structure of the spine shows rotation in scoliosis. The rotation causes the pedicles or indentations of the vertebrae to shift closer to the midline drawn on the X ray. The relative shift is described as a rotation of +1, +2, and so on.

TREATMENT AND THERAPY

Scoliosis can result from many different causes—each of which demands specific treatment. For the idiopathic variety, however, prevention is impossible due to the lack of a known cause, and there are enormous difficulties in predicting the course of the disease. As a result, the most that can be achieved in idiopathic cases is satisfactory correction.

A diagnostic examination for scoliosis requires careful attention to accurate family history. Particularly important is information concerning the first recognition and previous treatment of the condition. Subsequently, a detailed evaluation of the nature and extent of the curvature must be made. The examining physician should make certain that the patient is standing straight with the knees unflexed. A simple plumb line is used to examine the patient's back to determine any curvature in the spine. Then the forward bending test is conducted. This observation is considered one of the most reliable diagnostic tools. Various forms of curvature, including scoliosis, can be seen by the trained observer. When viewed at eye level from both front and back, one side of the thoracic or lumbar regions is higher. An accurate measurement of the degree of difference can be made with a level. The use of X-ray photographs also forms a vital part of the diagnostic data.

Even with the best diagnostic skill, training, and experience, the decision concerning the treatment of scoliosis is hardly straightforward. One important consideration is the patient's bone age. Because people grow and mature at such different rates, chronological age may not correspond well to the degree of maturity of that person's skeleton. Many clues are used to determine the bone age, including the degree of fusion observed in the individual vertebrae or the bony pelvic girdle. A catalog of hand x-rays is readily available and provides a useful measure of the bone age. The central concern is that curvature is more likely to progress if the growth and development of the patient's skeleton is still incomplete.

The treatment of scoliosis varies from simple observation to extensive surgical procedures. In general, treatment is undertaken for the prevention of further curvature or for the correction of the curvature already present. Some treatments, such as exercise, are of benefit to the patient as a whole, but only minimally arrest or correct spinal curvature. Preliminary research has also suggested that copper supplementation could potentially find a role in scoliosis treatment, though applicability of the available animal data to human treatment or prevention remains in question.

Of all the methods proposed, the use of braces and casts is certainly the oldest and the most common. Irrespective of the design or material employed, the central purpose of these interventions is to promote a straight alignment of the spine. The evolution of the brace has reached the point of an active or kinetic apparatus called the Milwaukee brace, developed by Walter Blount and Albert Schmidt. It is a carefully designed assembly of a molded plastic pelvic girdle and three metal bars which keep the wearer erect and allow a neck ring to be attached. The neck ring and its associated axillary sling keep the torso balanced and prevent listing to the right or left.

In order for the Milwaukee brace to be effective, it must be worn day and night and until the growth period of the patient is complete. It is also imperative that exercise be carried out on a daily basis. There are many advantages of the modern brace over older systems. For example, it can be removed for showering and swimming, and much greater activity is allowed. The value of the brace is that it can, with good use and exercise, maintain the already present curvature and prevent further progression. One serious caveat is that a patient cannot expect correction of the scoliosis. Additionally, a recent long-term (23+ years) follow-up study in female adolescent idiopathic scoliosis patients indicates that even with the brace, back pain associated with the condition is difficult to mitigate, as are declines in bone mineral content.

Only in certain cases will braces be of benefit to the patient. With curves of 40 or 50 degrees, pain unresponsive to treatment, or cases of failed bracing, surgery is the most reasonable approach. Surgery can offer some degree of correction, but it is important to recognize that only a partial correction is possible. Even with the safest techniques, pressure must be applied to the spine, creating a serious risk of damage to the spinal cord. Authorities typically estimate reasonable correction to be about 60 percent.

Once it is agreed that surgery is the proper route of treatment, a wide range of methods are available. The most common and safest method is arguably the Harrington rod technique. The incision is from the back (as opposed to front or side entries), and metal hooks are inserted at the highest and lowest points in the curve. These hooks hold metal rods used to straighten the spine and then to hold it in place. Small chips of bone are then taken from the hip or

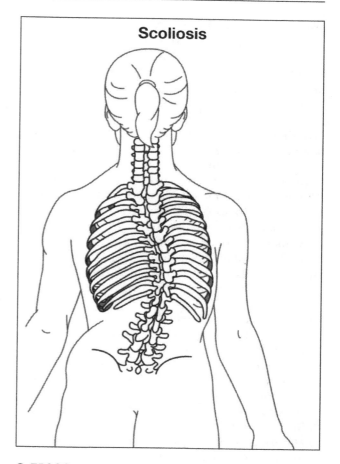

Scoliosis

© EBSCO

ribs and inserted between especially prepared vertebrae. In a period of six to eight months, solid bone will grow and fuse the vertebrae. After the surgery, the patient is usually placed in a brace or cast for four to six months.

The success of the Harrington rod technique has inspired several modifications, such as the use of two rods to achieve more balance and greater correction. With a patient who has unusually soft bones, a system of wires can be used to hold the rods in place. This method is considered superior insofar as the normal hooks are prone to breaking off. Several variants of the wire technique are also available. Some surgeons thread the wires through the neural canal, and others drill small holes to avoid coming near to the spinal cord.

Another technique which is growing in popularity avoids the use of a Harrington rod. Many small wires are herein attached through the neural canal and twisted around two thin rods, one on either side of the curvature. This Luque method provides greater stability, and usually there is no need to wear a cast after surgery. These advantages must be balanced, however, against a significantly greater risk of paralysis and a smaller amount of room for new bone growth in fusion. Another modern technique which is showing some promise involves placing small electrodes near the spine and transmitting tiny electrical impulses to nerve endings periodically during sleep. This electronic bracing, or electrosurface stimulation, appears to stop scoliosis curves from progressing in the majority of documented cases. These devices have about the same limitations as do conventional braces, with curves exceeding 40 degrees and certain types of lumbar curves typically failing to benefit from this treatment.

PERSPECTIVE AND PROSPECTS

One finds the beginning of serious study of the spine in the writings of Hippocrates (c. 460-c. 370 BCE). He described the curves of both the normal and the abnormal spine. He may not have been as clear in his description of scoliosis as with those of the clubfoot or epilepsy, but he was well aware of the difficulty of its treatment and recognized its possible relationship to pulmonary disease. Another celebrated physician of antiquity, Galen (129-c.199 CE), first suggested the medical term for this deformity, scoliosis, in the late years of the second century. Among the complications faced by early medical science were the inadequate methods and equipment available for making subtle diagnoses. Thus it was not until the sixteenth century that Ambrose Pare carefully described the various types of spinal curves. He also noted for the first time that scoliosis is largely a condition of children. Over the centuries, many men and women added to the array of methods and instruments as well as the store of knowledge and thoughtful speculation about scoliosis. Many possible causes were presented on the basis of observation and research. Many approaches to the treatment of these deformities were described and tested. Yet, despite all this research, scientists are just beginning to appreciate the complexity of the problem of scoliosis.

—K. Thomas Finley, Ph.D.
Updated by Ariel Choi, ScB

FOR FURTHER INFORMATION

Dewan, Michael C., et al. "The influence of pregnancy on women with adolescent idiopathic scoliosis." *European Spine Journal.* 2018. 17(2):253-263.

Freidel, Klaus, et al. "Quality of Life in Women with Idiopathic Scoliosis." *Spine.* 2002. 27(4):E87-E91.

Griesse, Rosalie. *The Crooked Shall Be Made Straight.* Atlanta: John Knox Press, 1979.

Misterska, Ewa, et al. "Back and neck pain and function in females with adolescent idiopathic scoliosis: A follow-up at least 23 years after conservative treatment with a Milwaukee brace." *PLoS One.* 2017. 12(12):e0189358.

Nasreen, Akseer, et al. "Does bracing affect bone health in women with adolescent idiopathic scoliosis?" *Scoliosis.* 2015. 10:5.

National Scoliosis Foundation. http://www.scoliosis.org.

Neuwirth, Michael, and Kevin Osborn. 2d ed. *The Scoliosis Sourcebook.* New York: McGraw-Hill, 2001.

Parker, James N., and Philip M. Parker, eds. *The 2002 Official Patient's Sourcebook on Scoliosis.* San Diego, Calif.: Icon Health, 2002.

Schommer, Nancy. *Stopping Scoliosis: The Whole Family Guide to Diagnosis and Treatment.* Rev. ed. New York: Putnam, 2002.

Urrutia, Julio, et al. "Scoliosis in Postmenopausal Women: Prevalence and Relationship With Bone Density, Age, and Body Mass Index." *Spine.* 2011. 36(9):737-740.

Sexual assault aftercare

CATEGORY: Social issue

WHAT WE KNOW

Sexual assault is any type of sexual activity that is nonconsensual (including when one is unable to provide consent), including physical, verbal, visual (e.g., being forced to view pornography), or any other type of unwanted sexual contact or attention. Sexual assault includes inappropriate touching, voyeurism (i.e., when someone watches private sexual acts), exhibitionism (i.e., when someone exposes him/herself in public), incest (i.e., sexual contact between family members), unwanted sexual advances (i.e., unwelcome sexual gestures, requests for sexual favors), and rape (i.e., nonconsensual vaginal, anal, or oral penetration).Sexual assault includes acts perpetrated within marriage or dating relationships, acts perpetrated by acquaintances or strangers, gang rape (i.e., rape involving two or more perpetrators), and systematic rape (i.e., mass rapes that occur during armed conflicts).

Sexual assault is both a criminal and a public health problem.

Lifetime prevalence rates of sexual assault vary from country to country, ranging from 4.2 percent in Singapore to 38.9 percent in Mexico. Approximately 1 in 5 women in Australia, the United States, and the United Kingdom experience sexual assault at some point in their lives.

A 2012 study by the U.S. Centers for Disease Control and Prevention (CDC) on sexual assault in the United States reported that:

1. 1 in 5 women reported experiencing rape at some time in their lives
2. 1 in 20 women experienced sexual violence other than rape (such as sexual coercion or unwanted sexual contact)
3. 37.4 percent of female rape victims were first raped between ages 18 and 24

The majority of sexual assault victims know their attacker. In a United States study that investigated subtypes of sexual assault, researchers found that:.

1. 27 percent of high-violence assaults, 18 percent of alcohol-related assaults, and 46 percent of moderate-severity assaults were committed by intimate partners
2. 33 percent of high-violence assaults, 55 percent of alcohol-related assaults, and 32 percent of moderate-severity assaults were committed by acquaintances
3. 19 percent of high-violence assaults, 15 percent of alcohol-related assaults, and 4 percent of moderate-severity assaults were committed by strangers

Women's decisions to report and/or seek care after a sexual assault are influenced by a variety of personal and environmental factors.

Personal factors include emotional states (i.e., shame, embarrassment, humiliation, and self-blame); fear of negative consequences of reporting (i.e., not being believed, retaliation, lack of confidentiality, poor treatment by law enforcement, public exposure, stigma, and unfair treatment); being assaulted by someone known to the victim (i.e., intimate partner, family member, acquaintance); and lack of knowledge (i.e., not knowing what services are available and how they are paid for).

Investigators in a 2014 study also found that post-traumatic stress disorder (PTSD) symptomatology was linked with likelihood of reporting sexual assault; re-experiencing and hyperarousal symptoms were associated with increased likelihood of reporting whereas avoidance symptoms were associated with decreased likelihood of reporting an assault.

Environmental factors include organizational and structural barriers (i.e., limited services, services that are difficult to access, inadequate funding, staff who are inexperienced or uncomfortable with sexual assault cases) and societal myths (i.e., biases based on race, gender, and sexual orientation, doubts about the authenticity of sexual assault).

The effects of sexual assault on women are well documented in research, and include:

1. *physical effects*: pregnancy, chronic pelvic pain, migraines, gynecological complications, pain;
2. *psychological effects*: shock, denial, fear, guilt, depression, PTSD, sleep disturbances, attempted suicide;
3. *social effects*: strained relationships with family members and friends, decreased contact with family members and friends, lower likelihood of marriage; and
4. *health effects*: engaging in high-risk behaviors (e.g., unprotected sex, trading sex for food or money), substance use, unhealthy diet-related behaviors (e.g., overeating, abusing diet pills, fasting, self-induced vomiting).

The impacts of sexual assault vary among survivors based in part on factors such as preexisting personality characteristics, history of childhood sexual abuse, and characteristics of the assault.

In a United States study, researchers found that women who experienced severe, forceful assault experienced higher levels of trauma symptoms, depression, and anxiety than women who experienced contact assault or attempted rape, or women who were incapacitated by intoxication rather than by violence.

Researchers in a longitudinal study in the United States found that women who experienced severe violence or alcohol-related assaults had more PTSD symptoms than those who experienced moderately severe assault. Victims who experienced severe violence initially had the highest level of PTSD symptoms, but victims of alcohol-related assaults experienced an increase in PTSD symptoms over time, which was attributed in part to self-blame and negative social reactions.

Certain risk factors may predispose women to react to sexual assault in specific ways; for instance, women who tend to act more impulsively when distressed have been found to have higher levels of externalizing dysfunction (e.g., increased alcohol and/ or drug use) following sexual assault, whereas those with a predisposition to depression and anxiety have higher levels of internalizing dysfunction.

Self-stigma, or perceiving oneself in a negative light based on perception of social stereotypes of sexual assault victims, is associated with more severe trauma symptoms.

Sexual assault victims who have a history of childhood sexual abuse are at higher risk of PTSD and depression, in part as a result of having maladaptive coping strategies and difficulties with emotional regulation.

Emergency assessments and interventions generally take place immediately for sexual assault victims who report sexual assault to police or go to an emergency room setting. These address the victim's injuries and usually include a forensic sexual assault exam, a medical evaluation of the individual who has been raped to collect information and forensic evidence for potential use in a law-enforcement investigation.

The goals of the sexual assault exam include the treatment of injuries, prophylactic treatment to prevent pregnancy and infection, crisis intervention, and safety planning. Sexual assault exams usually are conducted in the emergency department of a hospital and are time sensitive: they must take place no more than 72-96 hours after the rape because of the potential loss of forensic evidence (e.g., pubic hair, bodily fluids, bruising, lacerations).

A sexual assault response team (SART) is responsible for timely response to a victim of rape, including completion of a sexual assault exam. A SART is a collaborative effort of personnel including a victim service provider/advocate, sexual assault forensic examiner (SAFE) and/or a sexual assault nurse examiner (SANE), law enforcement officer, crime laboratory specialist, and the prosecutor. As a result of the creation of sexual assault response teams at the initial point of care (emergency departments of hospitals), most rape victims now receive prompt medical treatment, forensic evidence collection, thorough documentation of the sexual assault, crisis counseling, and safety planning.

Most victims of sexual assault need further support, known as aftercare. Crisis centers, individual or group therapy, and support groups can provide support and therapeutic interventions.

Crisis hotline services often are utilized by sexual assault victims. These hotlines usually are accessible 24 hours a day. The goals of crisis hotlines are to help the caller cope effectively with the crisis, to educate the caller on facts of sexual assault as well as possible short-and long-term impacts, and to inform the caller of safety resources as well as possible medical and legal resources.

The crisis-line provider should be nonjudgmental, use active listening skills, help the victim identify and clarify her feelings, help the victim explore all of her options, provide empathic responses, and provide referrals to community resources for ongoing support.

Victims may seek individual therapy after a sexual assault. Several therapeutic interventions have been noted to be beneficial for individuals who have experienced the trauma of sexual assault.

Psychodynamic therapy (also known as insight-oriented therapy) targets the client's avoidance symptoms and resolution of any inner conflicts. The therapist helps the client to understand the conscious and unconscious meanings of the symptoms she may be experiencing as a result of the trauma of sexual assault.

Eye-movement desensitization and reprocessing (EMDR) is a treatment often used within psychodynamic therapy. The therapist asks the client to produce images, thoughts, and feelings related to the sexual assault and to evaluate their distressing qualities. The client is then asked to generate alternative pleasing thoughts and images while using specific eye movements to follow the therapist as he or she waves his or her finger rapidly in front of the client's face.

Cognitive behavioral therapy (CBT) is a type of psychotherapy in which the client and therapist work together to examine the relationship between the client's thoughts, feelings, and behaviors. There are several subtypes of CBT:

1. In *exposure therapy* (also known as flooding) the client repeatedly confronts fearful images and thoughts of the traumatic sexual assault in order to lessen her fear and anxiety. It is believed to be the most effective of the CBT treatments for victims of sexual assault.
2. *Stress inoculation therapy* involves the therapist teaching the client concrete skills to manage anxiety and fear as they relate to the incident of sexual assault.
3. *Multiple channel exposure* therapy educates the client on panic and trauma and uses breathing exercises to help in reducing panic and anxiety.
4. *Cognitive processing therapy* (CPT) helps victims process the sexual assault by confronting cognitive distortions and maladaptive beliefs concerning the sexual trauma (e.g., No one will ever love me now that I have been raped). CPT for sexual assault survivors usually consists of 12 weekly hour-and-a-half long sessions. One study reported that at the conclusion of CPT treatment none of the participants in the study, all of whom had a diagnosis of PTSD, met the full criteria for PTSD; this was maintained at 6 months following treatment.
5. *Psychopharmacological treatment* may also be utilized to treat symptoms of depression and PTSD.

Researchers have examined the benefits of therapy for sexual assault victims, who were not victims of intimate partner violence, that includes their spouse or partner.

One study used CBT not only to address the PTSD diagnosis of the sexual assault victim but also to improve the support offered by the victim's spouse. Results at the conclusion of treatment and 3-month follow-up indicated that the victims no longer met the criteria for PTSD and that all reported significant improvement in the ways they were receiving support from their spouse as well as increased satisfaction in their overall relationship.

In another study investigators examined the use of solution-oriented therapy (SOT) (also called solution-focused therapy) with sexual assault survivors and their spouses/partners who had both disclosed negative impacts on their sexual functioning as a result of the sexual assault. The research suggests that SOT empowers the victim as well as the partner to regain a sense of control, improves mutual sexual functioning, and decreases the victim's PTSD symptoms.

SOT is brief (several sessions only), goal oriented, and is focused on solutions rather than problems or symptoms. SOT uses "the miracle question" (How would your future look different if the problem was no longer present?), scaling questions, coping questions, and problem-free talk (in which the client talks about problem-free areas of her life). These types of questions are intended to help the victim envision what she wants to change in her life and then use those desired changes as goals to work on in therapy.

Sexual assault group therapy is another effective therapeutic intervention for victims of sexual assault. Groups provide a sense of normalcy for victims as well as a safe place in which they may experience and share empathy and encouragement.

A study of a psychoeducational group model of therapy for sexual assault victims in a university setting in the Midwestern United States reported that participants experienced a decrease in PTSD symptoms and a lessening of their initial sense of isolation.

In this model the group is closed (i.e., no new members are accepted after the group is formed), consists ideally of 7-10 participants, and lasts 10-12 weeks. Goals of the group include empowerment, reduced isolation, increased self-esteem, learning about and modeling healthy relationships, and participants regaining a sense of control over their lives.

These goals are attained through group discussion as well as hands-on activities (e.g., an imagined older version of oneself writing a letter to one's current self that shares what the current self can and will overcome; sharing a meaningful song or piece of poetry with the group).

A controlled trial of psychotherapy for survivors of sexual violence in the Democratic Republic of Congo indicated that the improvements experienced by participants in group therapy were far greater than those experienced by participants in individual therapy. After 6 months of treatment, only 9 percent of the group therapy participants met the criteria for anxiety and/or depression versus 42 percent of the participants in individual counseling. Researchers have found that many victims of sexual assault do not receive needed services.

In a study in London, approximately half of sexual assault victims followed through with recommended medical care following the initial sexual assault exam, and only 33 percent of victims who were prescribed HIV preventive treatment completed the regimen.

Researchers in a United States study found that 43.5 percent of sexual assault victims utilized mental health services at 1.5 months after the assault, decreasing to only 31.4 percent at 6 months post-assault. Victims who had received previous mental health services and victims who abused alcohol were more likely to participate in mental health services following sexual assault.

—*Melissa Rosales Neff, MSW*

FOR FURTHER INFORMATION

Centers for Disease Control and Prevention. Sexual violence: https://www.cdc.gov/violenceprevention/sexualviolence/.

Deitz, M. F., Williams, S. L., Rife, S. C., & Cantrell, P. (2015). Examining cultural, social, and self-related aspects of stigma in relation to sexual assault and trauma symptoms. *Violence Against Women, 21*(5), 598-615. doi:10.1177/1077801215573330

Morgan, L., Brittain, B., & Welch, J. (2015). Medical care following multiple perpetrator sexual assault: A retrospective review. *International Journal of STD & AIDS, 26*(2), 86-92.

Munro, M. L. (2014). Barriers to care for sexual assault survivors of childbearing age: An integrative review. *Women's Healthcare, 2*(4), 19-29.

Price, M., Davidson, T. M., Ruggiero, K. J., Acierno, R., & Resnick, H. S. (2014). Predictors of using mental health services after sexual assault. *Journal of Traumatic Stress, 27*(3), 331-337. doi:10.1002/jts.21915

Ullman, S. E., Peter-Hagene, L. C., & Relyea, M. (2014). Coping, emotion regulation, and self-blame as mediators of sexual abuse and psychological symptoms in adult sexual assault. *Journal of Child Sexual Abuse, 23*(1), 74-93. doi:10.1080/10538712.2014.864747

World Health Organization. "Violence Prevention." https://www.who.int/gho/violence/en/.

Sexual assault emergency assessment

CATEGORY: Social issue

WHAT WE KNOW

Sexual assault is any type of sexual activity that is non-consensual (including when one is unable to provide consent), including physical, verbal, visual (e.g., being forced to view pornography), or any other type of unwanted sexual contact or attention.

Examples include rape within marriage or dating relationships, rape by acquaintances or strangers, gang rape (i.e., rape involving two or more perpetrators), systematic rape (i.e., mass rapes that occur during armed conflicts); and inappropriate touching, voyeurism (i.e., when someone watches private sexual acts), exhibitionism (i.e., when someone exposes him-/ herself in public), incest (i.e., sexual contact between family members), unwanted sexual advances (e.g., unwelcome sexual gestures, requests for sexual favors).

In 2013 the United States Federal Bureau of Investigation began using a more inclusive definition of rape (formerly defined as "the carnal knowledge of a female forcibly and against her will"): "the penetration, no matter how slight, of the vagina or anus with any body part or object, or oral penetration by a sex organ of another person, without consent of the victim."

Sexual assault is a global criminal and public-health problem. According to the World Health Organization (WHO),in 2013 the lifetime prevalence of sexual assault by an intimate partner reported by women ages 15 to 49 years old ranged from 6 percent in Japan to 59 percent in Ethiopia. Rates in other countries included 46.7 percent in Peru, 28.9 percent in Thailand, and 14.3 percent in Brazil. WHO reported that 0.3 percent–12 percent of women reported being forced after age 15 to have sexual intercourse or perform a sexual act with someone other than their partners. The wide range is due to the variance from country to country of reported rapes.

A 2012 study by the U.S. Centers for Disease Control and Prevention (CDC) on sexual assault in the United States reported that.

1 in 5 women experienced rape at some time in their lives

1 in 20 women experienced sexual violence other than rape (such as sexual coercion or unwanted sexual contact)

37.4 percent of female rape victims were first raped between ages 18 and 24

A literature review of 12 articles and 4 national surveys about barriers to seeking care after a sexual assault in the United States identified personal and environmental factors.

Personal factors included emotional states (i.e., shame, embarrassment, humiliation, and self-blame), fear of negative consequences of reporting (i.e., not being believed, retaliation, lack of confidentiality, poor treatment by law enforcement, public exposure, stigma, and unfair treatment), and lack of knowledge (i.e., not knowing what services are available and how they are paid for).

Environmental factors included organizational and structural barriers (i.e., limited services, services that were difficult to access, inadequate funding, staff members who are inexperienced or uncomfortable with sexual assault cases) and societal myths (i.e., biases based on race, gender, and sexual orientation; doubts about the authenticity of sexual assault).

The effects of sexual assault on women are well documented in research, including:

1. *physical effects*: pregnancy, chronic pelvic pain, migraines, gynecological complications, back pain, facial pain;
2. *psychological effects*: shock, denial, fear, guilt, depression, posttraumatic stress disorder, sleep disturbances, attempted suicide;
3. *social effects*: strained relationships with family members and friends, decreased contact with family members and friends, lower likelihood of marriage; and
4. *health effects*: engaging in high-risk behavior (e.g., unprotected sex, trading sex for food or money), substance use, unhealthy diet-related behaviors (e.g., overeating, abusing diet pills, fasting, self-induced vomiting).

A forensic sexual assault exam is a medical evaluation of an individual who has been raped. Information and forensic evidence are collected in the exam for potential use in a law enforcement investigation.

The goals of the sexual assault exam are treatment of injuries, prophylactic treatment to prevent pregnancy and infection, crisis intervention, and safety planning. Sexual assault exams typically are conducted in the emergency department of a hospital and are time-sensitive: They must take place no more than 72–96 hours after the rape because of potential loss of forensic evidence (e.g., pubic hair, bodily fluids, bruising, lacerations).

A sexual assault response team (SART) is a support team responsible for timely response to a victim of rape, including completion of a sexual assault exam. A SART is a collaborative effort of personnel including a victim service provider/advocate, a sexual assault forensic examiner (SAFE) and/or sexual assault nurse examiner (SANE), a law enforcement officer, a crime laboratory specialist, and the prosecutor who is assigned to the case at the time. As a result of the creation of sexual assault response teams at the initial point of care (emergency departments of hospitals), most rape victims now receive prompt medical treatment, forensic evidence collection, thorough documentation of the sexual assault, crisis counseling, and safety planning.

A primary goal of the SART is to provide victim-centered care throughout the entire sexual assault examination process. This process consists of:

1. giving sexual assault victims priority care in the hospital emergency department. The longer a victim waits, the greater the potential for loss of evidence and the greater possible emotional and physical trauma;
2. providing necessary means of ensuring victims' privacy. Victims should not be left in the main emergency department waiting room, but should be given a private room in which to wait for the sexual assault exam;
3. accommodating victims' requests to have a relative, friend, or other personal support person present during the exam (unless considered harmful by staff);
4. accommodating victims' requests for staff of a specific gender throughout the exam; and
5. providing information that is easy for victims to understand, in lay terms and in their native language. An interpreter should be used if needed.

Although SART evidence-collection protocols may vary slightly from place to place, they typically include:

1. a history in which the victim is questioned about the following aspects of the assault. It is important for the entire sexual assault response team to be present so that the victim need share this information only once, to prevent further possible trauma;
2. circumstances of the assault (date, time, location);
3. physical description of the alleged perpetrator;
4. areas of trauma (specifically, details of oral, vaginal, or anorectal contact or penetration);
5. condom use or ejaculation (absence or presence of);
6. presence of bleeding in victim or perpetrator;
7. recent consensual sexual activity prior to the assault;
8. whether the victim has showered, bathed, or changed clothes since the assault;
9. physical examination performed by a sexual assault forensic examiner or a sexual assault nurse examiner.

This exam can take 3-6 hours to complete. The exam includes; a) physical examination of entire body. Individuals who have experienced assault can feel revictimized by the exam. It is vital to allow the victim to have control whenever possible during the exam (e.g., to control who is in the room); and b) forensic evaluation and treatment. A sexual assault evidence collection kit is used that contains necessary items for specimen collection based on evidence requirements of the local crime laboratory.

Samples of vaginal or cervical secretion, anal secretion, pubic hair, blood, and urine are taken from the victim. Clothing (if unchanged after the event) samples also are taken.

Once complete, the forensic examiner or nurse examiner must complete, sign, and date the sexual assault evidence collection kit form, which indicates that the examination is complete and sealed.

Gonorrhea and chlamydia testing are recommended for all victims; human immunodeficiency virus (HIV), hepatitis B, and syphilis tests also are recommended.

Retesting is recommended at 6 weeks, 3 months, and 6 months after the assault.

Pregnancy risk is estimated to be 5 percent per rape in women ages 12–45.

Emergency contraception should be offered in all cases.

—*Melissa Rosales Neff, MSW*

FOR FURTHER INFORMATION

Centers for Disease Control and Prevention. *Sexual violence.* https://www.cdc.gov/violenceprevention/sexualviolence/.

Chisolm, S. L. (2014). Sexual assault. In F. F. Ferri (Ed.), *2014 Ferri's clinical advisor: 5 books in 1* (16th ed., p. 1010). Philadelphia, PA: Elsevier Mosby.

Federal Bureau of Investigation. (2013). Frequently asked questions about the change in the UCR definition of rape. Retrieved October 11, 2015, from http://www. fbi.gov/about-us/cjis/ucr/recent-program-updates/ new-rape-definition-frequently-asked-questions

Sexual violence: Consequences. (2014). *Centers for Disease Control and Prevention.* Retrieved October 11, 2015, from http://www.cdc.gov/violenceprevention/sexualviolence/consequences.html

Sexual assault examination. In E. Eckman (Ed.), *Lippincott's nursing procedures and skills* (6th ed., pp. 648-650). Philadelphia, PA: Wolters Kluwer Health/Lippincott Williams & Wilkins, 2013.

World Health Organization. "Violence Prevention." https://www.who.int/gho/violence/en/.

Sexual differentiation

CATEGORY: Biology

KEY TERMS:

differentiation: the process of gradual remodeling of tissues in the embryo or fetus; in this context, the process of formation of the male or female reproductive organs

external genitalia: in the male, the penis and scrotum; in the female, the clitoris, the vaginal opening, and the folds (labia) around it

gender identity: the mental view of oneself as a girl or woman or as a boy or man

gonad: the internal organ in either sex that produces the reproductive cells (ova and sperm): the ovary in the female and the testis in the male

hormone: a chemical that is produced by a gland in the body and secreted into the blood; hormones act as coordinating signals

hormone receptor: a molecule contained in or on a cell that allows it to respond to a hormone; if receptors are not present, the hormone will have no effect

Müllerian ducts: the pair of tubes in the early embryo that will develop into the internal female organs (uterus, oviducts, and upper vagina)

urethra: the tube that drains the bladder; the urethra opens in front of the vagina but does not have a reproductive function

Wolffian ducts: the pair of tubes in the early embryo that will develop into the internal male organs (the epididymis, vas deferens, and seminal vesicles)

X and Y chromosomes: the chromosomes that determine genetic sex; females carry an XX pair, and males carry an XY pair

FUNDAMENTALS

The chromosomal sex of a human is determined at the time of conception, when the ovum from the mother is fertilized by a single sperm from the father. All ova (eggs) produced by a female contain one chromosome, denoted X. Sperm from the male can carry either an X or a Y chromosome. The Y chromosome is smaller than the X and contains fewer genetic codes. Men normally produce equal numbers of X- and Y-bearing sperm. The type of chromosome carried by the one sperm that fertilizes the ovum will determine the sex of the embryo. A Y-bearing sperm joining with the ovum will result in an embryo with one X and one Y; this embryo will develop as a male. If the ovum is fertilized with an X-bearing sperm, the embryo will have two X's and will develop as a female.

Although the genetic sex is determined at conception, male and female embryos initially look alike, both internally and externally. For the first seven weeks of development, each human embryo has the anatomical potential to develop in either a male or a female direction: This period is referred to as the sexually indifferent stage. Internally, the gonads, which lie in the kidney region, cannot yet be identified as ovaries or testes. The other internal reproductive organs are represented in every embryo by two pairs of ducts: the Müllerian ducts, which will later develop in the female but will be lost in the male; and the Wolffian ducts, which will later develop in the male but will regress in the female. Externally, male and female embryos possess the same rudimentary genital organs, which will later be remodeled to become either male or female genitalia.

The first organ to differentiate in the embryo is the gonad. Starting at about seven weeks of development

in a male embryo, the cells within the gonad are reorganized to form a testis. This reorganization is brought about by the presence of the Y-chromosome, which contains the codes for the production of a substance called testis-determining factor (TDF). The chemical nature of TDF has not yet been determined, but its existence is clear from experimental evidence. TDF acts on the gonad to cause it to become a testis. In the absence of a Y chromosome and TDF in a female embryo, the gonad develops into an ovary at about twelve weeks of development. If an individual has only one X chromosome (a condition known as Turner syndrome), the gonads will develop into ovaries, but these ovaries will not contain ova and so the person will be infertile.

The development of the other reproductive organs is not directly determined by the X and Y-chromosomes, but rather by hormones secreted by the gonads. In the male, the fetal testes begin to produce testosterone by the tenth week of development, and this testosterone acts on the Wolffian duct system to cause it to develop into the epididymis, vas deferens, and seminal vesicles. The Müllerian duct system in the male regresses under the influence of another hormone from the testes, called Müllerian-inhibiting hormone (MIH). In the female, MIH is not produced, and the Müllerian ducts develop into the oviducts, uterus, and upper part of the vagina. The Wolffian ducts in the female regress in the absence of testosterone. Normal female development does not, at this stage, require any hormone produced by the ovaries, but instead occurs spontaneously in the absence of testicular hormones. Thus, the presence or absence of the Y-chromosome determines which type of gonad develops, and the presence or absence of gonadal hormones determines which type of internal reproductive organs develop.

Similarly, the development of the external genitalia is hormonally directed. In the male, testosterone is converted by the action of the enzyme 5-alpha-reductase to 5-alphadihydrotestosterone (DHT). DHT acts on the undifferentiated external genital tissue, causing it to take on a male appearance: A pea-shaped structure (the genital tubercle) at the front of the crotch area grows to become the penis, a slit-like opening (the urethral groove) is enclosed within the penis to become the urethra when two folds behind the genital tubercle fuse together, and two swellings on the sides of the urethral groove become enlarged as the scrotum. In the female, it is the absence of DHT that causes development in the female direction: The genital tubercle remains as the relatively small clitoris; the folds do not fuse, allowing the urethral groove to remain as an open area where the vagina and urethral openings are located; and the swellings that become the scrotum in the male remain separated as the labia in the female.

Hormones also cause sexual differentiation of the brain, but the mechanism is not fully understood in humans. The most obvious result of brain differentiation is the difference in adult hormone production patterns. In the adult male, hormone production is relatively constant from day to day, and this results in constant production of sperm in the testes. In the female, hormone production changes in a monthly cycle that is associated with ovum maturation and ovulation. The difference in the pattern of hormone release in adult males and females appears to be attributable to hormonal programming of the fetal brain. Animal studies indicate that the development of the male pattern results from exposure of the fetal brain to testosterone or one of its derivatives. The female pattern of development is prevalent when testosterone is absent. In humans, testosterone also affects brain differentiation, but the effect appears to be less permanent than in animals.

It is not known for sure if there is any direct influence of the chromosomes or prenatal hormones on male and female behavior. Most researchers agree that human behavior is heavily influenced by social and cultural factors, so the importance of prenatal programming is difficult to assess. Indeed, it appears that gender identity, the internal view of oneself as male or female, is so heavily influenced by learning that a child with a disorder of sexual differentiation can be successfully reared in the gender that is opposite to that of the chromosomes. For example, a child born with female-appearing genitalia, but with XY chromosomes and internal testes, can be reared as a girl and will firmly adhere to this identity even if some masculinization occurs at the time of puberty.

DISORDERS AND DISEASES

Disorders of sexual differentiation result from errors in the signaling systems that normally direct male and female anatomical development. There are several different classes of these disorders, some of which result in a mixture of male and female reproductive organs. These disorders are rare, with the number of documented cases numbering only in the hundreds for most types.

True intersex individuals are defined as individuals who possess both ovarian and testicular gonadal tissue. There may be one ovary and one testis, two gonads in which ovarian and testicular tissue are combined (ovotestes), or an ovotestis on one side and a normal ovary or testis on the other. An intersex condition can result from several distinct genetic anomalies. Some intersex people have been shown to be chimeras: individuals that develop from the fusion of two separate embryos at an early stage. These individuals possess two distinct cell populations, one with an XX pair of chromosomes and one with XY. It is thought that expression of both of these chromosome pairs leads to the mixture of ovarian and testicular tissue seen in intersex individuals. A similar condition is mosaicism, in which the mixture of XX and XY cells is caused by errors of chromosome replication in a single early embryo. Other intersex people are neither chimeras nor mosaics; they appear to have a normal pair of XX or XY chromosomes, but on closer examination, one of the chromosomes is found to have a defect. For example, a Y chromosome may be missing a tiny piece, or an X chromosome may contain a portion of a Y.

There is much variation in the anatomical features of intersex individuals. One basic guideline is that the effects of the presence of testicular tissue are local. Thus, an intersex person with a testis on the left side and an ovary on the right will have Wolffian duct-derived (male) organs on the left side but Müllerian duct-derived (female) organs on the right. The external appearance depends on the relative levels of estrogen and testosterone but might include a typical male penis along with enlarged breasts. There are documented cases of ovulation and even pregnancy in intersexual people. Successful sperm production appears to be less frequent than ovulation, and sperm production and ovulation are not seen in the same individual.

Pseudo-intersex individuals have external reproductive organs that do not match their gonadal sex. Pseudo-intersex males have testes but external organs that appear to be female; pseudo-intersex females have ovaries and varying degrees of external male development. Female pseudo-intersex has only one basic cause: the exposure of an XX fetus to masculinizing hormones. These hormones might come from the fetus itself, as in certain disorders involving the adrenal gland, or synthetic hormones given to a pregnant woman may have a masculinizing effect on a female fetus. The extent of masculinization depends on the timing of the hormone exposure, with earlier exposure leading to more extensive male-like appearance of the external genitalia, including fusion of the urethral folds and enlargement of the clitoris. The internal organs are normal female.

Pseudo-intersex in males arises from a wide variety of causes. There may be failure of testosterone production, or the reproductive organs may lack testosterone receptors, causing them to fail to respond to the hormone. Because of the hormonal abnormalities, the Wolffian duct organs may fail to develop, and the external genitalia will appear female to some extent. If MIH production is normal, internal female organs will not be present. The appearance at puberty is variable, depending on the exact hormonal deficiency. Some individuals undergo the typical male responses of increased muscle mass, deepening of the voice, and growth of beard and chest hair; others do not. Most pseudo-intersex males are infertile because of the hormonal problems.

For intersex individuals, the choice of sex for rearing sometimes depends on the predominant appearance of the external genitalia. If the genital tubercle has remained small, like a clitoris, a female sex assignment may be determined; if the tubercle appears more penis-like, the individual might be reared as a male. In some cases, typically only if the issue is harmful to the baby's health, the gonadal tissue that does not correspond to the sex of rearing will be removed. Appropriate hormone treatment and surgery can enhance the body form of the chosen sex. For example, testosterone treatment will cause beard growth, and estrogen treatment will cause breast development. It is usually not medically necessary to perform surgery immediately, if at all.

PERSPECTIVE AND PROSPECTS

Anatomical descriptions of people with disorders of sexual development are found in writings beginning in the pre-Christian era. The word "hermaphrodite," a term that has largely been deemed inappropriate and stigmatizing, derives from the Greek myth about Hermaphroditos, the son of Hermes and Aphrodite,

whose body was permanently merged with that of a nymph in a loving embrace. The myth probably arose from a desire to explain the existence of intersex individuals. Although the existence of this condition was known long ago, there was no understanding of the mechanism of sexual differentiation until modern times. During the nineteenth century, embryological studies firmly established the concept that the early human embryo is sexually indifferent anatomically. In the twentieth century, genetic and hormonal studies revealed the controlling factors in male and female development.

It was in the 1920s that the X and Y chromosomes were first discovered and recognized to be important in sex determination. Since the 1960s, researchers have had the ability to pinpoint the exact chromosome sites associated with many disorders of sexual differentiation. Ongoing efforts deal with the identification of the TDF coded by the Y-chromosome and the mechanism by which TDF causes testicular development. The nature of the hormonal control of sexual differentiation was determined by experiments such as those performed on rabbit embryos by A. Jost in the 1940s and 1950s. Jost systematically removed or transplanted embryonic testes and ovaries, and treated the embryos with estrogen and testosterone, in order to demonstrate the importance of hormones from the testis on the development of the internal and external reproductive organs.

Jost's conclusions for rabbits were confirmed in humans by studying individuals with disorders of sexual differentiation caused by genetic factors. Additional confirmation came from observations of the offspring of pregnant women treated with synthetic hormones as a possible preventive for miscarriage. Such treatment was later found to be ineffective in preventing miscarriage.

Discovery of the causes of true intersex and pseudo-intersex conditions have allowed physicians to make important distinctions between these disorders, with a clear physical cause and manifestation, and the psychological disorders of sexuality that were previously confused with them. For example, until the middle of the twentieth century, the term "hermaphrodite" was used to refer not only to people with a mixture of male and female reproductive organs but also to those with a psychological confusion of gender identity. The latter individuals are now called transgendered; they identify themselves by the gender that does not conform to the gender indicated by their reproductive organs. Transgendered individuals possess a complete set of normal reproductive organs and have no known chromosomal or hormonal abnormality. Gender is now understood to be a psychological, social and cultural feeling rather than biology.

—*Marcia Watson-Whitmyre, Ph.D.*

FOR FURTHER INFORMATION

Henry, Helen L., and Anthony W. Norman, eds. *Encyclopedia of Hormones.* 3 vols. Boston: Academic Press, 2003.

Kronenberg, Henry M., et al., eds. *Williams Textbook of Endocrinology.* 11th ed. Philadelphia: Saunders/ Elsevier, 2008.

Moore, Keith L., and T. V. N. Persaud. *The Developing Human.* 8th ed. Philadelphia: Saunders/Elsevier, 2008.

Morland, Iain, ed. *Intersex and After.* Durham, N.C.: Duke University Press, 2009.

Simpson, Joe Leigh, and Sherman Elias. *Genetics in Obstetrics and Gynecology.* 3d ed. Philadelphia: W. B. Saunders, 2003.

Sexual dysfunction

CATEGORY: Disease/Disorder

KEY TERMS:

etiology: the science of causes or origins, especially of diseases

neuropathy: malfunction of the nerves

organic disease: a disease caused or accompanied by an alteration in the structure of the tissues or organs

psychogenic: psychologic in origin

CAUSES AND SYMPTOMS

It is evident from the term "performance anxiety" that sexual anxiety is more easily recognized when it involves performance (that is, erections and orgasms) than when it involves subjective arousal. The most extreme example of this way of thinking is the familiar notion that women do not experience performance anxiety because it is only men who have to perform. When researchers searched for a corresponding term that refers not to performance but to subjectively felt arousal, they devised the oxymoronic-sounding term "pleasure anxiety." Performance anxiety refers to the fear of not being able to perform, while pleasure anxiety refers to the fear of feeling pleasure. Sex therapists have traditionally been much more concerned with the fear of not being able to perform.

To explain this blind spot in the field, it is clear that, historically, lack of desire has been considered a female disorder, whereas lack of performance has been considered a male disorder. From the male-identified point of view, the failure to perform is relatively understandable; it is often treated with humor, sympathy, or indulgence. Traditionally, however, the same indulgence has not been extended toward a woman when she cannot fulfill the role expected of her.

If there are any doubts that "frigidity" is a more accusatory term than "impotence," "impotence" as a diagnostic term retains its currency, whereas "frigidity" has largely been dropped. Researchers William H. Masters and Virginia E. Johnson were the first authorities to drop the term, and as a result of their influence it is rarely used in the field of sex therapy and research. It is still used, however, in the psychoanalytic literature.

The category of "inhibited sexual desire" in the American Psychiatric Association's *Diagnostic and Statistical Manual of Mental Disorders: DSM-III* (3d ed., 1980) indicated the difficulty in finding a nonjudgmental means of referring to the lack of erotic arousal: The term "inhibition" implies that the conditions for desire are present, but that desire is being withheld. One of the implied accusations in the term "frigidity" is that the woman who does not experience erotic arousal is a cold, unfeeling, or withholding person. The work group on psychosexual disorders for the revision of the DSM-III-R published in 1987 first recognized this difficulty and recommended that "inhibited sexual desire" be renamed "hypoactive sexual desire disorder," arguing that this more awkward term is necessary because it reflects greater neutrality in terms of etiology. The DSM IV used the terminology "hypoactive sexual desire disorder." The DSM V split the diagnosis based on gender and uses the terminology " male hypoactive sexual desire disorder" and "female sexual interest and arousal disorder."

In the 1970s researchers noted that the diagnosis of low sexual desire among couples seeking help with sexual dysfunction increased from approximately one-third of couples in the early 1970s to more than one-half of couples by the early 1980s. Men as well as women were identified with low sexual desire, or frigidity. Most of the knowledge of the causes of low sexual desire is based on clinical experience, rather than on more empirical and objective research. It has become clear that there is no single cause for low sexual desire. Rather, many cases involve several causal factors working simultaneously. But lack of sexual desire need not always be pathologized. Asexuality is an expression of sexuality that is characterized by a lack of interest in sexual activity. People who identify as asexual are distinct from those who identify as sexual but are experiencing a lack of desire. Asexual people do not need therapeutic or medical interventions to change their sexuality. It can be complicated for a medical professional to distinguish a person who has an asexual identity from a person who has sexual dysfunction, but it is important and necessary to do so.

Virtually every standard work on sexual dysfunction lists religious orthodoxy as a major cause of sexual dysfunction. Some patients suffer from low sexual desire because they essentially lack the capacity for play (the obsessive-compulsive personality). Specific sexual phobias or aversions also may cause low sexual desire. Low-desire men almost uniformly have some degree of aversion to the vagina and female genitals. Women who have been sexually molested as children, or raped as adults, often have specific aversion reactions.

Some patients fear that if they allow themselves to feel any sexual desire at all, they will lose all control over themselves and begin acting out sexually in ways that would have disastrous consequences. Fear of pregnancy is often a "masked" cause of low sexual desire among women. Depression, hormonal issues, the side effects of medication, relationship problems, lack of attraction to one's partner, fear of closeness, and an inability to fuse feelings of love and sexual desire are among the many causes of low sexual desire in both men and women.

TREATMENT AND THERAPY

Before beginning treatment, it is important to understand the etiology of the concern. In the female patient it is important to rule out pain with sex, or dyspareunia, first. Changes associated with menopause cause vaginal dryness and may lead to painful sex, this can be addressed with medication. If the lack of desire is secondary to a medication, then that may be addressed. If the lack of desire is secondary to depression, then the depression needs to be addressed. If the lack of desire is not concerning to the woman, then it need not be addressed at all. However, if the lack of sexual desire cannot be attribute to other factors, it may be psychogenic. In such cases psychotherapy is indicated. However, there are several difficulties inherent in devising a treatment program for low sexual desire. While most of the behavioral exercises devised by Masters and Johnson may enhance arousal and orgasm, they often fail in increasing sexual desire or motivation, since they were not designed to deal specifically with low sexual desire. A second problem is that many cases of low sexual desire not only are quite complex but are diverse in apparent etiology and maintenance factors as well. Each case of low desire must be examined on its own terms, and treatment must be tailored to the specific needs of the individual.

Behavior therapy and social learning theory contributed most of the effective techniques that constituted sex therapy in the 1980s. Other therapeutic approaches, however, have been used as adjunct techniques or proposed alternatives. One broad-spectrum approach attempts to integrate interventions from many theoretical orientations into a comprehensive treatment program, while remaining sensitive to the need to fine-tune the program to the individual.

The first step in this broad-spectrum approach is experiential/sensory awareness. Many patients with low sexual desire are unable to verbalize their feelings and are often unaware of their responses to situations involving sexual stimulation. The goal of this phase of therapy is to help patients recognize, using bodily cues, when they are experiencing feelings of anxiety, pleasure, anger, or disgust.

The second stage is the insight phase of therapy, in which patients, with the help of the therapist, attempt to learn and understand what is causing and maintaining their low desire. Frequently, patients with low sexual desire have misconceptions and self-defeating attitudes about the cause of the problem. Patients are helped to reformulate attitudes about the cause of the problem in a way that is conducive to therapeutic change.

The third stage, the cognitive phase of therapy, is designed to alter irrational thoughts that inhibit sexual desire. Patients are helped to identify self-statements that interfere with sexual desire. They are helped to accept the general assumption that their emotional reactions can be directly influenced by their expectations, labels, and self-statements. Patients are taught that unrealistic or irrational beliefs may be the main cause of their emotional reactions and that they can change these unrealistic attitudes. With change, patients can reevaluate specific situations more realistically and can reduce negative emotional reactions that cause low desire.

The final element of this treatment program consists of behavioral interventions. Behavioral assignments are used throughout the therapy process and include basic sex therapy as well as other sexual and nonsexual behavior procedures. Behavioral interventions are used to help patients change nonsexual behaviors that may be helping to cause or maintain the sexual difficulty. Assertiveness training, communication training, and skill training in negotiation are examples of such behavioral interventions.

The treatment of psychogenic impotence includes supportive psychotherapy and behavior-oriented tasks. If, during the course of evaluation, symptoms of depression such as loss of libido and appetite or sleep difficulties are present without a physical basis, the patient is often treated with an antidepressant medication. As mental depression lessens, sexual interest and potency will often return. Depression is the most common mental disorder detected when impotent patients undergo psychological studies.

PERSPECTIVE AND PROSPECTS

Anthropologists have found that impotence (erectile dysfunction) and frigidity (inhibited or low sexual desire) have been observed in both primitive and highly developed societies. During most of human history, it was taken for granted that women attain sexual gratification in the same manner as men. Little attention was paid to the failures.

One of the most significant social changes affecting attitudes toward these sexual dysfunctions has been the altered status of women in contemporary society. During the Victorian era, whether they

worked or not, women were legally the wards of men and had virtually no civil rights. Many of the Victorian attitudes toward sex-fears, prejudices, taboos, and superstitions-remained powerful influences into the late twentieth century. Researchers, however, have learned that they cannot understand the problem of impotence in women by comparing it with impotence in men, since the dynamics as well as the treatments for each disorder differ greatly. With the women's movement and the Masters and Johnson research into human sexuality, the archaic terms "impotence" and "frigidity" were called into question. More gender-neutral terms were used, and, particularly in the case of erectile insufficiency, organic as opposed to psychogenic etiologies were acknowledged. By the late twentieth century, erectile insufficiency had become a disorder more often treated by urologists than by psychiatrists.

With this changing attitude toward these sexual dysfunctions among the medical community as well as the public at large, more research was devoted to treating the problems effectively and to reassuring the patients. Age-old stereotypes came under attack, such as the notion that performance anxiety affects only men and that frigidity or low sexual desire is a disorder that affects only women. As more organic etiologies for both erectile dysfunction and low sexual desire are acknowledged, patients feel increasingly comfortable seeking medical attention, and the stigma of sexual dysfunction being purely psychological is slowly beginning to vanish.

—*Genevieve Slomski, Ph.D.*
Updated by Julia Lockamy, RN

FOR FURTHER INFORMATION

Crooks, Robert, and Karla Baur. *Our Sexuality.* 10th ed. Belmont, Calif.: Wadsworth, 2010.

Lefkowitz, Eva S., et al. "How Gendered Attitudes Relate to Women's and Men's Sexual Behaviors and Beliefs." *Sexuality & Culture*, vol. 18, no. 4, Mar. 2014, pp. 833–846.

Mayo Clinic Staff. "Female Sexual Dysfunction." *Mayo Clinic*, Mayo Foundation for Medical Education and Research, 6 Sept. 2018, www.mayoclinic.org/diseases-conditions/female-sexual-dysfunction/symptoms-causes/syc-20372549.

Miller, Karl E. "Treatment of Antidepressant-Associated Sexual Dysfunction." *American Family Physician* 61, no. 12 (June 15, 2000): 3728.

Phillips, Nancy A. "Female Sexual Dysfunction: Evaluation and Treatment." *American Family Physician* vol. 62, no. 1 (July 1, 2000): 127-136.

Sexual reassignment

CATEGORY: Procedure

KEY TERMS:

cisgender: a person whose sense of gender identity corresponds to the designation given at birth

feminizing genitoplasty: male-to-female surgical procedures including penectomy, orchiectomy, and vaginoplasty

gender: the properties of organisms based on their reproductive roles

gender dysphoria: discomfort or anxiety that arises with discontent with one's biological sex, with desire for another sex's physical characteristics and role

intersex: genitalia that are not absolutely identifiable as either male or female

masculinizing vaginoplasty: female-to-male surgical procedures including metoidioplasty and phalloplasty

trans man: a person born female who has transitioned to male

trans woman: a person born male who has transitioned to female

transition: the process of assuming the sexual identity that is congruent with one's own private and subjective experience; this process may or may not include medical assistance such as cross-gender hormone replacement or surgery

transgender: an umbrella term for anyone whose sense of gender identity does not correspond to the designation given at birth (gender-variant people); includes transsexual people

transsexual: one who wishes to assume a sexual identity different from that assigned at birth, or someone who has undergone surgery to change the sexual organs; pertains to sexual characteristics but not necessarily to sexual activities

INDICATIONS AND PROCEDURES

At or before birth a baby's sex is assigned based on the child's external genitalia. When a child's genitals are ambiguous, sometimes called intersex, generally a sex is assigned based on the sex that appears to be predominant. Even in the absence of ambiguity and even well before puberty, some people feel a gender identity that differs from the sex that was biologically assigned. The unease that this disparity evokes is called gender dysphoria.

People whose gender identity differs from their anatomic sex are transgender people, sometimes known as transgendered. When a woman feels that the sex she was assigned at birth is not who she is, she may either dress and act as a man or elect to undergo surgery known as female-to-male reassignment to bring her body more into line with her sexual identity; a man whose sexual identity is female may identify as female or undergo male-to-female surgical procedures. When people transition from one sex to another, they are considered transsexual. The process of sexual reassignment is known as gender-confirmation surgery or sex-reconstruction surgery.

Although many transgendered people report that they felt gender dysphoria in childhood, one study found that most do not disclose these feelings to their families until later in their teens. Living with such unspoken disparity is hard, and mental illness rates are higher in the transgendered than in the cisgendered. In addition, transgendered people are often targets of violence—which may be self-inflicted. According to a 2010 study, transgender people attempt suicide at a rate 25 times higher than do the cisgendered. Childhood can be a time of trial for anyone. For the transgendered, support from the family is particularly important yet is available only for the fortunate. It is noteworthy that mental health has been shown to improve in young transgendered people who transition surgically. People who experience gender dysphoria may elect to undergo sex-reassignment surgery (SRS, also called by a variety of terms including gender-reassignment surgery, gender-affirming surgery, sex-realignment surgery, sex-reconstruction surgery, or gender-confirmation surgery). The procedure (singular or several) seeks to alter physical appearance and existing sexual organs to more closely resemble those of the gender with which the transgendered person identifies.

In 1931 Berlin Dora Richter had the first known vaginoplasty, which consisted simply of removing the penis; other such surgeries followed suit. The limits of this disfigurement soon became apparent, and surgeons began to develop more complex and, for the patient, satisfying SRS procedures. The process was technically complex, but also hampered by reluctance on the part of many medical practitioners, in effect, to fix that which wasn't broken. Over time, however, the medical community and families of the transgendered began to be convinced that, to the afflicted, gender dysphoria is all too real and, in fact, might be capable of being 'fixed'.

As demand for the surgeries continued, a 1992 study found that 98.5% of those undergoing male-to-female surgeries, and 99% of those undergoing female-to-male surgeries, did not regret their decisions. It may be preferable, when possible, to transit earlier in life, prior to puberty, as trans people may experience considerable distress as their bodies begin to show characteristics that they feel are alien. Transgender surgery in people past puberty is also complicated by the difference in pubic bones between the sexes, as to accommodate childbirth a biological woman's pelvis is wider and larger and set at a more obtuse angle than a man's. Many variations in surgical procedures have been tried and are as yet being devised. Although most transgender surgeries go as planned, surgeons are human and surgical mishaps do occasionally occur. Even when all goes as planned SRS is in almost every case a lifetime commitment that before being undertaken must be thoroughly considered and understood. With or without surgery, hormone-replacement therapy has its own impacts, some of which are noted below.

MALE-TO-FEMALE SRS

Any procedure to construct a vagina is called vaginoplasty (including surgical reconstruction following removal of growths or to correct prolapse or congenital defects). Genital reconstruction for trans women often involves surgical inversion of the penis to create a vagina. Inversion techniques using segments of the sigmoid colon or small intestine rather than the penis may produce a better semblance to genitals of cisgender women. Skin flaps from the penis and scrotum, sometimes in combination with a urethral flap, or nongenital skin grafts from other body parts may also be used. The neovagina may be lined with skin from the inferior pedicle or abdomen. The urethra is shortened and reoriented.

Ancillary procedures to more closely align with cisgender women include removal of testes (orchiectomy) and, if not inverted, penis (penectomy).

Trans women may choose aesthetic procedures such as breast augmentation and hair implants, and surgeries to feminize their facial contours.

Complications. Sex differences in pubic architecture, noted above, can make it difficult to allow sufficient septal thickness between the rectal wall and the neovagina; resultant weakness can cause fistula (tearing). When a vagina has been constructed, without sufficient post-surgical dilation the inner skin graft can shrink or collapse. In shortening the urethra, stricture (narrowing) may occur but is usually reparable.

FEMALE-TO-MALE SRS

Genital reconstruction for trans men entails formation of a penis through phalloplasty or metoidioplasty. Phalloplasty involves extending the urethra with a tubed flap of tissue from another part of the body. During a second surgery, an erectile prosthesis may be implanted.

For metoidioplasty (sometimes known as metaoidioplasty), provision of testosterone gradually enlarges the clitoris to the point where it can be removed from the labia minora and lowered to the position occupied by the penis. Erectile tissue in the enlarged clitoris functions normally, as the clitoris develops from the same embryonic tissue as does the penis. The urethra need not be extended for metoidioplasty and thus is less expensive and has fewer complications, but then standing urination is no longer an option.

Technically, metoidioplasty is less complex and less expensive than phalloplasty. But, once recovered from surgery, people who have undergone phalloplasty are often more able to complete sexual penetration. This may be in part because the enlarged clitoris may not be capable of attaining the rigidity of a penis.

Medically assisted transition for trans men may include mastectomy and further surgical shaping of a male-contoured chest. Trans men may also undergo hysterectomy and removal of ovaries and Fallopian tubes (salpingo-oophorectomy).

Complications. Because the urethra of a trans man must be lengthened significantly, complications are more likely to occur. Postoperatively, about a quarter of patients in one study who had had their urethrae elongated had transient swelling that caused some urine dribbling, but this subsided without medical intervention. Trans men who had had the urethra extended had small changes of strictures, or narrowing of the urethra, or of a fistula, or hole in the urethra, needing minor repair. Chest surgery to remove breasts will leave scarring. The nipples may have reduced sensation, and their placement may be asymmetrical.

HRT EFFECTS

For transitions accompanied by hormones (hormone-replacement therapy), trans men will probably use testosterone in one of its forms, be it injectable, topically as a cream or gel, applied via patch, or by a pellet subcutaneously inserted; trans women may block their testosterone with an antiandrogen, commonly called a "t-blocker", while receiving estrogen and progesterone.

Although hormones have effects in everyone, often we overlook or minimize them. Sex hormones are the same for men and women, but their ratios differ across genders as well as being affected by time. Receiving hormones from the identified sex can ease the path of transition, but the unaccustomed influx can also rock one's psychic boat.

Some generalities apply. For trans men, previously unexperienced testosterone levels can affect the emotions, pushing anger up the roster of options. For trans women, as breasts develop they may not only be tender, but may leak milky fluid as well. Testosterone may cause hair to sprout in unexpected and perhaps inconvenient places, or familial baldness may wreak havoc on the hairline. For anyone receiving cross-gender HRT, acne may be worse this second time around and may even appear in places never before afflicted. Finally, when produced by hormones from a whole new quadrant, sexual desire may feel bafflingly unfamiliar.

PERSPECTIVE AND PROSPECTS

Regardless of age, most people feel that they belong to a particular gender. Is that feeling of gender determined by the shape of our sex organs or by chemicals such as enzymes and hormones? If not, what causes it?

Because despite individual variations the structure of male and female brains varies slightly, some have questioned whether the brains of transgender people are more like their gender identities than their assigned gender. When Spanish investigators in one small study made MRI investigations of brains of a

small number of female-to-male and male-to-female people, both before and after cross-sex hormonal treatment, results indicated that even before being treated the brains of transgendered people were in some ways more resembled the brains of their identified gender than those of their assigned gender. Subcortical areas, which tend to be thinner in men, were relatively thin in female-to-male subjects, while male-to-female subjects showed thinner right-hemisphere cortices, more characteristic of female brains. After hormonal treatment, these effects became more evident. But these researchers believe it an oversimplification to say that one sex is improperly housed in a body of the wrong sex. Instead, they propose that transgender people have transsexual brains.

The idea that being transgendered arises from hormonal imbalance has been debunked. A recent study in young people who do not identify with their assigned sex showed congruence between inatally assigned sex and hormonal status; in other words, their sex hormones were in alignment with their anatomical sex. So if someone assigned to be female at birth because of possessing female genitalia has the same mix of estrogen, progesterone, and testosterone as did her mother, yet feels and has always felt male, it is not because of hormones.

Has a transgender gene been found? The short answer at this time is no. As embryos we all start as both genders with two sets of undeveloped (or ambiguous) gonads. Around the sixth week of development one of two things happens. Either a gene turns on and the female organs fade away, or that gene is silent and the female organs flourish; in either case the male organs do the converse. In most cases, that is. Mutations in engaged genes or chromosomes may subvert the process. Other mishaps may occur; receptors may not bind the sex hormones that should dock there, enzymes that ignite sex characteristics may misfire, a hormonal cascade may be torrential or constrained. From without, drugs and chemicals not intended for fetal acquaintance may find their way in and wreak changes. How these and other potentialities are timed and interact cannot but introduce uncertainties.

Not everyone considers sexuality a polarity of male or female; black to white encompasses an infinity of shades. The term transgender includes not only people whose gender identity differs from their assigned sex, but also those occupying various places along the spectrum of one sex to its opposite; big-ender, pangender, agender. To be transgendered (the sex that one is) is not the same as sexual orientation (the sex that one prefers sexually); it differs as well from intersexed, which describes people born with ambiguous sex organs. Being transgendered may be more congruent with one's identity as heterosexual, homosexual, bisexual, asexual, or any variant. Or maybe it deserves a category of its own. But there is nothing physiologically wrong; there is nothing to 'cure'. (It is well to be mindful that, while transitioning to one's gender identity may solve one big problem, others may stubbornly persist.) All the same, the courage and openness of people like Caitlin Jenner, Chaz Bono, and Chelsea Manning has helped to bring awareness of the gender-atypical experience to the gender-typical population.

Although the mysteries behind our differences are yet to be unraveled, in the end only we can decide who we are.

—*Jackie Dial, PhD*

FOR FURTHER INFORMATION

Lewis, Ricki. "Is Transgender Identity Inherited?" DNA Science Blog, March 2, 2017. http://blogs.plos.org/dnascience/2017/03/02/is-transgender-identity-inherited/

Olson, Johanna et al. "Baseline Physiologic and Psychosocial Characteristics of Transgender Youth Seeking Care for Gender Dysphoria." Journal of Adolescent Health, October 2015, 57:4: 374-380. http://www.jahonline.org/article/S1054-139X(15)00216-5/fulltext

Rogers, Ashley Lauren. "Eight Things That Really Happen When Transgender People Start Hormone Therapy." Cosmopolitan, September 29, 2015. http://www.cosmopolitan.com/sex-love/news/a46391/things-that-really-happen-when-trans-people-start-hormone-therapy/

Russo, Francine. "Is There Something Unique about the Transgender Brain?" Scientific American, January 1, 2016. https://www.scientificamerican.com/article/is-there-something-unique-about-the-transgender-brain/

Wanjek, Christopher. "Being Transgender Has Nothing to Do with Hormonal Imbalance." LiveScience, July 23, 2015. https://www.livescience.com/51652-transgender-youth-dont-have-hormonal-imbalance.html

Sexual trauma in female veterans

CATEGORY: Social issue
Disease/Disorder

DESCRIPTION

Women make up approximately 16.4 percent of active-duty military forces in the United States, a percentage that is expected to increase. Female members of the military may now serve in combat situations, which increases their risk for combat exposure and increases the likelihood that they will be part of units that are predominantly male. Female service members have significantly higher rates of sexual assault than civilian women. With the increase in female active-duty personnel, the U.S. Department of Veterans Affairs (VA) recognizes the need to focus research and programs on the needs of female service members and veterans.

The VA defines military sexual trauma (MST) as "sexual harassment that is threatening in character or physical assault of a sexual nature that occurred while the victim was in the military, regardless of geographic location of the trauma, gender of the victim, or the relationship to the perpetrator." The perpetrator may be either a military service member or a civilian. Regardless of whether the victim was working or not at the time of the incident or was on or off base, if the individual was on active duty then the VA considers the incident to be MST. It is important to note that the term *military sexual trauma* encompasses both the harassment/assault and the trauma associated with harassment/assault.

The physical, psychological, and emotional trauma of MST is magnified in the unique context of the military. In situations of rape in the military, the female victim often knows the perpetrator and has to have continued contact with the perpetrator, who may be a peer or a superior. Alcohol often is involved in situations of unwanted sexual contact (USC). As a result, incidents of USC in the military may be surrounded by the same ambiguity and self-doubt on the part of the victim as occur with civilian acquaintance rape. This type of sexual trauma—when the perpetrator is known, and alcohol is involved—has been found to increase the risk for posttraumatic stress disorder (PTSD) and intensify PTSD symptoms.

Core military values of loyalty, teamwork, discipline, collectivism, unit cohesion, and mission success are highly valued and can lead victims to fear retribution if they report the USC. Reporting USC can also disrupt career advancement for the victim. She may need to leave the military for her own well-being. If the victim was engaged in illegal conduct during the episode of sexual contact (such as underage drinking or fraternization), she may be subject to disciplinary action. The military provides two methods for reporting USC: restricted and unrestricted reports. A restricted report allows the service member to maintain anonymity, but she forfeits her right to seek punishment for the perpetrator. As a result, many perpetrators remain on active duty because service members and veterans are not willing to go public with their MST. Unrestricted reporting triggers a formal investigation and filing of charges, so the victim will not remain anonymous.

Complications of MST include increased risk for mental health and behavioral issues such as PTSD, substance abuse, compulsive eating, risky sexual behaviors, and suicide as well as physical health issues such as sexually transmitted diseases (STDs), physical injuries, unwanted pregnancy, obesity, and chronic pain. MST has been linked to a 2 to 3 times greater risk for a mental health diagnosis. The association between MST and mental health distress is greater in female veterans than in male veterans. PTSD is the most prevalent diagnosis accompanying MST, followed by mood disorders and adjustment disorders.

The VA requires that all veterans seen in VA facilities be screened for MST. Every VA facility is to have a designated MST coordinator who assists identified patients with access to services. Some facilities have outpatient mental health services for MST while others have more intensive inpatient programs. Any veteran who feels that she was a victim of MST can apply for and receive counseling and medical treatment through the VA regardless of whether the MST-related problems are rated as being a disability or service connected (when physical or mental health problems are considered a direct result of military service and the veteran is then entitled to disability benefits at a specified percentage). Veterans receive assistance for MST independently of their VA benefits.

Social support has been shown to be the best predictor for recovery after a trauma, yet the culture of the military can limit the availability of social support. Deployed service members are geographically separated from friends and family members who would typically provide support. Female active-duty service members are less likely to be married than their male counterparts, which removes a potential support system for returning female veterans. Furthermore, service members returning from a deployment often face stressors such as difficulty reentering the family unit; these may be intensified for female veterans who experienced MST.

Treatment for female veterans who have experienced MST includes psychiatric evaluation and therapy, pharmacology, and close monitoring for suicide and self-injurious behavior.

FACTS AND FIGURES

The Department of Defense (DOD) produces an annual report on sexual assault and sexual assault prevention in the military. According to this report, in fiscal year 2014, 4.3 percent of women in the military reported experiencing USC, down from 6.1 percent in 2012. While overall numbers of USC have gone down, the number of reports filed has increased 16 percent in the same time period. This increase is believed to represent improvements made by the military in reporting procedures. However, there is still much work to be done. The same survey found that of the 4.3 percent of active-duty women who experienced USC, 62 percent reported experiencing some sort of professional or social retaliation, adverse administrative action, or punishment associated with their report. The VA found that between 15 percent and 36 percent of women seeking treatment from the VA screened positive for MST. Researchers investigating veterans who had screened positive for MST and had been to the VHA at least once in the previous year found that 75.9 percent had at least one visit to the VHA that was MST-related, and 55.4 percent had an average of four mental health visits related to MST treatment. There is also a significant association between eating disorders and MST.

Results from another study indicated that victims of MST were 3 times more likely to attempt suicide and 2 times more likely to have suicidal ideations than their military counterparts who had not experienced

MST. Researchers further found that female veterans who are victims of MST have higher levels of anxiety, drug use, and difficulties after returning from deployment such as homelessness, social phobia, and suicidal ideations than female veterans who are not victims of MST.

RISK FACTORS

Female service members are at a higher risk for unwanted sexual contact while on active duty than their male counterparts. Younger military service members are more vulnerable than older military service members. A history of childhood or adult sexual or physical maltreatment increases the risk for MST. Other risk factors include enlisted rank, lack of a college degree, and being impaired as a result of substance use.

SIGNS AND SYMPTOMS

Psychological signs include mood instability, anger, depression, anxiety, irritability, suicidal ideation, self-blame, emotional numbing, concentration difficulties, memory problems, shame, eating disorders, hallucinations, and flashbacks.

Physical symptoms include chronic pain, sexual dysfunction, irritable bowel syndrome (IBS), headaches, back pain, chronic fatigue, and gynecological issues including pelvic pain and menstrual problems. MST also creates an increased risk for arthritis, obesity, diabetes, hypertension, hyperlipidemia, heart disease, lung disease, miscarriage, and infertility.

Behavioral problems include avoidance of interpersonal contact, self-isolation, difficulty trusting others, substance use, high-risk behaviors, sleep and appetite disturbances, spiritual crisis, hallucinations, and flashbacks.

ASSESSMENT AND SCREENING TOOLS

Professionals may perform some of the following assessments for a person with MST: completing a bio-psycho-social-spiritual assessment of the veteran or active-duty military member, utilizing a depression screening instrument, screening for PTSD, assessing for risk of suicide or self-harm, screening for substance and/or alcohol or addiction issues, and screening for intimate partner violence (IPV).

If the assessment is being performed by someone in the VA system, certain specific questions are asked:

"While in the military, did you receive uninvited and unwanted sexual attention, such as touching, cornering, pressure for sexual favors, or verbal remarks?" and "Did someone ever use force or the threat of force to have sexual contact with you against your will?"

Screening tools that are specific to MST or other trauma may also include the Trauma Questionnaire (TQ), the Post-Deployment Readjustment Inventory (PDRI), the Sexual Experiences Questionnaire (SEQ-DOD), the Brief Symptom Inventory (BSI), the Beck Depression Inventory (BDI), and/or the Posttraumatic Checklist – Military Version (PCL-M).

Laboratory tests may include screenings for STDs and substance abuse.

TREATMENT

The most common treatment strategies used with veterans who have experienced MST are primarily PTSD-focused: psychoeducation, pharmacotherapy, psychodynamic therapy if there are childhood traumas that need to be addressed along with the MST, and cognitive behavioral therapy (CBT). The unique needs of female veterans who have experienced MST must be recognized. Professionals without military experience should become familiar with military culture through continuing education or training workshops. Female veterans frequently report having received little support during their deployments, which can intensify MST.

Psychoeducation consists of teaching the veteran about responses to trauma and reducing self-blame. Pharmacotherapy may include medications for anxiety, sleep disturbances, and managing symptoms of depression. Psychodynamic therapy may be utilized for the veteran who experienced childhood trauma or other victimization prior to the MST to help uncover any unconscious conflicts that are serving to place the veteran into situations that increase her vulnerability to revictimization. CBT has two components. Cognitive interventions address and try to alter the dysfunctional beliefs related to the MST while increasing positive beliefs that promote improved coping. Behavioral interventions teach coping skills and techniques to manage emotions, anger, communication, and physical symptoms of stress. Common CBT techniques are stress inoculation training (SIT), prolonged exposure therapy

Problem	Goal	Intervention
Veteran discloses that she experienced USC while on active duty and is experiencing MST.	Veteran will feel supported after disclosure and have a plan in place for treatment/counseling/VA assistance.	Assist in application for services through the VA. Validate the experience and show empathy. Educate on MST and its effects. Assess current safety, health, and mental health. Assess available support systems. Advocate for treatment and counseling.
Veteran has symptoms consistent with PTSD (sleep disturbances, self-blame, memory issues) and depression and disclosed during her initial assessment that she experienced USC.	Veteran will have a reduction in negative symptoms.	Ensure connection with available and appropriate resources and services, including peer support. Monitor support system and enhance if possible. Begin counseling interventions that are appropriate for the situation (SIT, CPT, PE). Screen for substance use and refer for assistance with any substance use disorder if present. Evaluate for risk for self-harm
Veterans disability claim for MST-related PTSD is denied, which is common with female veterans.	Veteran will feel supported and assisted in appeal.	Assist with appeal for MST-related PTSD service connection. Provide advocacy and support. Educate staff within the VA healthcare system regarding the realities of MST and its effects. Advocate with the Veterans Benefits Administration.

(PE), cognitive processing therapy (CPT), and eye movement desensitization and reprocessing (EMDR). SIT is a three-phase behavioral treatment: education, skill building, and skill application. In PE the veteran repeatedly reimagines the trauma in a controlled environment to lessen the power of the traumatic memories. CPT, developed specifically for sexual assault survivors, combines cognitive therapy with exposure therapy. EMDR utilizes elements of exposure therapy and CBT along with techniques that involve eye movements or hand tapping to move the veteran's attention back and forth across the midline.

Substance use problems among veterans with MST very likely are a means of coping with PTSD symptoms resulting from the unwanted sexual contact. Therefore, it is important to treat PTSD before substance abuse interventions. Female veterans benefit from therapeutic interventions such as Seeking Safety, which is a CBT therapy designed for the coexistence of a substance use disorder and PTSD. It emphasizes development of present-focused coping skills along with psychoeducation.

APPLICABLE LAWS AND REGULATIONS

VA benefits arising from Public Laws 102-585, 103-452, and 106-117 provide a counseling and treatment benefit for MST and potentially MST compensation by providing the veteran with a disability rating that is directly connected to her military service and will be reflected in her pension benefits.

The National Defense Authorization Act (NDAA) for 2015 contains provisions related to military sexual assault and harassment. The act authorizes physicians, nurse practitioners, and registered nurses to be assigned as sexual assault forensic examiners (SAFEs) and requires the secretary of each service branch to ensure that an adequate number of SAFEs are available and to maintain a SAFE training and certification program.

Professionals working with veterans who disclose MST must be respectful of the veterans' wishes regarding confidentiality; they must educate those retired from the military that to pursue charges against perpetrators, they must file unrestricted reports (a complete and public report to military and legal authorities).

In the United States, each state has its own criteria that must be met to place someone on an involuntary psychiatric hold when he or she is a danger to self or others. Professionals must be aware of the laws that pertain to their veterans and understand the legal mandates that apply when a veteran is making threats of self-harm or harm to others.

FOOD FOR THOUGHT

In a sample of active-duty female service members, PTSD was more significantly associated with MST than with combat experience stressors.

Researchers have found that female veterans with MST-related PTSD are showing heart rate variability at a younger age than other females. This variability increases the risk of cardiovascular disease.

Researchers have found that women with a depressive disorder and PTSD resulting from an interpersonal trauma (such as unwanted sexual contact) were at risk for future intimate partner violence. However, this risk was reduced with CBT.

Lesbian and bisexual veterans were found to be more likely to have experienced USC.

Male veterans with MST are receiving higher disability compensation ratings (70 to 100 percent) than female veterans (10 to 30 percent) when filing MST-related PTSD disability claims. In PTSD claims, the trigger for the PTSD must be identified; female veterans who filed a restricted report or, more likely, no report at all, are at a disadvantage in proving their claims.

Avoidance coping strategies are common among women veterans who have experienced MST. Often these take the form of behaviors that are carried out in isolation (compulsive spending, overexercising, bingeing and purging, and abusing prescription medications), which serve as a cognitive avoidance strategy.

Veterans who have experienced MST are at an increased risk for suicide and suicidal ideation. All veterans who have a positive screen for MST should be assessed on an ongoing basis for risk of self-harm.

MST has been shown to increase the risk of homelessness for female veterans.

—*Jessica Therivel, LMSW-IPR*

FOR FURTHER INFORMATION

Baltrushes, N., & Karnik, N. S. (2013). Victims of military sexual trauma—you see them, too. *The Journal of Family Practice, 62*(3), 120-124.

Burgess, A. W., Slattery, D. M., & Herlihy, P. A. (2013). Military sexual trauma: a silent syndrome. *Journal of Psychological Nursing, 51*(2), 20-26. doi:10.3928/02793695-20130109-03

Department of Defense. (2015). *Department of Defense annual report on sexual assault in the military: Fiscal year 2014*. Washington, DC: Author.

Klingensmith, K., Tsai, J., Mota, N., Southwick, S., & Pietrzak, R. (2014). Military sexual trauma in US veterans: Results from the National Health and Resilience in Veterans Study. *Journal of Clinical Psychiatry, 75*(10), e1133-1139. doi:10.4088/JCP.14m09244

Stander, V., & Thomsen, C. (2016). Sexual harassment and assault trends in the U.S. military: A review of policy and research trends. *Military Medicine, 181*(1), 20-27. doi:10.7205/MILMED-D-15-00336

Sexuality

CATEGORY: Biology

KEY TERMS:

bisexuality: the capacity to be sexually attracted to and aroused by both genders; the term also implies a significant and consistent capacity for such arousal and does not refer to occasional attraction to or activity with both genders

celibacy: originally meaning "unmarried," it also refers to the willful or circumstantial refraining from sexual intercourse and, by implication, erotic behavior; though sometimes misconstrued as asexual, celibates are no less sexual than noncelibates

erogenous zones: bodily areas that are especially sensitive to touch, leading to sexual arousal; although a dozen or so such zones are common (for example, the clitoral glans and labia, penile glans and shaft, breasts, buttocks, inner thighs), these zones can differ from person to person

erotic: referring to sensory perceptions that are sensual (gratifying or pleasurable) and sexual; the context in which they occur will determine whether the perceptions become erotic (for example, breast and testicle examinations are typically not erotic, while caressing these same body parts in romantic settings typically is)

gender: strictly speaking, the behavioral and social aspects of being either a girl/woman or a boy/man; the term is more loosely used to refer to the biological and physical aspects of being male or female as well

gender identity: a person's inner sense and feeling of maleness/ masculinity or femaleness/femininity, or both; it implies that one clearly identifies with one gender more than the other, although some people identify with both genders equally or near equally

gender role: behaviors and self-presentations that are associated with being a boy/man or a girl/woman and that one uses to identify or recognize others as a boy/man or a girl/ woman; the term also implies the sociocultural expectations of boys/men and girls/women

heterosexual: being principally attracted to and aroused by a person of the opposite gender; a synonymous term, "straight," refers to persons of either gender who are primarily Heterosexual

homophobia: obsessive fear of and anxiety about homosexuals and their social and sexual activities; while several causes of homophobia are known, the most common is a homophobe's private, often unconscious fear and doubt about his or her own sexuality and sense of sexual adequacy

homosexual: being principally attracted to and aroused by persons of one's own gender; two synonymous terms are "gay," which can refer to all homosexuals or to homosexual boys/men exclusively, and "lesbian," which refers only to homosexual girls/women

HISTORICAL OVERVIEW

Sexuality is usually manifested and experienced as orientation toward and attraction to people of the same gender, the opposite gender, or both. Sexual orientation is also referred to as "sexual preference." The term "preference," however, can imply that sexual attraction and orientation are chosen and voluntary, that one can will oneself to find another person sexually appealing. In fact, most research suggests the opposite: People find themselves attracted to an individual or a particular gender without having thought about that attraction or having consciously willed it. The attraction and orientation are not chosen. People can wish not to be attracted in the ways that they are, and they may choose not to act on these feelings, but the attraction felt and experienced is outside voluntary control.

A female athlete may wish not to have the sexual feelings she does for her teammates. A male chemistry major may want himself not to find a female classmate as distracting as she is. A female attorney who is happily married may want the sexual feelings she experiences for her male client to cease. A celibate priest may desire the sexual feelings that he has toward some male and female members of his congregation to go away. As much as these individuals may want to will such feelings away, success in this endeavor is unlikely. Each, instead, must choose how to cope with the feelings, from acting on them directly, to carrying on in spite of them, to pretending that the feelings are not there.

The historical evidence suggests that the prevailing belief in most societies was that people had either a homosexual or a heterosexual orientation; regardless of what made people attracted to their own or to the opposite gender, sexual orientation was "either-or." In the twentieth century, most social scientists and sex researchers came to think about sexual orientation as lying on a continuum marked by degrees of likelihood of finding one's own or the opposite gender attractive. Sexologist Alfred C. Kinsey and his associates published their landmark works, *Sexual Behavior in the Human Male* in 1948 and *Sexual Behavior in the Human Female* in 1953, in which they used a continuum of sexual orientation to quantify a range of attraction, from those who found only members of the opposite gender attractive (whom they defined as "heterosexual") to those who found only members of the same gender attractive (whom they defined as "homosexual"). Between the two extremes were the majority of people, who find both genders attractive and arousing in varying degrees-and thus are defined as "bisexual."

In determining sexual orientation, researchers once focused on the gender of sex partners, which also was the criterion on which laypersons generally focused. If a male usually had female partners, they would consider him heterosexual; if a female usually had female partners, they would consider her homosexual. Yet sexual orientation, how one is attracted by and toward others, is more accurately considered to be primarily the subjective experience of how one feels inside, not the overt behavior that one demonstrates outside.

Research has shown that, in any given individual, there can be a large discrepancy between the gender of one's actual partners and the gender to which one is more attracted and drawn. Social and cultural circumstances often affect, even determine, whether one will behave the way one feels. People who are primarily attracted to opposite-gender persons may be influenced to have, and even pursue, same-gender partners by particular religious beliefs, certain restricted environments (such as prison), or the sense that this behavior is or is not permissible. Orientation is better understood in the minds and feelings of persons themselves: which gender attracts, how often, and how much. Personal histories that include procreating children, marriage, homosexual activities, and bisexual experimentation should not be used to identify sexual orientation.

Although many studies followed the early work of Kinsey, most experts believe that Kinsey and his colleagues produced the most valid observations about sexuality and sexual orientation. Conducting research in this field is difficult. Different studies use different survey tools, and not all are equally reliable. In addition, many people will not candidly or honestly discuss their sexual attitudes, attractions, or behaviors. Nevertheless, the best estimates that rely and build on the Kinsey group's earlier work suggest that about 10 percent of the population in Western countries is primarily gay or lesbian and that an additional 10 percent of the population is primarily bisexual. (There is less research available on non-Western nations, and much of what is available is methodologically less reliable.) In the United States, 60 million people are likely to be homosexual or bisexual. Far more important than the numbers, however, is the reality that gay, lesbian, and bisexual orientations are neither unusual nor peculiar. This remains true even though heterosexuality is the more common pattern of most people, most of the time—a finding true for all societies ever studied. Yet a minority pattern of attraction cannot, simply on the basis of numbers, be considered abnormal.

Expert and lay opinions about how sexual orientation develops differ, often considerably. Yet expert, if not lay, opinions do converge about when it develops: at about age four or five, which is a year to two earlier than when experts believe an individual's personal traits and characteristics emerge intact as an identifiable personality. Because erotic behavior and erogenous stimuli do not usually become an important part of one's personal world until puberty begins (the developmental marker used to interpret when childhood ends and adolescence begins), many do not learn what their orientation is until late adolescence or even well into adulthood. People who eventually come to have nearly exclusive heterosexual fantasies, attractions, and sexual affiliations often have had earlier, adolescent homosexual experiences. Likewise, people who eventually come to discover that their orientation is strongly homosexual have often married, borne children, and had long periods of gratifying heterosexual dating experiences.

Most people eventually come to identify their orientation, at least implicitly, in terms of direction and strength. Direction refers to the direction of sexual orientation, toward one's own or one's opposite gender. Strength refers to the degree of exclusivity associated with the direction of one's orientation: attracted only by the same or opposite gender, sometimes attracted by each, always attracted to each. Bidirectional orientation is the least researched and least understood of sexual orientations. As with homosexual and heterosexual behavior, bisexual encounters, even if gratifying, do not in themselves mean that someone is bisexually oriented, and therefore bisexual. All sexual orientation is internal, not behavioral.

Some people, while learning about their sexual selves and their accompanying orientation, engage in experimental bisexual behavior. Some, with limited access to the gender toward which they are more predominantly or exclusively oriented, become sexually active with the gender toward which they are not oriented, but which is more available. Some are sexually active with both genders for money. Some are sexually stimulated and aroused regardless of gender. (William H. Masters and Virginia E. Johnson, perhaps the leading sex researchers and sex educators of all time, label this group "ambisexual.") Some indicate that they have a definite orientation toward sexual activity with both genders. Among this last group, there are those who report having long-term, one-gender relationships that followed long-term, other-gender relationships, and there are others who report having concurrent sexual relationships with partners of both genders.

Although descriptions of active bisexuality are readily available in the research, the sheer variety of patterns substantially challenges research-based understandings of how sexual orientation originates and develops. What is known is that people with bisexual orientations are neither poorer nor better psychologically adjusted than heterosexuals or homosexuals, and that bisexuality, while poorly understood, reflects a comfortable and fulfilling sexual life and identity for a significant percentage of the general population.

THEORIES OF SEXUAL ORIENTATION

No other area of sexuality has generated more interest, theory, or research than orientation and how it originates. No one theory stands alone as proven, and not-yet-explained data shake the foundations of even the most useful theories. Nevertheless, scientific inquiry has disproven many earlier theories. The most promising theories fall into several categories, some of which can overlap to a degree: genetic, hormonal, psychodynamic, parental, familial, behavioral, societal, and cultural.

The first significant study of genetic causality for sexual orientation was published in 1952. The research compared one group of male identical twins with one group of male fraternal twins. In both groups, one twin was known to be homosexually oriented. Reasonably assuming that both twins of a pair would be exposed to essentially the same environments, the study counted how many second twins, whose sexual orientations were unknown at the start of the study, were also gay. If the rate of homosexuality for twins was higher among the group of identical twins than in the group of fraternal twins, it would be evidence that genetic makeup, which is virtually the same between identical twins, the main cause of sexual orientation.

Twelve percent of fraternal twins who were homosexual had a homosexual twin. Because male fraternal twins are genetically as similar and dissimilar as any pair of brothers, and the rate of homosexuality among the fraternal set was close to the rates that the Kinsey group found in the general population, the results

were initially considered a breakthrough. The study also showed, however, that the twin of every known homosexual in the identical set was also homosexual. One hundred percent concordance rates are rare in studies of identical twins (even studies which might compare heights or weights between identical twins would not achieve 100 percent concordance) and are almost nonexistent in all other social groups on any variable ever studied. This particular study and its unique finding needed replication to be believed. Two later studies, published in 1968 and 1976, had quite different results, and the view that sexual orientation was principally a product of genetic conditions and variability was abandoned, though most researchers still believe genetics provides contributory influence.

Investigation into the role that hormonal factors play in sexual orientation divides between research on animals and research on humans. Studies clearly show that altering prenatal hormone exposure leads to male or female homosexual behavior in at least several animal species. Among humans, a number of studies have had findings that link prenatal exposure to specific sexual orientation outcomes. For example, females who were exposed to male hormones (androgens), especially testosterone, were more likely to develop lesbian orientations; males with Klinefelter syndrome, a chromosomal abnormality marked by a deficiency in androgens, are known to develop gay orientations at a greater frequency than the population average.

Other research on humans has shown that there are different hormone levels between adult homosexuals and heterosexuals. Some studies have found lower testosterone in homosexual males, some have found higher levels of estrogens (though present in both sexes, they are usually considered female hormones) in homosexual males, and other studies have found both. At least one study found higher blood testosterone in homosexual females than heterosexual females. While this evidence seems illuminating on the surface, it is far from conclusive. First, although many studies show different hormone levels between heterosexual and homosexual persons, several studies have also found hormone levels to be the same in both groups. Second, administering sex hormones to adults does not affect their orientation in any way.

Third, prenatal overexposure or underexposure to sex hormones is relatively rare. It would not account for the differences in orientation that are observed in the general adult population, nor is it beyond reason to view cases of abnormal hormonal prenatal environments as extraordinary and unrepresentative of how sexual orientation usually develops.

Fourth, while animal studies often describe processes in particular species that are readily analogous to processes in humans, this does not seem to be the case with human sexuality in general or human sexual orientation in particular. What seems clear is that there is no one-to-one link between sex hormones and sexual orientation. Prenatal hormones, which are known to influence brain development in many ways, may play an indirect role in predisposing individuals toward adapting certain adult sexual behavioral patterns of greater or lesser bisexuality.

Psychodynamic explanations focus on the nature of parent-child relationships and how parents encourage or discourage the growth of their children. Several studies showed homosexual males to have been reared in homes where mothers were dominant and overprotective and fathers were weak, passive, or emotionally uninvolved, a family constellation seen with less statistical frequency among heterosexual males. Other studies, however, showed strained, distant relationships between homosexual men and their fathers but could not find evidence of maternal dominance and overprotectiveness. One study even described the fathers of homosexual males as underprotective, generous, good, and dominant, while the mothers were not found to be overly protective or bossy. Another study simply found no differences in family constellation and dynamics between psychologically well-adjusted heterosexual and homosexual males and females. Given the varied results, the research outcomes from psychodynamic, parental, and familial studies lack cohesive evidence that homosexuality or any orientation results from poor parent-child relationships or dysfunctional family environments.

Behavioral, societal, and cultural theories assume that orientation is primarily learned as people become culturally assimilated and psychologically conditioned (rewarded and punished) for specific sexual feelings, thoughts, and behaviors. Therefore, in an environment where homoerotic feelings were accepted and valued, people would be more likely to develop homosexual, and perhaps bisexual, orientations. In an environment where homophobic attitudes were considered the norm, homoerotic feelings would more likely be abandoned. While these theories have utility in explaining certain sociological phenomena such as atypical gender role behavior (for example, tomboys) and observed shifts toward lesbian sexuality among some female rape victims, they seem to have less utility in explaining how orientation develops in the majority of the population.

Researchers have noted that if sexual orientation occurs along a spectrum of acts and self-identification, women are more likely than men to fall somewhere in the middle of the spectrum. One theory that explains this "heteroflexibility" has been advanced by evolutionary psychologists: Flexibility in women made good evolutionary sense, for women who were raped or whose male partners either died or abandoned them would enjoy better success in raising children if they paired up with another woman. Data from the National Longitudinal Study of Adolescent to Adult Health, which began tracking about 14,000 teenagers in 1994, can be compared with data from 2001–2002 and 2007–2008. These comparisons show that fewer women reported being either 100 percent homosexual or heterosexual. The data also suggests that women are three times as likely as men to switch sexual orientations as they enter early adulthood. Men, it is believed, have a relatively fixed, biologically determined sexual orientation that is not affected by context. Women have a more variable sexual orientation, one that is more responsive to context. Further, women's sexuality is more likely to be impacted by such cultural factors as education, religion, and the attitudes of peers and parents.

In recent years, researchers and academics who study issues involving sexual orientation have focused attention on bisexual and "queer" women. The word *queer* was long used as a derogatory term for homosexuals, but in the twenty-first century the word has been reclaimed by those who reject the binary distinction between homosexuality and heterosexuality and who emphasize the fluidity of sexual attraction. Queer identification is common among women who are members of a sexual minority (e.g., transgender), in part because it is difficult to describe this sexual orientation. Otherwise, many women who are transgender or who self-identify as queer embrace the label because it more closely describes their sexual experiences. Some research points to significant differences between women who identify as bisexual and those who identify as queer. Queer women, for example, are more likely to have sex with transgender or other queer persons; bisexual women, on the other hand, are likely to report a limited number of sexual partners. Further, bisexual women are more likely to report being equally attracted to men and transgender men and to women and transgender women. In contrast, queer women report being more attracted to one of these genders. For this reason, they believe that identification of their sexuality is not captured by conventional definitions of bisexuality. The result of all these complexities is that researchers are left exploring the multiple ways in which the queer label is used among women and the term's overlap with bisexuality.

PERSPECTIVE AND PROSPECTS

Although answers to the question of how orientation develops are complex, researchers Alan P. Bell, Martin S. Weinberg, and S. K. Hammersmith published the two-volume work *Sexual Preference: Its Development in Men and Women* (1981) in an attempt to reveal the causal chain of sexual orientation development in more than thirteen hundred adult homosexual, heterosexual, and bisexual men and women. They based their findings both on lengthy face-to-face interviews with every person in their study and on a sophisticated and reliable statistical technique called path analysis.

Bell, Weinberg, and Hammersmith's research represents the most extensive collection of data on a large number of people in existence, and most experts are taking at least some of their findings to be conclusive. These results show that sexual orientation is strongly established in most people by late adolescence and that sexual feelings rarely undergo directional changes in adulthood. Atypical gender role behavior in childhood, such as boys preferring to play with dolls and not having an interest in more competitive activities, was found to be more likely than not to proceed homosexual orientations in adolescence and adulthood. Adult homosexuals and bisexuals had, on average, the same amount of heterosexual experience as heterosexual adolescents, though their heterosexual experiences were less rewarding and enjoyable than either their own homosexual experiences or the heterosexual

experiences of heterosexuals. The study found that girls choosing their fathers as role models does not cause these girls to become lesbian (as several theories had maintained) and that the parental combination of a domineering, powerful mother and a weak, inadequate father does not cause homosexuality in males (as was once believed). Although their study was methodologically well planned and statistically sound, Bell, Weinberg, and Hammersmith could not find solid support for any of the prevailing theories about the causality of sexual orientation. Some theories explain some of the observed data, and some theories seem to enhance understanding of the origins of sexual orientation in some elements of the population, but no theory or combination of theories explains all the data.

If this research has moved medical science along to some degree, it also serves to remind everyone, professional and nonprofessional alike, that the very complexity of human experience and how humans develop their identity warrants caution if it is ever to be accurately understood. The evidence is not complete. It is known that some aspects of the theories of the origins of sexual orientation are true and that others are false. Learning one's own sexual orientation is a complex process requiring self-observation, self-reflection, and self-recollection. People discover what they like and who they like; the content and orientation of their sexual fantasies; and which gender feels closer to their sexual identity as persons (rather than the gender role that they feel a societal obligation to play). It is their own experiences of what is, and is not, sexually gratifying that teaches people how they are oriented sexually.

—*Paul Moglia, Ph.D.*
Updated by Michael J. O'Neal

FOR FURTHER INFORMATION

Berzon, Betty. *Permanent Partners: Building Gay and Lesbian Relationships That Last.* Rev. ed. New York: Plume, 2004.

Corinna, Heather. *S.E.X.: The All-You-Need-to-Know Progressive Sexuality Guide to Get You Through High School and College.* New York: Marlowe, 2007.

Dibble, Suzanne L., and Patricia A. Robertson. *Lesbian Health 101: A Clinician's Guide.* San Francisco: UCSF Nursing Press, 2010.

Katz, Jonathan Ned. *The Invention of Heterosexuality.* Chicago: University of Chicago Press, 2007.

Mereish, E. H., S. L. Katz-Wise, and J. Woulfe. "We're Here and We're Queer: Sexual Orientation and Sexual Fluidity Differences between Bisexual and Queer Women." *Journal of Bisexuality* 17 no. 1 (2017): 125–39.

Strong, Bryan, et al. *Human Sexuality: Diversity in Contemporary America.* 6th ed. Boston: McGraw-Hill, 2008.

Sexually transmitted diseases (STDs)

CATEGORY: Disease/Disorder
Also known as: Venereal diseases

KEY TERMS:

antibody: a protein found in the blood and produced by the immune system in response to contact of the body with a foreign substance

asymptomatic: an infection without any symptoms

bacteria: microscopic single-celled organisms that multiply by means of simple division; bacteria are found everywhere, and most are beneficial - only a few species cause disease

immunity: the capacity to resist a disease caused by an infectious agent

infertility: the inability to produce offspring by a person in the childbearing years who has been having sex without contraception for twelve months

inflammation: a response of the body to tissue damage caused by injury or infection and characterized by redness, pain, heat, and swelling

latent: lying hidden or undeveloped within a person; unrevealed

pelvic inflammatory disease (PID): an extensive bacterial infection of the pelvic organs, such as the uterus, cervix, Fallopian tubes, and ovaries

protozoan: a single-celled organism that is more closely related to animals than are bacteria; only a few drugs are available that will kill protozoa without harming their animal hosts

virus: a noncellular particle of protein and nucleic acid; viruses, which can reproduce only inside cells, usually cause damage to their hosts by killing the cells they enter

CAUSES AND SYMPTOMS

Sexually transmitted diseases, or STDs (formerly called venereal diseases), have plagued humankind for centuries. The most prevalent, serious STDs are syphilis, gonorrhea, nongonococcal urethritis, trichomoniasis, genital herpes, genital warts, viral hepatitis, and HIV/AIDS. Others, troublesome but not as serious, include lice, scabies, and vaginal yeast infections.

They are passed on from one person to another mostly by sexual contact, although some of these diseases may be acquired indirectly through contaminated objects or blood. In addition, nearly all these diseases can be passed on from an infected mother to her fetus, which may cause birth defects, severe and damaging infections, or even death. A person can acquire several STDs at the same time, and since recovery from an STD does not confer immunity, a person can get them again and again. Many of these diseases are asymptomatic, which allows them to spread and cause serious complications before a victim is aware of being infected. Finally, some STDs are treatable and some are not.

Syphilis is caused by *Treponema pallidum.* This bacterium normally infects the vagina or cervix, but it can also enter through a cut on the mouth or other parts of the skin. Once inside, the bacteria grow at the site of entry, then spread throughout the body through the lymph and blood vessels. The symptoms of syphilis are caused by the efforts of the immune response of the patient to fight off the infection.

The disease occurs in three stages: primary, secondary, and tertiary. There also may be latent stages in between each stage where the person infected is asymptomatic. In primary syphilis, a flat, firm, painless, red sore called a chancre appears at the site of entry two to ten weeks after infection. Secondary syphilis is characterized by a red rash that appears two to ten weeks after the disappearance of the primary lesion. The rash will disappear in a few weeks. Without treatment, 40 percent of patients will progress to the tertiary stage within three to ten years. Tertiary syphilis is characterized by the formation of severe lesions called gummas on the skin, bones, or internal organs. Gummas on the spinal cord, brain, or heart can lead to seizures, insanity, or death. Almost all pregnant women with untreated primary or secondary syphilis will transmit the bacteria through the placenta to the developing baby, who will develop congenital syphilis.

Many babies with congenital syphilis are spontaneously aborted or stillborn. Many others are born with characteristic birth defects, secondary or tertiary syphilis, or neurological damage, and may die shortly after birth.

Gonorrhea is caused by the *Neisseria gonorrhoeae* bacterium (also known as gonococcus). The bacterium infects the cervix, vagina, or urethra in females. Between 20 and 80 percent of women infected with gonococcus are asymptomatic or show only mild symptoms. Symptoms include burning or high frequency of urination, vaginal discharge, fever, and abdominal pain. In 20 to 30 percent of untreated women, gonococcus will spread to the Fallopian tubes and cause pelvic inflammatory disease (PID), which can lead to infertility. Infected mothers can transmit the bacteria to their babies as they pass through the birth canal, causing ophthalmia neonatorum, a type of conjunctivitis (inflammation of the eye) that can cause blindness if untreated.

Most cases of nongonococcal urethritis (NGU) are caused by *Chlamydia trachomatis* types *d* through *k*. This bacterium infects the the cervix or urethra in females. The symptoms of chlamydia infection are often mild and go unnoticed. Women are either asymptomatic or experience mild cervicitis (inflammation of the cervix) or urethritis. Complications include PID and infertility in females. Infants born to mothers with cervicitis can develop eye (inclusion conjunctivitis) or lung (infant pneumonia) infections.

Trichomoniasis is caused by the protozoan *Trichomonas vaginalis*. In both sexes, the disease is often mild or asymptomatic. In women, the organism can infect the vulva, vagina, and cervix. Women may suffer from severe vaginitis, which includes a tender, red, and itchy genital area, and a profuse, frothy, foul-smelling, greenish-yellow discharge. Newborns may acquire the infection from an infected mother during delivery.

Most genital herpes infections are caused by herpes simplex virus type 2, but some are caused by herpes simplex virus type 1. The virus infects the the cervix, vulva, vagina, or perineum in females. Two to seven days after infection, painful blisters appear in the genital area that ulcerate, crust over, and disappear in a few weeks.

Herpes viruses are unique in that they can remain latent in the nerves and cause a recurrent infection at any time in the future. Fever, stress, sunlight, or local trauma may trigger the virus to come out of hiding and cause a recurrent infection. The virus can be transmitted from an infected mother to her baby either congenitally, through the placenta, or neonatally, as the baby passes through the birth canal. In congenital or neonatal herpes, the virus can infect all parts of the body, the death rate is high, and survivors commonly have long-term neurological damage and recurrent infections.

Viral hepatitis is also an STD. At least three variants of the virus-hepatitis A virus (HAV), HBV, and HCV-are known to be transmitted sexually. HBV is the form most commonly transmitted sexually. Vaccines are available to immunize persons at risk for HAV and for HBV.

Genital warts are caused by human papillomaviruses (HPVs). They are found on the vagina, cervix, perineum, and anus in women. The warts themselves may be removed, but the infection remains for the life of the patient. HPV infection seems to increase a woman's risk for cervical cancer. There are three vaccines FDA approved: Gardasil, Cervarix and Gardasil 9. All of these vaccines vaccinate against HPV 16 and 18, but Gardasil protects against 2 other strains, and Gardasil 9 protects against nine total strains. As of 2017, Gardasil 9 is the only available HPV vaccine in the United States.

AIDS is caused by the human immunodeficiency virus (HIV). This virus is acquired through sexual contact as well as through intravenous drug use and blood transfusions. HIV infects and inactivates the T helper cells that are needed by the immune system to respond to and fight off infections. Without T helper cells, the immune system eventually becomes nonfunctional, and the affected person becomes susceptible to every type of infection possible. Two-thirds of all AIDS patients get pneumonia caused by *Pneumocystis carinii*. Other common diseases associated with AIDS patients are tuberculosis and other mycobacterial infections, viral infections such as those caused by cytomegalovirus and herpesviruses, fungal infections, cancers such as Kaposi's sarcoma, and neurological disorders. HIV can also be transmitted from an infected mother to her baby through the placenta. Virtually every person infected with HIV will eventually die of AIDS.

TREATMENT AND THERAPY

Sexually transmitted diseases can be diagnosed in several ways. One way is by observing the symptoms and case history of the patient. Characteristic sores or symptoms can lead a doctor to suspect a particular disease, and a sample of a scraping from a lesion or an unusual discharge can be examined under a microscope to identify the infecting organism. The syphilis, gonorrhea, chlamydia, and trichomoniasis organisms all have unique shapes that a doctor can recognize.

For those STDs with mild symptoms or no symptoms, a doctor can try to grow the organism in the laboratory from samples taken from appropriate sites on the body. All organisms that cause STDs can be grown in the laboratory, and since these organisms are not normally present in humans, isolation of the organism from the body is a sign that the body has been infected by that organism. Finally, there are many blood tests that have been developed to test whether a person has specific antibodies in his or her blood that bind to one of these organisms. The presence of antibodies to an organism implies that one has been or is currently infected with that organism. In many cases, doctors will use several of these methods to confirm a diagnosis of an STD.

Specific treatment recommendations for each sexually transmitted disease are subject to periodic revision. Current recommendations are reviewed by the Centers for Disease Control and are published in the *Morbidity and Mortality Weekly Report* every three or four years. It is important for physicians to review these recommendations in order to prescribe the best method for treating STDs. All the bacterial and the protozoal STDs can be treated and cured with antibiotics. It is important to seek early diagnosis and treatment of these diseases for three reasons: First, to prevent the disease from spreading; second, to prevent the various complications associated with the diseases; and third, to prevent the infection of infants by pregnant mothers. There is no cure for STDs caused by viruses; there are only drugs that slow the progress of the infection.

Syphilis is commonly treated with penicillin, or alternatively with erythromycin, doxycycline, or ceftriaxone. In most patients receiving appropriate therapy during primary or secondary syphilis, the active disease is totally and permanently arrested. Treatment during the latent stage stops the development of symptoms of the tertiary stage. There is no successful treatment for patients in tertiary syphilis.

A combination of an intramuscular injection of ceftriaxone and a single dose taken orally of azithromycin are the agents used to treat gonorrhea. Quinolones, such as ciprofloxacin, and azithromycin are other antibiotics that can be effective treatment for gonococcal infections. Doxycycline or azithromycin are used to treat NGU caused by chlamydia, and trichomoniasis is treated with metronidazole or tinidazole.

Genital herpes is treated with antiviral agents such as acyclovir. Topical application of acyclovir is helpful in reducing the duration of primary, but not recurrent, infections. The use of oral acyclovir to suppress recurrent infections may cause more severe and more frequent infections once the therapy has stopped. Neonatal herpes is treated with acyclovir or vidarabine, which can reduce the severity of the infection but cannot reverse any herpes-related neurological damage or prevent recurrent infections. Genital warts can be removed by chemicals, freezing, electrocautery, or laser therapy. Antiviral drugs are useful in treating some STDs: acyclovir for genital herpes and interferon for hepatitis virus. They slow the progress of the disease in some persons, but they do not cure it. There is now antiretroviral therapy (ART) that is recommended for all HIV-infected individuals regardless of CD4 cell count that helps decrease viral load and decreases serious adverse outcomes of HIV including death. There are also Pre-exposure prophylaxis (PrEP) medicines that are given to people at high risk of getting HIV such as Truvada and post-exposure prophylaxis (PEP) medications that are given to those who do not have HIV, but have been exposed to HIV within 72 hours of exposure.

As with any disease, prevention is the most desirable means of controlling STDs. With the exception of viral hepatitis and HPV, there are no vaccines for STDs; although much research is being done and many potential vaccines have been developed and tested, none is yet satisfactory for general and routine use. Therefore, behaviors resulting in disease avoidance are the only means of preventing most STDs. The only 100 percent effective way to prevent a sexually transmitted disease is abstinence. Abstinence means to refrain voluntarily from engaging in sexual activity. Since many of these diseases can be spread through sexual activity other than intercourse, abstinence must include all sexual activity.

Information on Sexually Transmitted Diseases (STDs)

Causes: Infection through sexual contact; also from contaminated blood or from infected mother to fetus

Symptoms: Varies; may include skin lesions or rash in genital area, itching, abdominal pain, painful urination, vaginal or penile discharge, birth defects, infertility

Duration: Acute to chronic with recurrent episodes

Treatments: Antibiotics, antiviral agents

Choosing to exercise one's sexuality within a monogamous relationship for life can also help prevent sexually transmitted disease. The use of a condom or any other barrier method is only somewhat helpful in the prevention of STDs. Prevention of transmission of STDs from infected mothers to their babies involves early diagnosis and treatment of the mothers before birth and preventive medication of the babies after birth. In the past, ophthalmia neonatorum was the cause of blindness for half of the children admitted to schools for the blind. Therefore, the government made it mandatory to treat all newborns' eyes with silver nitrate, tetracycline, or erythromycin, to prevent this disease. The instillation of silver nitrate in babies' eyes does not prevent chlamydia eye infections, so babies born to mothers with chlamydia need additional antibiotic treatment. Prevention of neonatal herpes may involve delivery by cesarean section to avoid infection of the child as it passes through the birth canal. Preventing the spread of AIDS includes screening blood supplies, organ donors, and semen donors and avoiding contact with infected body fluids through sexual contact, blood transfusions, or intravenous drug use.

Control of STDs in a population is complex, since it is both a medical and a social problem. First, it is important that persons who contract a sexually transmitted disease receive early diagnosis and adequate treatment that will prevent further spread of the disease, serious complications, and infection of infants. This is difficult because many STDs are asymptomatic; therefore, people do not know they have the disease and have no reason to seek treatment. Many persons contract STDs from asymptomatic carriers. In addition, social stigma or embarrassment reduces the motivation of a victim to seek prompt medical care. Adequate treatment of STD victims is difficult if they do not want to return for subsequent treatment or will not take all their medication.

Finally, people often contract several STDs at the same time, so detection of one STD should routinely instigate testing for other STDs. Not only does the person with an STD need to be treated, but all the sexual contacts of that person need to be contacted, tested, and treated as well. Public health officials interview victims of STDs to determine the names and addresses of contacts and then try to find and treat the contacts. This is difficult if a victim does not remember who those contacts are, if he or she does not want to discuss his or her sexual activity, or if the contacts do not want to be bothered by the health department. In addition, many private physicians do not report cases of STDs to the public health department; therefore, in many cases, the sources of STDs are never interviewed.

A reduction in risky sexual behavior, such as unprotected sex, would aid in the control of STDs. Effective education to change sexual behavior must be predicated upon the motivation and cognitive development of the student. One-third of all cases involve teenagers and young adults; sexual activity in this age group is on the rise, and members of this group are more likely to have multiple sex partners. Prostitution for money or drugs also increases the incidence of STDs. Other control measures include development of vaccines for these diseases, mandatory reporting of all STDs, and education of the population regarding the dangers and risks involved in acquiring these diseases.

Perspective and Prospects

Syphilis was first recognized at the end of the fifteenth century in Europe, where it rapidly reached epidemic proportions and was called the "great pox." Gonorrhea was described and given its present name by the Greek physician Galen in 150 CE. From the fifteenth century to the eighteenth century, there was much confusion as to the nature of syphilis and gonorrhea, and many persons thought they were different stages of the same disease. In 1767, an English physician named John Hunter inoculated himself with a urethral discharge from a patient with gonorrhea in order to determine once and for all whether they were one disease or two. Unfortunately, that patient also had syphilis, so when Hunter developed symptoms of both gonorrhea and syphilis he concluded they were a single disease. It was not until 1838 that it was clearly proved that they were two separate diseases. Traditionally, 95 percent of all cases of sexually transmitted disease were either syphilis or gonorrhea. Since the late twentieth century, however, there has been a dramatic increase in the incidence of several other sexually transmitted diseases, such as genital herpes, NGU, AIDS, genital warts, and trichomoniasis.

The rise in incidence of STDs is of epidemic proportions. Worldwide in the 1990s, about 250 million new cases of STDs occurred annually. In the United States, about 12 million new cases, including 3 million in teenagers, occurred annually. By 1997, chlamydia had become the most frequently diagnosed STD in the United States, estimated at more than 4 million annually. Other STDs with high incidence included gonorrhea (1.3 million new cases annually) and genital herpes (0.5 million annually). Because there is no cure for genital herpes, it may be present in 20 percent of Americans.

As of 2002, about 1 million North Americans were HIV-positive; only a portion of these had AIDS. By the late twentieth century, the U.S. government announced that the incidence of new cases of AIDS, about 56,000 at that time, had begun to decline. A decline in the numbers of persons dying from AIDS was also announced. It is estimated that there are 3 to 5 million new cases of NGU per year. One in five couples in the United States is infertile, and much of that infertility is caused by the complications associated with STDs, with chlamydial infection being the primary preventable cause of sterility in women. In the United States, it is estimated that 25 percent of all women are infected with trichomoniasis and more than 20 million people are infected with herpes simplex virus type 2. Despite the fact that most STDs can be controlled, the incidence of many of the diseases is still quite high; thus, STDs obviously present a social as well as a medical problem. An increase in education concerning the signs and risks of these diseases, a reduction in promiscuity, and development of vaccines would help in controlling these destructive and fast-spreading diseases.

IMPACT ON WOMEN

For a variety of reasons, women are more commonly affected by STDs than men are. STDs are believed to be a major public health concern in the United States, especially among women. Women's anatomy puts her a higher risk for STDs, based on the delicate lining of the vagina, however women are actually less likely to have obvious symptoms as compared to men. Women are more likely to seek treatment, therefore there is more record of women experiencing STDs. STDs in women can also lead to greater issues such as infertility and they have the chance of passing the infection or illness to their baby. Women are more likely to contract HPV, which is the leading cause of cervical cancer. Luckily women are more likely to seek treatment from their doctors for these conditions. Parents of young women should be sure to give their daughters the vaccine to prevent HPV. It is extremely important to educate young girls about how STDs are transmitted, in order to help them learn about how to engage in safe sexual activity.

—*Vicki J. Isola, Ph.D.*
Updated by Armand M. Karow, Ph.D.
and Stephanie Marie Ong, RN
and Kimberly Ortiz-Hartman, Psy.D., LMFT

FOR FURTHER INFORMATION

"10 Ways STDs Impact Women Differently from Men", *Centers for Disease Control and Prevention*, 14, March 2019, https://www.cdc.gov/std/health-disparities/stds-women-042011.pdf

Berek, Jonathan S., ed. *Berek and Novak's Gynecology.* 14th ed. Philadelphia: Lippincott Williams & Wilkins, 2007.

Biddle, Wayne. *A Field Guide to Germs.* 2d ed. New York: Anchor Books, 2002.

"Condom Fact Sheet in Brief," *Centers for Disease Control and Prevention*, 4 March 2019, https://www.cdc.gov/condomeffectiveness/brief.html

Larsen, Laura. *Sexually Transmitted Diseases Sourcebook.* Detroit, Mich.: Omnigraphics, 2009. Little, Marjorie. *Sexually Transmitted Diseases.* Rev. ed. Philadelphia: Chelsea House, 2000.

Morse, Stephen A., Ronald C. Ballard, and King K. Holmes. *Atlas of Sexually Transmitted Diseases and AIDS.* 3d ed. New York: Mosby, 2003.

"PEP." Centers for Disease Control and Prevention, 4 March 2019, https://www.cdc.gov/hiv/basics/pep.html

Sexually transmitted diseases risk factors

CATEGORY: Disease/Disorder

KEY TERMS:

chlamydia: a sexually transmitted infection caused by the bacterium Chlamydia trachomatis; often asymptomatic

genital herpes: a disease characterized by blisters in the genital area, caused by a variety of the herpes simplex virus

gonorrhea: a venereal disease involving inflammatory discharge from the urethra or vagina

human papilloma virus (HPV): a virus with subtypes that cause diseases in humans ranging from common warts to cervical cancer

Pap smear: a test carried out on a sample of cells from the cervix to check for abnormalities that may be indicative of cervical cancer

CAUSES AND RISK FACTORS

Many factors can increase a woman's risk of acquiring a sexually transmitted disease (STD), including both individual characteristics or behaviors and broader environmental conditions. Younger age is a recognized risk factor for STDs. Nearly 50 percent of the 19 million new STD cases in the United States each year occur in 15- to 24-year-olds. Individuals in this age group are more likely to engage in risky sexual behaviors, to be less comfortable negotiating condom use or discussing sexual matters with partners, and to lack the self-confidence needed to refuse to have unprotected intercourse. Women in this age range make up the highest percentage of persons impacted by gonorrhea. Being in an age-discordant relationship (specifically, a relationship between a younger adolescent female and an older adult male) is also a risk factor for adolescent STD infection.

There are biological differences between men and women that increase a women's risk for contracting an STD. The vaginal wall is thinner than the skin of the penis, making it easier for bacteria and viruses to pass into the body. The lining of the vagina is susceptible to tearing during penetration, increasing the likelihood of bacterial infection. The vagina is also a breeding ground for bacteria, due to moisture created by glands in the cervix and vaginal wall.

There are racial and ethnic disparities in rates of STDs among female young adults. Black females between the ages of 15 and 24 are 8.7 times more likely to contract chlamydia and 20.5 times more likely to contract gonorrhea when compared to white females of the same age. Hispanic females are twice as likely as whites in this age category to acquire gonorrhea or chlamydia.

Certain sexual behaviors increase the risk of acquiring STDs. These include lack of condom use/unprotected sex; having multiple sex partners; concurrent sexual relationships; anonymous sex partners; engaging in sex in exchange for money; engaging in anal intercourse, with receptive anal sex carrying the highest risk for acquiring HIV; having unprotected sex with a partner who has unhealed lesions or a known STD; serosorting, or engaging in unprotected anal sex with partners thought to have the same HIV status; and having forced sexual intercourse.

Environmental and social factors that have been associated with an increased risk of acquiring STDs include a history of substance and/or alcohol use, which lowers a women's decision-making skills and inhibitions and can lead to risky sexual behavior. It is estimated that binge drinkers are 77 percent more likely than non-binge drinkers to report engaging in high-risk sexual behaviors. Intravenous drug use and the sharing of needles can cause STD transmission. In addition, having unprotected sex with an intravenous drug user is associated with an increased risk for STD infection. Unprotected sexual intercourse and the sharing of needles are estimated to both take place in approximately 29 percent of relationships in which both partners are injection drug users.

Lower socioeconomic status increases the risk of acquiring STDs because of the greater likelihood of inadequate preventive care or education on reducing STD risk. The lack of appropriate preventive care or education regarding STD risk is especially common among homeless persons. Homelessness is associated with increased risk for sexual victimization and with survival sex (i.e., trading sexual acts in exchange for shelter or food), which may expose the victim to STDs.

Homeless young women have been found to be at greater risk for STDs than homeless young men are. Having been in foster care is associated with increased risk for STDs in young adulthood. A history of exposure to sexual, verbal, and physical abuse increases the chances that an individual will experience anxiety, depression, and posttraumatic stress disorder (PTSD), all of which may increase the risk for unsafe sexual behavior. Victims of intimate partner abuse also are at increased risk for STD infection.

Childhood sexual abuse survivors report higher rates of unprotected sex and STDs than do individuals who were not abused. One in four females will be sexually abused by the time they turn 18, putting them at the greater risk of forced unprotected sex. Relationships that lack an equal distribution of power can render individuals unable to negotiate for safe sex practices or without the perceived right to refuse to have unprotected intercourse. Male-to-female transgender persons who experienced gender abuse (i.e., abuse related to their transgender status) and had depressive symptoms were found to be more likely to engage in high risk sexual behaviors and had a higher incidence rate of HIV and other STDs.

Victims of sexual assault and sexual abuse are at a high risk of contracting an STD. Women are disproportionally the victims of sexual assault, with 91% of all victims being female. Men are overwhelmingly the common perpetrator. Men who perpetrate sexual coercion or rape are less likely to routinely wear condoms than are men who do not engage in aggressive sexual behavior. One in five women will be the victim of rape in their lifetime, making the risk of forced unprotected sex amongst females high.

Sex workers are at an increased risk of contracting an STD. It is estimated that there are 40-42 million sex workers worldwide, with 80% being female. Though prostitution is illegal in the United States in all states (with the exception of Nevada), illegal prostitution occurs throughout the country. Sex workers are less likely to use protection and more likely to engage in risky sexual behaviors, increasing the risk of contracting an STD.

Women with mental illness diagnosis and symptoms are at increased risk of acquiring STDs. Presence of STDs have been associated with mental health disorders such as schizophrenia, bipolar disorder, psychotic disorder, depression, and anxiety disorder among indigent, homeless, publicly insured, and institutionalized populations. Clients with mental health problems often display poor judgment and impulsive behavior, leading to risky sexual behaviors. Low self-esteem accompanying mental illness is a barrier to taking responsibility for behavior and taking care of personal health needs. Cultural values and accepted behaviors among various ethnic and cultural groups regarding healthcare, drug and alcohol use, and sexual behavior can place individuals at risk for STDs. For example, Hispanic adolescents are less likely than black or white adolescents to use condoms during sex. Lack of regular healthcare due to poverty, mental illness, or cultural beliefs may contribute to a lack of education regarding safe sex practices.

Human papillomavirus (HPV) is the most common STD in the United States with around 79 million people currently infected. Almost all sexually active adults will be infected by HPV and along with being the most common STD in the United States, it is also the most common STD for women. The immune system normally combats HPV, but it is particularly important for women to get routine testing as HPV is the one of the main causes of cervical cancer. The one of the greatest risks for straight, sexually active women contracting HPV is the lack of a medically approved HPV test for men. Since HPV is typically asymptomatic, women who are in a non-monogamous relationship, have multiple sexual partners, practice risky sexual behaviors or are starting a relationship with a new partner, are at a high risk for contracting HPV.

Psychological barriers to STD screening and treatment can increase risk for STD infection and lead to advanced disease progression or death. These include mistrust of the healthcare system, lack of culturally or linguistically appropriate treatment or education, stigma and shame related to STDs and STD care, and social pressures. Misinformation and misunderstandings about STD screening can increase risk for STD infection. Approximately one quarter of subjects across three samples were found to have an incorrect understanding of the purpose of a Pap smear, for instance. The Pap smear tests for cervical cancer, yet 82 percent to 91 percent of study subjects believed it tested for HPV, 76 percent to 92 percent thought it tested for vaginal infections, 65 percent to 86 percent thought it tested for yeast infections, 55 percent to 81 percent thought it tested for gonorrhea, 53 percent to 80 percent thought it tested for herpes, 22 percent to 59 percent thought it tested for HIV/AIDS, and 17 percent to 38 percent thought it was a pregnancy test. Such beliefs may lead women with negative Pap smears to think that they do not have an STD.

Pregnant women face the same risks of contracting an STD as non-pregnant women. It is especially important to get tested if considering pregnancy or are in the early stages of pregnancy, as STD's can pose serious health risks to both the mother and infant. STD's such as genital herpes, HIV and gonorrhea can be transferred to the unborn baby during pregnancy. STD's can also complicate pregnancy, and in some cases can be life threatening.

SYMPTOMS

One of the biggest challenges in identifying STD's in women is that women are less likely to have visible symptoms when compared to men. Two of the most common STD's for women, besides HPV, are gonorrhea and chlamydia. There has been an increase in the number of reported cases of both in recent years, increasing the risk of becoming infected. This presents a problem as most cases of gonorrhea and chlamydia in women are asymptomatic, making detection without regular testing extremely difficult. Untreated, these STD's can cause pelvic inflammatory disease, along with other major health issues. Symptom's such as ulcers and bumps, which can occur with STD's such as herpes, can be difficult to identify as they may not be visible on the outside of the vagina.

Another difficulty with identifying STD's for women is that many of the symptoms associated with STD's are commonly mistaken for other health issues, such as urinary tract infections and yeast infections. Some of the most common symptoms women with STD's experience are abnormal or unusual vaginal discharge, acute pain during intercourse, appearance of genital warts, frequent urination, painful urination, itching in the vaginal area, irregular bleeding between menstrual cycles, and vaginal rashes or sores.

TREATMENT AND THERAPY

Social workers can learn about the risk factors for STDs and use this knowledge to fully assess individual clients and their healthcare and educational needs. Social workers should provide respectful and empathic client care and avoid negative, judgmental attitudes that can alienate clients and reduce the likelihood they will pursue follow-up care for STD treatment.

Social workers can encourage a multidisciplinary approach to sexual health treatment and prevention by requesting referrals to various specialist services (e.g., mental health clinicians, drug and alcohol treatment programs, primary care clinicians, licensed social workers).

Social workers may provide behavioral counseling and prevention education to all sexually active women who are at increased risk of contracting an STD. Social workers should screen clients for abusive relationships and, if appropriate, provide counseling and information on community resources for safety and STD prevention. Social workers and medical professionals treating sexually active adolescents should become familiar with state and local laws governing the age of consent and reporting of abuse and neglect. Facility and professional protocols for mandated reporting of criminal activity and abuse and neglect should be followed.

Social workers should inform adolescent female clients that testing and treatment for STDs is confidential and parental consent for treatment is not required in the United States. Medical professionals should provide routine screening for STDs to all sexually active clients and their partners and, if necessary, refer for treatment.

—*Carita Caple, RN, BSN, MSHS,*
and Tanja Schub, BS
Updated by Michael Moglia, BA

FOR FURTHER INFORMATION

Daley, E., Perrin, K., Vamos, C., Hernandez, N., Anstey, E., Baker, E. Ebbert, J. (2013). Confusion about Pap smears: Lack of knowledge among high-risk women. Journal of Women's Health, 22(1), 67-74. doi:10.1089/jwh.2012.3667

Pflieger, J. C., Cook, E. C., Niccolai, L. M., & Connell, C. M. (2013). Racial/ethnic differences in patterns of sexual risk behavior and rates of sexually transmitted infections among female young adults. American Journal of Public Health, 103(5), 903-909. doi:10.2105/AJPH.2012.301005

Rosenthal, L., & Levy, S. R. (2010). Understanding women's risk for HIV infection using social dominance theory and the four bases of gendered power. Psychology of Women Quarterly, 34(1), 21-35. doi:10.1111/j.1471-6402.2009.01538.x

Villar-Loubet, O., Jones, D., Waldrop-Valverde, D., Bruscantini, L., & Weiss, S. (2011). Sexual barrier acceptability among multiethnic HIV-positive and at risk women. Journal of Women's Health, 20(3), 365-373.

Workowski, K. A., & Berman, S. (2010). Sexually transmitted diseases treatment guidelines, 2010. MMWR. Morbidity and Mortality Weekly Report. Recommendations and Reports, 59(RR-12), 1-110.

Skin cancer

CATEGORY: Disease/Disorder

INTRODUCTION

Cancer is the common term used to describe the large class of diseases called neoplasms. Neoplasms, which occur only in multicellular organisms, develop and function in an autonomous way that does not abide by the biological mechanisms that govern the growth and metabolism of the individual cells and the reactions that take place in a living organism. When such neoplasms grow at a rate faster than the tissues from which they arise, while at the same time invading those tissues, they are called malignant and are commonly described as cancerous. Benign neoplasms, which do not invade surrounding tissues, generally are not as dangerous as malignant ones.

Sun radiation is life-sustaining, but the higher-energy part of the sunlight spectrum brings the danger of skin cancer. When living tissue is irradiated, its molecular structure is disrupted, thus initiating a chain of reactions, many of which are not the usual ones associated with the living organism. Therefore, a change in the chromosomal composition and the development of unwanted cells is likely to occur. Such changes take place because of the formation of free radicals in the deoxyribonucleic acid (DNA) molecules that constitute the genetic code. The result is skin cancer, the most common form of cancer in both men and women in the United States.

Skin cancer usually presents in older patients, but the number of diagnosed young women in the United States has risen in recent years. Women under 50 are being diagnosed with skin cancer more often than men. It is possible that tanning, both indoors and outdoors, has contributed to this rise, as well as to the change in style of swim wear. With the invention of the bikini, body exposure rose to 92% and tan skin was promoted in fashion media. Young women tend to be more concerned about their health and appearance during these years than men, and often suffer more psychological distress as a result of their diagnosis.

TYPES OF SKIN CANCER

Skin neoplasms may be benign or malignant, acquired or congenital, although the majority are benign and acquired. The common mole (the medical term for which is melanocytic nevus) is a neoplasm of benign melanocytes. These are often seen at birth, but may develop throughout the lifespan. Such moles are generally harmless unless they are large in size, in which case they may have up to a 10 percent chance of becoming malignant. Other melanocytic nevi are strawberry hemangiomas and port-wine stains, which are of vascular origin.

The most common forms of skin cancer are the basal cell and squamous cell carcinomas, which arise from the corresponding part of the keratinocytes of the epidermis and are caused by the cumulative effects of ultraviolet radiation on the skin. They are generally localized, however, and rarely metastasize. These

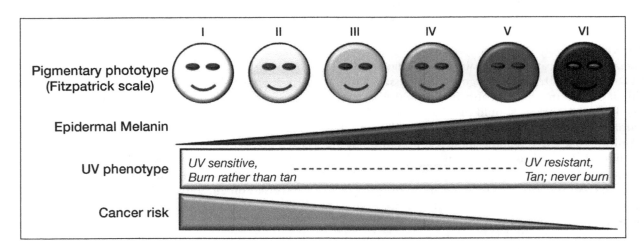

The risk of skin cancer decreases with higher levels of melanin. (John D'Orazio via Wikimedia Commons)

Information on Skin Cancer

Causes: Genetic factors, ultraviolet radiation from sun exposure

Symptoms: Lesion that increases in size and turns several colors (black, blue, white, brown); in later stages, itching, bleeding, and pain

Duration: Short-term to recurrent

Treatments: Surgical removal, chemotherapy, radiation therapy

cancers are easily identified as persisting sores or crusting patches that grow mostly on sun-exposed parts of the body such as the hands, neck, arms, and nose. They can be treated with routine surgical procedures.

A malignant melanoma is formed from the pigment-forming melanocyte, is very aggressive and commonly undergoes metastasis. It should therefore be removed surgically at the earliest possible stage. If the melanoma is detected at a later stage, chemotherapy, radiation or immune therapy are considered for disease conrol. A malignant melanoma appears as a lesion that increases in size and turns several colors, such as black, blue, white, and brown. Symptoms such as itching, bleeding, and pain are not as common at first but are encountered at the later stages of development.

There are two additional skin malignancies that may be fatal: mycosis fungoides and Kaposi's sarcoma. Mycosis fungoides is a skin lymphoma that may be confined to one location for ten or more years before it metastasizes to internal organs, with death following. As a result, it is difficult to track this skin cancer, both clinically and histologically, and several biopsies (skin histological examinations) may be required to ascertain its presence. On the other hand, Kaposi's sarcoma occurs either as lesions (commonly among older Mediterranean men) or as skin abnormalities in HIV-infected people. The sarcoma is derived from skin blood vessels and appears as violet patches or lesions. As long as it is contained only in the skin, it is not fatal. Once the inner organs are affected, however, death is imminent, even though the lesions may be treated with irradiation and chemotherapy.

The effects of sunlight on skin. Extensive skin exposure to sunlight, such as at the beach, leads to the polymerization of skin chemicals (known as catecholamines) and the subsequent formation of different types of epidermal pigmentation (the melanins), which are responsible for tanning. Tanning occurs only if there is gradual exposure to sunlight; otherwise, a sunburn will arise. Photoprotection is believed to be one of the major biological functions of the melanin pigment. It appears that melanin formation can participate effectively in reducing the harmful effects of sunlight by an array of photoinduced chemical reactions, which result in the consumption of scavenging active oxygen species such as the superoxide anion and hydrogen peroxide. It has been determined that in biological systems, superoxide and hydrogen peroxide are formed in small quantities during normal processes.

Both species are known to produce several biological effects, most of which are harmful to tissues. It should be pointed out, however, that although melanin may act as a free radical scavenger, it may also become energetically overloaded and may change to a toxic state. Evidence exists that melanin increases the radiative damage to cells, which leads to sunlight-induced skin cancer. In other words, melanin formation is good only when moderate exposure to sunlight occurs.

In the atmosphere 12 to 48 kilometers above the earth's surface lies a small layer of ozone. Although this layer does not contain much ozone-it is estimated to be about 3 millimeters thick under normal conditions of temperature and pressure- it has a profound effect on life. The ozone layer absorbs the harmful ultraviolet radiation from the sun, thus providing the mechanism for the heating of the stratosphere. A reduction in the ozone layer would lead to a large increase of ultraviolet rays intruding into the atmosphere, thus increasing the incidence of skin cancer. F. S. Rowland and M. J. Molina declared in 1974 that the presence of the volatile chlorofluorocarbons would eventually reduce the ozone layer. Some measurements done by scientists in 1979 showed a decrease in the layer, which led to the action taken by several governments to decrease and replace the chlorofluorocarbons commonly used in aerosols.

As the average life span steadily increases, the incidence of skin cancer will increase as well. The use of effective sunscreens and sunglasses with high ultraviolet blocking is recommended for people who are exposed to large amounts of sunlight.

—*Soraya Ghayourmanesh, PhD*
Updated by Patrick Richardson

FOR FURTHER INFORMATION

Dollinger, Malin, et al. *Everyone's Guide to Cancer Therapy.* 5th ed. Kansas City, Mo.: Andrews McMeel, 2008.

James, William D., Timothy G. Berger, and Dirk M. Elston. *Andrews' Diseases of the Skin: Clinical Dermatology.* 10th ed. Philadelphia: Saunders/Elsevier, 2006.

McClay, Edward F., and Jodie Smith. *One Hundred Questions and Answers About Melanoma and Other Skin Cancers.* Boston: Jones and Bartlett, 2004.

Skin Cancer Foundation. http://www.skincancer.org.

Weedon, David. *Skin Pathology.* 3d ed. New York: Churchill Livingstone/ Elsevier, 2010.

Sleep apnea

CATEGORY: Disease/Disorder
Also known as: Obstructive sleep apnea

KEY TERMS:

apnea: lack of airflow for more than ten seconds

apnea-hypopnea index (AHI): the average number of apneic and hypopneic episodes in one hour

CPAP: Continuous Positive Airway Pressure; a constant flow of air pressure to ensure that the airway stays open during sleep

hypopnea: a decrease in airflow greater than 50 percent

oxygenation: the process of getting oxygen into the bloodstream

oximeter: noninvasive device worn over a finger that measures the oxygen level in the bloodstream

polysomnography: a sleep study used to diagnose a variety of sleep disorders

uvulopalatopharyngoplasty: surgical removal of excess soft tissue including the tonsils in the back of the mouth

uvulopalatoplasty: procedure in which a laser is used to remove parts or all of the uvula

CAUSES AND SYMPTOMS

Obstructive sleep apnea (OSA) is caused by upper airway obstruction. Soft tissue in the back of the mouth collapses during sleep and temporarily obstructs airflow into the lungs.

People with sleep apnea experience many periods of apnea and hypopnea. During such periods, the oxygen level in the bloodstream can decline significantly. Since these episodes happen throughout the night, sleep pattern is interrupted, and the person will feel sleepy during the day. Symptoms of OSA may include morning headaches, fatigue, difficulty with concentration, and daytime sleepiness (somnolence). The person might doze off while watching television, reading, or, more dangerously, driving. The person may not be aware of apnea or the resultant snoring. However, a sleeping partner will frequently notice these symptoms. It should be noted, however, that snoring alone, without apnea, is very common and does not indicate sleep apnea.

Risk factors for the development of OSA include obesity, large neck circumference, small jaw, deviated septum of the nose, big tongue, and enlarged tonsils. Smokers are also at higher risk of developing sleep apnea. The clinical triad of snoring, apneic episodes, and daytime somnolence suggests OSA.

The classic depiction of a patient with sleep apnea is an obese forty-year-old man with a short, thick neck and a loud snore. While this image often fits the profile of a sleep apnea patient, it does not capture the widespread demographics of those with sleep apnea, and can lead to missed diagnoses. For example, women with OSA often present differently than men. Some women with OSA are young and thin, and present with fatigue or irritability as their only symptoms, leading to a misdiagnosis of insomnia or fatigue rather than OSA. Additionally, women are less likely to report loud snoring, and men are less likely to be attentive to their partner's sleep patterns. Furthermore, many of the symptoms of OSA overlap with that of menopause, such as frequent nighttime awakenings, night sweats, daytime sleepiness, depressed mood, and poor concentration. In fact, a recent study showed that 50% of all women 20 to 70 years of age in a random sample of 400 women in Sweden tested positive for OSA.

Undiagnosed and untreated OSA can lead to increased blood pressure and increased strain on the heart, ultimately leading to an increased risk of developing more ominous medical complications such as heart failure, stroke, and pulmonary hypertension. In pulmonary hypertension, the lungs become stiff and fail to provide normal oxygenation. Furthermore, in obese pregnant women, undiagnosed and untreated OSA is associated with a higher risk of preeclampsia, neonatal intensive care unit admissions, and cesarean delivery. Therefore, it is extremely important to recognize and treat sleep apnea.

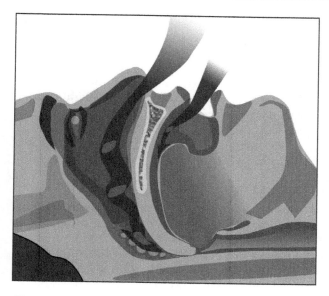

Shows airway obstruction found in cases of sleep apnea. (Habib M'henni via Wikimedia Commons)

A diagnosis can be made by an overnight oximeter or by a formal sleep study (polysomnography). An oximeter is a noninvasive device worn over a finger that measures the oxygen level in the bloodstream. It can be worn overnight at home and is useful for detecting any drop in oxygen level caused by apneic or hypopneic episodes. A formal sleep study requires an overnight observation in a sleep center where multiple monitors record brain waves, heart rate, breathing rate, abdominal muscle movement, and oxygen level. Based on these measurements, an apnea-hypopnea index (AHI), the average number of apneic and hypopneic episodes in one hour, is reported. An AHI of 5 to 20 is considered mild sleep apnea. An AHI of 21 to 50 is moderate, and an AHI of greater than 50 is considered severe.

TREATMENT AND THERAPY

Obese individuals with OSA should lose weight, quit smoking, and avoid sedating medications and alcohol because they may impair breathing even further.

Initial OSA treatment consists of a nasal continuous positive airflow pressure (CPAP) machine. A triangular mask fits over the nose and is hooked up to a machine that pushes air under pressure into the upper airway to keep it open. A repeat sleep study using a CPAP machine can determine the level of pressure necessary to prevent apneic and hypopneic episodes. Such a device can be very effective in treating OSA. Side effects may include anxiety from using the mask, nasal congestion, nosebleeds, dry mouth, and irritation of the skin from the mask.

Some individuals require surgical treatment, especially those who cannot tolerate the use of a CPAP machine. The procedure, called uvulopalatopharyngoplasty, involves surgical removal of excess soft tissue including the tonsils in the back of the mouth. Laser-assisted uvulopalatoplasty, in which a laser is used to remove the soft tissue, can be performed in the office. Other surgeries can move the tongue and jaw forward in order to open up the airway in the back of the mouth. For very severe cases of sleep apnea, an opening can be made in the trachea (the windpipe in the upper neck) to bypass the obstruction in the mouth and nose.

PERSPECTIVE AND PROSPECTS

Accounts of what may have been sleep apnea date back to 305 to 30 BCE and involve eleven members from seven generations of the Egyptian royal family. These individuals were obese and were reported by contemporary philosophers and historians to have a tendency toward falling asleep during social and political events.

Sleep apnea has sometimes made an appearance in literature. In the late sixteenth century, symptoms of OSA were suggested in characters created by William Shakespeare for this plays *Richard II* and *Henry IV*. In *Richard II*, the obese Sir John Falstaff snores and sleeps much of the day, interrupted by an apneic breathing pattern. In *Henry IV*, King Henry IV has trouble sleeping, with periods of not breathing in his sleep. Lewis Carroll described a character with sleep apnea in his book *Alice's Adventures in Wonderland* (1865). At the Mad Hatter's tea party, the Dormouse suffers from daytime sleepiness. The other characters try to help the Dormouse by putting him into a tight teapot, which would serve as a positive pressure to assist his breathing.

The famous composer Johannes Brahms (1833-1897) was thought to have developed sleep apnea in his later years when he gained weight. He was known to his friends to snore loudly at night. He also fell asleep during a performance by another famous composer, Franz Liszt.

—*Veronica N. Baptista, M.D.*
Updated by Shiliang Alice Cao, B.A.

FOR FURTHER INFORMATION

Goldman, L., Ausiello, D. *Cecil Textbook of Medicine.* 23d ed. Philadelphia: Saunders/Elsevier, 2007.

Iftikhar I.H., Valentine, C.W., Bittencourt, L.R., et al. Effects of continuous positive airway pressure on blood pressure in patients with resistant hypertension and obstructive sleep apnea: a meta-analysis. J Hypertens, 2014.

Lavie, P. *Restless Nights: Understanding Snoring and Sleep Apnea.* Translated by Anthony Berris. New Haven, Conn.: Yale University Press, 2003.

Louis J, A. D., Miladinovic, B., Shepherd, A., Mencin, P., Kumar, D., et al. Perinatal outcomes associated with obstructive sleep apnea in obese pregnant women. Obstet Gynecol. 2012;120(5):1085–92.

Mason, R.J., et al., eds. *Murray and Nadel's Textbook of Respiratory Medicine.* 5th ed. Philadelphia: Saunders/Elsevier, 2010.

Randerath,W. J., Bernd, M. S., and Virend, K.S. *Sleep Apnea: Current Diagnosis and Treatment.* New York: S. Karger, 2006.

Rock, P., ed. *Obesity and Sleep Apnea.* Philadelphia: Saunders/ Elsevier, 2005.

Terris, D.J., and Goode, R.L. *Surgical Management of Sleep Apnea and Snoring.* Boca Raton, Fla.: Taylor & Francis, 2005.

Sterilization

CATEGORY: Procedure

KEY TERMS:

contraception: the prevention of pregnancy

corpus luteum: a yellow cell mass produced from a Graafian follicle after the release of an egg

endometriosis: a disease of the female reproductive system that occurs when cells of the uterine lining (endometrium) grow outside the uterus and cause severe pain

Fallopian tubes: the two tubes that connect the ovaries to the uterus and through which an egg travels during ovulation

Graafian follicle: any of the ovarian follicles that produce eggs

hormone: a substance made by a body organ and carried through the blood to a second (or target) organ in order to optimize the operation of that target organ

hysterectomy: a surgery that removes part or all of the uterus

laparoscopy: a surgical procedure in which a small incision is made near the navel and the organs of the abdominal cavity, including the uterus and Fallopian tubes, are viewed with a lighted tube called a laparoscope

ovariectomy: the removal of the ovaries

peritoneal cavity: the abdominal cavity that contains the visceral organs

INDICATIONS AND PROCEDURES

Sterilization a woman, is a permanent method of surgical contraception that renders her incapable of conceiving children. Female sterilization involves the blockage or removal of the Fallopian tubes, the ovaries, or the uterus. Sterilization procedures performed on women are considered irreversible. Although the most frequently utilized types of female sterilization possess the potential for reversal at a later date, attempted reversals are often unsuccessful.

Therefore, a woman choosing this type of contraception should be quite sure that she does not want another child. By the beginning of the twenty-first century, sterilization was the most prevalent form of contraception worldwide, with an estimated one hundred million women choosing the procedure. In the United States, approximately 700,000 women are sterilized each year. One reason that female sterilization is a popular form of contraception with women is because it represents a onetime effort that is usually both simple and the cause of only mild side effects. Another advantage of sterilization over the use of birth control pills is its high success rate: Less than a tenth as many sterilized women will become pregnant (as a result of improperly performed or incomplete procedures) as will women who rely on birth control pills for their contraception. The use of condoms, diaphragms, and all the other barrier pregnancy prevention devices are even less effective than birth control pills.

Before considering the various aspects of sterilization, it is useful to describe the female reproductive system and its biological operation. This organ system consists of two ovaries connected to paired Fallopian tubes that open up into the uterus. The entire system passes through a monthly menstrual cycle that is controlled by the female hormones progesterone and the estrogens. During each menstrual cycle, an ovary produces one egg (sometimes more) in a Graafian follicle. The egg then enters one of the Fallopian tubes, which carries it to the uterus. If an egg is fertilized, it then implants in the endometrial tissue that lines the interior of the uterus and subsequently develops into an embryo.

Egg formation and uterus preparation for implantation are controlled by the female hormones. Once an egg implants, the uterus is kept in a state that optimizes pregnancy with the production of progesterone and related hormones, first by the corpus luteum (originally the Graafian follicle that yielded the egg) and then by the placenta that forms from commingled uterine and fetal tissue. In the absence of fertilization, the menstrual cycle continues, most of the endometrium breaks down into the monthly menstrual flow, and the process begins over again.

Menstruation stops between forty-five and fifty-five years of age in most women, causing them to undergo a process called the menopause. After hundreds of repeated menstrual cycles since puberty, the Graafian follicles stop producing eggs. Cessation of the menstrual cycle means that female hormone production stops almost entirely. Therefore, the menopause is accompanied by gradual atrophy of the sex organs and possible related symptoms, including hot flashes, depression, and irritability. When ovariectomy or hysterectomy is performed to achieve sterilization, these symptoms of the menopause may be induced prematurely.

For pregnancy to occur, then, a woman must have at least one functional ovary that produces eggs, an intact and operational Fallopian tube to transport the egg, and a functional uterus. The surgical methods that are used for sterilization must, therefore, make one of these reproductive organs nonfunctional. Most often, sterilization cuts and then blocks or removes the Fallopian tubes. Such interruption of the Fallopian tubes is the preferred form of female sterilization surgery for three reasons. First, these operations are relatively minor surgical procedures and are unlikely to be very risky. In addition, premature menopausal symptoms are not produced because the menstrual cycle continues. Finally, when carried out appropriately, interruption of the Fallopian tubes can sometimes be reversed if the patient changes her mind as a result of altered marital arrangements, lifestyle, or financial circumstances.

In many cases, a 1-centimeter to 1.5-centimeter section in the middle of each Fallopian tube is removed surgically or burned away via electrocoagulation. Alternatively, plastic or metal clips are used to close off each tube, or similar tube closure is effected by making a loop in each Fallopian tube and closing it off with a tight plastic ring or band.

Very frequently, the method that is used to damage the Fallopian tubes is a form of surgery called a laparoscopic procedure. The patient is given a general anesthetic, a very small incision is made close to the navel, and a flexible lighted tube laparoscope-is inserted into the incision. The laparoscope is equipped with fiber optics and enables an examining physician to see into the abdominal (peritoneal) cavity. Visibility of the Fallopian tubes and the other abdominal organs with laparoscopic examination is enhanced by pumping harmless carbon dioxide gas or nitrous oxide gas into the abdomen, to distend it. This process is called pneumoperitoneum.

After laparoscopic examination identifies the operation site in the peritoneal cavity, the surgical tools for cauterization, cutting, banding, and other aspects of interrupting the Fallopian tubes are passed through the laparoscope, and the chosen surgical interruption procedure is carried out. An entire laparoscopic procedure often takes less than thirty minutes, which is one of the reasons for its great popularity. In addition, women who choose to undergo such surgery can usually go home in a few hours and are fully recovered after only one to two days of postoperative bed rest, followed by a week or so of curtailed physical and sexual activity.

Despite the popularity of the laparoscopic procedure for sterilization, some physicians prefer to carry out sterilization by use of a larger surgical incision through which the tubes are altered directly. Despite the larger size of the incision, the physicians who use this method believe that it is safer and more successful, and has a greater potential for reversibility.

Other methods for sterilization through Fallopian tube surgery are culdoscopy and chemical means. Culdoscopy, in which an optical instrument and surgical tools reach the Fallopian tubes through the uterus, has a somewhat lower success rate than do the laparoscopic procedure and the direct method. Chemical methods for tubal closure have also been attempted and are not viewed as viable

In the News
Sterilization of Native American Women

On the phone, during long marches, occupying federal surplus property, in court fighting for treaty rights – wherever Indian activists gathered during the "Red Power" years of the 1970s, conversation inevitably turned to the number of women who had had their tubes tied or their ovaries removed by the Indian Health Service. Communication spurred by activism provoked a growing number of Native American women to piece together what amounted to a national eugenic policy, translated into social reality by copious federal funding. They organized WARN (Women of All Red Nations) at Rapid City, South Dakota, as Native women from more than 30 tribes and nations met and decided, among other things, that "truth and communication are among our most valuable tools in the liberation of our lands, people, and four-legged and winged creations.

WARN and other women's organizations publicized the sterilizations, which were performed after pro-forma "consent" of the women being sterilized. The "consent" sometimes was not offered in the women's language, following threats that they would die or lose their welfare benefits if they had more children. At least two fifteen-year-old girls were told they were having their tonsils out before their ovaries were removed.

"They took away our past with a sword and our land with a pen. Now they're trying to take away our future with a scalpel," one Native American woman told Arlene Eisen of the *London Guardian* (March 23, 1977, 8). She continued: This total disregard for the health and dignity of Native American women is the I.H.S. version of smallpox-infested blankets [and] the forced marches and massacres of Native peoples. Racism continues because it is so deeply entrenched – even 'enlightened professionals do not see Indian people as human (Johansen and Maestas, 1979, 71).

Native Americans were far from the only victims of eugenic thinking into the 1970s. Beginning in 1929 and ending in 1978, the state of North Carolina sterilized as many as 7,600 people, "to reduce welfare costs and cleanse the gene pool" (Severson, 2011, A-13). California sterilized about 20,000 people for the same purposes. In 2012, 34 years after North Carolina's program ended, the state became the first three-dozen states that had had such programs to put a price on the practice, deciding that each living survivor of the program should be paid $50,000. That figure was set by a state task force, subject to approval of the governor and legislature. The bill could reach $100 million for the 1,500 to 2,000 living victims, mostly minorities and people of limited income and low intelligence.

No one even today knows exactly how many Native American women were sterilized during the 1970s. One base for calculation is provided by the General Accounting Office, whose study covered only four of twelve IHS regions over four years (1973 through 1976). Within those limits, 3,406 Indian women were sterilized, according to the GAO (Johansen and Maestas, 1979, 71). Another estimate was provided by Lehman Brightman, who is Lakota, and who devoted much of his life to the issue, suffering a libel suit by doctors in the process. His educated guess (without exact calculations to back it up) is that 40 per cent of Native women and 10 per cent of Native men were sterilized during the decade. Brightman estimates that the total number of Indian women sterilized during the decade was between 60,000 and 70,000.

because of a low success rate and frequent, serious postoperative complications. The other avenues available for sterilization are ovariectomy (removal of the ovaries) and hysterectomy (removal of the uterus). Both of these types of sterilization surgery are much more serious and riskier. In addition, ovariectomy and hysterectomy are totally irreversible. Ovariectomy, a more complicated procedure than the one inactivating the Fallopian tubes, is usually utilized only when both ovaries are diseased. This procedure produces an early menopause because most of a woman's female hormones are made by the ovaries' Graafian follicles.

Hysterectomy is the most uncommon form of female sterilization because it requires even more extensive surgery and can have fatal complications. While the operation is sometimes carried out when a woman has completed her desired family, most hysterectomies are curative. They are performed in cases of very severe and widespread endometriosis and in the presence of other serious gynecological problems.

USES AND COMPLICATIONS
The most popular method of female sterilization is to block or damage both Fallopian tubes so that eggs

cannot pass through them to the uterus. In some cases, the tubes are removed completely. While removal ensures successful sterilization, it is irreversible and considered too drastic by women who might someday wish to reverse the operation. Several popular alternatives to removal are the methods that interrupt the tubes, retaining the potential for reversal at a later date. Women undergoing this type of surgery are warned, however, that such reversal may be impossible.

When the Fallopian tubes are damaged but not entirely closed off, they may reconnect and cause an ectopic pregnancy, in which a fertilized egg implants in one of the tubes and begins to grow into a fetus. Ectopic pregnancy can be fatal to the pregnant woman, and when identified, it is corrected by surgical removal of the fetus. Although the cause of this problem is not clear, there is some thought that alteration of the interior wall of the tube or slowed passage of an egg through the tube may be the causative agent. Fortunately, ectopic pregnancy is relatively uncommon.

Whether the laparoscopic method or the direct approach is utilized, the best time to carry out female sterilization is at the end of a menstrual cycle; at this time, early pregnancies cannot be compromised. It is advised that the patient discontinue intercourse and the use of birth control pills for at least a month prior to the surgery. The cessation of intercourse eliminates the chance of unexpected pregnancy at the time of surgery, while stopping the use of birth control pills decreases the possibility of blood-clotting problems.

The complications of all types of Fallopian tube surgery can include internal bleeding, blood-clotting problems, injury to the intestines and the other abdominal organs, and abnormal postoperative menstrual cycles. It is estimated, however, that these complications occur in less than 1 percent of patients. A more frequent problem is the difficulty of restoring fertility by reconnecting the Fallopian tubes (with only a 20 to 40 percent success rate).

Hysterectomy is never a highly recommended female sterilization operation. Rather, it is used mostly in those cases where other uterine health problems are sufficiently severe to make the process sensible. These problems may include recurrent and heavy vaginal bleeding, severe endometriosis, and chronic pelvic inflammatory disease (PID). This extensive surgery results in a high rate of complications and a significant number of deaths.

A woman may seek sterilization when she is having an abortion or soon after giving birth to an undesired child. Such a decision, perhaps made hastily at a time of intense emotional stress, is not advisable. It is essential that a sterilization operation be performed only after careful reflection. Divorce or the death of a spouse and subsequent remarriage may cause a sterilized woman regret should she desire more children. Severe psychological problems for both the patient and her family may accompany female sterilization. Therefore, it is highly recommended that these women, their families, and both partners in married couples consult a gynecologist and a psychological counselor before proceeding with female sterilization surgery.

In contrast to the complications associated with female sterilization, with vasectomy a day of bed rest and a week of avoidance of all strenuous physical activity usually produce complete recovery. Health complications occur in less than 5 percent of vasectomy patients. In addition, these problems are usually minor and almost never lead to fatalities. Skin discoloration, swelling, and oozing of clear fluid from the scrotum incision are common symptoms immediately following the surgery, but they spontaneously disappear as the healing process continues. Less frequently, inflammation and a condition called sperm granuloma can occur when sperm leak out of the cut portion of the vas deferens closest to the testicle. A granuloma produces severe inflammation, pain, and swelling. When this condition does not subside spontaneously, the granuloma must be removed surgically.

Perspective and Prospects

While surgical sterilization was first described in the nineteenth century, it was not widely available for contraception until the 1920's, nor did it become popular immediately. Though voluntary sterilization began slowly in the 1950s, its use accelerated until it became a popular form of fertility control in the industrial and developing nations of the 1970s.

A source of discontent with the sterilization techniques that are available is their total or poor reversibility when fertility reinitiation is desired later in life. This discontent has occurred because, with passing time, an unexpectedly large segment of sterilized men and women have come to regret their decisions regarding sterilization. All hysterectomies and Fallopian tube removals are forever irreversible, and a low reversibility rate is seen even in the two most popular- and potentially reversible-sterilization methodologies: Fallopian tube interruption and vasectomy.

Consequently, the development of sterilization surgery has been directed toward devising methods that will enable much larger incidences of reversibility, where desired. One direction has been to expand the understanding of Fallopian tube and vas deferens anatomy and functionality. Particularly useful results obtained include the realization that destruction of the nerves that control the operation of these organs can make the recovery of fertility incomplete or impossible even when excellent corrective surgery reverses the original interruption of continuity. This discovery has led to the development of more sophisticated interruption surgery that is less likely to damage the vas deferens or Fallopian tube nerve integrity. Some improvement of the reversibility of these operations has been obtained in this manner, but the overall results are still far from satisfactory.

Consequently, many other surgical techniques have been attempted, including the placement of removable plugs in the Fallopian tubes or of tiny, faucet like valves in the vas deferens that allow or stop the ejaculation of sperm. Other useful methods to ensure reversible sterilization may include hormones, vaccines against eggs and sperm, and chemical treatments. It is hoped that improved anti-fertility methodologies will be developed that combine more reversible surgical sterilization, vaccines, chemicals, and various contraceptives.

—*Sanford S. Singer, Ph.D.*
Updated by Bruce E. Johansen, PhD

FOR FURTHER INFORMATION

Ammer, Christine. *The New A to Z of Women's Health: A Concise Encyclopedia.* 6th ed. New York: Checkmark Books, 2009.

Connell, Elizabeth B. *The Contraception Sourcebook.* Chicago: Contemporary Books, 2002.

Gotter, Ana, et al. *What Every Woman Should Know About Female Sterilization.* HealthLine, 27 Sept. 2018, www.healthline.com/health/birth-control-female-sterilization.

Office of Population Affairs. "Female Sterilization." *HHS.gov,* US Department of Health and Human Services, 28 Nov. 2017, www.hhs.gov/opa/pregnancy-prevention/sterilization/female-sterilization/index.html.

Planned Parenthood. *Tubal Ligation Procedure.* Planned Parenthood, www.plannedparenthood.org/learn/birth-control/sterilization.

Sherwood, Lauralee. *Human Physiology: From Cells to Systems.* 7th ed. Pacific Grove, Calif.: Brooks/Cole/Cengage Learning, 2010.

Stillbirth

CATEGORY: Disease/Disorder

KEY TERMS:

antiphospholipid syndrome: also known as Hughes syndrome, a disorder of the immune system that causes an increased risk of blood clots

cholestasis: any condition in which substances normally excreted into bile are retained; bile flow is decreased due to impaired secretion by hepatocytes or by obstruction of bile flow though intra- or extrahepatic bile ducts

fetoscopy: an endoscopic procedure during pregnancy to allow surgical access to the fetus

isoimmunization: the development of antibodies against antigens from the same species

karyotyping: test to determine the presence of chromosomal abnormalities

placenta abruptio: the premature separation of the placenta from the uterus

preeclampsia: a pregnancy complication characterized by high blood pressure and signs of damage to another organ system, most often the liver or kidneys

thrombophilias: an abnormality of blood coagulation that increases the risk of blood clots in blood vessels

ultrasonography: a technique using echoes of ultrasound pulses to delineate objects of different density in the body

CAUSES AND SYMPTOMS

There are many causes of stillbirth, but in many cases, the precise cause of a fetal death is not known. The causes of stillbirth can be grouped into general categories such as fetal asphyxia; hematologic, chromosomal, or developmental problems with the fetus; and maternal illness. Fetal asphyxia occurs when the blood supply to the fetus is reduced or cut off, such as in cases

Information on Stillbirth

Causes: Often unknown but may include lack of oxygen to fetus (umbilical cord entanglement, placenta abruptio); hematologic factors (isoimmunization, thrombophilias); chromosomal or developmental problems with fetus; maternal illnesses (diabetes, infections)

Symptoms: Absence of fetal movement or heartbeat, sometimes bleeding and contractions in mother

Duration: Acute

Treatments: Grief counseling, induction of labor, minimization of trauma to mother during labor, control of any maternal illnesses, investigation into cause (fetal autopsy, karyotyping)

of umbilical cord entanglement or placenta abruptio (abnormal detachment of the placenta from the uterus caused by such factors as maternal high blood pressure or preeclampsia, trauma, or certain drugs). Hematologic causes of stillbirth include isoimmunization (in which maternal antibodies attack fetal blood cells) or thrombophilias (abnormalities in blood clotting). Maternal illnesses such as diabetes, infections (such as listeria), cholestasis, and antiphospholipid syndrome are also associated with increased risk of stillbirth.

The primary symptom of fetal demise is the absence of fetal movement. The death can be confirmed on ultrasonography or fetoscopy, which reveals the absence of a fetal heartbeat. Stillbirth may be associated with other symptoms, depending on its cause. For instance, if it results from placenta abruptio, then the woman may experience bleeding and contractions.

TREATMENT AND THERAPY

Once a stillbirth has been confirmed, treatment is directed at helping the woman and her family cope with the loss. Grief counseling is an important component of therapy. If the patient is already in labor, then minimizing obstetric trauma to the mother is of prime concern. If the patient is not in labor, then plans regarding the induction of labor are made, since prolonged retention of the dead fetus and placenta may result in disseminated intravascular coagulation (DIC), a dangerous blood condition. The patient also receives treatment aimed at controlling any maternal illnesses, such as diabetes or preeclampsia. If no obvious conditions contributed to the stillbirth, then the patient may

be offered an investigation into causes of the demise. This investigation may involve tests on maternal blood for abnormalities of blood clotting, infections, abruption, diabetes, and liver abnormalities. With appropriate consent, witnessed sampling, and chain of custody handling, a urine specimen may be evaluated for the maternal ingestion of toxic substances. The stillborn fetus may be sent for autopsy and karyotyping.

No effective means exist for preventing stillbirth, although with advances in medical care, by 2003 the stillbirth rate in the United States had fallen to about 7.5 per 1,000 births, about half of what it was in the mid-1940s. If a pregnant woman has conditions putting her at increased risk of fetal demise or a history of stillbirth, then increased surveillance using ultrasonography and fetal heart tone monitoring may be indicated.

—*Anne Lynn S. Chang, M.D.*

FOR FURTHER INFORMATION

Creasy, Robert K., and Robert Resnik, eds. *Maternal-Fetal Medicine: Principles and Practice.* 8th ed. Philadelphia: W. B. Saunders, 2018.

Cunningham, F. Gary, et al., eds. *Williams Obstetrics.* 25th ed. New York: McGraw-Hill, 2018.

Gabbe, Steven G., Jennifer R. Niebyl, and Joe Leigh Simpson, eds. *Obstetrics: Normal and Problem Pregnancies.* 5th ed. Philadelphia: Churchill Livingstone/Elsevier, 2007.

Kohner, Nancy, and Alix Henley. *When a Baby Dies: The Experience of Late Miscarriage, Stillbirth, and Neonatal Death.* Rev. ed. New York: Routledge, 2001.

Stress

CATEGORY: Disease/Disorder

KEY TERMS:

alarmone: a type of intracellular hormone which alerts the cell to various chemical imbalances in the cellular environment

anxiety: a type of stressful condition in which heightened neural activity accentuates an individual's anticipation of a stress-producing event

cellular transformation: carcinogenesis; the biochemical conversion of a cell from a normal state to a cancerous one of uncontrollable proliferation

chaos: a disorderly shift from predictable, linear

behavior to nonlinear randomness, a situation which often occurs in stress and homeostatic breakdown

fight-or-flight response: a stressful biochemical reaction in animals, usually involving the adrenal hormone epinephrine, that prepares the animal for confrontation with predators or competitors

homeostasis: the maintenance of constant, linear conditions within a system, such as the maintenance of human body temperature, pH, and hormonal levels at stable states

hormone: a gene regulatory molecule which is produced in one body tissue region and which targets or controls cells in another region

nonlinear system: a process which is unstable and unpredictable in nature; such a process often results from a disturbance to a linear, predictable system

tend-and-befriend response: a neuroendocrine-linked stress response observed in females characterized by a tendency to respond to stressful situations by protecting self and young through nurturing behaviors and forming alliances with a larger social group

type A behavior: a psychological behavior classification for individuals who exhibit stressful, time-conscious lifestyles

type B behavior: a psychological behavior classification for individuals who exhibit unstressed, relaxed lifestyles

CAUSES AND SYMPTOMS

Stress is a psychophysiological response, within an individual animal, to a perceived danger. Stress involves a complex interplay of nervous and hormonal reactions to internal and external stimuli. All living organisms respond to stimuli, usually by means of gene-regulating chemical messengers called hormones.

Chemistry of stress. Hormones are produced in certain cells within the individual and then target tissues elsewhere in the body; these hormones control by controlling the gene regulation within their target cells. Hormones will activate certain genes within target tissue cells while inactivating other genes. If a hormone activates the control region of a gene so that the gene is "on," then it can be "read" by an enzyme (RNA polymerase), thereby leading to RNA and protein production. The produced protein may affect cellular chemical processes or may affect the expression (the on/off status) of other genes. In the latter case, the protein would be a type of intracellular hormone called an alarmone.

If a hormone inactivates the control region of a gene so that the gene is "off," then RNA polymerase will be unable to read the DNA nucleotide sequence of the gene. Therefore, no RNA and no protein will be produced. In this fashion, a hormone may activate certain genes while inactivating others. Consequently, a hormone controls what happens within the cell.

Such control is critical within complex multicellular organisms such as animals. Different cells specialize to become different tissues and organs (such as eyes, ears, hair, intestines, the heart, and so on) under the specific influence of hormones. Additionally, changes in the development of an organism over time involve changes in gene expression caused by hormones. Critical developmental changes in an individual must occur at precise times when a hormone is produced and acts correctly upon the proper array of genes in target cell tissues. When a hormone does not act correctly or issues incorrect instructions to genes, the homeostatic stability of the organism becomes disrupted. Incorrect proteins are produced in the wrong cells at the wrong times, thereby disturbing development and possibly threatening the organism's survival.

In higher functioning animals, including humans, the body is regulated by hormones and by complex nervous systems that evolved from hormones. Most hormones are produced and secreted from the glands of the endocrine system, including the pituitary, thyroid, and adrenal glands as well as numerous organs, tissues, and cells throughout the body. The nervous system is an array of several trillion nerves concentrated in the brain and spinal cord and extending peripherally to virtually every cellular region of the body. The two systems are tightly interconnected. Both the endocrine and nervous systems at some point involve the secretion of hormones. Nerve tissue secretes hormones called neurotransmitters between electrically conducting cells called neurons.

Physiological responses to stress. Stress is therefore a biochemical response to danger that occurs within animals. The nervous system detects danger from internal or external stimuli, usually external stimuli such as predators, competitors, or life-threatening events. Increased electrical conductivity along millions of nerve cells targets various tissues to prepare the body for maximum physical activity. Among the tissues affected will be the skeletal muscles, the heart muscle, the hormone-secreting glands of the endocrine system, the immune system, the stomach, and blood vessels. Under nerve activated stress, skeletal muscles will be poised for contraction.

The heart will beat faster, thereby distributing more blood and nutrients to body cells, in the process accelerating the breathing rate to distribute more oxygen. Blood vessels will constrict. The stomach and other intestinal organs will decrease their activity, including a decreased production of mucus that protects against acid.

Heightened nerve activity also will trigger the production of various hormones from the immune system, specifically hormones that influence bodily metabolism such as thyroxine and epinephrine (adrenaline). These hormones target body tissue cells to prepare the body for increased output in the face of danger. Massive production of epinephrine will trigger maximum physical readiness and extraordinary muscular output, a phenomenon often referred to as the fight-or flight response.

These physiological changes within an animal facing danger are important survival adaptations that evolved very early in the history of animal life on earth. Stress is a fact of life for animals because they must eat to survive. Competition for available food resources and avoidance of predators must be faced by all animals, including humans. While predation by larger animals is of little worry to current-day modern humans, the struggle for available resources remains. Furthermore, human technology has created stresses of an entirely different character.

The fight-or-flight stress response and other evolutionary stress adaptations endure within the individual for only seconds or minutes. Such natural stresses are to an individual's advantage, ensuring survival. The stresses that humans face are based on these behavioral adaptations. Much human stress is artificial, however, and lasts not for minutes but for hours, days, weeks, months, and years. Such stresses involve the same nervous and endocrine system responses, but they are usually brought about by perceived danger, not true danger.

Human societies impose norms and rules for the behavior of the individuals who compose the society. People must adhere to the societal norms or face punishment. In fast-paced technological societies, increasing bureaucratization and organization place less emphasis on the individual and more emphasis on process and productivity. People must face deadlines, be on time, produce quotas, generate company profit, and meet the demands of family, colleagues, and administration simultaneously. The result is a continuous fight or- flight response in which individuals fear losing their jobs and thus the means of supporting themselves and their families.

The physiological manifestations of prolonged stress are devastating. Continued hyperactivity of nerve impulses and overproduction of hormones at incorrect developmental stages lead to the abnormal functioning of internal organs. The stomach under secretes mucus, thereby leading to ulcers. The heart muscle contracts too rapidly, leading to higher pulse and respiration rates. The blood vessels constrict for lengthy periods of time, thereby causing the heart to pump harder and leading to high blood pressure and heart disease. Hormone overproduction leads to incorrect cell instructions and gene activation/inactivation, causing abnormal tissue functioning and cellular transformation leading to cancer. The immune system weakens under abnormal signaling by hormones, thereby decreasing the body's ability to defend itself from disease.

Newer research on stress response in women has uncovered a mechanism of stress response that is of interest given this upswelling of constant stress. *Work by Shelley E. Taylor has documented an alternative to "fight or flight" known as "tend and befriend." Potentially linked to oxytocin, such tend-and-befriend behavior may help to facilitate relaxation and interpersonal bonding in response to stress. The potential stress response promises longer-lasting benefits, adaptively connecting humans to their social groups.*

Stress and disease. A wide variety of human illnesses and disorders have been associated with stress. Heart disease, cancer, stroke, mental illness, allergies, accidents, asthma, chronic fatigue, depression, suicide, and deviant behavior are among the many illnesses and disorders that are considered by scientists to be stress-related illnesses. These stress-related diseases and disorders are responsible for the majority of deaths, hospitalizations, and visits to physicians by people in highly technological societies such as the United States, Japan, and Western Europe. In the United States alone, several billion dollars are spent each year for medications to treat stress-related illnesses that otherwise could be prevented by anti-stress methodologies.

Before the advent of industrialization in Europe and North America, the leading killers of humans were bacterial and viral diseases, which continue to be the principal killers of humans in the pretechnological and emerging technological countries of the Middle East, Asia, Africa, Latin America, and Oceania. European and North American industrialization has been accompanied by prodigious advances in medical science and the eradication or control of many microorganismal diseases. The psychological demands of fast-paced living and the dehumanized expectations of technological societies, however, have produced a plethora of stress-generated diseases and disorders, some of which had been masked by microorganismal diseases.

There still is some debate concerning the causal relationship between stress and illness, despite overwhelming scientific evidence demonstrating bodily responses to stressful situations. Abnormal nerve hyperactivity and prolonged, abnormal secretions of gene regulatory hormones from various endocrine glands disrupt the balanced homeostasis of many different body systems. Immune system reduction often occurs during stress, thereby making a stressed individual more susceptible to contracting infectious bacterial and viral diseases.

A clear linkage exists between the occurrence of stress in people and their subsequent susceptibility to infectious disease. Furthermore, there is a tendency for strokes, heart attacks, cancer, and sudden death to occur in individuals who recently have experienced major traumatic events in their lives. Too little attention has been given to the effects of everyday living upon the physical well-being of people. Environmental stimuli, nervous and endocrine systems, and physiological rhythms within the body are intricately connected.

Most bodily processes follow a self-regulatory, homeostatic pattern that is rhythmic, linear, stable, and predictable. For example, the beta cells of the islets of Langerhans in the pancreas secrete the hormone insulin in response to elevated blood glucose levels, whereas the alpha cells in these same islets secrete the hormone glucagon in response to low blood glucose levels. Likewise, the body chemically maintains a constant blood temperature (37 degrees Celsius), pH (7.35 to 7.45), calcium levels, and so on. The heart muscle requires an electrical stimulus approximately once per second to trigger a wave of muscular contractions throughout the myocardium via the sinoatrial and atrioventricular nodes.

Linear, balanced physiological rhythms are sensitive to subtle chemical changes in the cellular and organismal environment. An orderly, homeostatic process in the body can collapse into disorderly, nonlinear, and unpredictable chaos because of the slightest disturbance. Stress is a disturbance that imbalances the nervous and endocrine systems, which subsequently imbalance cells and organ systems throughout the human body. Physiological systems become unstable, and disease or cancer may ensue.

IMPACT ON WOMEN

Both men and women are impacted by stress. Due to female hormones and a difference in biological, relational and societal pressers on women they may face stress at a higher level. Although it has been suggested by some research that women are more sensitive to stress, it also is believed that due to their specific hormones they are better able to handle stress. Women may be more likely to verbalize their stress and deal with it in a logical way, making them more successful at coping with stress than men.

In modern American society many women are managing a work and home life balance. Although women have been in the workplace for many years now, the burden of household management and caring for children still falls primarily on the mother. According to research done in the book, *The Second Shift*, by Arlie Russell Hochschild women will actually work about a month more a year than their husbands This book suggests that managing the work/family balance causes increased stress for women, due to the increase of work load outside the home without a reduction of family responsibilities. Many women work throughout their pregnancies and soon after they have children, creating little time for healing and focusing on parenting. This has been linked to increase emotional struggles around prenatal and postpartum times.

The medical impact of stress on women may include headaches, acid reflux, stomach issues, nausea, aches and pains, chronic fatigue, increased need to urinate, lack of sexual drive, changes in menstruation, anxiety, depression, insomnia, immune system issues, constipation or diarrhea, skin problems, and hair loss. Since stress in women in intensified by the demand placed on them by society, it is important for women to seek support in their daily lives. Self-care, including taking time for their physical health, healthy eating and emotional support are all very important.

TREATMENT AND THERAPY

Psychologists, psychiatrists, physicians, and other medical professionals are becoming more aware of the physiological effects of stress. Through this awareness, professionals have sought to examine whether there are any characteristic styles of stress response. In response, psychologists have identified two principal behavioral types when it comes to stress among humans: type A behavior pattern and type B behavior pattern.

Type A individuals are highly anxious, task-oriented, time conscious, constantly in a rush to accomplish their jobs and other objectives, and somewhat prone to hostility. Research indicates that type A individuals may have a higher incidence of heart disease. Increasingly, the hostility component of type A behavior is seen as a very important contributing factor. the other hand, type B individuals are more relaxed and experience less stress. Nevertheless, it should be emphasized that behavior is a continuum: Different people may exhibit varying degrees of type A and B behavior patterns. Given this discovery, it is not uncommon for professionals to recommend to their stressed clients to monitor their participation in type A behavior and to try behaving more in kind with type B behavior patterns.

Another important focus for health care has become the prevention, management, and treatment of stress itself. Health education programs emphasize the importance of physical fitness and stress reduction in everyday living. Stress-reducing methodologies for the individual include time management, peer counseling and support, spending longer amounts of time relaxing, strengthening family bonds, improving self-esteem, exercise, and learning to reframe how daily life events are interpreted, such as may be done through psychological therapy. These approaches greatly enhance an individual's quality of life and help the individual to cope positively with stressful events. All these stress reduction techniques emphasize an individual's personality and the more efficient use of an individual's free time. Relaxation, social interaction, and physical activity help the body to return to normal physiological rhythms following the numerous stressful events that every person faces daily. Individuals in American and Western societies are coming to

***

Information on Stress

Causes: Nervous system and hormonal reactions to internal and external stimuli

Symptoms: Hormonal imbalances; immune system collapse; increased susceptibility to disease, cancer, ulcers, high blood pressure, and heart disease

Duration: Temporary to chronic

Treatments: Lifestyle modification, relaxation, time management, peer counseling and support, strengthening family bonds, improving self-esteem, exercise

***

realize that a slower, more relaxed living pace is essential for reducing stress and the millions of cases of stress-related disease that occur each year.

PERSPECTIVE AND PROSPECTS

Because stress is a major contributor to illness and disease in American and Western societies, a major objective of health care professionals in these countries is the identification of stress initiators and the reduction of stress in the general population. Stress cannot be eliminated entirely in any individual. Humans always will experience stress as a result of their continuous interactions with one another and with the environment. Stress is an important survival adaptation for animal life on earth. Nevertheless, stressful events in an individual's life serve as negative environmental stimuli that hyperactivate the human nervous and endocrine systems to create a fight-or-flight response. When this fight-or-flight response is maintained for abnormally long periods of times, prolonged elevations in nervous and hormonal activity modify body tissues and the developmental gene expression within cells to produce abnormal growths (such as cancers) and abnormal system functioning (such as diabetes mellitus).

Breakdown of the human immune system under stress makes the body less capable of fighting spontaneous tumors, cancers, and infectious disease. The net result from physiological stress is illness, disease, rapid aging, and death. Stress reduction should be a prime focus of medical research and education. The simplicity of educating the public with respect to stress can yield incredible savings in terms of lives saved, quality of lives improved, length of human life spans increased, and money saved. Some researchers propose that stress reduction not only can yield enormous health benefits but also can produce greater industrial productivity, happier people, and considerably less crime. It is expected that additional research into oxytocin, the tend-and-befriend response, and yet undiscovered mechanisms of stress response will contribute meaningfully to decreased stress and increased mental and physical well-being.

—*David Wason Hollar, Jr., Ph.D.*
Updated by Nancy A. Piotrowski, Ph.D.
and Kimberly Ortiz-Hartman, Psy.D., LMFT

FOR FURTHER INFORMATION

Balhara, Yatanpal Singh, et al. "Gender Differences in Stress Response: Role of Developmental and Biological Determinants." *Industrial Psychiatry Journal*, vol. 20, no. 1, 2011, p. 4., doi:10.4103/0972-6748.98407.

"Gender and Stress." *American Psychological Association*, www.apa.org/news/press/releases/stress/2010/gender-stress.

Krantz, David S., et al. *How Stress Affects Your Health*. American Psychological Association, 2013, HYPERLINK "http://www.apa.org/helpcenter/stress" www.apa.org/helpcenter/stress.

Mayor, Eric. "Gender Roles and Traits in Stress and Health." *Frontiers in Psychology*, vol. 6, 2015, p. 779., doi:10.3389/fpsyg.2015.00779.

Montero-Marin, Jesus, et al. "Coping with Stress and Types of Burnout: Explanatory Power of Different Coping Strategies." *PLoS ONE*, vol. 9, no. 2, 13 Feb. 2014, doi:10.1371/journal.pone.0089090.

"Stress and Your Health." *Womenshealth.gov*, Office on Women's Health, 2017, www.womenshealth.gov/mental-health/good-mental-health/stress-and-your-health.

Stress reduction

CATEGORY: Treatment

KEY TERMS:

hypnosis: the induction of a state of consciousness in which a person apparently loses the power of voluntary action and is highly responsive to suggestion or direction

palliative treatments: therapies that reduce symptoms without completely eradicating a disorder

psychotherapy: treatment using the mind to remedy problems related to disordered behavior or thinking, emotional problems, or disease

stress: physical, environmental, or psychological strain experienced by an individual that requires adjustment

INDICATIONS AND PROCEDURES

Stress can exacerbate difficulties in daily functioning, slow recovery from mental or physical problems, and impede immunological functioning. Stress reduction techniques represent a cluster of procedures that share the goal of reducing bodily and emotional tension: drug and physical therapies, exercise, biofeedback training, meditation, hypnosis, psychotherapy, relaxation training, and stress reduction therapy.

The drugs used in stress reduction are designed to provide overall bodily relaxation, to induce rest, or to decrease the anxious thinking that exacerbates stressful experiences. Sedatives, tranquilizers, benzodiazepines, antihistamines, betablockers, and barbiturates are examples of such drugs. Similarly, physical therapies and exercise are recommended for these purposes. Baths (hydrotherapy), massages, and moderate exercise can also be part of a stress reduction program.

Psychotherapy is a common treatment for stress implemented by psychiatrists, psychologists, social workers, psychiatric nurses, and counselors. Not only does it help individuals to sort out their problems mentally, but it is also an effective stress management strategy. When individuals analyze their lifestyles and life events, stress-inducing behaviors and life patterns can be explored and targeted for modification.

Biofeedback training, meditation, hypnosis, and relaxation training all focus on inducing relaxation or altered consciousness by shifting a person's attention. Biofeedback uses monitoring devices attached to the body to provide visual or aural feedback to the trainee. Such devices include the electromyograph (EMG), which measures muscle tension, and the psychogalvanometer, which measures galvanic skin response (GSR). An EMG involves placing sensors on various muscle groups to record muscular electrical potentials. GSR also relies on sensors, but these sensors record bodily responses caused by sweat gland activity and emotional arousal. The feedback from such

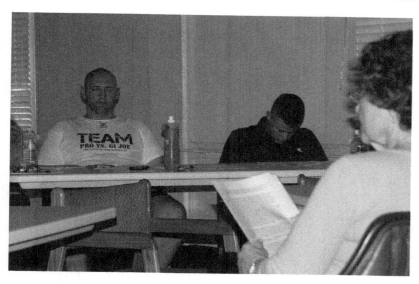

Linda Stark a certified clinical hypnotherapist, reads to a stress hypnotherapy class aboard Marine Corps Recruit Depot San Diego to help people find calmness. The two-hour class provided tools necessary to live a more enjoyable, stress-free life. First participants had to address and identify their stressors. Then Stark talked them through hypnotherapy which was intended to make the participants feel refreshed and calm. (Wikimedia Commons)

devices allows a trainee to learn to control certain bodily processes (for example, muscle tension, brain waves, heart rate, temperature, and blood pressure). Biofeedback training is used to treat headaches, temporomandibular joint (TMJ) syndrome, high blood pressure, and tics, and it can also facilitate neuromuscular responses in stroke patients.

Meditation is a focused thinking exercise involving a quiet setting and the repetition of a word or phrase called a mantra. By blocking distracting thoughts and refocusing attention, meditation reduces anxious thinking. It is useful for mild anxiety, minor concentration difficulties, and daily relaxation.

Hypnosis involves the use of suggestion, concentrated attention, and/or drugs to induce a sleeplike state, or trance. Hypnosis can be induced by a hypnotist or via self-hypnosis. Hypnotic states are characterized by increased suggestibility, ability to recall forgotten events, decreased pain sensitivity, and increased vasomotor control. The ability to be hypnotized varies from person to person based on susceptibility to suggestion and psychological needs. Hypnosis is used as a brief therapy targeting such problems as insomnia, pain, panic, and sexual dysfunction. In addition, hypnosis is sometimes used when drugs are contraindicated for anesthetic use, particularly for dental procedures.

Relaxation training involves three primary methods: autogenic training, which involves such techniques as head, heart, and abdominal exercises; progressive relaxation, which involves becoming aware of tension in the various muscle groups by relaxing one group at a time in a specific order; and breathing exercises. Relaxation training is best learned when a therapist trains an individual in person and then the exercises are practiced independently. Relaxation can be practiced several times daily, as well as in response to stressful events. High blood pressure, ulcers, insomnia, asthma, drug and alcohol problems, spastic colitis, tachycardia (rapid heartbeat), pain management, and moderate-to-severe anxiety disorders are treated with relaxation training. Stress inoculation therapy is a specific type of psychotherapy involving techniques that alter patterns of thinking and acting. It comprises three steps: education about stress and fear reactions, rehearsal of coping behaviors, and application of coping behaviors in stress-provoking situations. It is useful for treating anxiety disorders related to stress.

IMPACT ON WOMEN

Women may seek out different stress reduction techniques than men do and tend to be more open-minded to some. Women tend to seek out mental health therapy and support groups more often then men do. This is beneficial for women, since emotional expression and gaining coping is a healthy way to engage in stress reduction. Women may also be more likely to seek medical help for stress and utilized medications. There is some research that suggests that men are better at getting physical exercise and are more physically active than women are.

Women are in general the primary caregivers for their children and do a lot to maintain their household. This can cause increased stress for women and provides little time for women to engage in the self-care needed for stress reduction. Therefore, women may not be as good at finding time for stress reduction activities due to the increased economic demand on them. It is very important for women to be supported in finding time to manage their stress in order to ensure it does not have a negative impact on their physical and emotional health.

USES AND COMPLICATIONS

Individuals should not apply stress reduction procedures without proper consultation; medical conditions that might be causing symptoms should be assessed or ruled out first. Biofeedback training for headaches, for example, would be unwarranted until other, more serious causes of headaches had been eliminated from consideration. Similarly, exercise, drug, and physical therapies could actually worsen conditions such as high blood pressure, alcohol and drug problems, and chronic pain if applied incorrectly. For example, where stress or pain is chronic, drug therapies might encourage the development of drug dependence.

Instead, skilled providers should administer these procedures. Training via self-help materials alone or by an unskilled provider may provide no benefit or create difficulties. Poor training could result in frustration, hypervigilance, heightened anxiety, depression, or pain caused by over attention to symptoms or conflicts. In fact, some individuals are prone to these effects even with good training. Therefore, ongoing assessment is necessary. Finally, interpretation of any memories provoked by hypnosis should be done with caution because of the suggestibility that is characteristic of hypnotic states.

PERSPECTIVE AND PROSPECTS

Stress reduction techniques evolved from ancient meditation practices and simpler methods of pain management predating the development of modern anesthetics. The palliative and preventive effects of these techniques have given these procedures a sure hold in future medical practice, while benefits such as decreased absenteeism and increased feelings of wellness in employees have secured these strategies in the workplace. The expanded use of stress reduction procedures in prenatal care and with the elderly is likely.

—*Nancy A. Piotrowski, Ph.D.*
Updated by Kimberly Ortiz-Hartman, Psy.D., LMFT

FOR FURTHER INFORMATION

Davis, Martha, Elizabeth Robbins Eshelman, and Matthew McKay. *The Relaxation and Stress Reduction Workbook.* 5th ed. Oakland, Calif.: New Harbinger, 2000.

Pelletier, Kenneth. *The Best Alternative Medicine.* New York: Fireside, 2002.

Schafer, Walt, and Sharrie A. Herbold. *Stress Management for Wellness.* 4th ed. Belmont, Calif.: Thomson/Wadsworth, 2000.

Seaward, Brian Luke. *Managing Stress: Principles and Strategies for Health and Well-Being.* 6th ed. Sudbury, Mass.: Jones and Bartlett, 2009.

Stroke rehabilitation: Taking care of the caregiver

CATEGORY: Treatment

WHAT WE KNOW

Worldwide, in 2013, strokes were responsible for 6.5 million deaths worldwide and were the second leading cause of death and a primary source of disability. In the United States, in 2013, 6.8 million people were living after having experienced a stroke.

In the United States there are 34.2 million unpaid, nonprofessional caregivers (e.g., family, friends) providing care to an adult over the age of 50. Nearly 1 in 10 of these caregivers is over the age of 75. Twenty-three percent of the caregivers are providing more than 40 hours of care per week. These nonprofessional caregivers are often the primary caregiver for individuals who have had a stroke.

An individual who has experienced a stroke will typically move from having 24-hour medical care and an intensive therapy program to being at home with little or no professional support, with the expectation that family or friends will provide any needed supportive care. These nonprofessional caregivers will often describe their experience in this transition process as being difficult or traumatic.

Preparing caregivers (e.g., in using medical equipment, providing mouth care, feeding, managing medication) before the stroke survivor is discharged from the hospital helps prepare them to deal with the physical, emotional, and cognitive needs of the stroke survivor and improves the caregiver's self-efficacy.

In recognition that excessive caregiver burden can affect not only stroke survivors but also the caregivers' quality of life (QOL), increasing attention has been drawn to the needs of nonprofessional caregivers, or individuals who care for disabled individuals.

Because stroke often results in persistent functional and cognitive deficits, survivors commonly require comprehensive assistance from caregivers. Individuals who become caregivers may find their social lives, occupational and financial situations, and emotional health threatened by their new roles and responsibilities.

The majority of caregivers (62 percent) are nonprofessional caregivers (typically the spouse and other family members) who lack medical or nursing experience yet provide challenging physical care for stroke survivors who need day-to-day assistance with eating, bathing, dressing, ambulation, and transfer from one place to another (e.g., bedroom, bathroom, doctor's appointments). Caregivers may also face the burden of handling their loved one's financial and legal matters.

Because stroke is a sudden, unanticipated event, caregivers are thrust into their new roles with little preparation, training, or support. As a result, caregivers typically face high levels of stress, burden, and feelings of helplessness and hopelessness. The impact of stroke reaches beyond functional outcomes for affected clients. Caregivers report feeling particularly overwhelmed by emotional, cognitive, and behavioral changes that may persist after the stroke client regains physical functionality.

Stroke survivors typically need the most assistance during their first year of recovery; thus, caregivers often are most burdened during this time period. An early hospital discharge poststroke is associated with improved functional ability in clients but may result in increased caregiver burden.

There are specific factors that can influence the success of care at home and ease the stress on the caregiver. These include the strength of the caregiver–client relationship, the caregiver's understanding of and willingness to provide care, the caregiver's preexisting health issues, pre-stroke roles and responsibilities, accessibility of the home, availability of informal support resources for the caregiver, financial resources, pre-stroke caregiver experiences, a

sustained ability to provide care over the long term and having strategies for self-care.

The ability of caregivers to adapt to and cope with their caregiving role is important to both their own well-being and the well-being of the stroke survivor. An active coping style, or using problem solving and information gathering to deal with a stressful life event, is associated with positive outcomes for the caregiver. Passive coping, also referred to as avoidance or escape coping, is a negative predictor of caregiver QOL.

Formal interventions for caregivers often include structured courses on improving coping ability; assistance with daily tasks, including housekeeping, meal preparation, and grocery shopping; respite for the caregiver; and emotional support via telephone, the Internet, nurse-led support groups and/or nurse home visits, and psychological counseling.

Investigators who processed a systematic review found that psychosocial interventions alone often failed to reduce the burden on caregivers because the impact on the caregiver is physical, emotional, social, and financial. For persons newly assuming the role and responsibilities of caregiver, the Internet has become a primary means of education and informal help and support. Internet discussion groups, blogs, message boards, social networking sites, and educational websites have become widely used resources that provide avenues for caregivers to share their feelings, glean practical advice, and receive social support, which has been cited by caregivers as their greatest need.

There are various conceptual theories and models that are related to caregiver stress and stroke survivors, which affect the interventions that are provided. Family systems theory presumes that a change in any part of the family system alters the entire system. Therefore, the changes experienced by the stroke survivor have an impact on all the members of the family, especially the caregiver. The stress and coping theory suggest that stressful events will trigger a coping process to try to restore balance. This theory also incorporates the concept of contextual factors (e.g., background, socioenvironmental factors, illness) that can affect coping processes and outcomes. The psychoeducational model will combine providing information on stroke and caregiving, while also taking a psychological approach to any survivor or caregiver stress.

Although caregivers face numerous challenges in providing care and assistance for stroke survivors, evidence shows that most caregivers are less likely than survivors to be depressed or to focus on the survivors' functional deficits (e.g., limited mobility, difficulty with self-care, speech). Stroke survivors often exhibit emotional, behavioral, and cognitive impairment that can alter the relationship between themselves and their caregivers. Yet evidence shows that although survivors tend to perceive a loss of intimacy with their caregivers, caregivers tend to perceive their relationship as strengthened despite increasing challenges.

Stroke survivors tend to feel uncomfortable with their need for assistance and may equate dependence with inadequacy. Conversely, caregivers generally are comfortable in their role and are willing to provide more assistance with tasks than care recipients are willing to accept.

Researchers in the Netherlands found that when stroke survivors were anxious and had lower life satisfaction, there was an increase in the strain on the caregivers. Research indicates that the QOL of the care recipient is in part dependent upon the QOL of the caregiver. Depression in caregivers is associated with poor stroke survivor function, communication, and social participation. In Canada, the healthcare community has released guidelines for physicians, nurses, and any other allied health professionals to screen for depression for all clients who are living with stroke and those clients' caregivers.

If the caregivers have high levels of mastery in their caregiving skills, are in good physical health, and provide higher levels of assistance to the survivor, they typically report improved mental health and quality of life. These caregivers may feel needed and appreciated, seeing that there is a positive outcome to providing care.

—*Laura McLuckey, MSW, LCSW*
Updated by Oi-Lee Tiffany Wong, RN, MS

FOR FURTHER INFORMATION

Cameron, J. I., et al. "What makes family caregivers happy during the first 2 years post stroke?" *Stroke*, 45, no. 4, 2014, 1084-1089.

Canadian Stroke Network. https://www.heartand-stroke.ca/heart/risk-and-prevention.

Centers for Disease Control and Prevention. "Stroke Facts." *Stroke*. 6 September 2017. http://www.cdc.gov/stroke/facts.htm.

Cheng, H. Y., et al. "The effectiveness of psychosocial interventions for stroke family caregivers and stroke survivors: A systematic review and meta-analysis." *Patient Education and Counseling*, 95, 2014, 30-44.

Feigin, V.L., et al. "Global burden of stroke." *Circ Res.* 120, no. 3, 2017, 439-448.

Go, A. S., et al. "Heart disease and stroke statistics – 2013 update: A report from the American Heart Association." *Circulation*, 127, no. 1, 2014, e6-e245.

Oosterveer, D. M., et al. "Anxiety and low life satisfaction associate with high caregiver strain early after stroke." *Journal of Rehabilitation Medicine*, 46, no. 2, 2104, 139-143.

Young, M. E., et al. "A comprehensive assessment of family caregivers of stroke survivors during inpatient rehabilitation." *Disability and Rehabilitation*, 33, no. 22, 2015, 1892-1902.

Stroke risks and protective factors

CATEGORY: Disease/Disorder

KEY TERMS:

atrial fibrillation: a quivering or irregular heartbeat (arrhythmia) that can lead to blood clots, stroke, heart failure and other heart-related complications

hemorrhagic stroke: stroke caused by the rupture of a blood vessel in or on the surface of the brain with bleeding into the surrounding tissue

ischemic stroke: stroke caused by a blood clot that blocks or plugs a blood vessel in the brain

statin: any of a group of drugs that act to reduce levels of fats, including triglycerides and cholesterol, in the blood

WHAT WE KNOW

Stroke is a medical emergency that occurs as a result of cerebral ischemia (i.e., insufficient blood flow to the brain as a result of clots or events such as heart attacks) or cerebral hemorrhage (i.e., bleeding inside the brain), both of which lead to permanent damage to brain cells. Stroke is the fifth leading cause of death in the United States and a leading cause of disability. Approximately 7 million American adults have had a stroke, and 795, 000 new or recurrent strokes occur each year. Ischemic stroke is more common than hemorrhagic stroke, occurring in about 87 percent of stroke cases. By 2030 it is projected that an additional 3.4 million adults will have a stroke, which is a 20.5 percent increase in prevalence from 2012.

Numerous factors have been identified that increase an individual's risk for stroke. Risk factors for a stroke include nonmodifiable risk factors (those that cannot be changed), modifiable lifestyle factors (those that can be changed), cardiovascular and metabolic conditions, and certain biomarkers.

Nonmodifiable risk factors for stroke include sex, age, and ethnicity/race. In general, women have a higher lifetime risk of stroke than men. The lifetime risk of stroke among women between the ages of 55 to 75 was 1 in 5 versus the risk for men is 1 in 6. However, women in the younger and middle-age groups who have a lower age-specific incidence rate of stroke than men in the same age range. The risk for stroke doubles every 10 years after age 55, with an estimated 20 percent of deaths from stroke occurring after age 65. Worldwide, rates of stroke are higher among Blacks, Hispanics, and Native Americans than among Whites. This discrepancy is likely due to the greater incidence of diabetes mellitus and hypertension in these groups.

Modifiable lifestyle factors include tobacco use, unhealthy diets, lack of physical activity, alcohol or drug abuse, and the use of oral contraceptives. Tobacco use doubles the risk for stroke. Diets low in fruits and vegetables and high in saturated or trans-unsaturated fatty acids, cholesterol, and sodium are associated with an increased risk for stroke. Physical inactivity increases the risk for stroke by 50 percent. Alcohol and drug abuse can increase blood pressure (BP), thereby increasing the risk for stroke. The use of oral contraception has been linked to an increase in risk for ischemic stroke but not hemorrhagic stroke.

Cardiovascular, metabolic, and other medical conditions that may increase an individual's risk for stroke. Hypertension (i.e., BP over 130/80 mmHg) increases the risk for stroke. Diabetes mellitus increases stroke risk 1.8-fold in clients older than 75 years and 5.6-fold in those aged 30–44 years. Clients with both conditions, diabetes and hypertension, have a risk for stroke that is increased approximately fourfold. Pregnancy-related stroke from hypertensive disorders during pregnancy has increased dramatically. From 1994–1995 to 2010–2011, pregnancy-related stroke increased almost 65 percent.

Obesity, usually defined by a body mass index (BMI; i.e., a measurement of body fat based on height and weight) over 30, can be a risk factor for stroke. Furthermore, ischemic stroke risk is increased twofold in people with a BMI over 32 kg/m. Benign paroxysmal positional vertigo (BPPV) is a common type of vertigo that results from changes in head position. Investigators found in a recent study that risk for ischemic stroke was increased for clients with BPPV. Individuals who have had a transient ischemic attack (TIA) or prior stroke have up to a 17 percent increased risk for stroke, especially within the first 90 days after the initial event. Sleep apnea has been found to increase risk in men. Sleep duration, both too short and too long, can increase stroke risk. The underlying mechanisms as to how sleep is related to the risk of stroke have not been clearly defined, but research has indicated that sleep duration should be included as behavioral risk factor for stroke.

Atrial fibrillation (i.e., an irregular rapid heartbeat) is responsible for approximately 20 percent of all strokes, increasing an individual's stroke risk fivefold. Other cardiovascular conditions that increase stroke risk include coronary artery disease, history of myocardial infarction, left atrial enlargement, heart failure, and carotid or peripheral artery disease. A parental history of ischemic stroke can result in a threefold increase in stroke risk for adult children, increasing as the adult child ages. Chronic kidney disease also increases risk of stroke. Septicemia, which is infection throughout the body, creates systemic inflammation. Both infection and inflammation are associated with higher stroke risk. Clients under age 45 with a history of septicemia are at the greatest risk, particularly in the first 6 months after the septicemia occurs. Clients who have had a stroke and cancer have an increased risk for recurrent stroke and cardiovascular mortality, with a recurrence rate of 13.94 percent a year compared to only 4.65 percent a year with no cancer history.

Biomarkers for increased stroke risk include cholesterol levels. Abnormal cholesterol levels are associated with an increased risk for stroke, particularly ischemic stroke. Specifically, high levels of low-density lipoprotein (LDL, "bad cholesterol") and low levels of high-density lipoprotein (HDL, "good cholesterol") increase the risk for stroke Other risk factors for stroke include sickle cell disease. Hormone replacement therapy (HRT) in high risk population increases ischemic stroke risk by 44 percent. Further, high number of births of live children and migraine headaches are associated with a doubling of ischemic stroke risk.

Protective factors include medication and lifestyle modifications. Treatment of high BP with antihypertensive medications (e.g., angiotensin-converting enzyme [ACE] inhibitors, angiotensin receptor antagonists), treatment of high cholesterol with statins lovastatin), and treatment of coronary heart disease or atrial fibrillation with antithrombotic medications (e.g., clopidogrel [Plavix], warfarin [Coumadin]) are associated with a significant reduction in the risk for stroke. Treatment of hypertension can reduce stroke risk by up to 50 percent. Statin therapy has been shown to reduce the risk for a fatal stroke or a hemorrhagic stroke but may increase the risk for stroke in clients who have had a renal transplant, undergone regular dialysis treatment, or have already experienced a TIA or stroke. Warfarin therapy is associated with a 70 percent decrease in stroke risk in clients with atrial fibrillation. Although warfarin is highly effective, it has numerous limitations (e.g., narrow therapeutic window, drug–food interactions) that have led researchers to develop alternative agents for long-term oral anticoagulant therapy; oral direct thrombin inhibitors (e.g., dabigatran) and factor Xa inhibitors (e.g., rivaroxaban) that may prove to be suitable alternatives.

Cessation of smoking, weight loss if overweight, use of HRT only as indicated, and avoidance of excess consumption of alcohol can significantly decrease the risk for stroke. Routine physical exercise can also reduce stroke risk. Recent studies have found that physical exercise protects against all types of stroke with the reduction of risk in both women and men. Researchers who evaluated the effects of walking as physical exercise found that, especially for older adults, it was the total time spent exercising more than the intensity of the activity that was important for stroke prevention.

—*Carita Caple, RN, BSN, MSHS*
Updated by Oi-Lee Tiffany Wong, RN, MS

FOR FURTHER INFORMATION

Clayville, L. R., et al "New options in anticoagulation for the prevention of venous thromboembolism and stroke." *Pharmacy & Therapeutics*, vol. 36, no. 2, 2011, 86-88, 93-99.

Furie, K. L., et al. "Guidelines for the prevention of stroke in patients with stroke or transient ischemic attack: A guideline for healthcare professionals from the American Heart Association/American Stroke Association." *Stroke*, vol. 42, no. 1, 2011, 227-276.

Ge, B., & Guo, X. "Short and long sleep durations are both associated with increased risk of stroke: A meta-analysis of observational studies." *World Stroke Oraganization*, *10*, 2015, 177-184.

Benjamin, E.J., et al. "Heart disease and stroke statistics-2019 update: A report from the American Heart Association." *Circulation*, 139, 2019, e226-e238.

Lau, K. K., et al. "Stroke patients with a past history of cancer are at increased risk of recurrent stroke and cardiovascular mortality." *PLoS One*, 9, no. 2, 2014, e88283.

Leffert, L. R., et al., "Hypertensive disorders and pregnancy-related stroke: Frequency, trends, risk factors, and outcomes." *Obstatrics & Gynecology*, 125, no. 1, 2015, 124-131.

Strokes

CATEGORY: Disease/Disorder
Also known as: Cerebrovascular accidents (CVAs)

KEY TERMS:

amaurosis fugax: temporary blindness in one eye

angiography: radiological modality to visualize the arteries in the body; involves the placement of a catheter in an artery and the injection of dye

embolus: a small piece of atherosclerotic plaque, thrombus, or other debris that breaks off and lodges in a blood vessel

endarterectomy: a surgical technique in which an atherosclerotic plaque is excised

hemorrhagic: weakened blood vessel ruptures, as a result of aneurysm or arteriovenous malformation

infarct: tissue death resulting from lack of blood flow

ischemia: lack of blood in a particular tissue

revascularization: procedures to reestablish the circulation to a diseased portion of the body

thrombosis: the aggregation of platelets and other blood cells to form a clot

transient ischemic attacks (TIAs): commonly known as mini strokes; associated neurological deficits last less than twenty-four hours and usually only minutes

CAUSES AND SYMPTOMS

According to the National Stroke Association, the third leading cause of death in women is stroke. Stroke kills two times more women than breast cancer, in part because women do not perceive stroke as a threat. Because women tend to live longer than men, more women than men have strokes and more often die, but men are at greater risk. Stroke risk increases after age 55. African-Americans have a higher risk of stroke than people of other races. Living alone when having a stroke may lead to a delay in care, the need for long-term care or aggressive rehabilitation, and poor outcomes.

Predisposing factors to strokes include hypertension (high blood pressure), diabetes, obesity, high cholesterol, smoking, atherosclerotic disease in other portions of the body (such as the heart or legs), and a previous or family history of strokes or transient ischemic attacks. Gender and age are also associated with the incidence of strokes. Generic risk factors are prevalent for both men and women, but women have additional risk factors. Stroke risk during normal pregnancy due to body changes, birth control pills combined with generic risk factors, taking hormone replacement therapy (HRT) during menopause, and having migraine headaches with aura are all unique risk factors for women.

Strokes produce damage to portions of the brain as a result of decreased blood supply due to occlusion or hemorrhage. Strokes are commonly known as cerebrovascular accidents (CVAs). Symptoms of strokes will vary depending on the part of the brain that is affected. Rapid intervention is critical to management of stroke. The American Stroke Association has developed a guide to recognizing stroke symptoms to encourage the public to seek immediate emergency care. Using the word "FAST" to represent facial drooping, arm weakness, speech difficulty and time to call 911, allows individuals to recognize the symptoms of stroke and seek immediate treatment. Other symptoms of stroke may include trouble speaking, difficulty seeing out of one or both eyes, confusion, difficulty understanding simple commands such as "raise your right arm", trouble walking and weakness, especially on one side of the body, loss of balance and severe headache.

Resulting speech disorders may include aphasia (loss of the ability to speak) or dysarthria (difficulty in speaking). A sudden weakness or numbness of one side of the body is known as hemiparesis or hemiplegia. The eyes can also be involved. A dimness or transient loss of vision, particularly in one eye, is called amaurosis fugax. Occasionally, it can involve the same portion of the visual field in both eyes. Other symptoms of stroke may include dizziness, unsteadiness, sudden falls, headaches, confusion, or stupor. Coma is less commonly involved in a stroke.

In cerebrovascular disease, atherosclerosis affects the arteries that circulate blood to the brain. The brain receives blood from two major sets of arteries. The carotid arteries, in the front of the neck, supply the anterior (front) portions of the brain. The vertebral arteries travel through the transverse processes of the spine and join the basilar artery to provide blood to the posterior (back) portion of the brain. Both circulatory systems are joined within the brain in a structure known as the circle of Willis, a composite of arteries that join to form an anatomical circle. The various arteries supply the necessary blood flow to different areas of the brain. Only 25 to 50 percent of people have a complete circle of Willis; this anatomical variance may be a factor in the severity of the stroke.

In atherosclerotic disease, fat, cholesterol, and calcium deposits are laid down along the walls of the arteries, primarily at sites where arteries divide and natural turbulence tends to occur. These components build up to form plaques, which may cause stenosis (narrowing) and occlusion (closure) of the arterial lumen. Accumulation of platelets and other blood cells can form a thrombus (blood clot) along with plaque buildup, which also may obstruct the arteries. Pieces of plaque or thrombotic material may break off and cause emboli to lodge acutely in the main vessels or their more distant branches.

The most common components of cerebrovascular disease are transient ischemic attacks (TIAs), also referred to as ministrokes. By definition, TIAs last less than twenty-four hours; usually, they last only a few minutes or hours. Most TIAs are produced by emboli. An embolus occurs when a piece of plaque from the lining of a major artery breaks off and temporarily blocks the blood flow to a particular area of the brain. If the symptoms last for more than twenty-four hours, a cerebrovascular accident, cerebral infarct, or stroke has occurred. A reversible ischemic neurological deficit (RIND) is similar to a stroke in that it is an event that lasts for more than twenty-four hours but resolves in about seventy-two hours.

The majority of strokes in the United States (85 percent) are the result of impaired blood flow (ischemia) to the brain. Atherosclerosis in the cerebrovascular system will cause similar symptoms of ischemia in other portions of the body. There is increasing narrowing, or stenosis, of blood vessels. Eventually, they will close off completely and become occluded. The development of new, small vessels that bypass a diseased artery is called collateralization. This process requires weeks or months to occur. Collateralization seems to be especially prominent in the cerebrovascular system, since the brain is an organ that requires constant blood flow at all times. Eventual occlusion or thrombosis of a major vessel causes the majority of CVAs, producing significant ischemia in a portion of the brain. In certain cases, the blockage is acute, having resulted from an embolus or thrombus that blocks an artery. If collateralization has not developed, the damage to an affected structure is more severe. A thrombus or embolus can also arise from the heart. This is most common in individuals who have had a recent heart attack, who have disease that involves the mitral valve, or who have atrial fibrillation, a variety of irregular heartbeat.

Another cause of stroke is cerebral hemorrhage, or bleeding into the brain, resulting in loss of consciousness or incapacity. An older term rarely used now for cerebral hemorrhage is apoplexy. Hypertension is the most common cause of intracranial bleeding and accounts for 10 to 15 percent of cases. Other causes of strokes are cerebral aneurysms (5 to 7 percent), tumors that have developed blood supplies (3 to 5 percent), and genetic bleeding tendencies (1 to 2 percent). A cerebral aneurysm occurs when the wall of an artery becomes weak and enlarges like a balloon. These aneurysms often rupture. With a ruptured cerebral aneurysm and subsequent hemorrhage, byproducts of red blood cell degeneration may produce a condition called vasospasm, wherein the arteries will constrict. This often leads to ischemia. One or more thrombi are often formed in an aneurysm. If they break loose, they can become emboli, float until they become lodged in a small blood vessel, block the flow of blood, and cause ischemia. This can ultimately lead to a stroke.

Stroke refers to the disease process that is mainly produced by atherosclerotic changes in the arteries to the brain. Contributing or significant risk factors in the development of atherosclerosis include hypertension (high blood pressure), hyperlipidemia (high levels of cholesterol in the blood), smoking, diabetes mellitus, and a family history of similar incidents. Evidence of atherosclerotic disease in other portions of the body, such as the heart or legs, increases the risk of stroke. Atherosclerosis is a generalized disease process that affects arterial beds throughout the body.

Symptoms of TIAs in structures near the front of the brain, the area supplied by the carotid arteries, include hemiparesis, a numbness or loss of function in half of the body. Hemiplegia, a weakness of an arm or leg (or both), can be attributable to disease in the carotid artery on the side of the body opposite to the affected body part. Another relatively common problem usually caused by disease in the left carotid artery is aphasia, a speech disorder. Disease in either carotid artery can cause amaurosis fugax, or blindness in one eye. Victims often describe this condition as a shade being drawn over the eye.

Other, more generalized symptoms are the result of problems in the vertebral arteries or the blood vessels at the base of the brain, which supply the back portions of the brain. Associated symptoms include dizziness, a loss of orientation often produced by decreased blood flow to the brain. Dizziness is frequently caused by abrupt positional changes, in which blood pressure will suddenly fall with rapid standing or sitting, or by cardiac arrhythmias (irregular heartbeats), which prevent adequate amounts of blood flow from being delivered during certain cardiac cycles.

Vertigo is different from dizziness. Individuals suffering from vertigo experience a spinning sensation that may be accompanied by nausea. A common cause for vertigo is a condition known as subclavian steal, in which atherosclerotic disease affects the arteries of the arms just prior to the point where the vertebral arteries branch off. As an arm is used, or with abrupt changes in head position, blood will flow out of the vertebral arteries in a reverse manner (the so-called steal) to aid circulation in the arm (via the subclavian arteries) and vertigo will ensue. In addition, imbalance and other visual disturbances may be associated with problems in the vertebral arteries. These symptoms may also result from cerebrovascular disease in which inadequate blood supply to multiple areas of the brain can produce diverse symptoms. In the majority of strokes,

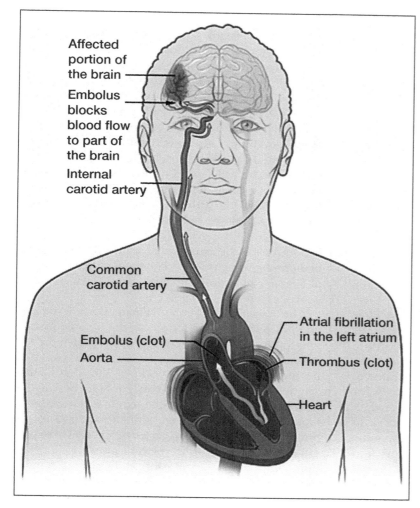

Affected portion of the brain

Embolus blocks blood flow to part of the brain

Internal carotid artery

Common carotid artery

Embolus (clot)

Aorta

Atrial fibrillation in the left atrium

Thrombus (clot)

Heart

This illustration shows how a stroke can occur during atrial fibrilation. blood clot can form in the left atrium of the heart. If a piece of the clot breaks off and travels to an artery in the brain, it can block blood flow through the artery. The lack of blood flow to the portion of the brain fed by the artery causes a stroke. (US Marine Corps via Wikimedia Commons)

symptoms last twenty-four to seventy-two hours. Approximately 25 percent of patients will develop permanent deficits that will affect them for the rest of their lives. Approximately 20 percent of individuals who have strokes will experience no symptoms (be asymptomatic) and not know that they have had a stroke. They are unlikely to even develop TIAs. Such unheralded events result from occlusion or thrombosis of the blood vessels in the brain. This causes ischemia that leads to infarction or cell death in a particular section of the brain.

Asymptomatic cerebrovascular disease, however, can often be detected by the presence of a bruit, a French word meaning "noise." Stenosis in arteries can be compared to rapids in a river. Blood will flow very quickly through the narrow area and create turbulence, producing a bruit that can be heard with a stethoscope. Patients with narrowing in the carotid arteries ranging from 20 to 80 percent may possess a bruit. The absence of a bruit does not mean that the carotid arteries are disease-free. Once the stenosis reaches critical proportions, the flow is diminished and turbulence may be negligible, indicating a severe stenosis or an occluded artery. Often, doctors will recommend elective surgery to patients with coronary artery stenosis between 60 and 80 percent in an effort to reestablish blood flow and prevent eventual occlusion and possible stroke. About 75 percent of strokes are caused by ischemia that results from the above process. Crescendo TIAs, in which multiple TIAs occur in a brief period of time, and evolving strokes require immediate medical treatment. Appropriate diagnosis and treatment may prevent a stroke or decrease its severity.

Although disease caused by an aneurysm is a separate entity, it may be associated with atherosclerotic disease in certain cases. Most aneurysms within the brain produce no symptoms. As aneurysms increase in size, the probability of rupture increases; therefore, elective surgery may be recommended. Occasionally, diagnoses of cerebral aneurysms are made during investigations of other cerebral events, such as headaches. Acute onset of severe headaches or stiff neck should mandate immediate medical attention, since rupture of a cerebral aneurysm often manifests itself in this manner.

TREATMENT AND THERAPY

Strokes and TIAs often occur quickly and without warning. The best treatment for them is preventive behavior to avoid the atherosclerotic disease leading to such events.

Immediate medical care is critical to managing stroke and minimizing the long-term effects of the event, including the potential to prevent death. Medical advances in radiological imaging and stroke treatments have improved survival rates over the past decade. When a stroke is caused by a clot, Alteplase IV r-tPA may be administered in an attempt to dissolve the clot. As the only FDA-approved treatment for ischemic stroke, Alteplase IV r-tPA is a tissue plasminogen activator that works to improve blood flow by dissolving the clot and restoring blood flow to the brain. It must be administered within 4.5 hours of initial stroke symptoms if given in a vein. Often patients delay seeking hospital care resulting in permanent disability reflected by the tissues in the brain deprived of oxygen. If a patient experiences a stroke during the night or has no recollection of when symptoms began, the use of r-tPA is limited. Continued research may allow longer periods of time from onset to drug delivery. An endovascular procedure may be used to send a catheter to the site of blockage in an attempt to remove the clot and r-tPA may be injected intra-arterially into the clot in some instances. The best clinical protocols for endovascular procedures are still being researched.

When a stroke or TIA is suspected upon arrival to the Emergency Room, it is imperative to determine the time of onset of symptoms. A brief history and physical examination followed by a CT scan follows to determine the type of stroke and the patient's eligibility for r-tPA. Because of the three-hour time window for administration, determining symptoms and noting significant risk factors and findings upon physical examination will help a physician determine the primary area of the brain affected, schedule the appropriate tests for further diagnosis, and choose the best course of therapy. If the patient is documented to be well outside the three to 4½ hour accepted window, a more comprehensive work-up may be acceptable. The National Institutes of Health Stroke Scale (NIHSS) was developed by national and international panels to provide a quantitative measure of stroke-related neurologic deficit. It provides baseline data for a comprehensive clinical assessment of stroke patients and may be a predictor of outcomes in stroke patients.

Stroke care has evolved over time and continues to be the focus of research due to the debilitating and costly impacts on the patient. Because of the high incidence of death and disability associated with strokes, a variety of diagnostic tests have been developed since the 1950s. One of the oldest noninvasive methods is the directional Doppler test. A Doppler device employs a probe with one or two piezoelectric crystals. An ultrasonic signal using a frequency of 2 to 5 megahertz (MHz) is sent into the body. Movement of red blood cells causes a shift in the frequency of the signal that is transmitted back. The amount of shift is proportional to the speed of blood flow. This device can also be used to determine the direction of blood flow. By listening with a continuous-wave Doppler over a branch of the ophthalmic artery at the corner of the eye and performing certain compression maneuvers on the arteries that supply the face, information regarding possible collateral pathways can be obtained concerning internal carotid artery blockages of greater than 75 percent.

The vascular surgeon William Gee developed another device, called an ocular pneumoplethysmograph (OPG). The OPG utilizes cups placed in the eye to measure the ocular pressure. A vacuum is applied to the eyes, effectively blocking the ophthalmic arteries, which are the first major branches of the internal carotid artery. As the vacuum is released, the blood flow is reestablished, and the appearance of arterial pulsations is noted on a strip chart. These pulsations denote systolic blood pressure in the ophthalmic arteries. A pressure difference of 5 millimeters of mercury (mm Hg) between the two eyes or an index of less than 0.66 (comparing the systolic blood pressure in the ophthalmic artery with that in the brachial artery) is consistent with carotid artery blockage of more than 50 to 75 percent.

Both of these methods are indirect tests, in which significant internal carotid artery disease is implied if the test is positive. Deficiencies in the test procedures include quantification of the percentage of carotid artery disease or differentiation of significant stenosis from occlusions. They also may be wrong if the vertebral or basal arteries contribute significant collateral blood flow. The OPG is still used in certain situations as a quick screening tool, but the directional Doppler has lost favor as an accurate diagnostic test. Duplex ultrasound machines, first employed in the early 1980s, utilize B-mode (brightness-mode) ultrasound to visualize the vessels and type of plaque. In comparison, Doppler ultrasound can audibly evaluate the blood flow in the vessels. Using real-time spectrum analyzers, the Doppler signals are then analyzed in terms of velocity (speed of the blood flow) and waveform characteristics. The greater the velocity, the greater the amount of stenosis. Absence of blood flow will denote occlusions.

Much research has been done in evaluating plaque morphology and its association with the incidence of TIAs, but results have been controversial using the standard gray-scale duplex devices. The use of color duplex ultrasound, in which the Doppler signals are color-coded in terms of flow direction and speed to denote the various flow patterns in normal and diseased vessels, has enhanced the diagnostic accuracies of the examinations. The use of color Doppler in many ultrasound machines is allowing more rapid detection of arterial lesions in blood vessels both inside and outside the skull. Transcranial Doppler uses a MHz pulsed Doppler probe through various normal anatomic windows (holes) in the skull. Measurements can be made through the side of the head (transtemporal), from the back of the head (transoccipital), and through the eye (transocular). The purpose of the examination is to assess the blood circulation in the circle of Willis. The transcranial Doppler gives information concerning various collateral pathways established when significant disease is present in blood vessels outside the skull. It is also useful when there is stenosis of arteries inside the skull. It is extremely accurate in detecting and monitoring early vasospasm in individuals with bleeding inside the skull. Additional research with this device is ongoing in other areas, such as in the detection of cerebral aneurysms and arteriovenous malformations in which there is an abnormal connection between the arteries and the veins.

Computed tomography (CT) scanning is a radiological technique that provides a three-dimensional picture of the brain and its structures. Occasionally, a contrast medium is also used in this examination. CT scanning is especially useful in the diagnosis of cerebral aneurysms and areas of infarct. Magnetic resonance imaging (MRI) is a nonradiological technique that also provides exceptional three-dimensional images of the soft tissue structures of the brain. MRI can detect cerebral infarcts at an earlier stage than can CT scanning. Arteriography or angiography is an invasive procedure that is performed in a hospital setting. A catheter is placed in one of the arteries, and dye containing iodine is injected. Multiple X rays are then taken to visualize the circulation. Arteriograms are considered to be standard in diagnosis. The delineation of the blockages and collateral pathways is then used primarily to plan surgical procedures.

Aspirin is often prescribed to alleviate symptoms of TIAs and to help protect patients from strokes or heart attacks. Although it is a powerful drug in decreasing the incidence of embolus formation, a national study has demonstrated that patients with a history of TIAs and carotid artery stenosis of greater than 60 percent should undergo surgical revascularization to protect against major strokes. The chances of having a stroke after suffering a TIA are approximately 40 percent greater.

Endarterectomy is a surgical technique in which the inner wall and part of the middle wall of the carotid artery are excised, effectively scraping out atherosclerotic plaques. Although used in other arterial segments, endarterectomy is the most common surgical procedure used to revascularize the carotid arteries. Occasionally, procedures are performed to bypass diseased segments of the cerebral vessels. Long-term research has shown that they have limited effectiveness. Consequently, many have been abandoned.

Other techniques for intervention have been developed. Percutaneous balloon angioplasty involves placing a balloon catheter in the diseased segment during an angiogram. When the balloon catheter is inflated, it opens up the area of stenosis or small segment of occlusion. This method has been employed in the coronary arteries as well as in the vessels leaving the aorta, the iliac arteries, and arteries in the lower extremities. It is not used often in the treatment of atherosclerotic plaques in the cerebral circulation because of the possibility of emboli traveling to the more distant blood vessels of the brain or eye. Some success in the use of balloon angioplasty has been reported in the treatment of vasospasm.

STROKE PREVENTION

Practicing healthy lifestyle behaviors such maintaining weight, not smoking, eating correctly and exercising routinely can help prevent strokes. Additionally, women who have migraines with aura should immediately stop smoking. Blood pressure monitoring during prenatal care is critical. Atrial fibrillation, especially in women 75-80, should be monitored and treated as indicated. Blood pressure screening prior to beginning birth control is important. Any woman with a family history and any risk factors should know the signs of stroke and seek care immediately if they present. Working with a primary care physician to maintain health may prevent stroke.

PERSPECTIVE AND PROSPECTS

Stroke is the third-leading cause of death in the United States, with approximately 158,000 deaths annually. There are 700,000 strokes annually, and about one-fourth of all nursing home patients are permanently impaired from strokes. Women have approximately 60,000 more strokes than men annually. These statistics have a great impact on the amount of money spent annually on care for victims of strokes.

Since the 1960s, the death rate from strokes in the United States has decreased significantly, by about 60 percent. Control of blood pressure and diet, the development of new drugs and diagnostic techniques, and the advent of cardiovascular surgery in the early 1950s have contributed to these results. Unfortunately, strokes are still prevalent given the extent of atherosclerotic disease in the American population, which is largely attributed to a high-fat diet. Autopsies of U.S. soldiers killed in the Korean and Vietnam Wars demonstrated evidence that atherosclerosis begins at a very early age, often by age eighteen. Atherosclerosis is more prevalent in males. Females have more protection until the onset of the menopause. Within five years of the menopause, however, the stroke and death rates of men and women tend to equalize.

High-salt diets, which contribute to hypertension, also contribute to the development and progression of atherosclerosis, as well as hemorrhagic strokes. Ethnic African and Asian populations appear to be at greater risk in this respect. Since the 1960s, however, extensive education of the American public concerning diet and the control of blood pressure has had a favorable impact. More recently, the increase in individuals who have stopped smoking and who have undertaken regular exercise has helped to lower stroke rates further.

Since the 1950s, a number of both noninvasive and invasive procedures have been developed to diagnose atherosclerotic disease. Cardiovascular surgical techniques were developed in the 1950s. The first bypass surgery (arterial autograft) probably occurred during the Korean War. The development of ultrasound devices in the 1950s initiated the research into using these noninvasive devices to diagnose cerebrovascular disease. The duplex devices introduced commercially in the late 1970s and early 1980s have spurred the development of new diagnostic devices for detecting atherosclerotic disease. These devices allow for visualization of plaque morphology (composition of the plaque, such as thrombus, calcium, hemorrhage, and other particulate matters) and blood flow characteristics for a better understanding of the disease process. Future developments in the field of ultrasound include holographic imaging for the three-dimensional visualization of plaques. These noninvasive technologies will also allow physicians to monitor the effects of new drugs and techniques in the treatment of atherosclerosis. Advances in digital subtraction and computer enhancement of angiographic techniques, along with new contrast media, have made arteriograms safer and more accurate.

Color duplex devices are utilizing low-frequency probes to visualize and produce color scans of blood vessels that lie inside the skull. By analyzing the blood flow direction and velocity in the circle of Willis and within the blood vessels of the skull, physicians will come to a better understanding of the formation of collateral pathways and will learn how to detect other pathological conditions that lead to cerebrovascular disease. Magnetic resonance imaging (MRI) is also being utilized to measure actual flow in individual arterial segments of the body.

Carotid endarterectomies, which lost favor for a period of time, have become the preferred therapeutic treatment for individuals with episodes of TIAs and severe atherosclerotic plaques in the carotid arteries. Additional studies will further delineate which other patient populations may benefit from this surgery. Aspirin still remains a potent drug in the treatment of TIAs in patients with lesser degrees of disease and in post surgery patients. Recognition and prompt treatment of symptomatic cerebrovascular symptoms remain the key to better survival rates.

—*Silvia M. Berry, M.Sc., R.V.T.;*
L. Fleming Fallon, Jr., M.D., Ph.D., M.P.H.;
Updated by Bradley R. A. Wilson, Ph.D.
and Patricia Stanfill Edens, PhD, RN, LFACHE

FOR FURTHER INFORMATION

American Medical Association. *American Medical Association Family Medical Guide.* 4th rev. ed. Hoboken, N.J.: John Wiley & Sons, 2004.

American Stroke Association. http://www.stroke association.org.

American Stroke Association. "Women and Stroke." https://www.stroke.org/understand-stroke/impact-of-stroke/women-and-stroke/.

Marler, John R. *Stroke for Dummies.* Indianapolis, Ind.: John Wiley & Sons, 2005.

National Institutes of Health Stroke Scale. http://www.nihstrokescale.org/

Rao, Paul R., Mark N. Ozer, and John E. Toerge, eds. *Managing Stroke: A Guide to Living Well After Stroke.* Washington, D.C.: ABI Professional, 2000.

Senelick, Richard C., and Karla Dougherty. *Living with Stroke: A Guide for Families.* 3d ed. Albany, N.Y.: Delmar, 2001.

Wiebers, David O., Valery L. Feigin, and Robert D. Brown, Jr. *Handbook of Stroke.* Philadelphia: Lippincott Williams & Wilkins, 2006.

Zamanlu M, et al. "Recent advances in targeted delivery of tissue plasminogen activator for enhance thrombolysis in ischemic stroke." *J Drug Target.* 26, no. 2, 2018, 95-109.

Substance misuse treatment

CATEGORY: Disease/Disorder

WHAT WE KNOW

The *Diagnostic and Statistical Manual of Mental Disorders,* fifth edition (*DSM-5*), was published in 2013, replacing the *DSM-IV.* The *DSM-IV* chapter "Substance-Related Disorders" included substance dependence, substance abuse, substance intoxication, and substance withdrawal and then discussed specific substances (e.g., alcohol, amphetamines).

The *DSM-5* divides these disorders into two categories: substance use disorders and substance-induced disorders (intoxication, withdrawal, and other substance- or medication-induced mental disorders). Thus, it removes the distinction between abuse and dependence and instead divides each disorder into mild, moderate, and severe subtypes. Drug craving has been added as a criterion for substance use disorder, whereas "recurrent legal problems" has been removed. In the *DSM-5*, substance abuse is referred to as *substance use disorder* or *substance dependence*, whereas in the research literature it is still commonly referred to as *substance abuse*. When there is a pattern of continued use of a substance (e.g., alcohol, cannabis, opioids, sedatives) that cause cognitive, physiological, and behavioral symptoms, resulting in problems in various areas of functioning, that use may be classified as moderate(i.e., 4 to 5 symptoms) to severe (i.e., 6 or more symptoms). The pattern of use is pathological. The individual may experience impaired behavioral control, continued use even in the face of risks to the self, and social impairment. There also may be tolerance and withdrawal. This problematic pattern of use must take place for at least 12 months to be classified as substance use.

In 2013, the Substance Abuse and Mental Health Services Administration (SAMHSA)determined that 24.6 million people over the age of 12 estimated that 24.6 million people over the age of 12 were current users of illicit drugs; 21.6 million people over the age of 12 in the United States were classified as being dependent on substances or meeting the *DSM-IV* criteria for substance abuse.

- 2.6 million met the criteria for both alcohol and illicit drug dependence or abuse (e.g., marijuana; cocaine; heroin; hallucinogens; inhalants; and the nonmedical use of prescription-type pain relievers, tranquilizers, stimulants, and sedatives).
- 4.3 million met the criteria for illicit drug dependence or abuse alone.
- 14.7 million met the criteria for alcohol dependence or abuse alone.

Rates of substance dependence and substance use vary by gender: in 2013, 10.8 percent of men over the age of 12 in the United States met the criteria for substance use or dependence, whereas 5.8 percent of women over age 12 did.

Nationwide, women made up approximately 32 percent of the population in treatment for substance use. Only 6 percent of substance use treatment facilities in the United States in 2012were for women only.

There is a general disparity between the number of people needing treatment and the number of people receiving treatment. Women seeking substance use treatment often are experiencing multiple issues (e.g., intimate partner violence, financial issues, childcare needs)that increase their vulnerability to substance use and will have an impact on their treatment.

In 2013, only 2.5 million people received specialty substance use treatment out of the 22.7 million who needed treatment. Some 908,000 respondents reported needing treatment but did not receive treatment. The most common reason given for not receiving treatment was being uninsured or unable to afford treatment at 37.3 percent,and not wanting to stop using accounted for 24.5 percent.

Women can be reluctant to recognize that their substance use is problematic; professionals (e.g., physicians, social workers, nurses) may be more reluctant to screen female clients for substance use.

Women who become pregnant while using substances are more likely to delay their first healthcare visit because of their substance use.

There is significant evidence for a connection between trauma exposure/trauma history and substance use disorders, which can be difficult to treat systemically.

Researchers found that approximately 50 percent of a sample of women who had completed a community substance use program reported childhood abuse, 87 percent reported psychological victimization by an intimate partner, 79 percent reported physical abuse by an intimate partner, and 47 percent reported physical victimization by a stranger.

Sixty-two percent of these women reported at least one symptom from each of the clusters for posttraumatic stress disorder (PTSD).

Researchers for a second study found similar results, with 51 percent of women in a substance treatment program reporting sexual abuse and 69 percent reporting physical abuse.

Dual substance dependence can further increase risk for PTSD. Participants in a study who had lifetime comorbidities of alcohol and cocaine dependence had a higher number of traumatic events in their trauma histories, were more likely to have experienced violence, and were more likely to have PTSD.

Abuse may increase the risk of substance use and addiction if the client is using substances to relieve emotional pain. There may be a higher risk for relapse if any underlying trauma is not addressed during treatment.

Childcare, child custody, and parenting issues may strongly influence the commitment and ability of substance-abusing women to undergo treatment. As a result, a stepped care model may be the most appropriate where the lowest-intensity/least invasive option is offered first and if that level of care is not sufficient, the client is stepped up to the next level.

Social support networks are critical for women seeking treatment for substance use. Such networks provide both emotional and informational support and the practical help (e.g., with childcare, financial assistance, housing) that women often need in order to complete treatment.

Researchers found that women in residential treatment had less supportive environments and more substance users in their personal networks than women in outpatient treatment did.

Substance-abusing women may report a greater severity of problems as a result of addiction and develop severe problems with addiction more quickly than men do, which is referred to as the telescoping effect (i.e., acceleration in the progression from substance use to substance use).

Depression and anxiety are common comorbidities with substance use in women. Researchers found that all of the women in a community-based treatment sample reported a history of depression, and approximately 80 percent were currently using antidepressant medication.

Researchers also found that women with high psychiatric symptom severity made greater reductions in their substance use after 12 weeks of single-gender, women-focused group therapy treatment than did participants who were in mixed-gender group drug counseling. The women assigned to single-gender treatment also had more continued improvement at 6-month follow-up than those in mixed-gender treatment did.

Conceptual models that attempt to explain why substance use develops advocate and outline interventions and desired outcomes that fit those models. Social workers need to be aware of the interventions and outcomes related to the theoretical basis for treatments that they choose to use.

The most commonly researched and utilized models are the disease model, psychological model, motivation and change theories, transtheoretical model/stages of change, and harm reduction (i.e., the public health model).

The *disease model* is most commonly associated with Alcoholics Anonymous (AA) and other 12-step programs that view substance use and substance use as a disease rather than a moral failing. The theory that substance use is a medical condition recognizes the influence of biological, environmental, behavioral, and genetic factors in addiction.

The *psychological models* focus on the cognitive and behavioral reasons individuals use substances and advocate strategies for change that incorporate these perspectives. Addictive behaviors and traits are viewed as habits that can be studied and changed. Relapses are considered to be a likely occurrence and are not considered an abject failure on the part of the client.

Motivation and change theories emphasize examining the client's motivation for change and the nature and mechanics of change itself while working to establish a collaborative relationship between social worker and client. Motivational interviewing (MI) focuses on why people make changes in behavior.

According to the *transtheoretical model/stages of change*, behavior change typically proceeds through five stages: precontemplation, contemplation, preparation, action, and maintenance. This model has three key tenets: The change process can start even if the client has not started with a stage of precontemplation, relapse is a likely occurrence, and interventions must match the client's stage (e.g., a client in precontemplation is not ready for action-oriented interventions). In the last 10 years, studies of the effectiveness of this model and interventions based on it have shown mixed results.

Harm reduction does not dismiss abstinence as a goal if it is desired but prioritizes improvement over complete cessation of use.

Successful substance use treatment programs designed for women should incorporate prenatal care and childcare. They must also recognize and address the influence of gender roles on the physical and emotional health of the client.

Many women who are in treatment for substance use have a history of childhood use and sexual victimization, so single-sex treatment with a focus on empowerment may help them feel safe and comfortable to explore that history and its role in their addiction.

Women's needs may not be met in traditional treatment models that rely on confrontational interventions, demand strict attendance at 12-step meetings (which may be dominated by men), emphasize the individual's powerlessness, focus on substance use to the exclusion of psychiatric needs, and focus solely on abstinence.

Barriers to treatment that are internal (e.g., denial, shame, guilt, self-blame) and external (e.g., poverty, limited treatment options) are experienced by both men and women who use substances, but women face a higher number of external barriers, many of which are gender-specific.

The lack of childcare in treatment programs has a more significant effect on women; many women fear they will lose custody of their children if they enter residential treatment. Nationally, only 13 percent of substance use treatment facilities have childcare programs. Only 12 percent of substance use treatment facilities offer prenatal care.

Having an insufficient number of female staff members in a treatment program can alienate female clients and make establishing trust more difficult, especially for victims of trauma.

An emphasis on traditional models of treatment that were developed for male clients results in a scarcity of gender-specific treatments.

Some female clients fear that their male partner will leave them if they enter treatment because they will be absent from the home.

Women who live in rural areas face more barriers to treatment: They may have to travel greater distances for treatment, rural populations typically experience poorer health, and rural communities are more likely to be poor.

Women with children who are involved in the child welfare system may be caught in a conflict between the timeframe of the child welfare agency and that of substance use treatment: Treatment and recovery from addiction may take months or years, but child welfare agencies may terminate parental rights before treatment and recovery are concluded.

Substance use treatment programs and child welfare agencies may also view relapse differently: child welfare agencies often view relapse as evidence of treatment failure and grounds to remove the child from the parent's care, whereas most substance use treatment programs see relapse as a common occurrence in treatment and not a failure but an opportunity for learning and personal growth.

—*Jessica Therivel, LMSW-IPR*

FOR FURTHER INFORMATION

American Psychiatric Association. (2013). Substance-related and addictive disorders. *Diagnostic and Statistical Manual of Mental Disorders, fifth edition (DSM-5)*. Arlington, VA: American Psychiatric Publishing.

Brown, C. G., & Stewart, S. H. (2008). Exploring perceptions of alcohol use as self-medication for depression among women receiving community-based treatment for alcohol problems. *Journal of Prevention & Intervention in the Community, 35*(2), 33-47.

Cosden, M., Larsen, J. L., Donahue, M. T., & Nylund-Gibson, K. (2015). Trauma symptoms for men and women in substance abuse treatment: a latent transition analysis. *Journal of Substance Abuse Treatment, 50*, 18-25. doi:10.1016/j.jsat.2014.09.004

Haug, N. A., Duffy, M., & McCaul, M. E. (2014). Substance abuse treatment services for pregnant women. *Obstetrics and Gynecology Clinics of North America, 41*, 267-296. doi:10.1016/j.ogc.2014.03.001

Min, M. O., Tracy, E. M., & Park, H. (2015). Personal networks of women in residential and outpatient substance abuse treatment. *Counselor: The Magazine for Addiction Professionals, 16*(4), 66-71.

Successful aging

CATEGORY: Biology

BACKGROUND

Seniors are living longer and becoming a greater percentage of the population in the twenty-first century. Advances in medicine enable people to live longer and healthier lives. Since the early twentieth century, the average life span worldwide has increased from forty-seven to seventy-two years. In United States the average is 78.6 years. Women live longer than men do, with the average lifespan for American women at 79.1, French women at 80.9 and the highest are Japanese women at 82.5 years old. Traditional retirement age of sixty-five is no longer considered old, since many live into their eighties and nineties. Seniors may choose to delay their retirement into their late sixties or early seventies.

The growing number of seniors is redefining aging. Concerns have surfaced about society's ability to cope with an aging population that puts greater demands on health care and community caregiving resources. However, many individuals entering their later years are healthy, active, and involved in their communities. They are willing and able to contribute to society. Seniors are at the forefront of the movement to discover strategies for successful aging.

The perception of aging has changed since the beginning of the twentieth century. Retirement was for the rich only until Social Security was introduced in the United States in 1935. Everyone could expect to live decently in old age. Retirement communities sprang up to cater to the aging with the funds and leisure time to enjoy retirement. Today, many older adults continue to work and volunteer after retirement. Culture and genetics influence how people age. Scientists have discovered places in the world where people live a long time with a high quality of life, including Sardinia in Italy, Okinawa in Japan, and Loma Linda in California. Genetics, healthy eating habits, and a culture promoting freedom and well-being are factors in the successful aging process in these locations. Researchers studying centenarians have found that although health and life span are generally determined by genetics, genes can be influenced by lifestyle, diet, and environmental factors. The mapping of the human genome promises new possibilities to extend life expectancy and promote healthy aging.

Healthy aging is a combination of physical, mental, and social well-being. In general, older individuals today are in better physical shape than their predecessors. In the United States, chronic diseases are affecting people later in life. According to a study conducted by Pew Research, older individuals do not feel "old." One-third of respondents between the ages of sixty-five and seventy-four felt ten to nineteen years younger than their chronological age. Seniors who continue to maintain an active social life with family, friends, and community feel free to remain independent as they age successfully.

Although men and women share many aspects of aging, women face unique physical and psychological challenges. For example, the life expectancy of women (81.1 years) exceeds that of men (76.1 years) by five years. About 40% of women age 65 and older have lost a spouse to death. Widows may experience grief with depression and anxiety for some time before moving forward with the support of family and friends. Healthy aging includes focusing on positive memories and maintaining social connections. Physically, women experience hormonal changes with menopause and have evolving health care needs. Health screening and testing, such as pap smears, mammograms, bone density tests, blood pressure checks, diabetes screening, skin cancer screening, hearing and vision testing, and colorectal cancer screening, can uncover a health problem early so women can seek treatment. Women should remember that it is never too late to adopt and benefit from positive lifestyle changes.

OVERVIEW

Successful aging begins with intentional effort to continue participating in life. In *Living the Good Long Life* (2013), lifestyle specialist Martha Stewart says, "The quality of the rest of your life is more within your control than you think." Many chronic diseases can be prevented or managed by making positive lifestyle choices. Healthy habits such as staying physically active, reducing stress, maintaining a healthy weight, not smoking, and drinking moderately have been proven to improve the quality of life and reduce the incidence of chronic diseases. Physical activity in the form of daily exercise totaling at least two and a half hours a week keeps both the brain and the body healthy.

Another effective aging strategy is to challenge the brain by working on stimulating mental activities, such as solving puzzles, learning a language, or traveling. Giving the gift of time as a volunteer benefits others but also keeps older citizens engaged in their community. More wealthy individuals are reinventing themselves as they age. For example, Bill Gates left Microsoft to devote his time to combating malaria and solving the world's energy problems through the Bill and Melinda Gates Foundation.

Having an active social life reduces loneliness and being involved also alleviates symptoms of depression and other mental illnesses. Engaging with active social groups is essential to successful aging. Social interaction improves life at all ages, but is particularly important for older individuals who need the support of a circle of friends to provide counsel, affection, and the freedom to interact with others. According to Pew Research, 70 percent of respondents over sixty-five enjoy spending time with family members.

Perhaps the most important strategy for successful aging is having a positive attitude about life. Staying curious about the world and finding one's passion promotes joy in life. Acceptance of life's challenges reduces stress. Sharing this positive attitude with others is an important aspect of aging. Passing on knowledge, compassion, and beliefs to the younger generation unites the generations and builds a better world. When older individuals engage in their community, they are leaving a valuable legacy to the world as well as creating a blueprint for successful aging.

—Myra Junyk, MA, Med
Updated by Marylane Wade Koch, MSN, RN

FOR FURTHER INFORMATION

Arrison, Sonia. *100 Plus: How the Coming Age of Longevity Will Change Everything, from Careers and Relationships to Family and Faith.* New York: Basic, 2011. Print.

Cornforth, Tracee. Must Have Medical Test and Screenings for Women. *Verywell Health: Healthy Aging.* March 14, 2017, https://www.verywell-health.com/must-have-medical-tests-for-women-3522624

Cravit, David. *The New Old: How the Boomers Are Changing Everything—Again.* Toronto: ECW, 2008. Print.

"Growing Old in America: Expectations vs. Reality." *Pew Research Center.* Pew Research Center, 29 June 2009. Retrieved from http://www.pewsocialtrends.org/2009/06/29/growing-old-in-america-expectations-vs-reality/

Gurian, Michael. *The Wonder of Aging: A New Approach to Embracing Life after Fifty.* New York: Atria, 2013. Print.

Horstman, Judith. *The Scientific American Healthy Aging Brain.* San Francisco: Jossey, 2012. Print.

Reichstadt, J., Sengupta, G., Depp, C. A., Palinkas, L. A., & Jeste, D. V. (2010). Older Adults' Perspectives on Successful Aging: Qualitative Interviews. *The American Journal of Geriatric Psychiatry: Official Journal of the American Association for Geriatric Psychiatry, 18*(7), 567–575. https://www.ncbi.nlm.nih.gov/pmc/articles/PMC3593659/

Stewart, Martha. *Living the Good Long Life: A Practical Guide to Caring for Yourself and Others.* New York: Clarkson Potter, 2013. Print.

Stibich, Mark, PhD. How is Aging Different for Men and Women? *Verywell Health: Healthy Aging.* October 5, 2018. https://www.verywellhealth.com/is-aging-different-for-men-and-women-2224332

Sudden infant death syndrome (SIDS)

CATEGORY: Disease/Disorder

KEY TERMS:

apnea: absence of breathing

bradycardia: slowness of the heartbeat

hyperthermia: environmentally influenced elevated body temperature

hypothermia: environmentally influenced lower-than-normal body temperature

hypoxemia: subnormal oxygenation of arterial blood

neonatal: the period of time succeeding birth and continuing through the first twenty-eight days of life

prone: lying face-downward

supine: lying face-upward

tachycardia: rapid beating of the heart

thermolabile: unstable when heated

CAUSES AND SYMPTOMS

The distribution of sudden infant death syndrome (SIDS) is worldwide. Incidence rates vary from 0.12 to 3.0 for every thousand live births. In the United States, rates range from 1.6 to 2.3 for every thousand live births, with considerable ethnic variation: 0.5 among Asians, 1.3 among whites, 1.7 among Latinos, 2.9 among African Americans (5.0 for those of low socioeconomic status), and 5.9 among American Indians.

Cultural practices may make the incidence rate vary. In England, a Birmingham study found that 22 percent of Asian babies were put to sleep on their backs, compared with 3 percent of white babies. Sleeping prone is significantly more common in infants dying of SIDS than in controls. In the same study, 98 percent of Asian babies slept in the same room as their parents for the first year, 34 percent in the same bed. Only 65 percent of white infants slept in the same room as their parents. Perhaps the risk of sudden infant death increases in proportion to the amount of time an infant spends asleep out of parental earshot. In Zimbabwe, SIDS practically does not exist. According to English pediatrician Duncan Keeley, who served in that country for two years, black Zimbabwean infants almost invariably sleep with their mothers, at least until they are six months old and often until they are a year old.

The cause of sudden infant death syndrome is unknown, but a variety of genetic, environmental, and social factors have been associated with an increased risk of SIDS. Besides sleeping in the prone position, other associations include cold weather, overheating, the hours of the day from midnight to 9:00 a.m., and poor socioeconomic conditions, including overcrowding. The young, unmarried mother, especially if she has had no prenatal care, is more likely to have an infant with SIDS; so is the mother who smokes (either before or after the birth), is anemic, or ingests narcotics. Prematurity, especially with a history of apnea or damage to the immature lungs from elevated levels of inspired oxygen while on a respirator, also increases the risk.

Males are at a higher risk for SIDS than are females; so are the brothers and sisters of infants with SIDS. Likewise, a previously aborted episode of SIDS (that is, a "near miss") increases risk. On average, Apgar scores (a measure of infant health immediately after birth) are lower in infants with SIDS than they are in surviving peers. In a family that has lost an infant to SIDS, the risk for the next or subsequent child is about five times the usual risk. Most risk factors, however, are associated with only a twofold or threefold elevation of incidence. Therefore, predicting which infants will die unexpectedly is extremely difficult. Recent immunization is not a risk factor. Breastfeeding is not associated with a decreased risk, as was originally thought. Although the peak incidence of SIDS is around three months of age and coincides with normally low levels of circulating immunoglobulins, the syndrome is not associated with any known pathogen.

Pathologists report a wide variety of findings in their postmortem reports-especially changes in the brain and other parts of the body that suggest chronic or intermittent hypoxemia. Yet pathologists also fail to find an increase in the number of cells in tissue of the carotid bodies, a chemoreceptor that responds to decreases in blood oxygen tension; such a finding weighs against the presence of chronic hypoxia.

Like many other aspects of this disease, the mechanism or mechanisms of death in SIDS are unknown. Does the infant stop breathing, or does some cardiac irregularity occur? An immature cardiorespiratory control mechanism involving the nervous system is the most common hypothesis. D. P. Davies and Madeleine Gantley of the University of Wales College of

Medicine believe that an important mechanism underlying SIDS is failure of respiratory control at a vulnerable stage of development-more a physiological syndrome than a disease in the accepted sense. These doctors hypothesize that the disturbance to this delicate equilibrium might upset the regulation of breathing, sometimes leading to death. Epidemiological risk factors, such as an upper respiratory infection (which is not uncommon), are somehow linked with destabilizing influences to breathing. By avoiding or modulating these factors, the risk of death can be reduced.

Although the pathogenesis of SIDS remains unclear, Anne-Louise Ponsonby and her colleagues at the University of Tasmania in Australia propose that SIDS be considered as a biphasic event, with the first set of factors operating to predispose the infant and the second set of factors acting as loading factors that operate at a critical stage of the infant's development. The Australian doctors believe that a warm environment could lead to sudden infant death through direct hyperthermia; a thermolabile, sudden fall in blood pressure leading to a diminished oxygen supply to the brain; impaired respiratory control; altered sleep state; or depressed arousal. An asphyxial mode of death would also be more likely, particularly in heavily dressed infants found prone (face down). Concern for the confusion of SIDS with child abuse should not be ignored, nor should the efforts of the National Sudden Infant Death Syndrome Foundation to provide information about psychosocial support groups and counseling for families of SIDS victims.

TREATMENT AND THERAPY

Since the causes and mechanisms of death from SIDS may continue to be unknown, strategies that might reduce the incidence of this syndrome seem imperative. Cold weather and the hours of midnight to 9:00 a.m. bring increased risks for SIDS. A closer look explains that other risk factors are involved. Overheating as a response to cold weather and leaving the infant alone at night (particularly in Western countries) may be more important. Babies sleeping alone might lose external sensory stimulation that may help stabilize breathing patterns. Davies and Gantley, citing experimental work with mothers and infants co-sleeping in sleep laboratories, have shown how patterns of breathing may interact. They say that the alertness of the babies' caregivers to early symptoms of illness might also be important.

French doctors studied the seasonal variation of death from SIDS in their country for a two-year period in the early 1980s. They concluded that for babies born in the spring, the third month of age was not necessarily associated with the highest SIDS risk. Babies born during other seasons, however, exhibited a normal pattern of increasing risk between the first and third months. Age was an especially critical factor among babies who reached three months of age during the winter months. If they reach this age in July or August, they are less susceptible to SIDS.

This finding, then, leads to a consideration of the risk of overheating. Explanations for the association between cold weather and SIDS include hypothermia, increased viral illness, and indirect hyperthermia. New Zealand doctors looked at the role of thermal balance in SIDS by investigating the death scene. They found that infants who died of SIDS were significantly more likely to be overdressed for the room temperature at the death scene and in the prone position, when compared to control infants. They also suggest that parents may have responded to infections in their babies by increasing the amount of clothing and bedding or by otherwise warming the infant.

The government of New Zealand initiated a program of education for parents recommending that the prone sleeping position be avoided, that mothers not smoke, and that breastfeeding be encouraged. (Most experts believe that breastfeeding itself does not reduce risks for SIDS. Rather, closer and more frequent contact with mothers is the operative factor.)

A similar education program for parents in Avon, England, was initiated, but it omitted advice on breastfeeding and included suggestions to avoid overheating after a retrospective case-control study that suggested a nearly nine fold relative risk for SIDS from infants sleeping prone. New Zealand and Avon both reported fewer deaths from SIDS after their parental education programs were introduced. The Department of Health extended Avon's campaign nationally.

In an editorial note in 1986, the National Center for Health Statistics acknowledged that "the rapid decline of infant mortality rates in the 1970s has been attributed largely to the advent of medical technology in the area of premature and other clinically ill newborns." Yet, "in the 1980s, this decline has slowed considerably-partly because of a lack of progress in primary prevention of conditions which lead to infant death." Undoubtedly, the United States would benefit from a massive, national program of education for parents. For example, cigarette packages carry a warning of the harmful effects of smoking on the fetus; perhaps they should also include a warning about the dangers to infants of maternal smoking.

Another possibility for intervention exists in the area of infections: Pertussis (whooping cough) could be prevented by the immunization of infants under six months of age. In the long term, all nations should work toward improving the socioeconomic status and health care of the poor.

Finally, improved medical technology will be less important over the long haul than will efforts to educate parents in infant care practices. The ability of parents and other members of the household to monitor infants and respond appropriately to both true and false alarms is crucial, as is appropriate training in infant CPR (cardiopulmonary resuscitation) and the proper use of monitory equipment. Even if all SIDS is eliminated in at-risk children, there will continue to be cases among children not known to have been at risk.

PERSPECTIVE AND PROSPECTS

The term "sudden infant death syndrome" was popularized by Abraham Berman's book on SIDS in 1969, which grew out of a conference on that subject. Since then, recognition of the syndrome has led to the creation of organizations dealing with it. The Sudden Infant Death Foundation merged, on January 1, 1991, with the National Center for the Prevention of SIDS to form one organization, the Sudden Infant Death Alliance.

There are things that expecting mothers can do to lower their children's risk for SIDS, including getting adequate medical care within the first three months of pregnancy. Regular follow-up visits, a nutritionally balanced diet, and avoiding smoking cigarettes can also lower the risk of SIDS. SIDS is more common among young mothers under the age of 20 and the risk increases with each birth the young mother experiences. Even in older women, having babies back-to-back can increase the risk for SIDS. Though some women choose not to breastfeed or are unable to, breast milk makes babies less vulnerable to diseases and infections that might result in SIDS.

Information on Sudden Infant Death Syndrome (SIDS)

Causes: Unknown; may involve interrelated genetic, environmental, and social factors (sleep disorders, sleep position, cold weather, overheating, poor socioeconomic conditions, premature birth)

Symptoms: Varies and often has no warning signs or symptoms; may include sleep apnea, slow heart rate, low body temperature

Duration: Acute, with little warning

Treatments: Parent education, placing infants to sleep on their backs

---

In dealing with SIDS, one factor looms most important: Education of parents makes all the difference. In 1991, for example, England's Scarborough district reported a 50 percent fall in the SIDS death rate after parents were advised not to overwarm their small infants. That same year, four other districts in England reported a similar reduction after parents were advised not to let their infants sleep in a prone position. The Foundation for the Study of Infant Deaths and the Department of Health recommend both procedures: a supine sleeping position and prevention of overwarming.

These successes raise two issues: the overall decline in rates of SIDS worldwide in industrial countries and parental guilt. For a number of years, the incidence of SIDS was generally falling. This decline slowed considerably in the 1980s. How much, then, did the parental education programs actually lower the incidence rate in these English districts? No one can say with certainty, but one thing is clear: If doctors make recommendations regarding sleeping positions and warming, they run the risk of inducing guilt in parents who have not followed their recommendations or, alternatively, who have followed the recommendations but have still lost an infant to SIDS.

Parents who have lost a child to SIDS are grief-stricken. They are not prepared for such a tragedy, and their grief is compounded by guilt, because no definitive cause for SIDS has been identified and, as a result, parental behavior seems to be implicated. Investigations conducted by police, social workers, or others who become involved only add to this guilt. Parents may be confronted by questions of whether they positioned their infant correctly or overdressed the child. Regardless of these behaviors, however, the factors causing the death may not have been under the parents' control. Parents who have experienced this loss should seek immediate and ongoing mental health therapy, including loss support groups. This loss impacts the entire family, therefore marital, couple and family therapy may be indicated as well.

SIDS will continue to occur until the exact etiologies of the syndrome, its mechanisms, and its correct treatment-based on fact, not simply risks alone-are identified. Until that time, it is expected that incidence rates will continue to go down, based on what is now known of the risk factors and recommendations against prone sleeping positions and overwarming.

—*Wayne R. McKinny, M.D.*

FOR FURTHER INFORMATION

Beers, Mark H., et al., eds. *The Merck Manual of Diagnosis and Therapy.* 18th ed. Whitehouse Station, N.J.: Merck Research Laboratories, 2006.

Behrman, Richard E., Robert M. Kliegman, and Hal B. Jenson, eds. *Nelson Textbook of Pediatrics.* 18th ed. Philadelphia: Saunders/ Elsevier, 2007.

Byard, R. W., and H. F. Krous. "Sudden Infant Death Syndrome: Overview and Update." *Pediatric and Developmental Pathology* 6, no. 2 (March/April, 2003): 112-127.

Samuels, M. "Viruses and Sudden Infant Death." *Pediatric Respiratory Reviews* 4, no. 3 (September, 2003): 178-183.

SIDS Network. http://sids-network.org.

Suicide

CATEGORY: Disease/Disorder

KEY TERMS:

"no suicide" contract: an agreement, verbally or in writing, that a suicidal person will not act on his or her urges to commit suicide and instead will take other more adaptive action

psychosomatic: referring to physical symptoms interacting with psychological problems

rational suicide: suicide to avoid suffering when there is no underlying cognitive or psychiatric disorder

ritual suicide: a formal, ceremonial, and proscribed form of suicide performed for social reasons in Japanese history

serotonin: an abundant neurotransmitter in the brain that affects many emotional states

suicide cluster: the occurrence of several suicides immediately following a much-publicized suicide

suicide gesture: a superficial suicidal action in which the intention is not to die but to solicit help

NATIONAL SUICIDE PREVENTION LIFELINE
1-800-273-8255

CAUSES AND SYMPTOMS

Suicide is the deliberate taking of one's own life. Most often, suicidal individuals are trying to avoid emotional or physical pain that they believe they cannot bear; sometimes, they are very angry and take their lives to lash out at others. Suicide is seen as a solution to an otherwise insoluble problem. In 2017 there were about 575,000 self-inflicted injuries (based on emergency room visits) and more than 47,000 completed suicides, with about 280,000 family survivors in the United States. Women attempt suicide more often than men, but men complete suicide more often than women because men tend to use more lethal means, such as a gun. Men die from suicide at a rate of 3.54 times that of women, according to the American Foundation for Suicide Prevention. It should also be noted that adolescents and the elderly are two high-risk groups. A 2017 Youth Risk Behavior Survey reported that 7.4 percent of youths in grades nine through twelve had made at least one suicide attempt in the previous twelve months, with female students attempting nearly twice as often as male students.

Overall, suicide is the tenth leading cause of death in the United States, but in 2016 it became the second leading cause among persons ages ten to thirty-four. What is disturbing is that in recent years the suicide rate has been trending upward across all age groups and among women. The increase in the suicide rate among women rose sharply from 2000 to 2016; for years, the average annual rate of increase in suicides among women had been 2 percent, a figure that jumped to a 3 percent average increase from 2007 on. Among women in the forty-five to sixty-four age range, the rate of suicide deaths increased from 6.2 per 100,000 women in 2000 to 9.9 per 100,000 in 2016.

Researchers have struggled to find an explanation for the increase among women in this age group. The American Psychological Association cites increased stress levels among middle-aged women in recent years. Middle-aged women are members of the "sandwich generation," caught between caring for their own children and for aging parents. Feeling the intense pressures of work and home responsibilities, many become depressed and some see suicide as the only way out. Adding to the stress and depression problem is the growing number of single-parent families headed by women.

Differences between men and women, and among age groups, exist in methods of committing suicide. Girls ages ten to fourteen employ suffocation in 70 percent of cases. For women in the twenty-five to forty-four age bracket, firearms are the most common method, accounting for 32 percent of suicides. For women age forty-five and older, poisoning was the most common method (40 percent), followed by firearms (32 percent). Another important difference between women and men has to do with the risk of suicide based on one or more previous attempts. About 62 percent of women who succeed in suicide have made a previous attempt; in contrast, 62 percent of men who successfully commit suicide have not made a previous attempt. Women, in comparison with men, use a greater variety of suicide methods: drug poisoning, exsanguination (i.e., bleeding, as from slit wrists), drowning, and hanging, as well as firearms, although women are 73 percent less likely to use a gun than men.

In 2015, 283 women veterans committed suicide; in 2016, the number was 257. The suicide rates among women veterans for those two years were 15.5 per 100,000 and 13.9 per 100,000, respectively. In response to this rate, in 2016, the Female Veterans Suicide Prevention Act was passed by Congress and signed into law by President Barack Obama on June 30. The law requires the Department of Veterans Affairs (VA) to identify programs and approaches for reducing the number of suicides among female veterans. One of the sponsors of the bill, Senator Richard Blumenthal of Connecticut, stated: "Our bipartisan bill will help literally save lives by ensuring VA is providing the care, counseling, and outreach our women veterans need to combat the invisible wounds of war. This measure will help address the staggering rate of suicide among female veterans by ensuring that VA's mental health and suicide prevention programs meet the gender-specific needs of our nation's women veterans."

When an individual contemplates suicide to avoid the physical pain of a terminal illness and does not have a mental disorder, that form of suicidal thought is often called "rational" suicide. This does not imply that this form of suicide is appropriate, moral, or legal but merely that the suicidal thoughts do not arise from a mental disorder (nonrational). Social views on rational suicide vary by culture. For example, many Dutch people consider rational suicide to be acceptable, whereas most Americans do not.

Most suicidal people encountered by physicians, psychologists, social workers, and other mental health professionals experience suicidal thoughts as a result of a mental disorder. The suicidal thoughts and impulses are seen as symptoms of the underlying disorder and require treatment just as any other symptom. The treatment may involve protecting the person against his or her suicidal actions, even to the point of involuntary commitment to a mental hospital.

The rationale behind society's willingness temporarily to deny suicidal individuals' usual civil rights by involuntary commitment is that they are considered to be not "acting in their right mind" by virtue of their mental illness. Thus, they deserve the protection of society until their illness is treated. In fact, suicidal thoughts usually do abate when suicidal patients are treated. The vast majority of these individuals are appreciative afterward; they are glad that they were prevented from killing themselves, as they no longer wish to do so.

The most common mental illness that causes suicidal thoughts is depression. In fact, suicidal thoughts are considered to be a symptom of clinical depression. Other mental disorders associated with suicidal ideation include anxiety disorders such as panic disorder, psychotic disorders such as schizophrenia, substance use disorders such as alcohol dependence, and certain personality disorders such as borderline personality disorder.

Although suicide may occur at any time of the year, there is a seasonal variation in its peak incidence. Suicides are most common in both men and women in May; women have a second peak around October and November. This seasonal variation may be attributable to seasonal differences in the incidence of depression.

Suicide appears to have multiple factors involved in its etiology. There are biological, psychological, social, and contextual factors that interact in a complex way to contribute to the causes of suicide in any given individual. The biological factors include genetic contributions to the development of mental disorders such as clinical depression. This may be attributable in part to problems in the neurotransmitter systems in the brain, such as those that control levels of serotonin and dopamine.

Alcohol and other substances of abuse may also cause suicidal ideation. Suicidal thoughts may occur while the individual is using, intoxicated, or in withdrawal. Paradoxically, suicidal thoughts may also arise while the patient is taking antidepressant medications. Fortunately, this side effect is uncommon. and most antidepressant medications do not have such effects. The fact that suicidal thoughts may occur even when on medication, however, underscores the need for individuals taking medications to stay in regular contact with the prescribing physician and to never discontinue their medication without medical consultation. If family members observe a depressed individual taking medication become more depressed, hostile or angry, or suddenly happy or relieved, or if the individual has no apparent response to the medication, then it would be wise to consult with the prescribing physician. This is especially true for family members of children or elders on antidepressant medication.

Psychological factors contributing to suicide include a depressed and/or anxious mood, hopelessness, and a loss of normal pleasure in life activities. Chronically depressed people often have diminished problem-solving skills during periods of depression and can see no way out of their difficulties; suicide is seen as the only solution. There are also personality characteristics that contribute to suicide. In women, borderline personality disorder is often associated with suicide attempts. This disorder is characterized by widely fluctuating moods, rages, feelings of emptiness or boredom, and unstable relationships.

The social factors involved in suicide include cultural acceptance or rejection of suicide. Historically, Japanese people have accepted ritual suicide within their culture and somewhat sanction suicide as a response to a severe loss of face or social esteem. This does not mean that they embrace it, but rather that the history contributes to cultural norms where this is thought of as an option for dealing with shame. Similarly, the Dutch government has legalized rational suicide as an option for dying. In contrast, most Americans have a more negative view of the suicide act. Other social factors that increase the likelihood of suicide include social instability, divorce, unemployment, immigration, and exposure to violence as a child. In the United States, European Americans commit suicide more often than African Americans; white males accounted for almost 80 percent of suicides in 2017. Native Americans have a high incidence of suicide. In general, good social support reduces the risk of suicide.

Some patients engage in suicidal gestures; that is, they say they want to kill themselves and take actions such as swallowing some pills or superficially cutting their wrists, but there is no real intention to die. They act this way as a cry for help. For some, this may be the only way to receive attention for what troubles them. Unfortunately, the suicide gesture may go awry, and unintended death may occur. Anyone who speaks of suicide or engages in what may appear to be a gesture should be taken seriously.

Most people who are suicidal have ambivalent feelings: Part of them wants to die, part does not. This is one of the reasons that the majority of suicidal people tell others of their intention in advance of their attempts. Most have visited their personal physician in the months prior to the suicide. Adolescents sometimes hint at their wish to die by giving away their prized possessions just prior to an attempt.

Contextual factors, or the circumstances in which people find themselves, can also contribute to individuals attempting suicide. Access to means of self-harm, such as weapons or drugs, can increase the likelihood of a suicide attempt. Similarly, physical isolation from others can also increase the odds, as there is no one to readily intervene. Even painful emotional or physical states, such as exhaustion or those that might be brought on by substance use, can set the stage for impulsive behavior to increase the likelihood of suicide attempts. In contrast, simply talking to someone about suicidal thoughts will not cause someone to commit suicide and instead may be a way to get help from a professional.

Anyone experiencing suicidal thoughts should be thoroughly evaluated by a professional trained in the assessment of suicidal patients. If the risk of suicide is considered to be high enough, the patient will have to be protected. This may require hospitalization, either voluntary or involuntary. It may mean removing suicidal means from that person's environment, such as removing guns from the home. Having someone stay with the patient at all times may be required. These steps should be individualized, considering the patient's situation.

Treatment of the underlying cause of the suicidal ideation is very important. Depression and anxiety can be treated with medications and/or psychotherapy. There are treatment programs for alcoholism and drug abuse. Usually, successful treatment of the underlying mental disorder results in the suicidal thoughts going away.

While they await the resolution of the suicidal ideation, patients need to be offered support and hope. Sometimes, a "no suicide" contract is helpful. This is simply a commitment on the part of the patient not to act on any suicidal thoughts and to contact the health professional if the urges become worse. While this contract may be written down, it is usually verbal.

Suicide prevention includes the early detection and management of the mental disorders associated with suicide. Because social isolation increases the risk of suicide, patients should be encouraged to develop and actively maintain strong social supports such as family, friends, and other social groups (church, clubs, and sports teams).

It may also be helpful to provide counseling to teenagers after an acquaintance has committed suicide, as this may prevent social contagion and suicide clusters. A suicide cluster is when several individuals (often teenagers) commit suicide after learning of the suicide of an acquaintance or a person who is attractive to them, such as a music or film star. Suicide clusters have increased among the young.

Family members of a suicide victim often go through a grieving process which is more severe than that which occurs after death from other causes. The stigma of suicide and mental illness is strong, and surviving family members often have greater feelings of both guilt and abandonment. Family survivors also have increased psychosomatic complaints, behavioral and emotional problems, and risk of suicide themselves. Referral to a suicide survivor group may be helpful.

TREATMENT AND THERAPY

An understanding of the causes, detection, and treatment of suicide has led to the development of a number of suicide hotlines and suicide prevention centers. There is evidence that, after these support groups are introduced into a community, the suicide rate for young women decreases. It is not yet known if they have any effect on other groups, such as young men or the elderly.

Most people who contemplate suicide do not seek professional treatment even if they tell people around them of their suicidal ideas. Thus, it is important for physicians, clergy, teachers, parents, and mental health workers to remain alert to the possibility of suicidal thoughts in those in their care. Someone who is depressed or very anxious should be asked about suicidal thoughts. Such a question will not plant the idea in his or her head, and the person may feel relieved after being asked. Once someone with suicidal ideation is identified, evaluation and treatment should proceed quickly. The following sample composite cases illustrate the application of the concepts described in the overview.

Mary is a seventeen-year-old senior in high school. She is from a broken home and was severely abused by her father prior to her parents' divorce ten years ago. Her teachers think that she is a bright underachiever who has a rather dramatic personality. Her friends see her as moody and easily angered. Her relationships with boyfriends are intense and always end with deep feelings of hurt and abandonment. Her mother is best described as cold, aloof, and preoccupied with herself.

Mary is brought to the school counselor by one of her friends when Mary threatens to kill herself and superficially scratches her wrists with a safety pin. The counselor learns that Mary has just broken up with her boyfriend, a young man at a local junior college. She is devastated. When she tried to tell her mother about it, her mother seemed uninterested and said that Mary always makes too much of such little things. It was the next morning that she scratched herself in front of her friend.

While more information is needed, this case illustrates a suicide gesture. In this case, Mary does not want to die but instead wants someone to realize how distressed she is. She feels rejected by her boyfriend and then by her mother. One can suspect a gesture rather than a serious suicide attempt by the superficial, nonlethal means (scratching with a safety pin) and by the likelihood of discovery (done in front of a friend).

Here is a second case. Theresa is a forty-eight-year-old accountant. She is separated from her husband and three children and lives alone in an apartment. She has no real friends, only drinking buddies. Like her mother and two aunts, Theresa is an alcoholic. Each day after work, she stops at her favorite bar and drinks between five and eight glasses of wine.

She is brought to the emergency room of the local hospital by the police, who found her sitting on the steps of a church sobbing. She threatened to kill herself if she wasn't allowed to see her children. The emergency room doctor noted the strong odor of alcohol on her breath and ordered a blood alcohol test, which showed that she was legally intoxicated. Theresa insisted that she would kill herself by running in front of a moving bus if she could not be with her family. The emergency room doctor had Theresa's belt and other potentially dangerous items taken from her and arranged for a staff member to sit with her until she was sober. Six hours later, her blood alcohol had returned to near zero. Theresa no longer felt despondent and had no more suicidal thoughts. She was embarrassed by her statements a few hours before. An alcoholism counselor was called, and outpatient treatment for her alcoholism was arranged.

This case illustrates suicidal ideation caused by alcohol intoxication. As often happens, the suicidal ideation resolves when the patient becomes sober. The primary treatment is for the underlying addictive disorder.

Here is a third case. Sally is a fifty-three-year-old married mother of two. She is a part-time hairdresser and normally a very active, happy person. For the past three weeks, however, she has gradually lost all interest in her job, her children, her home, and her hobbies. She feels irritable and sad most of the time. Although she is tired, she does not sleep well at night, waking up very early each morning, unable to return to sleep. She is worried by the fact that she is having intrusive thoughts of killing herself. Sally imagines she could end all this dreariness by overdosing on sleeping pills and never waking up. She is a strict Catholic and knows it is against her religion to commit suicide. She calls her parish priest.

After a brief conversation, her priest meets her at the office of a psychiatrist who acts as a consultant for the diocese. The psychiatrist diagnoses major depression as the cause of Sally's suicidal ideation. She has a

---

Information on Suicide

Causes: Psychological and emotional factors, depression, mental disorders, substance abuse

Symptoms: Depressed and/or anxious mood, hopelessness, loss of normal pleasure in life activities, diminished problem-solving skills, borderline personality disorder, unstable relationships

Duration: Temporary or recurrent

Treatments: Psychotherapy, counseling, drug therapy

---

good social support network, so the psychiatrist decides to treat her as an outpatient and has her agree to a "no suicide" contract. Sally is also started on antidepressant medication, which gradually lifts her depression over a period of two to three weeks. Simultaneously, her suicidal thoughts leave her.

This case illustrates suicidal thoughts caused by depression. If Sally had been more depressed or her suicidal urges stronger, she would probably have needed hospitalization. If she had required hospitalization and had refused to go voluntarily, the psychiatrist could have had her committed according to the laws of the state where he practiced. Most states require a signed statement by two physicians or one physician and a licensed clinical psychologist. They must attest that the patient is a danger to himself or herself and that no less restrictive form of treatment would suffice.

Finally, here is a fourth case. Harriet is a sixty-seven-year old resident of a hospital, where she has been for the past two years. She has a serious neurological disorder called amyotrophic lateral sclerosis (also called Lou Gehrig's disease). It has caused progressive weakness such that she cannot even breathe on her own. Harriet is permanently connected to a respirator attached to a tracheotomy tube in her throat. She has few visitors and mostly stares off and thinks.

Harriet tells her nurse that she is "sick of it all" and wants her doctors to disconnect her from the respirator and let her die. Her neurologist requests a psychiatric evaluation. The psychiatrist confirms the patient's wish to die. There is no evidence of dementia or other cognitive disorder, nor is the patient showing any evidence of a mental illness. Subsequently, a meeting is called of the hospital ethics committee to make recommendations. Membership on the committee includes physicians, nurses, an ethicist, a local minister, and the hospital attorney.

This case illustrates a difficult example of rational suicide request. The patient has a desire to die and is not suffering from any mental disorder. In this case, she is requesting not to take her own life actively but to be allowed to die passively by removal of the respirator. Some people do not consider this to be suicide at all. They make a distinction between passively allowing a natural process of dying to occur and actively taking one's own life. If this patient requested a lethal overdose of potassium to be injected into her intravenous tubes, such action would be considered suicide and ethically different. In either event, these matters are more ethical, social, and legal than psychiatric.

PERSPECTIVE AND PROSPECTS

Throughout history, there have been numerous examples of suicide. In Western culture, early views on the subject were mainly from a moral perspective and suicide was viewed as a sin. Mental illness in general was poorly understood and often thought of as weakness of character, possession by evil spirits, or willful bad behavior. Thus, mental illness was stigmatized. Even though society now has a better medical understanding of mental illness, there is still a stigma attached to mental illness and to suicide. This stigma contributes to under diagnosis and under treatment of suicidal individuals, as many sufferers are reluctant to come forth with their symptoms.

Suicide remains an important public health problem. In 2017, it was the tenth most common cause of death in the United States (although it was third for adolescents and young adults). Each year, there are more than forty thousand known suicides in the United States. The actual incidence may be higher because an unknown number of accidental deaths or untreated illnesses may actually be undiagnosed suicides. For every suicide death, between eight and twenty-five other individuals attempt suicide. Unfortunately, most cases of suicidal ideation never come to the attention of health professionals. Therefore, when someone talks of suicide, a high index of suspicion should be maintained. Those people who express suicidal thoughts should be taken seriously and thoroughly evaluated. Increased levels of awareness of suicide may help to improve detection and treatment of this potentially preventable cause of death. Research in this area continues to focus on prevention and early identification and treatment for individuals who are distressed.

—*Peter M. Hartmann, M.D.;*
Updated by Nancy A. Piotrowski, Ph.D.
and Michael J. O'Neal

FOR FURTHER INFORMATION

DePaulo, J. Raymond, Jr., and Leslie Alan Horvitz. *Understanding Depression: What We Know and What You Can Do About It.* New York: Wiley, 2003. A leading expert on depression examines the disease's nature, causes, effects, and treatments.

Jamison, Kay Redfield. *Night Falls Fast: Understanding Suicide.* New York: Alfred A. Knopf, 2000.

Kolf, June Cerza. *Standing in the Shadow: Help and Encouragement for Suicide Survivors.* New York: Baker Books, 2002.

Koplewicz, Harold S. *More than Moody: Recognizing and Treating Adolescent Depression.* New York: Penguin, 2003.

Roesch, Roberta. *The Encyclopedia of Depression.* 2d ed. New York: Facts On File, 2001.

Suicide Awareness Voices of Education. http://www.save.org.

Supplements

CATEGORY: Treatment

KEY TERMS:

nutraceutical: a food or part of a food allegedly containing health-giving additives and having medicinal benefit

photonutrient: a substance found in certain plants which is believed to be beneficial to human health and help prevent various diseases

phytochemicals: chemical compounds produced by plants, generally to help them thrive or thwart competitors, predators, or pathogens

THE ROLE OF SUPPLEMENTS

Adequate nutrition is the foundation of good health. Everyone needs the four basic nutrients: water, carbohydrates, proteins, and fats. It is important to choose the proper foods to deliver these nutrients and, as necessary, to complement the diet with supplements.

Health-conscious adults have heard the message repeatedly that they can get the vitamins they need from the foods they eat, but surveys have shown that people in many countries fail to eat adequate amounts of fruit, vegetables, whole grains, and low-fat dairy foods. Should public health officials or registered dieticians recommend that people take supplements to compensate for poor eating habits? The answer to this question can be found in a discussion of vitamin supplements.

The 1990s brought to light much new information about human nutrition, its effects on the body, and the role that it plays in disease. The fuel for the body's engine comes directly from the food that one eats, which contains many vital nutrients. Nutrients come in the form of vitamins, minerals, enzymes, water, amino acids, carbohydrates, and lipids (fats). These nutrients provide people with the basic materials that human bodies need to sustain life.

One of the latest types of dietary supplements are nutraceuticals. These supplements are obtained from naturally derived chemicals in plants, called photonutrients, that make the plants biologically active. They are not nutrients in the classic sense. They are what determine a plant's color, ability to resist disease, and flavor.

Nutritionists have discovered that fruits and vegetables, grains, and legumes contain other healthful nutrients called phytochemicals. Researchers have identified thousands of phytochemicals and have the ability to remove these chemical compounds and concentrate them into pills, powders, and capsules. Phytochemicals are believed to be powerful ammunition in the war against cancer and other cellular mutations. In simple terms, cancer is a mutation of body cells through a multistep process. Phytochemicals are hypothesized to fight that disease by stopping one or more of the steps that lead to cancer. For example, a cancer process can be kindled when a carcinogenic molecule invades a cell, possibly from foods eaten or from air breathed. Sulforaphane, a phytochemical commonly found in broccoli, is then hypothesized to activate an enzyme process that removes the carcinogen from the cell before harm is done.

Researchers and pharmaceutical companies sell concentrated forms of various phytochemicals found in such vegetables as broccoli, brussels sprouts,

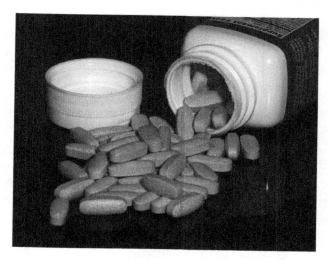

Vitamin B supplements. (Wikimedia Commons)

cauliflower, and cabbage. Because no single supplement can possibly compete with nature, some nutritionists recommend a shopping basket full of fruits and vegetables, as opposed to using expensive bottled supplements. Tomatoes, for example, are believed to contain an estimated ten thousand different phytochemicals.

Natural food supplements can be high in certain nutrients. Examples are aloe vera, bee pollen, fish oils, flaxseed, primrose oil, ginseng, ginkgo biloba, garlic, and oat bran. In general, natural food supplements are composed of byproducts of foods that can provide a multitude of health benefits. One caution, however, is that supplements of this type may not have the same kind of quality control or oversight as medications prescribed by a doctor and bought from a pharmacy. As such, the effects of supplements may vary from pill to pill and bottle to bottle.

THE PROMISE OF ANTIOXIDANTS

No discussion of supplements would be complete without mention of antioxidants. They are a group of vitamins, minerals, and enzymes that help to protect the body from the formation of free radicals. Free radicals are groups of atoms that can cause damage to cells and thus impair the immune system. This damage is also thought to be the basis for the aging process. Free radicals are believed to be formed through exposure to radiation and toxic chemicals such as cigarette smoke, as well as overexposure to the sun's rays. Some common antioxidants are vitamin A

In the News:
Dietary Supplement Crackdowns by the FDA

In the past, the dietary supplement industry has been loosely regulated. Even though the Food and Drug Administration (FDA) required all the ingredients to be label-listed, there were no rules that limited the manufacturers' recommendations regarding serving sizes or the actual content amount of the nutrients. Moreover, no proof was required to guarantee product safety. However, as a result of the increasing problem of cross-contamination and misleading labeling of dietary supplements, coupled with adverse health outcomes, in March, 2003, the FDA proposed new labeling and manufacturing standards. A final rule was announced in June, 2007, indicating that the current Good Manufacturing Practices (cGMPS) would apply to the dietary supplement business. These standards were already in effect for the pharmaceutical and veterinary industries. The new rulings will establish industry- wide standards to guarantee consistent manufacturing standards in order to assure the public that the dietary supplement industry is safe and provides pure products with known strengths and compositions.

The FDA had been averaging about 550 supplement-related adverse event reports yearly since 1993; however, that figure doubled in 2002. For instance, dietary supplements had to be recalled by one manufacturer because of excessive lead contamination. Another manufacturer of niacin supplements mistakenly marketed a product that contained ten times the safe limit of niacin, which was not reflected on the label. The product was recalled after health reports of nausea, vomiting, and liver damage were received. Dietary supplements containing ephedra, used for weight loss, increased energy, and athletic performance enhancement, have been linked to several deaths, resulting in the banning of ephedra-enhanced products. A sports supplement abuse case involved the use of vitamins by a world-class athlete who failed a drug doping test; the results were later reversed when the product was tested and found to be cross-contaminated by an anabolic steroid compound that was also manufactured at the same laboratory where the vitamins were packaged.

Under the cGMPS ruling, manufacturers are required to document the identity, composition, purity, quality, and strength of the ingredients in dietary supplements. If the product is found to deviate from what the manufacturer has claimed to be the ingredients, the FDA considers the product adulterated. The minimum standards require physical plants to be constructed to ensure proper manufacturing operations, facility maintenance and cleaning, the establishment of quality control procedures, final product testing before going to market, and better methods for handling and resolving consumer complaints. These rulings do not limit consumer's access to dietary supplements but rather ensure a safer product.

—Bonita L. Marks, Ph.D.

and its precursor, beta carotene; vitamin C; and vitamin E. Zinc and the trace mineral selenium are thought to play an important role in neutralizing free radicals. Each vitamin or mineral has a recommended daily allowance (RDA).

Some in the field of nutrition have recommended higher supplementation doses of antioxidants and specific use of four antioxidant supplements-vitamins C and E, selenium, and mixed carotenes-to protect the immune system even further. Recommendations such as this are numerous and related to different kinds of supplement use, and they must be weighed carefully against data obtained from controlled clinical trials. While many of the substances touted as beneficial to health may have some benefits, supplements can be harmful in the wrong person; at the wrong dose; if taken in combination with the wrong

medications or diet; or if taken in the presence of certain health conditions. For example, it is possible to overdose on vitamins such as A, B, and E, or on iron supplements. Some supplements, like St. John's wort, may create a side effect of light sensitivity, and discontinuing drugs such as valerian root can lead to heart problems. Also, it is easy to succumb to the temptation to seek "health in a bottle" instead of engaging in proven preventive practices. For these reasons, careful consideration and consultation with one's doctor should occur before embarking on any regimen of supplements.

WOMEN'S SUPPLEMENTS

Doctors and nutritionists recommend that all people should eat a balanced diet high in fruits, vegetable, legumes, and whole grains to get the nutrients they need. That said, for various reasons, women might be lacking one or more essential vitamins or minerals, with the result that taking a vitamin supplement makes good sense. In connection with supplements, nutritionists sometimes tell women that they need to think of "bones, babies, and bellies." Older women may need supplements to maintain bone density and reduce the risk of osteoporosis. Folates are essential for fertility and fetal development. And any supplement that keeps the waistline in check will reduce the risk of cardiovascular and other chronic diseases.

Among the supplements that a woman and her doctor might conclude she needs are iron, which might be taken by women with heavy periods to reduce the risk of anemia; calcium, which postmenopausal women might need to prevent osteoporosis; magnesium, which is involved in more than three hundred chemical reactions in the body and can help ward off a host of disorders; vitamin A, which can reduce the risk of cancer and improve immune function; folate, which, taken during the first trimester of pregnancy, can reduce the risk of neural tube defects like spina bifida and anencephaly in the developing fetus by 72 percent or more; biotin, which aids in metabolization; B vitamins, which can prevent a wide range of health problems, from depression to fatigue to birth defects; vitamin C, an immune system booster; vitamin D, which helps ward of brittle and thin bones, as well as other conditions; omega-3 fatty acids, which help prevent a number of chronic diseases; melatonin, which helps control the production and release of reproductive hormones; and others that can be ingested from green tea, flaxseed, and grape seed extract.

Some research suggests that older women should exercise extreme caution in the use of dietary supplements. One study found that several commonly used dietary and mineral supplements, including multivitamins, vitamin B6, folic acid, iron, magnesium, zinc, and copper, were associated with a *higher* risk of mortality in older women. In particular, the study found that iron could increase total morality risk. These cautions strongly suggest that women should consult with their doctors before taking dietary supplements.

PERSPECTIVE AND PROSPECTS

Use of supplements is based both on modern research and development and on discoveries by mainstream scientists about the benefits of various substances. Substances such as garlic and aloe vera are examples of home remedies that have shown some promise for different kinds of ailments. Natural supplements have been used for centuries in many parts of the world as alternative medicines.

Considered and careful examination of supplement regimens in controlled clinical trials will serve as the ultimate test on the utility of these substances for health purposes. Simultaneously, consumers must remain aware that personal use of these supplements may, at times, be somewhat experimental. Quality control concerns and interactions between supplements and prescribed medications are an important consideration.

Additionally, knowledge of the supplements found in pills or popular beverages and how they may interact with street drugs of different types is also important in order to avoid unnecessary harm. This is especially true for children and elders.

—*Lisa Levin Sobczak, R.N.C.;*
Updated by Nancy A. Piotrowski, Ph.D.
and Michael J. O'Neal

FOR FURTHER INFORMATION

Balch, James F., and Phyllis A. Balch. *Prescription for Nutritional Healing: A Practical A to Z Reference to Drug-Free Remedies Using Vitamins, Minerals, Herbs, and Food Supplements.* 4th rev. ed. Garden City Park, N.Y.: Avery, 2008.

Hendler, Sheldon Saul. *The Doctors' Vitamin and Mineral Encyclopedia.* New York: Simon & Schuster, 1990.

Murray, Michael. *The Pill Book Guide to Natural Medicines: Vitamins, Minerals, Nutritional Supplements, Herbs, and Other Natural Products.* New York: Bantam, 2002.

Mursu, Jaakko, Kim Robien, Lisa J. Harnack, et al. "Dietary Supplements and Mortality Rate in Older Women." *Archives of Internal Medicine.* 171, no. 18 (October 2011):1625–33.

The PDR Family Guide to Nutritional Supplements: An Authoritative A-to-Z Resource on the One Hundred Most Popular Nutritional Therapies and Nutraceuticals. New York: Ballantine Books, 2001.

Weil, Andrew. *Eight Weeks to Optimum Health: A Proven Program for Taking Full Advantage of Your Body's Natural Healing Power.* Rev. ed. New York: Ballantine Books, 2007.

Syphilis

CATEGORY: Disease/Disorder
Also known as: "Bad blood," bejel (endemic syphilis)

KEY TERMS:

chancre: a painless ulcer, particularly one developing on the genitals as a result of venereal disease such as syphilis

gumma: a soft, non-cancerous growth that results from the tertiary stage of syphilis

pathogen: a bacterium, virus, or other microorganism that can cause disease

CAUSES AND SYMPTOMS

Treponema pallidum (gram negative, spiral shaped bacteria belonging to the spirochete family) is the pathogen responsible for the syphilis infection. The transmission is through sexual contact and vertically from mother to child during pregnancy or at birth. The syphilis organisms (particularly during stages I/II) are highly contagious. Sexual contact with a partner who suffers from active syphilis will lead to infection in 30% of the cases

The history of the disease is unclear. Evidence exists that its origin may have been linked with a disease, yaws, found in the Western Hemisphere at the time of explorer Christopher Columbus (1451-1506). Yaws is a relatively mild disease generally transmitted through contaminated objects or open skin lesions, but not generally through sexual transmission; it results from infection by a subspecies of *Treponema* called *T. palladum ssp. pertenue.* The theory suggests that this may have been the form of the disease brought back to Europe on one of Columbus's ships. Mutation and sexual transmission in the population of Europe may have produced the more serious form of the disease.

The disease is characterized by several distinct stages. Initial exposure to the organism during sexual intercourse results in formation of a painless skin lesion called a chancre at the site of infection (primary syphilis), developing anywhere from a week to months after infection. Spirochete bacteria may be isolated from the lesion, as well as being found live inside white blood cells (macrophages and neutrophils) that infiltrate the area. These white blood cells may be a mechanism for systemic spread of the organism. The lesion generally heals spontaneously, leaving the impression that the disease has been eliminated.

During the weeks after formation of the chancre, the spirochetes multiply to large numbers and become disseminated throughout the body. A second stage (secondary syphilis) often appears within two months following regression of the chancre. Symptoms are often described as flulike, with malaise, headache, fever, and joint aches. A skin rash often appears, covering most of the body. Condyloma lata, or wart-like lesions on the anogenital region may occur. Sores may develop in the mouth and throat and on many of the mucous membranes in the body. Patchy alopecia and sore throat are also seen in this stage. The organism is highly transmissible during this period. The rash and other symptoms generally fade over a period of weeks.

In latent syphilis, there are typically no symptoms and can last months, years, or an entire lifespan. The disease may resolve itself, reactivate, or progress into tertiary syphilis.

Approximately 10 percent of untreated cases develop a third, or tertiary, stage of syphilis. The organism can infiltrate any organ or system in the body, resulting in soft tumors (gummas) in the eyes, lungs, bone, brain, or other organs. Symptoms are characteristic of the organ infected. For example, infection of the brain or other areas of the central nervous system are described as neurosyphilis or syphilitic dementia, characterized by memory loss, personality changes, and neurodegeneration. If neurosyphilis is symptomatic, it may lead to meningitis, subacute stroke, cranial neuropathies, frontotemporal dementia, psychosis, personality changes, cognitive dysfunction, Argyll Robertson pupil, tabes dorsalis (demyelination of dorsal columns and dorsal root ganglia – 25 – 30 years after infection), broad based ataxia, loss of sensation in lower extremities, sharp, shooting pain in legs and abdomen. Cardiovascular syphilis affects the heart and includes symptoms of aortitis, ascending aortic aneurysm, syphilitic mesaortitis, aortic root dilation. Even if tertiary syphilis is treated, prognosis for the patient at this stage is often poor.

Treponema has the ability to cross the placenta, and the infection of a pregnant woman may result in congenital syphilis, or infection of her unborn child. Infection may kill the fetus or cause it to be born with obvious deformities such as blindness or physical abnormalities. The infant may also be asymptomatic.

An undiagnosed infection will likely progress, with symptoms appearing within weeks after birth. It is common for a rash to appear, with evidence of tertiary stage neurosyphilis or cardiovascular syphilis.

DIAGNOSTICS AND SCREENING

Two separate serological tests are required for diagnosis: nontreponemal tests are used for screening purposes and treponemal tests confirm the diagnosis. In early primary syphilis, both types of tests may be nonreactive.

Nontreponemal tests are used for screening, evaluation of disease activity and monitoring response to treatment. Common tests are rapid plasma reagin (RPR) which is the test of choice. Venereal disease research laboratory (VDRL) is useful in evaluating neurologic involvement using cerebrospinal fluid (CSF). This test leads to many false – positive results due to cross reacting antibodies in viral infections, rheumatic fever, lupus, or leprosy.

Treponemal tests are confirmatory tests after positive or equivocal nontreponemal test. In this test antibodies used to detect treponemal antigens. Positive results indicate active syphilis or antibodies from previous infection. The commonly used tests are treponema pallidum particle agglutination (TPPA) or fluorescent treponemal antibody absorption test (FTA-ABS).

Definite tests to detect primary and secondary syphilis is another confirmatory diagnosis, but negative results do not rule out syphilis. Polymerase chain reaction (PCR) or darkfield microscopy can be used.

A diagnosis of syphilis can be made through microscopic examination of lesion exudates, noting the presence of spirochetes. However, *Treponema* is notoriously unstable, and the test must be made shortly after obtaining the specimen. More commonly, diagnosis is based upon serological testing for serum antibodies against the organism or tissue lipids released from infected or damaged cells.

TREATMENT AND THERAPY

Benzathine penicillin G is the preferred method of treatment for primary, secondary, or early latent syphilis. If the disease has progressed to the tertiary stage, then antibiotic treatment will still eliminate the organism, but it will not reverse organ damage that may have occurred. Weekly intramuscular injections are given for 3 weeks. If the patient has neurosyphilis,

she requires intravenous antibiotics for 10-14 days. Treatment for related organ involvement is symptomatic.

Alternative antibiotics, if the patient is allergic to penicillin, include doxycycline or ceftriaxone. However, only penicillin is effective during the tertiary stage or for use in pregnant women.

Prevention is key to stopping the spread of syphilis. Wearing condoms during sex usually prevents transmission. Syphilis is a nationally notifiable disease like chlamydia, gonorrhea, herpes, and HIV.

PERSPECTIVE AND PROSPECTS

Despite the long-time existence of effective therapy, penicillin or alternative antibiotics, and the absence of any reservoir for *T. pallidum* other than humans, syphilis remains the third most common sexually transmitted bacterial disease in the West. Only gonorrhea and chlamydia are more common.

As a result of effective therapy and the generally obvious symptoms of the disease, tertiary syphilis has largely disappeared. However, sexual practices continue to sustain spread of the disease, with approximately fifty thousand cases reported each year in the United States. Three factors are primary contributors to the resurgence of the disease: prostitution, the increase in riskier sexual practices among homosexual men, and general apathy toward a disease that is relatively easy to treat in its early stages. An increase in congenital syphilis also reflects the presence of the disease in women of childbearing years. In the absence of condom use, both unwanted pregnancy and the spread of STDs such as syphilis may result.

No vaccine currently exists for syphilis. For now, the best means of controlling syphilis remains the prevention of its spread through education and safer-sex practices, as well as early treatment of those infected.

—*Richard Adler, Ph.D.*
Updated by David Hernandez

FOR FURTHER INFORMATION

Centers for Disease Control and Prevention. *The National Plan to Eliminate Syphilis from the United States.* Atlanta: U.S. Department of Health and Human Services, 2006.

James WD, Berger T, Elston D. *Andrews' Diseases of the Skin: Clinical Dermatology.* Philadelphia, PA: Elsevier Health Sciences; 2015.

Kasper DL, Fauci AS, Hauser SL, Longo DL, Lameson JL, Loscalzo J. Harrison's Principles of Internal Medicine. New York, NY: McGraw-Hill Education; 2015.

Mandell, Gerald L., John E. Bennett, and Raphael Dolin, eds. *Mandell, Douglas, and Bennett's Principles and Practice of Infectious Diseases.* 7th ed. New York: Churchill Livingstone/ Elsevier, 2010.

Parker, James N., and Philip M. Parker, eds. *The Official Patient's Sourcebook on Syphilis.* San Diego, Calif.: Icon Health, 2002.

Patton ME, et al. "Primary and secondary syphilis: United States, 2005-2013." *Morbidity and Mortality Weekly Report,* 63, no. 18, 2014, 402–406.

Sutton, Amy L., ed. *Sexually Transmitted Diseases Sourcebook.* 3d ed. Detroit, Mich.: Omnigraphics, 2006.

Syphilis risk factors

CATEGORY: Disease/Disorder

KEY TERMS:

sexually transmitted disease (STD): a disease that is usually transmitted from person to person through contact between the vaginal or urethral discharges from an infected person and the genital mucous membranes of a person susceptible to infection

Treponema pallidum: spirochete bacterium visible only by using dark field illumination

CAUSES AND SYMPTOMS

Syphilis is an infectious bacterial disease caused by the bacterium Treponema pallidum. Syphilis is spread through contact of bodily fluids and is primarily contracted by sexual intercourse. The risk factors for syphilis include poverty in urban areas, illegal drug use, exchange of sex for drugs, unprotected oral sex, not using condoms, multiple sex partners, anonymous sex partners, HIV infection, incarceration, and exposure to infected body fluids such as blood. Newborns may be at risk for congenital syphilis as a result of untreated syphilis infections in their mothers. A newborn may also be at risk for syphilis through vertical transmission of the infection during passage through the birth canal of an infected mother. Signs and symptoms are generally the same in men and women. Syphilis may affect more men than women.

Syphilis has three distinct clinical stages: primary, secondary, and latent (also called tertiary). Primary syphilis, the initial stage, is characterized by the appearance of a primary chancre (i.e., a painless lesion at the site of the infection) on the genitalia, anus, lips, tongue or elsewhere in the mouth, or tonsils. The chancre tends to be ulcerated and painless and usually heals without treatment within a few weeks. If the chancre is left untreated, primary syphilis progresses to secondary syphilis, which is characterized by a maculopapular (i.e. red spots) rash on the trunk, extremities, soles, and palms of the individual. Latent syphilis develops from untreated secondary syphilis and is divided into two stages of latency, early latent and late latent.

In the early latent stage (having syphilis less than a year), the individual is usually asymptomatic (does not have any symptoms). Late latent stage syphilis (having syphilis longer than a year) may manifest as cardiovascular syphilis (i.e., infection of the heart and blood vessels with T. pallidum), neurosyphilis (i.e., infection of the brain or spine with T. pallidum), or gummatous syphilis (i.e., granulomatous lesions that affect the mucous membranes, skin, bones, and internal organs).

If syphilis is left untreated, complications resulting in additional medical conditions can develop, including cardiovascular disease, central nervous system disease, hepatitis, arthritis, periostitis, membranous glomerulonephritis, meningitis, hypertrophic gastritis, patchy proctitis, ulcerative colitis, recto-sigmoid mass, and irreversible organ damage. Other complications include severe ocular problems such as optic neuritis, retinitis pigmentosa syndrome, papillary abnormalities, iritis, and uveitis. In its latent stage, untreated syphilis can result in irreversible blindness, paralysis, heart disease, dementia, chronic bone and joint inflammation, and eventually death.

Ulcerated STDs, such as syphilis in its primary stage with sores, increase the risk of acquiring and transmitting HIV. According to the CDC, in the United States in 2000, the rate of reported primary and secondary syphilis cases was 2.1 in 100,000 adults. In 2005, it was 2.9; in 2008, it was 4.4; and in 2013, it was 5.3. For women, in 2005, the rate was 0.9; in 2008, it was 1.5; and in 2013, it was 0.9 again. For men, in 2005, the rate was 5.1; in 2008, it was 7.5; and by 2013, it had grown to 9.8. Rates of syphilis infection are highest in men 25–29 years of age.

Syphilis rates remain high among high-risk groups such as men who have sex with men (MSM), commercial sex workers, individuals who exchange sex for drugs, prison inmates, and certain minority groups.

TREATMENT AND THERAPY

Social workers should become knowledgeable about syphilis, including risk factors, signs and symptoms, treatment options, and possible psychological ramifications that an individual may experience if they are chronically infected. Social workers and medical professionals assisting clients with syphilis should use standard universal precautions including wearing gloves, masks, or gowns in all client care to help prevent the spread of the disease. Social workers and medical professionals can encourage clients, especially those who are HIV-positive, to be tested for STDs in order to identify healthcare needs early.

Social workers should educate clients to have a medical exam if they have lesions to determine the cause of the lesions since primary syphilis chancres may resemble ulcerated lesions caused by other sources such as the herpes simplex virus, chancroid, granuloma inguinale, carcinoma, trauma, lichen planus, fungal infections, or drug eruptions. The rash of secondary syphilis can be similar to rashes caused by pityriasis rosea, psoriasis, drug eruptions, lichen planus, scabies, or other acute febrile rashes. Other symptoms of secondary syphilis can mimic illnesses such as mononucleosis or hepatitis infections.

Social workers and medical professionals should advise a client with syphilis to abstain from sex until completion of the prescribed antibiotic regimen and until the infection has cleared, as made evident by laboratory test results interpreted by the treating clinician. Clients should be educated about the need for their sexual partner(s) to have an examination and receive medical treatment if the client is positive for syphilis. Clients should be encouraged to comply with the drug regimen and educated about the importance of completing their treatment to ensure treatment efficacy and prevent further complications.

Social workers can advocate for clients to make sure they are able to obtain the necessary medications to complete their drug regimen. Advocating

---

Information on Syphilis

Causes: *Treponema pallidum*

Symptoms: chancre, diffuse rash, neurological changes

Duration: Can remain in the body for years if left untreated

Treatments: Antibiotics such as Penicillin G

---

may include discussing coverage options with insurance companies or seeking financial support from the community. Social workers and treating medical professionals should provide clients with educational material on syphilis and the potential for HIV and other STDs. Written information, if available, on safe sex, including the use of condoms and other barrier methods may be helpful for further education about prevention techniques.

Social workers may assist clients in accessing community health services that can provide condoms or other materials related to safe sex. Social workers should encourage clients to follow mandatory reporting practices for partner notification of the client's positive STD test results. The social worker and medical professionals should be aware of and follow facility protocols for mandatory reporting of infectious disease.

—*Renee Matteucci, MPH, and Sara Richards, MSN, RN*
Updated by Christine Gamble, M.D.

FOR FURTHER INFORMATION

Badowski, M., & Patel, M. C. (2014). Syphilis. In F. J. Domino, R. A. Baldor, J. A. Grimes, & J. Golding (Eds.), The 5-minute clinical consult standard 2015 (23rd ed., pp. 1152-1153). Philadelphia, PA: Wolters Kluwer Health/Lippincott Williams & Wilkins.

Centers for Disease Control and Prevention (CDC). (2014). Primary and secondary syphilis – United States, 2005-2013. Morbidity and Mortality Weekly Report (MMWR), 63(18), 402-406.

———. (2017 June 8). Syphilis - CDC Fact Sheet. Retrieved February 20, 2019, from http://www.cdc.gov/std/syphilis/STDFact-Syphilis.htm

Hook, E. W., III. (2012). Syphilis. In L. Goldman & A. I. Schafer (Eds.), Goldman's Cecil medicine

(24th ed., pp. 1922-1929). Philadelphia, PA: Elsevier Saunders.

Mattei, P. L., Beachkofsky, T. M., Gilson, R. T., & Wisco, O. J. (2012). Syphilis: A Reemerging Infection. *American Family Physician,* 433-440.

Pletcher, S. D., & Cheung, S. W. (2003). Syphilis and otolaryngology. Otolaryngologic Clinics of North America, 36(4), 595-605, vi.

U.S. Preventive Services Task Force. (June 2016). Infection in Nonpregnant Adults and Adolescents: Screening. https://www.uspreventiveservicestaskforce.org/Page/Document/UpdateSummary-Final/

Systemic lupus erythematosus (SLE)

CATEGORY: Disease/Disorder
Also known as: Lupus

KEY TERMS:

antibodies: proteins manufactured by the body to attack and neutralize foreign substances, such as bacteria

antinuclear antibody (ANA): an unusual antibody that is directed against structures within the nucleus of cells

autoantibodies: antibodies that attack the body's own cells and tissues

autoimmune: a term describing a disease in which the body produces antibodies against its own cells

connective tissue: the substance holding the body and organs together

cytotoxic: having a damaging effect on cells

discoid rash: raised red patches

erythematosus: characterized by redness of the skin

hyperlipidemia: an excess of lipids (for example, cholesterol and triglycerides) in the blood

malar rash: a redness or rash on the face covering the cheeks and the bridge of the nose; also called butterfly rash

photosensitivity: a sensitivity to light or sunlight

Raynaud's phenomenon: discoloration and pain in the fingertips induced by cold

serositis: inflammation of the lining of the lung or heart

CAUSES AND SYMPTOMS

The cause of lupus is unknown, but scientists believe that both genetic and environmental factors are involved. Although there is a genetic predisposition to lupus, and researchers have identified an associated gene in some cases, only 10 percent of lupus patients have a familial connection and only 5 percent of children born to individuals with lupus will develop the disease. People of African, American Indian, Asian, and Hispanic origin seem to develop the disease more frequently than do non-Hispanic Caucasians. Lupus affects both men and women, but the incidence is ten to fifteen times higher in women and between 85 and 90 percent of patients are women. The majority of lupus diagnoses occur in young women in their late teens to thirties. It is possible that hormonal factors play a role in this disparity, because it is known that symptoms in women increase before menstrual cycles and during pregnancy. Environmental triggers include infections, exposure to ultraviolet light, and extreme stress, as well as antibiotic usage (particularly penicillin and those in the sulfa group). Certain other drugs, particularly hydralazine, procainamide, and isoniazid, can also cause lupus, but this type of drug-induced lupus usually disappears after the offending drug is discontinued.

Symptoms may begin suddenly with fever or may develop gradually over the course of months or years. The clinical course is usually marked by remissions, periods when symptoms are minimal or absent, and relapses (called flare-ups), when the patient experiences an aggravation of symptoms and general malaise.

SLE can affect all organ systems of the body. The production of autoantibodies is the underlying physiologic problem in lupus. These autoantibodies can appear in a great number and variety, differing from patient to patient, thus causing their varying symptoms. General symptoms include fatigue, fever, anemia, weight loss, Raynaud's phenomenon, and headaches. Joint inflammation and pain (arthritis) occurs in about 90 percent of patients and is often the earliest manifestation of the disease. It usually occurs intermittently and generally does not cause permanent joint damage or deformity.

Skin manifestations are present in most patients and include malar (butterfly) and/or discoid skin rashes; redness on the hands, fingertips, and nails;

mucous membrane ulcers in the mouth and nose; and photosensitivity. Inflammation of the sac around the lungs (pleurisy) or heart (pericarditis) is a frequent occurrence, resulting in pain upon deep breathing or chest pain. On rare occasions, there may be severe complications, such as bleeding into the lungs, which is life-threatening, or cardiac failure. Neurologic complications may also occur, including headaches, thinking impairment, personality changes, seizures, strokes, depression, dementia and psychosis.

Kidney involvement may be either minor or progressive, leading to severe nephritis that can be fatal. Ocular changes sometimes occur, causing conjunctivitis or blurred vision. In rare cases, retinitis, inflammation of the blood vessels at the back of the eye, can occur, leading to blindness if not treated quickly.

SLE is difficult to diagnose, due to its variety of symptoms and similarity to many other diseases. The constellation of symptoms appears and progresses differently for each patient and initially may seem vague and unrelated. Usually, patients will first see their family doctors. Upon diagnosis or the discovery of particular body system involvement, the family doctor may refer the patient on to one or more specialists.

There is no single test for lupus. A physician will perform several laboratory tests as part of the differential diagnostic process, including various blood and urine tests and biopsies of the skin and kidney. For a positive diagnosis of SLE, a patient must have at least four of the eleven criteria established by the American College of Rheumatology: malar rash, discoid rash, photosensitivity, oral ulcers, arthritis, serositis, renal disorder, neurologic disorder, hematologic disorder, immunologic disorder, and the presence of antinuclear antibodies (ANA).

TREATMENT AND THERAPY

There is no cure for lupus. Treatment is aimed at minimizing symptoms, reducing inflammation, and maintaining normal bodily functions. The treatment approach will vary according to the specific symptoms and organ involvement of the individual patient. Preventive therapy involves lifestyle strategies aimed at reducing the risk of flare-up episodes. Patients are advised to follow a healthy diet, get adequate rest, and participate in moderate weight-bearing exercise in order to combat fatigue and

muscle weakness. Counseling, support groups, and patient education help reduce stress and protect emotional wellbeing. Other recommendations include smoking cessation, limited alcohol intake, and adequate intake of vitamin D and calcium. Avoidance of excessive sun exposure through the use of protective clothing and sunscreens can reduce the occurrence of skin rashes and possibly systemic disease flares.

Patients can learn to recognize the warning signs of an impending flare-up, such as increased fatigue, headaches, dizziness, stomach upset, fever, or the appearance of a rash. Regular laboratory tests can also detect an imminent flare-up. Early treatment of flare-ups can make them easier to control, can prevent tissue damage, and may reduce the length of time that the patient is given high doses of drugs.

Medications are an integral part of the treatment of lupus, and fall into four main categories: nonsteroidal anti-inflammatory drugs (NSAIDs), corticosteroids, antimalarial drugs, and cytotoxic and immunosuppressive agents. NSAIDs are used to control symptoms and reduce muscle and joint pain and inflammation. Commonly used NSAIDs include acetylsalicylic acid (aspirin), ibuprofen, naproxen, indomethacin, sulindac, nabumetone, tolmetin, and ketoprofen. Since these drugs can cause stomach upset, patients are usually advised to take them with meals or to take antacids or prostaglandins as well. Some NSAIDs have a prostaglandin added to the capsule. Patients taking NSAIDs must be monitored because of the potential adverse effects to the liver, kidney, and central nervous system.

Corticosteroids are synthetic hormones that have excellent anti-inflammatory and immunoregulatory effects and reduce symptoms promptly. They are used to treat a spectrum of lupus manifestations, especially in cases when organs are threatened. Prednisone is the most commonly used, followed by hydrocortisone, methylprednisolone, and others. Topical formulations are used for skin rashes, and oral doses are given for systemic involvement. Dosages are monitored carefully and tapered after initial inflammation reduction is achieved in order to reduce possible side effects. Corticosteroids may also be administered by injection into the skin or joint. For severe cases, intravenous administration of large doses of methylprednisolone (called pulse steroids) for three days is given. Unfortunately, high doses of corticosteroids over long periods of time can produce unpleasant side effects, such as weight gain, rounded face, acne, emotional lability, hypertension, hyperlipidemia, increased risk of infection, diabetes, and osteoporosis.

Antimalarial drugs are frequently used in the management of skin rashes, joint inflammation, and serositis, though it may take months before their beneficial effects become apparent. They also help protect against the damaging effects of ultraviolet light. The most common agents are hydroxychloroquine (Plaquenil), chloroquine (Aralen), and quinicrine (Atabrine). These medications can be taken in combination with NSAIDs and other drugs to increase their effectiveness. They are particularly helpful when used with corticosteroids in order to decrease the amount of steroid needed. Damage to the retina is a potential side effect and is dose-related. Patients must be evaluated by an ophthalmologist twice a year.

Cytotoxic and immunosuppressive agents are potent drugs utilized in cases requiring aggressive therapy to protect major organs. They are used in conjunction with, or in place of, corticosteroids in order to spare the patient the side effects of the corticosteroids. Cytotoxics are not approved by the Food and Drug Administration (FDA) for use in the treatment of SLE; however, they are considered part of standard practice. These drugs target autoantibodies, thus suppressing the overactive immune response of lupus patients.

Cyclophosphamide (Cytoxin) and azathioprine (Imuran) are both used in the treatment of lupus nephritis and are also effective in combating blood cell deficiencies, pulmonary bleeding, vasculitis, and central nervous system disease. Imuran is less potent but causes fewer side effects than does Cytoxin. Methotrexate, mycophenolate mofetil (CellCept), cyclosporine, chlorambucil, and nitrogen mustard are other cytotoxic agents that have been used in the management of lupus. Intravenous immunoglobulin injections are given to some patients to increase the production of blood platelets. Side effects of cytotoxic drugs include nausea, hair loss, increased risk of certain cancers, increased risk of infection, sterility, and bone marrow suppression.

Pregnancy in a lupus patient requires special care. Even though more than 50 percent of lupus pregnancies follow a normal course, all lupus pregnancies are considered high risk. Doctors recommend planning pregnancy during times of remission. Recent studies contradict the traditional belief that pregnancy increases the chance of flare-ups and also suggest that most flare-ups during pregnancy are mild, consisting only of rashes, fatigue, and arthritis. Frequent doctor visits are a necessity in order to detect and treat any problems early. The obstetrician will regularly check the baby's growth and heartbeat in order to detect any abnormalities that might signal problems. Some lupus medications, such as prednisone, are safe to take during pregnancy because they do not cross the placenta. Others, such as cyclophosphamide, need to be used with caution or discontinued during the pregnancy. About 20 percent of women with lupus experience preeclampsia during their pregnancy. This is a serious condition in which there is a sudden increase in blood pressure and/ or protein in the urine requiring immediate treatment of the patient and delivery of the baby.

About one-third of women with lupus have antiphospholipid antibodies. These antibodies cause blood clots, which puts the patient at risk for developing them in the placenta, interfering with the nourishment of the baby. Since these blood clots usually form in the placenta in the second trimester, often the baby has developed enough to be delivered prematurely. The mother can be treated with heparin, which reduces the chance of clots and miscarriage.

About 50 percent of lupus pregnancies result in birth before full term. The majority of babies born between thirty and thirty-six weeks will grow normally with no problems. Those born before thirty-six weeks are considered premature. Approximately 3 percent of women with lupus will have a baby with a syndrome called neonatal lupus. This syndrome consists of a transient rash and blood count abnormalities and disappears by three to six months of age. Sometimes, a permanent abnormality in the heartbeat also occurs, but it is treatable and the baby is able to grow normally.

PERSPECTIVE AND PROSPECTS

The identification of lupus as a distinct medical entity dates back to the twelfth century, when the term "lupus" (Latin for "wolf") was used to describe ulcerative facial lesions, because they looked similar to either a wolf's bite or a wolf's facial markings.

Information on Systemic Lupus Erythematosus (SLE)

Causes: Unclear; possibly related to paramyxoviral infection
Symptoms: Red or purple facial lesions, joint pain and swelling, fatigue, low-grade fever
Duration: Chronic
Treatments: None; alleviation of symptoms

Other descriptions of the various dermatologic manifestations of lupus were noted by physicians over the next several centuries; the first medical textbook illustration occurred in 1856. The Viennese physician Moriz Kaposi, in 1872, was the first physician to recognize and describe the systemic manifestations of lupus, as well as the fact that there seemed to be two distinct forms of lupus, discoid and systemic.

This was soon expanded upon by Canadian physician Sir William Osler, who detailed the major organ manifestations. In the late nineteenth century, the usefulness of quinine and salicylates in the treatment of lupus was reported. In the mid-twentieth century, the discovery of the immunologic aspects of lupus were discovered, when the presence of antinuclear antibodies were identified. Around this same time, the first animal models were used for the study of lupus, and the genetic component of lupus was also recognized. A major advance was the discovery of the effectiveness of cortisone in the treatment of systemic lupus. Corticosteroids remain the primary treatment modality, complemented by antimalarials (for skin and joint involvement) and cytotoxic agents (for severe kidney manifestations and other lifethreatening complications).

The prognosis for lupus patients has improved dramatically as a result of earlier diagnosis and better treatment. The longterm prognosis for a given patient is still variable, however, and is often related to the severity and the controllability of the initial inflammation. Also, the morbidity patterns of lupus patients have changed because of the increased usage of corticosteroids and cytotoxic drugs. Infections, accelerated atherosclerosis, and osteoporosis have become significant risk factors. Overall, however, the outlook for survival and quality of life has greatly improved. As of 2005, more than 90 percent of lupus patients lived more than ten years postdiagnosis. Those with organ-threatening disease had a lower rate, with only 60 percent surviving fifteen to twenty years.

A proliferation of research into the treatment of lupus that began in the 1950s continues and brings much promise for additional insight into the pathogenesis of lupus as well as new treatment modalities and agents. Some focus areas of current research include investigations into patterns of gene activity, the role of the protein interferon-alpha in the progression of lupus, environmental factors, immune ablation, stem cell transplantation, and the targeting of destructive white blood cells. An intensified effort by the federal government, private industry, and nonprofit organizations, such as the Alliance for Lupus Research and the Lupus Foundation of America, fuels the hope that better treatments, prevention, and ultimately a cure for lupus will be found.

—*Barbara C. Beattie*
Updated by David Hernandez

FOR FURTHER INFORMATION

Kasitanon, Nuntana, Laurence S. Magder, and Michelle Petri. "Predictors of Survival in Systemic Lupus Erythematosus." *Medicine* 85, no. 3 (May, 2006): 147-156.

"Lupus and Women." *Womenshealth.gov*, Office on Women's Health, 12 July 2018, www.womenshealth.gov/lupus/lupus-and-women.

Lupus Foundation of America. http://www.lupus.org.

Meadows, Michelle. "Battling Lupus." *FDA Consumer* 39, no. 4 (July/August, 2005): 28-34.

Seppa, N. "Self-Help: Stem Cells Rescue Lupus Patients." *Science News* 169, no. 5 (February 4, 2006): 67-68.

"Unlocking the Reasons Why Lupus Is More Common in Women." *National Resource Center on Lupus*, Lupus Foundation of America, www.lupus.org/resources/unlocking-the-reasons-why-lupus-is-more-common-in-women.

Wallace, Daniel J. *The Lupus Book: A Guide for Patients and Their Families.* 3d ed. New York: Oxford University Press, 2005.

Zonali, M. "Taming Lupus." *Scientific American* 292, no. 3 (March, 2005): 70-77.

T

Thalidomide

CATEGORY: Treatment

KEY TERMS:

angiogenesis: the development of new blood vessels
phocomelia: a rare congenital deformity in which the hands or feet are attached close to the trunk, the limbs being grossly underdeveloped or absent
teratogen: an agent or factor which causes malformation of an embryo

INDICATIONS AND PROCEDURES

In 1961, a link was established between the use of thalidomide, a mild sedative, and an increase in the frequency of severe defects in newborn babies in Germany, Great Britain, and other countries around the world where the drug had been in use. The "thalidomide babies" had minor defects of the fingers or toes but had major malformations of the limbs, resulting in incomplete or even missing arms and legs. The defects resembled those of a rare genetic disorder known as phocomelia ("seal limb"). Since thalidomide was able to cross the placenta to the fetus it has historically affected mostly pregnant women. Following the tragic discovery that thalidomide is a potent teratogen (a substance that causes a birth defect), use of the drug was discontinued.

In recent years, however, it has been discovered that thalidomide may be a useful therapeutic agent in a number of conditions, including leprosy, several other dermatologic disorders, different types of cancer, and acquired immunodeficiency syndrome (AIDS). The Food and Drug Administration (FDA) in the United States has approved thalidomide for use in the treatment of leprosy. Studies have demonstrated that thalidomide can inhibit in vitro angiogenesis, the process of formation of new blood vessels. Since many types of cancers require development of new blood vessels for their continued growth, thalidomide may be especially useful in cases where conventional treatments have ceased to be effective. Its use may be indicated in patients either relapsing after high-dose chemotherapy or who are developing serious side effects and are not able to tolerate additional chemotherapy.

USES AND COMPLICATIONS

Since thalidomide is such a powerful angiogenesis inhibitor, it is being used in disorders requiring anti-angiogenic therapy. Successful treatments have been made in cases of ovarian cancer, breast cancer, gastrointestinal carcinoma, renal melanoma, chronic graft-versus-host disease, and multiple myeloma. In some cases, the effectiveness of thalidomide increased when accompanied by other treatments, including immunotherapy, chemotherapy, and surgery.

Thalidomide appears to have few side effects in its new applications, but its return to medical respectability has raised again the specter of "thalidomide babies." Adverse effects noted in a few patients have included lethargy, constipation, and peripheral neuropathy. The potential problems associated with thalidomide causing a new round of severe birth defects may be a more serious consequence.

PERSPECTIVE AND PROSPECTS

The outbreak of thalidomide-related birth defects in the 1950s and 1960s led to the creation of birth defect surveillance programs in many countries. Unfortunately, medical standards and safeguards are not uniformly good, and there already appears to be an increase in birth defects associated with the new applications of thalidomide in South America. It will be necessary to regulate and to monitor closely the prescription, dispensing, and use of the drug. Counseling of patients of childbearing age will be an especially critical component if the tragedy of thalidomide's history is not to be repeated.

—*Donald J. Nash, Ph.D.*

FOR FURTHER INFORMATION

Brynner, Rock, and Trent Stephens. *Dark Remedy: The Impact of Thalidomide and Its Revival as a Vital Medicine.* Cambridge, Mass.: Perseus, 2001.

Fanelli, M., et al. "Thalidomide: A New Anticancer Drug?" *Expert Opinion on Investigational Drugs* 12, no. 7 (July 2003): 1211-1225.

Patrias, Karen, Ronald L. Gordner, and Stephen C. Groft. *Thalidomide: Potential Benefits and Risks—January, 1963, Through July, 1997.* Bethesda, Md.: Department of Health and Human Services, 1998.

Perri, A. J., and S. Hsu. "A Review of Thalidomide's History and Current Dermatological Applications." *Dermatology Online Journal* 9, no. 3 (August, 2003): 5.

Thyroid cancer

CATEGORY: Disease/Disorder

INTRODUCTION

Thyroid cancer is a malignancy that originates in the cells of the thyroid gland. The thyroid is an endocrine organ located at the base of the anterior neck that produces hormones which serve a wide variety of functions in the body. These functions include regulation of heart rate, respiration, blood pressure, metabolism, and temperature. Therefore, cancer of the thyroid can cause dysregulation of these body functions. Thyroid cancer is categorized as papillary, follicular, medullary, or anaplastic depending on the appearance of the cancerous cells. More women than men develop thyroid cancer, most likely due to the differences in hormones.

RISK FACTORS

Approximately 2/3rd of thyroid cancers are diagnosed in patients younger than 55 years of age, and women are more likely to develop thyroid cancer than men. Exposure to excessive radiation, certain industrial chemicals, or tobacco use increase the risk of developing thyroid cancer. Certain thyroid cancer types may have a genetic component, so a family history of thyroid cancer is considered a risk factor. A diet that is deficient in iodine is also a risk factor for this disease, which is a greater concern in countries where iodine is not added to table salt.

SYMPTOMS AND DIAGNOSIS

Signs and symptoms of thyroid cancer include pain in the neck that can radiate to other areas of the head, a lump or swelling in the front of the neck, or in the lymph nodes of the head and neck. As thyroid tumors enlarge, patients may experience difficulty swallowing or breathing. Thyroid cancers may interfere with normal thyroid function, and therefore some patients may have unexplained changes in heart rate, blood pressure, temperature, or weight. A blood test revealing abnormal thyroid functions may be a warning sign of thyroid cancer. Around 80% of women experience thyroid nodules, but only 5-15% of those cases are malignant.

TREATMENT

If caught early, thyroid cancer usually responds well to surgery, and 5-year survival rates are nearly 100% for stage I or stage II disease. More aggressive thyroid cancers may be treated with drugs that suppress thyroid activity such as radioiodine or thyroid hormone supressors, or with a type of chemotherapy called multitargeted kinase inhibitors (MKIs). Treatment decisions should be made in consultation with an endocrinologist or an oncologist who specializes in head and neck cancer.

PREVENTION AND FUTURE RESEARCH

Current research is primarily focused on prevention of thyroid cancer and early diagnosis of inherited thyroid disease. Beyond avoiding tobacco use, there is a correlation between a healthy diet low in animal fat and reduced thyroid cancer incidence. Maintaining a healthy body weight and reducing alcohol consumption are also correlated with reduced cancer prevalence.

—Cherie Marcel, BS
Updated by Patrick Richardson

FOR FURTHER INFORMATION

Marinella, M. A. (2009). Refeeding syndrome: An important aspect of supportive oncology. *The Journal of Supportive Oncology, 7*(1), 11-16. Retrieved from Baldwin, C., Spiro, A., Ahern, R., & Emery, P. W. (2012).

Oral nutritional interventions in malnourished patients with cancer: A systematic review and meta-analysis. *Journal of the National Cancer Institute, 104*(5), 371-385. doi:10.1093/jnci/djr556

Boleo-Tome, C., Monteiro-Grillo, I., Camilo, M., & Ravasco, P. (2012). Validation of the Malnutrition Universal Screening Tool (MUST) in cancer. *British*

Journal of Nutrition, 108(2), 343-348. doi:10.1017/S000711451100571X

Dal Maso, L., Bosetti, C., La Vecchia, C., & Franceschi, S. (2009). Risk factors for thyroid cancer: An epidemiological review focused on nutritional factors. *Cancer Causes & Control, 20*(1), 75-86. doi:10.1007/s10552-008-9219-5

Ferri, F. F. (2014). Thyroid carcinoma. In F. F. Ferri (Ed.), *2014 Ferri's clinical advisor 5 books in 1* (pp. 1093-1095). Philadelphia, PA: Mosby, an imprint of Elsevier Inc.

National Comprehensive Cancer Network (NCCN). NCCN Clinical practice guidelines in oncology. https://www.nccn.org/professionals/physician_gls/pdf/aml.pdf

British Thyroid Association, Royal College of Physicians. Guidelines for the management of thyroid cancer, 2007. http://www.british-thyroid-association.org/news/Docs/Thyroid_cancer_guidelines_2007.pdf

Thyroid disorders

CATEGORY: Disease/Disorder

KEY TERMS:

isthmus: a narrow organ, passage, or piece of tissue connecting two larger parts

larynx: the hollow muscular organ forming an air passage to the lungs and holding the vocal cords in humans and other mammals; the voice box

parafollicular cells: neuroendocrine cells in the thyroid for which the primary function is to secrete calcitonin; also called C cells

parathyroid: a gland next to the thyroid which secretes a hormone (parathyroid hormone) that regulates calcium levels in a person's body

CAUSES AND SYMPTOMS

The thyroid gland is a small butterfly shaped gland. It normally weighs about twenty to grams and is located in the neck just below the larynx, or voice box. The gland is named for the shield-shaped "thyroid" cartilage that forms the front of the larynx. The thyroid has two lateral lobes that are connected by an isthmus that crosses in front of the trachea. By placing a finger on the trachea below the larynx it is possible to feel

---

Information on Thyroid Disorders

Causes: Tumors, iodine deficiency, autoimmune disorders

Symptoms: In hypothyroidism, intolerance of cold, low body temperature, tendency to sleep longer, lack of energy, infrequent bowel movements, constipation, possible weight gain, puffy face and hands; in hyperthyroidism, bulging eyes, intolerance of heat, weight loss, nervousness, increased or decreased skin pigmentation, more frequent bowel movements, hair loss, rapid heart rate

Duration: Several months to chronic

Treatments: Thyroxine, antithyroid drugs (propylthiouracil, methimazole), radioactive iodine, surgery

---

the ridge-like isthmus pass under the finger after swallowing. The bilobed (two-lobed) shape of the rest of the gland can be felt just under the skin of the neck on either side of the midline, although its boundaries are normally indistinct except to a trained examiner.

The thyroid produces the hormones known as T3 (triiodothyronine) and T4 (thyroxine). Thyroxine, a product of the follicular cells, is the major hormone produced by the thyroid that helps regulate metabolism. Within the thyroid are also parafollicular cells that produce calcitonin, an essential hormone involved in calcium metabolism. Calcitonin affects multiple different systems to lower the amount of calcium in the blood stream. it does so by increasing calcium absorption by the bones, decreasing the amount of calcium absorbed by the gut, and decreasing the amount of calcium excreted by the kidneys. In the event that serum calcium is too low, there is a mechanism that works to counteract calcitonin in the parathyroid glands.

On the posterior aspect of the thyroid lie four small glands known as the parathyroids. The parathyroid glands produce parathyroid hormone, PTH, or parathyroid hormone, which works to increase blood calcium levels. In the case of thyroid surgery, the surgeon has to be mindful of the location of the parathyroid glands. It may be necessary to resect some or part of the parathyroid. However, if all four glands are removed, there may be life-threatening tetanus—the sustained contraction of muscles, including those needed for breathing.

The normal functioning of the thyroid results from an elaborate physiological control system involving the hypothalamus of the brain, the anterior lobe of the pituitary gland, and the thyroid gland. The hypothalamus produces thyrotropic releasing hormone (TRH), which is passed by special blood vessels to the anterior lobe of the pituitary, the adenohypophysis. The TRH-stimulated cells in the adenohypophysis produce thyroid-stimulating hormone (TSH), which is released into the general circulation. When it reaches the thyroid gland, it stimulates the gland to produce thyroxine. Normally, thyroxine has a negative feedback effect on its own production; that is, thyroxine can inhibit the activity of the hypothalamus and the pituitary to maintain its concentration in the blood. Various thyroid disorders, which are more common in women than in men, can develop from tumors that either increase or decrease the hormones produced in these three interdependent structures.

The normal thyroid (or euthyroid state) produces mainly thyroxine, which is converted into triiodothyronine in the tissues of the body before it has its effects, which are generally to increase the metabolic rate of the body. Some triiodothyronine is directly produced by the thyroid. The thyroxine molecule contains iodide, the negative ion of iodine (I⁻); which is why iodine is an essential component of one's diet. If iodine is not available in the diet—as in the case of vegetables grown in geographical areas glaciated in the past, such as mountainous terrain and the American Midwest—then the body cannot produce thyroxine. Industrialized countries have iodine added to table salt to ensure an adequate supply of this element in the diet.

A lack of iodine, and therefore a lack of thyroxine, prevents the functioning of the negative feedback effect of thyroxine on the hypothalamus and pituitary, resulting in very low thyroxine levels and high TSH levels in the blood. High levels of TSH cause substantial growth of the thyroid, which will bulge from the neck as a goiter. A person with such a condition has hypothyroidism (that is, have lower-than-normal thyroxine levels in the blood) and may be affected by cretinism (mental impairment and

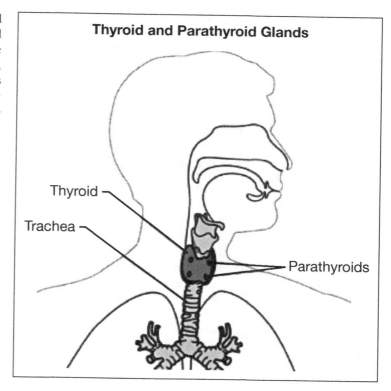

The thyroid is an important gland that produces thyroid hormone, the proper level of which is crucial to health; the inset shows the location of the thyroid gland. © EBSCO

stunted physical growth) if this condition occurs early in childhood. Women are eight times more likely to develop a hypothyroid condition than men. Symptoms of hypothyroidism include fatigue, depression, constipation, cold intolerance, weight gain, and dry skin and hair.

Hypothyroidism can arise in other ways as well. Hashimoto's thyroiditis is a common type of hypothyroidism that is caused by an autoimmune reaction whereby white blood cells known as lymphocytes infiltrate the thyroid and gradually destroy its tissue. The presence of antibodies against normal thyroid proteins can be detected with this condition.

Hypothyroidism can have serious effects during pregnancy and is associated with infertility and miscarriage. Hypothyroidism can cause complications such as preeclampsia, abruptio placenta (premature separation of the placenta from the uterus), premature labor, and postpartum hemorrhage. The infant may also be affected by low birth weight and neurodevelopment issues. Postpartum thyroiditis (PPT) affects 4-10% of women and occurs during the first year after delivery.

It is also possible to have too much thyroid activity, as is the case in hyperthyroidism. Graves' disease, the most common type of hyperthyroidism, is an autoimmune disorder in which antibodies mimic the action of TSH and therefore stimulate the thyroid to produce excessive thyroxine. Sometimes, nodules develop in the thyroid that may produce the excessive thyroxine. Although the presence of a nodule in the thyroid may cause a person to suspect cancer, the nodules are often benign. Graves' disease most often presents in women over the age of twenty and women have a seven times more likely chance to develop the disease. Hyperthyroidism may be associated with bulging eyes, but this orbitopathy does not always occur. Generally, there is an intolerance of heat, a loss of body weight, a high degree of nervousness, increased or decreased skin pigmentation, more frequent bowel movements, loss of hair, and a fast heart rate.

TREATMENT AND THERAPY

Patients suspected of having hypothyroidism or hyperthyroidism will have their blood tested for levels of TSH and thyroxine. Ultrasonography can be used to detect tumors or nodules and serve as an anatomical guide for potential surgery. In the case of hypothyroid, patients are managed with medication and do not require surgery. Hypothyroidism patients are prescribed an oral dose of thyroxine, which is adjusted until a euthyroid state is. Then the patient is maintained on thyroxine, with semi-annual or annual follow-up visits.

For hyperthyroidism patients, several modes of treatment are possible. Antithyroid drugs, such as propylthiouracil (PTU) or methimazole, can be given to inhibit thyroxine synthesis. Radioactive iodine is commonly given to destroy part of the thyroid gland and thus reduce its thyroxine output. Second or even third doses of radioactive iodine may be given if the blood thyroxine levels remain high. Radioactive iodine is not used during pregnancy because damage to the fetal thyroid is likely. Additionally, surgery can be performed to remove enough thyroid tissue to restore normal thyroxine levels. Following any of the treatments, a hypothyroidism may be induced that will require that the patient receive thyroxine supplements. If warranted, surgery can be used to reduce the bulging of the eyes caused by hyperthyroidism.

—John T. Burns, Ph.D.;
Updated by Matthew Berria, Ph.D.
and Julia Lockamy, RN

FOR FURTHER INFORMATION

Health Library. "Hyperthyroidism." *Health Library,* November 26, 2012.

Health Library. "Hypothyroidism." *Health Library,* March 15, 2013.

Kovacs, William J.., and Sergio R. Ojeda, eds. *Textbook of Endocrine Physiology.* 6th ed. New York: Oxford University Press, 2012.

MedlinePlus. "Thyroid Diseases." *MedlinePlus,* May 30, 2013.

Melmed, Shlomo, and Robert Hardin Williams, eds. *Williams Textbook of Endocrinology.* 12th ed. Philadelphia: Elsevier/Saunders, 2011.

Thyroid Disease & Pregnancy. Siemens Healthineers USA, 2015, usa.healthcare.siemens.com/clinical-specialities/womens-health-information/laboratory-diagnostics/thyroid-disease/thyroid-disease-and-pregnancy.

Women and Thyroid Disease. Siemens Healthineers USA, 2015, usa.healthcare.siemens.com/clinical-specialities/womens-health-information/laboratory-diagnostics/thyroid-disease/thyroid-disease-in-women.

Thyroid gland

CATEGORY: Anatomy

KEY TERMS:

cretinism: a severe hypothyroidism in which infants are born with insufficiently developed thyroid tissue

endocrine system: a series of ductless glands that deliver hormones to target cells directly through the bloodstream

Graves' disease: a common type of hyperthyroidism in which the thyroid gland produces an oversupply of hormone

hormones: chemicals, usually proteins or steroids, that carry messages regulating the body's chemical balance, responses to stimuli, and development

hypothyroidism: a condition in which the thyroid gland produces an insufficient supply of hormone

parathyroid: one of four small endocrine glands physically close to the thyroid that control the calcium balance of the body

pituitary: the endocrine gland responsible for the functioning of the thyroid, along with many other central control activities

thyroxine: the chief hormone of the thyroid gland, an iodine containing derivative of the amino acid tyrosine

STRUCTURE AND FUNCTIONS

The human body is, to an extraordinary extent, under the metabolic control of chemical secretions called hormones. These molecules are produced by the ductless, or endocrine, glands and carry messages that regulate the rate of production of necessary substances in remote parts of the organism. The endocrine glands in turn are largely controlled by the nervous system, which also uses chemical messengers to manage the multiple and interrelated systems of the body.

The thyroid gland was one of the earliest glands to be studied in detail. It synthesizes, stores, and secretes two principal hormones, thyroxine and triiodothyronine. These substances stimulate carbohydrate metabolism and protein synthesis or breakdown.

The first description of the thyroid that has been accepted as definite was given by Thomas Wharton in 1656; he also named the gland. In his studies of all the glands, he performed animal dissections and human autopsies. Although his written accounts were widely reprinted, it was more than two hundred years later before any serious further work was undertaken.

Nineteenth century clinical studies of goiter (swelling of the thyroid) and hyperthyroidism (the gland's overproduction of hormones) contributed little to an understanding of the thyroid. An exception is found in the study of the insufficient production of hormone by the thyroid, called hypothyroidism. English and Swiss physicians made discoveries that are considered by some medical historians to be as important as the demonstration that the element iodine is associated with thyroid action.

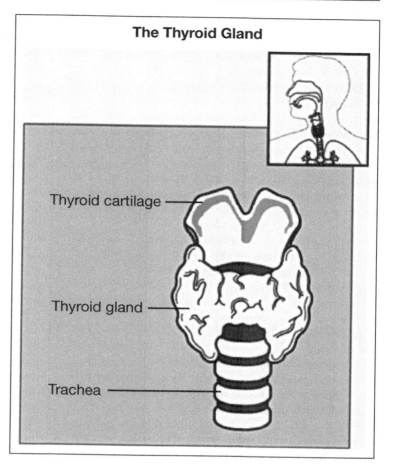

The Thyroid Gland

Thyroid cartilage

Thyroid gland

Trachea

© EBSCO

In the 1870s, the Swiss surgeon Emil Theodor Kocher began to describe the significance of the thyroid gland and its role in goiter formation. He was awarded the 1909 Nobel Prize in Physiology or Medicine for providing a fuller appreciation of the thyroid and associated glands. Kocher was neither a physiologist nor a pathologist by training or disposition, but he recognized that to be an effective surgeon it was essential to understand well the function of the thyroid and its role in the goiters so common in Bern. In this region, 80 to 90 percent of schoolchildren had a malfunctioning thyroid gland and the often-associated goiter. Kocher's drawings in books and papers show that such enlargements are extremely disfiguring and often interfere with normal breathing and speech.

In Kocher's day, little was known about any of the endocrine glands, of which the thyroid is the first to have been studied surgically. Such glands deposit chemical regulatory substances called hormones directly into the bloodstream, which carries them to the sites of their activity.

Later clinical observations provided evidence that the thyroid gland produces some material essential for good health. In 1896, Eugen Baumann made the key discovery that the thyroid contains an unusual amount of iodine. He also showed that this excess iodine is present in a protein that he could decompose with water to yield a new substance. During the next twenty-five years, technical progress was made to the point that the hormone thyroxine could be produced in a pure, crystalline form.

With the new tool of radioactive iodine, a powerful method for the study of thyroid functions and malfunctions became available. For example, overactive and underactive thyroid glands can be easily determined through the ingestion of a tiny amount of one of the radioactive isotopes of iodine and the later determination of the amount of the tracer present in the thyroid.

Although thyroid issues affect both men and women, women are more likely to have thyroid diseases. Approximately one in eight women will have an issue with her thyroid at one point in her life. This may be due to the link between the thyroid helping to control women's menstrual cycle. The most common thyroid issue in women in hypothyroidism, which is when the thyroid is underactive. The symptoms women should look out for include fatigue or weakness, weight gain, decreased appetite, change in menstrual periods, loss of sex drive, feeling overly cold, constipation, muscle aches, puffiness around the eyes, brittle nails or hair loss. Since some of these symptoms could also be associated with mood disorders, women should be sure to advocate for themselves to be checked for thyroid issues by their medical doctor.

DISORDERS AND DISEASES

It is possible for the thyroid to produce either too much (hyperthyroidism) or too little (hypothyroidism) of the hormone thyroxine, which plays a role in controlling metabolism and body growth. If an insufficient quantity of it is produced, the condition called Gull's disease results. In children, this condition limits both physical and mental growth and is known as congenital hypothyroidism or cretinism. In

Graves' disease and related conditions, the overactive thyroid gland produces too much hormone. Either of these conditions can produce an enlarged thyroid gland, or goiter. This imbalance existed in many different countries, but physicians designated it by various names, thus causing much misunderstanding and confusion.

Emil Kocher's studies presented the first organization of the field in the form of these basic definitions. In his first one hundred operations carried out between 1872 and 1883, Kocher completely removed the thyroid gland in thirty-four cases. After a report by his colleague Jacques Louis Reverdin indicating that removal of the thyroid was a causal factor in cretinism, Kocher made as detailed a follow-up of these patients as possible. His conclusion was that if the entire gland was removed, cretin-like symptoms almost always appeared. If at least some of the gland was left, it appeared to regenerate itself and supply the required hormone. He vowed never to remove a thyroid completely again except in the case of malignancy.

Only in the twentieth century did reliable diagnoses and treatments become available for thyroid disorders. Because of the variety of these conditions and their causes, accurate diagnosis is indispensable. Modern approaches that supplement radioactive iodine include ultrasound and the needle biopsy.

The principal difficulty in the treatment of a malfunctioning thyroid gland is the several variations often displayed. Hyperthyroidism can occur in forms that appear quite unrelated to the most common form, Graves' disease. For example, there may not be a heredity basis, the condition may not spread over the entire gland, the production of antibodies may not be involved, and there may be no progressive failure of the thyroid.

The causes of hypothyroidism are also less than uniform. The age at which the disorder begins is significantly related to its cause. Newborn children with this condition may have never developed the required amount of thyroid tissue. Others may have inherited a defect that prevents the thyroid from producing sufficient hormone. In developing countries, iodine deficiency remains a problem (although an overabundance of that element in the diet of expectant mothers can lead to infants with hypothyroidism and a goiter). Later in life, infection can be the cause of Hashimoto's disease and the loss of thyroid tissue.

Finally, the treatment of an overactive thyroid places a person at risk of later underproduction of hormone.

The most common symptoms associated with thyroid problems are a too rapid or too slow heartbeat, nervousness or a tired and run-down feeling, frequent bowel movements or constipation, and weight loss or weight gain. An excess of the hormones that direct the use of food and the production of energy might reasonably be expected to produce the first of each pair of contrasting observations, while a deficiency would lead to the opposite effects.

The treatment of Graves' disease falls into three distinct classes, and in modified application these techniques are employed with the other forms of hyperthyroidism. Since the early 1940s, a series of antithyroid drugs have been synthesized. They function by preventing the gland from making hormone, and the symptoms lessen in a short time. Unfortunately, only about 30 percent of patients remain well when the medication is stopped after six to twelve months. If antithyroid drugs fail to control the overactive thyroid, a radioactive isotope of iodine is often successful. Since the iodine goes directly to the thyroid and remains there for a period of time, it is able to irradiate and destroy a portion of the tissue. It is a demanding task to calculate the proper amount of iodine to administer, but a surprising 80 percent of patients find their condition under control after a single treatment.

Surgical treatment of Graves' disease and related hyperthyroid conditions became practical with Kocher's efforts, and it remains the method of choice in many cases. Kocher began his Nobel Prize lecture by describing the crucial importance of the work of Louis Pasteur, Joseph Lister, and others in making surgery on internal organs possible, and he suggested the future of thyroid research when he examined the effective use of extracts and the search for chemical means of providing substitutes for the gland's secretions. The standard treatment of hypothyroidism is oral thyroid hormone tablets. Typically, a synthetic form of thyroxine, called Levothyroxine, is given to compensate for low thyroid hormone levels. As is the case with Graves' disease, good follow- up is essential because the prescribed dosage will likely change with the patient's age. The administration of too much thyroxine can lead to hyperthyroidism.

Two notes should be made in concluding this discussion of malfunctions of the thyroid. First, there is a tendency to believe that iodine prevents and cures goiter. Statements to that effect, found in many general reference books, are both misleading and dangerous. Second, publications for laypersons tend to minimize the importance of thyroid blood tests, which is a serious disservice. Regular and complete physical examinations are essential in maintaining good health.

PERSPECTIVE AND PROSPECTS

Historians of medical history have attributed knowledge of the thyroid gland and the treatment of goiter to many significant figures. The works of Galen, Paracelsus, ancient Chinese writers, and other classical Roman and Greek authors, as well as medieval manuscripts, have been studied. In the twentieth century, the study of the thyroid and goiter illustrates central themes in the evolution of medical practice; these are shown clearly in the career of Emil Kocher. His being chosen as an early Nobel laureate is prophetic—first for his role in creating modern surgery, with its total reliance on a germ-free environment and its demand for detail, and second for successful synthesis of the roles of clinician and research scientist. He both possessed the necessary surgical skill to develop such a delicate procedure as thyroidectomy (removal of the thyroid gland) and appreciated the importance of understanding the role played by the thyroid in controlling distant and seemingly unrelated functions. Finally, Kocher kept abreast of any new discovery that might, in any way, be of significance to his surgical goals.

The study of the thyroid in many ways unlocked the secrets of other endocrine glands. As in many areas of scientific research, new medical knowledge follows quickly after the discovery of materials and techniques. At the same time, the search for knowledge provides both motivation and information driving the discovery of materials and techniques. The identification of iodine as an elemental substance by the French chemist Bernard Courtois in 1811 rapidly led to its indiscriminate use as a treatment for goiter, along with a wide variety of related conditions. Important work in the mid-nineteenth century by A. Chatin demonstrated the high correlation between goiter and low levels of iodine in the food and water supplies throughout central Europe. In the 1930s, with the creation of radioactive isotopes, including those of iodine, a vital and productive new phase of thyroid research began. A similar pattern is seen during World War II, when four independent research groups showed that sulfa drugs were capable of exerting a strong influence on the behavior of the thyroid. All these studies were conducted within a two-year period, and it was less than a year later that the therapeutic use of sulfa drugs was demonstrated.

While much knowledge and technical skill concerning the thyroid has been gained, the number of conferences and publications devoted to endocrinology attests to the continued importance of that general field of study. For example, while malignant tumors are rare in the thyroid, benign lumps or nodules are common. The reasons for this pattern and the role of endocrine glands in the development and spread of cancerous cells warrant detailed and continuing study.

In 2013, researchers analyzing data from the U.S. National Health and Nutrition Examination Survey linked exposure to perfluorinated chemicals (PFCs) to changes in thyroid function. PFCs are often found in fabrics, cosmetics, and carpets.

—*K. Thomas Finley, Ph.D.*
Updated by Kimberly Ortiz-Hartman, Psy.D., LMFT

FOR FURTHER INFORMATION

Bayliss, R. I. S., and W. M. Tunbridge. *Thyroid Disease: The Facts.* 4th ed. New York: Oxford University Press, 2008.

Burman, Kenneth D., and Derek LeRoith, editors. *Thyroid Function and Disease.* Philadelphia: Saunders/Elsevier, 2007.

Dallas, Mary Elizabeth. "Thyroid Disorders Tied to Complications in Pregnancy." *MedlinePlus.* May 29, 2013.

Holt, Richard I.G., and Neil A. Hanley. *Essential Endocrinology and Diabetes.* 5th ed. Malden, Mass.: Blackwell, 2007.

Marieb, Elaine N. *Essentials of Human Anatomy and Physiology.* 9th ed. San Francisco: Pearson/Benjamin Cummings, 2009.

Preidt, Robert. "Chemicals in Carpets, Cosmetics Tied to Thyroid Problems." *MedlinePlus.* May 29, 2013.

Preidt, Robert. "Iodine Supplements May Be Too Much of a Good Thing." *MedlinePlus.* June 12, 2013.

Rosenthal, M. Sara. *The Thyroid Sourcebook.* 5th ed. New York: McGraw-Hill, 2009.

Toxic shock syndrome

CATEGORY: Disease/Disorder

CAUSES AND SYMPTOMS

Toxic shock syndrome, an overwhelming and potentially life-threatening infection, is most commonly known for its association with tampon use in young women. Despite tampon use being associated with many of the TSS cases, it is important to remember that this is caused by an infection rather than appropriate tampon use. Though this is still the most commonly affected population, toxic shock syndrome can affect non-menstruating women, children and men as well.

Two distinct organisms can be responsible for toxic shock syndrome, each associated with a different constellation of symptoms. The bacteria *Staphylococcus aureus* (staph) causes all cases of menstrual toxic shock syndrome, and some non-menstrual cases as well. Non-menstrual cases can arise from an infected surgical wound or infections elsewhere in the body. The bacteria *Streptococcus pyogenes* (strep) is responsible for non-menstrual toxic shock syndrome only.

All patients with staph toxic shock syndrome have high fevers, light-headedness associated with low blood pressure, and a diffuse rash resembling a sunburn. The eyes, mouth, and vagina can become red and irritated, and several weeks following the initial illness, the skin on the palms and soles begins to

---

Information on Toxic Shock Syndrome

Causes: Bacterial infections with staphylococci (menstrual cases, associated with tampon use) or streptococci (nonmenstrual cases, as from injuries, surgical wounds, infections elsewhere in body)

Symptoms: In staph cases, high fever, lightheadedness, low blood pressure, diffuse rash, redness and irritation of eyes, mouth, and vagina, vomiting, diarrhea, muscle aches, jaundice, kidney failure, confusion; in strep cases, severe pain and swelling at injury site, fever, confusion, low blood pressure, tissue death (necrotizing fasciitis)

Duration: Acute

Treatments: Hospitalization, intravenous fluids, antibiotics, removal of cause (tampon, bandages or packing), sometimes surgery to remove infected tissue

In the News:
Sinus Infections Leading to Toxic Shock Syndrome in Children

A retrospective study at The Children's Hospital of Denver found that rhinosinusitis (infection of the nose and paranasal sinuses) can be a primary cause of toxic shock syndrome in young children. The study published in the June, 2009, issue of *Archives of Otolaryngology—Head and Neck Surgery* describes data from seventy-six pediatric patients admitted between 1983 and 2000 who were identified through medical records as having toxic shock syndrome. Of these patients, 21 percent had rhinosinusitis. Study authors, including Kenny Chan, chief of Pediatric Otolaryngology at Children's Hospital of Denver and professor of otolaryngology at the University of Colorado, suggest that physicians consider rhinosinusitis a primary cause of toxic shock syndrome when another site of infection cannot be identified. Because toxic shock syndrome can be fatal, quick treatment and identification of the source are critical.

Sinus infections have not been well reported as a potential primary source of toxic shock syndrome. A study published by Paul D. Gittelman from New York University Medical Center and colleagues found an association between toxic shock syndrome and rhinologic surgery and medical devices. The study, published in *Laryngoscope* in 1991, included 140 adult patients. Toxic shock syndrome was linked to circulating exotoxin of a toxigenic strain of *Staphylococcus aureus*. About 30 percent of patients in the study selected for surgery were *S. aureus* carriers, with toxin-capable isolates identified in 40 percent of those tested. The study also found users of cocaine, topical decongestants, and steroid sprays had a statistically higher rate of *S. aureus* compared to nonusers.

—*Sandra Ripley Distelhorst*
Updated by Kimberly Ortiz-Hartman, Psy.D., LMFT

slough. Other symptoms may include vomiting, diarrhea, muscle aches, jaundice, kidney failure, and confusion.

Strep toxic shock syndrome typically arises at a site of minor trauma to the skin, either an injury or a recent surgical wound. Severe pain at the site is the most common finding. The patient may have a fever, confusion, and low blood pressure. Severe swelling at the site of infection can lead to major damage to the skin and underlying tissues; this necrotizing fasciitis (so-called flesh-eating bacteria) is a well-known manifestation of strep toxic shock syndrome.

Women are the primary population affected by Toxic Shock Syndrome. It is most commonly associated with tampon use in menstruating women. However, tampon use itself does not cause this disorder, rather a bacterial infection. It was first recognized in women wearing super absorbency tampons, which got significant recognition. This is a rare syndrome affecting approximately one to three women in every 100,000. TSS is a life-threatening condition and immediate medical care is required for treatment.

TREATMENT AND THERAPY

Because of the severity of the illness, almost all patients with toxic shock syndrome require hospitalization. Intravenous fluids and other medications are administered to improve the blood pressure, and antibiotics are used to kill the bacteria and to decrease production of the toxins that they release. In cases of menstrual toxic shock syndrome, removal of the tampon is critical. For infected surgical wounds, removal of bandages and packing is required, as well as occasional removal of infected tissue with surgery. In cases of necrotizing fasciitis, surgical removal of infected tissue is necessary and may involve a loss of a significant amount of skin and underlying muscle.

PERSPECTIVE AND PROSPECTS

The initial association of toxic shock syndrome with highly absorbent tampons in the 1980s led to a withdrawal of such products from the market. Consequently, the number of cases of menstrual toxic shock syndrome has significantly declined; however, extended tampon use remains a risk factor for toxic shock syndrome. Frequent tampon changes and tampon use only on the heaviest days of bleeding should reduce this risk. Women who have had menstrual toxic shock syndrome or other problems with staph infections should avoid tampon use.

—*Gregory B. Seymann, M.D.*
Updated by Kimberly Ortiz-Hartman, Psy.D, LMFT

FOR FURTHER INFORMATION

Beers, Mark H., et al., eds. *The Merck Manual of Diagnosis and Therapy*. 19th ed. Whitehouse Station, N.J.: Merck, 2011.

Icon Health. *Toxic Shock Syndrome: A Medical Dictionary, Bibliography, and Annotated Research Guide to Internet References*. San Diego, Calif.: Icon Health, 2004.

Mandell, Gerald L., John E. Bennett, and Raphael Dolin, eds. *Mandell, Douglas, and Bennett's Principles and Practice of Infectious Diseases.* 7th ed. New York: Churchill Livingstone/ Elsevier, 2010.

National Institutes of Health. "Toxic Shock Syndrome." *MedlinePlus,* 07 March 2019, https://medlineplus.gov/ency/article/000653.htm.

Parker, James N., and Philip M. Parker, eds. *The Official Patient's Sourcebook on Toxic Shock Syndrome.* San Diego, Calif.: Icon Health, 2002.

Sheen, Barbara. *Toxic Shock Syndrome.* San Diego, Calif.: Lucent Books, 2006.

Wood, Debra. "Toxic Shock Syndrome." *Health Library,* November 26, 2012.

Transgender adults: Psychosocial issues

CATEGORY: Biology, Disease/Disorder

KEY TERMS:

gender dysphoria: a distressed state arising from conflict between a person's self-identified gender and the sex the person has or was identified as having at birth

gender-nonconforming: person whose behavior or appearance does not conform to prevailing cultural and social expectations about what is appropriate to their gender

BACKGROUND

Transgender is an umbrella term used to describe individuals whose gender identity and behaviors fall outside traditional gender norms and do not feel in line with their biological sex.

Transgender individuals may be transsexuals (who identify opposite to their assigned biological sex), bi-gendered persons (who exhibit both genders), intersex persons (whose chromosomal structure or sex organs are not distinctly male or female), or transvestites (i.e., men who dress as women or women who dress as men). *Gender-nonconforming* and *gender-variant* are also terms used to describe individuals whose gender identity does not conform to the binary of female or male. Transgender individuals may identify, and frequently are referred to in the literature, as either male-to-female (MTF) or female-to-male (FTM) transgender.

Experiences of being transgender vary with the age of the individual and should be placed in historical context of changing societal attitudes. The internal experience of masculinity and femininity for each individual increasingly is understood as an idiosyncratic experience that exists on a spectrum of gender identification, rather than being a fixed, binary characteristic.

Many transgender individuals are aware of their gender variance in childhood and describe feeling a "mind-body dissonance." One study showed that MTF transgender individuals were aware of their gender dissonance earlier in childhood than FTMs were.

Gender dysphoria, as outlined in the *Diagnostic and Statistical Manual of Mental Disorders 5* (*DSM- 5*), may be diagnosed in some transgender individuals. In the *DSM-5*, the disorder is now separate from other sexual dysfunctions and paraphilic disorders. Diagnosis in *DSM-5* requires that there be a marked difference between an individual's expressed or experienced gender and the gender that others wish to assign him or her, which must cause clinically significant distress or impairment in social, occupational, or other areas of functioning for at least 6 months. To ensure access to treatment, the *DSM-5* includes a post-transition specifier for individuals living full-time as their desired gender.

Some scholars emphasize the tendency to misdiagnose mental health problems in transgender individuals. One study showed no difference in physical and mental health between stably housed transgender adults and the overall U.S. population. Another study found that 9 of the 10 individual case studies researchers examined at a gender identity clinic demonstrated at least one significant pathology.

DISCRIMINATION AND VICTIMIZATION

Coming out as transgender can be a process that requires the individual to reestablish all of his or her relationships; because of this, it is an experience that is different from revealing oneself as gay, lesbian, or bisexual. Researchers who carried out a study of transgender individuals living in rural versus urban environments noted significant differences in access to mental healthcare, along with similar levels of alcohol and marijuana use.

Sexual identity and gender are related, but often are conflated and should not be confused: Being transgender does not imply a particular sexual orientation.

A study of the impact of testosterone treatment found that some participants changed their self-defined sexual orientation after starting treatments. Scholars, advocates, and transgender individuals have been critical of state and medical requirements that insist on sex reassignment surgery and hormone replacement treatment before establishing the preferred gender of the transgender individual.

In 2011 the United Nations High Commission for Human Rights adopted a resolution explicitly supporting the human rights of transgender individuals (as well as lesbian, gay, and bisexual individuals). The report expresses grave concern about the global abuse of and discrimination toward these populations.

Verbal and physical abuse of transgender individuals occurs frequently and may come from family, peers, and religious and other authority figures. Transgender identity is persistently over-sexualized by society, and transgender individuals are extremely vulnerable to sexual abuse.

Researchers of one study found widespread negative attitudes among heterosexual adults in the United States toward transgender individuals. More frequent negativity toward transgender individuals was reported by heterosexual men than by heterosexual women. Less frequent negativity was reported by heterosexuals who had contact with sexual minorities.

Discrimination in the housing market is reported by transgender individuals buying and renting homes: 1 in 5 have been homeless at some point since identifying as transgender. Two thirds of transgender adults report experiencing discrimination in the workplace.

Results from a review of 33 studies indicated that between 35 percent and 72 percent of transgender individuals had been arrested at some point. Transgender individuals are targeted by law enforcement with illegal police stops, abuse, and harassment; the abuse includes condoning violence toward transgender prison inmates by other inmates. Transgender individuals may not seek assistance when they are victims of crime because of fear of secondary victimization by law enforcement.

In California, transgender individuals are twice as likely to have a bachelor's degree than Californians overall, but they earn 40 percent less than other graduates. As a result of discrimination in California, transgender individuals are twice as likely to live below the poverty threshold as the general population is.

Transgender individuals have an elevated risk of poor mental health. Rates of depression and suicidal ideation among transgender persons are described as high; they are highest among younger transgender individuals. These rates may lessen with age due to improved coping mechanisms. Statistics from Europe, the United States and Canada reveal that 22 percent–43 percent of transgender individuals report a history of suicide attempts, 9 percent–10 percent having attempted suicide in the past year. Results from one study indicated that FTM transgender individuals were at a higher risk of attempting suicide in their lifetime compared to MTF transgender individuals.

Non-suicidal self-injury (NSSI) (when individuals intentionally harm themselves without lethal intent) is prevalent among transgender individuals. Examples of NSSI are cutting, burning, severe scratching, and hitting. Results from a study of transgender adults in the United States indicated that 41.9 percent of participants reported a history of NSSI. The mean age of NSSI initiation was 13 years of age, and the behaviors continued well into adulthood.

Results from a study of older transgender adults indicated that they had significantly poorer health (i.e., physical health, disabilities, symptoms of depression, and perceived stress) than non-transgender lesbian, gay, and bisexual older adults.

Transgender adults who experience more daily discrimination are more likely to participate in health-harming behaviors such as drug and alcohol abuse, smoking, and suicide attempts. In a U.S. study, quality of life was significantly lower among FTM transgender persons compared to the overall male and female population. Younger transgender individuals are at risk of being institutionalized and subjected to gender-conforming interventions.

Substance abuse and HIV reportedly are high among transgender individuals. HIV is highest among transgender women, specifically black MTF transgender persons. A significant connection has been shown between substance abuse and sexual risk-taking. Transgender sex workers are especially at risk for substance abuse and HIV infection.

Transgender individuals have difficulties accessing social and health services because of discrimination.

Researchers found that 42 percent of FTM transgender adults reported verbal harassment, physical assault or lack of access to equal treatment in a medical office setting or hospital.

THERAPY AND TREATMENT

A strong social support system, protection from transphobia, and undergoing a full medical transition (with hormone use and/or surgical procedures) are significant protective factors from suicide risk among transgender individuals.

Research indicates that many communities and mental health professionals lack knowledge and information about transgender individuals and therefore require educational interventions to prevent discrimination and victimization. Transgender parents and their children report experiencing a tremendous amount of stress: Parents feel stress from being rejected by their family and from job discrimination. Their children report feeling stressed from bullying, having to change their perception of their parents, and feeling like they are caught in the middle of family relationships and strife. Both transgender parents and their children report viewing therapy as a beneficial resource.

Physicians and mental health workers should learn about the psychosocial issues of transgender individuals and help create trans-positive environments by providing education and sensitivity trainings to colleagues.

Clinical practice and research should recognize the unique experience of transgender individuals and be alert to the convenience and oversimplification of consolidating all LGBT individuals together.

Learning about the discrimination and prejudice that transgender individuals experience, and advocating for legislation that prohibits it will go a long way to alleviating some psychosocial issues. Working closely with transgender individuals on developing healthy coping strategies to decrease stress associated with being transgender will give them more confidence in social interactions. Transgender individuals can practice self-soothing techniques to replace any present maladaptive coping mechanisms. It is the role of the mental health professional working with the transgender individual, to help them to seek support, validation and acceptance in the different systems involved in their lives, such as family, friendships, work, or school.

—*Jan Wagstaff, MA, MSW*

REFERENCES

Bauer, G., Scheim, A., Pyne, J., Travers, R., & Hammond, R. (2015). Intervenable factors associated with suicide risk in transgender persons: A respondent-driven sampling study in Ontario, Canada. *BMC Public Health, 15*, 525. doi:10.1186/ s12889-015-1867-2

Centers for Disease Control and Prevention. (2015). HIV among transgender people. Retrieved November 22, 2015, from http://www.cdc.gov/ hiv/ group/gender/transgender/

Davis, S. A., & Colton, M. S. (2014). Effects of testosterone treatment and chest reconstruction surgery on mental health and sexuality in female-to-male transgender people. *International Journal of Sexual Health, 26*(2), 113-128. doi:10.1080/19317 611.2013.833152

Dickey, L., Resiner, S., & Juntunen, C. (2015). Non-suicidal self-injury in a large online sample of transgender adults. *Professional Psychology: Research and Practice, 46*(1), 3-11.

Factor, R. J., & Rothblum, E. (2008). Exploring gender identity and community among three groups of transgender individuals in the United States: MTFs, FTMs, and genderqueers. *Health Sociology Review, 17*(3), 235-253. doi:10.5172/ hesr.451.17.3.235

Miller, L., & Grollman, E. (2015). The social costs of gender noncomformity for transgender adults: Implications for discrimination and health. *Sociological Forum, 30*(3), 809-831. doi:10.1111/ socf.12193

Motmans, J., Meier, P., Ponnet, K., & T'Sjoen, G. (2012). Female and male transgender quality of life: Socioeconomic and medical differences. *Journal of Sexual Medicine, 9*(3), 743-750. doi:10.1111/j.1743-6109.2011.02569.x

Trichomoniasis

CATEGORY: Disease/Disorder
Also known as: Trich

KEY TERMS:

asymptomatic: infected but with no discernable symptoms of disease

carrier: a person infected by an organism who can transmit that organism to other people but who is asymptomatic

Centers for Disease Control and Prevention (CDC): a government facility, located in Atlanta, which coordinates investigations of disease occurrence in the United States

protozoan: a unicellular organism with an organized nucleus

sexually transmitted disease (STD): a disease that is usually transmitted from person to person through contact between the vaginal or urethral discharges from an infected person and the genital mucous membranes of a person susceptible to infection

urethritis: inflammation and infection of the urinary tract

vaginitis: inflammation and infection of the vagina

CAUSES AND SYMPTOMS

A flagellated motile protozoan known as *Trichomonas vaginalis* causes trichomoniasis, which is the most common non-viral sexually transmitted disease (STDs). The disease is common among people with multiple sex partners, those who engage in unprotected sex, and those who seek services at STD clinics. Trichomoniasis in pregnant women can cause premature birth and babies born to infected mothers are more likely to have a low birth weight.

Some estimates suggest that 180 million people per year are infected with Trichomoniasis worldwide. The most common population found to be infected is females sixteen to thirty-five years old, which is prime childbearing age. This is an important epidemiological group, as Trichomoniasis infections are a leading cause of premature rupture of the placenta, premature birth, and low birth weight.

After infection, there is an incubation period of about seven days, with a range from about five to twenty-eight days. Although 70-85 percent of infected people remain asymptomatic, *T. vaginalis* infections may produce itching or irritation of genitals, discomfort with urination, discharge from the penis or discharge from the vagina. Women may experience vaginal discharge described as a frothy yellow or green vaginal discharge which may or may not have a foul smell. Sometimes, vaginal inspection shows a distinctive "strawberry cervix" (red patches on the cervix) and red spots on the vaginal walls. Men's symptoms sometimes include dysuria, a frothy or purulent urethral discharge, and, in rare cases, scrotal pain due to epididymitis.

The symptoms of infection by *T. vaginalis* are of questionable value in diagnosing the infection because many infected people remain asymptomatic for years.

Information on Trichomoniasis

Causes: *Trichomonas vaginalis*

Symptoms: dysuria, irritation of genitals, vaginal or urethral discharge

Duration: Can remain dormant for years if not treated

Treatments: Metronidazole or Tinidazole

Most existing diagnostic tests, such as microscopic viewing of wet mounts, Pap tests, and polymerase chain reaction (PCR), often fail to show the infectious agent even in people with symptoms. Culture of the vagina and urethra is considered to be the most effective way of detecting *T. vaginalis* infection. These factors add to the difficulty in reducing infection rates.

TREATMENT AND THERAPY

The CDC's *Sexually Transmitted Diseases Treatment Guidelines 2015*, which includes Trichomoniasis, focuses on microbiological cure, alleviation of signs and symptoms, prevention of sequelae, and prevention of transmission. The infection is treated with a single oral dose of either metronidazole or tinidazole. Any sex partner should be treated simultaneously even if he or she is asymptomatic. Patients should abstain from sex until they and the partner have completed treatment. Treatment is successful in 90 to 100 percent of cases but there is an as much as 17% reinfection rate within three months of receiving treatment, so some physicians recommend retesting for *T. vaginalis* after treatment.

Treatment during pregnancy is controversial, but no case of fetal malformation has been attributed to metronidazole. Studies have shown that Trichomoniasis is associated with low infant birth-weight, premature rupture of the membranes, and preterm births. However, studies of pregnant women with Trichomoniasis who are treated failed to show an improvement in preterm deliveries and even trended toward more preterm deliveries; therefore, treatment remains controversial.

PERSPECTIVE AND PROSPECTS

Many men and women infected by the organism remain asymptomatic for years, spreading the disease to other people through sex. Safe sex practices help decrease the rate of transmission. People with multiple sex partners should use latex or polyurethane condoms to help curtail the spread of this disease. It is crucial that sex education programs emphasize that people with any unusual genital symptoms, including dysuria, irritation of genitals, and vaginal discharge, seek medical treatment.

People infected by *T. vaginalis* may also be infected by other STD organisms, especially the bacterium that causes gonorrhea. Medical professionals believe that infection by the *Trichomonas* protozoan predisposes a person to infection by the human immunodeficiency virus (HIV) upon exposure through unprotected sex with infected partners. Trichomoniasis in young children may indicate sexual abuse, and health professionals may be obligated to report such infections, if local regulations require it.

—*Anita Baker-Blocker, M.P.H., Ph.D.*
Updated by Christine Gamble, M.D.

FOR FURTHER INFORMATION

Boston Women's Health Collective. *Our Bodies, Ourselves: A New Edition for a New Era.* 35th anniversary ed. New York: Simon & Schuster, 2005.

Centers for Disease Control and Prevention. 2015 Sexually Transmitted Diseases Treatment Guidelines. https://www.cdc.gov/std/tg2015/trichomoniasis.htm

Edwards, T., et al. "*Trichomonas vaginalis*: Clinical relevance, pathogenicity, and diagnosis." *Critical Reviews in Microbiology,* vol. 42, no. 3, 2014, 406-417.

Garber G. E. "The laboratory diagnosis of *Trichomonas vaginalis.*" *The Canadian journal of infectious diseases & medical microbiology,* vol. 16, no. 1, 2005, 35-8.

Heymann, David L., editor. *Control of Communicable Diseases Manual.* 19th ed. Washington, D.C.: American Public Health Association, 2008.

Paladine, H. L., & Desai, U. A. "Vaginitis: Diagnosis and Treatment." *American Family Physician,* vol. 97, no. 5, 2018, 321-329.

Tubal ligation

CATEGORY: Procedure

KEY TERMS:

culdoscopy: an endoscopic procedure performed to examine the rectouterine pouch and pelvic viscera by the introduction of a culdoscope through the posterior vaginal wall

colpotomy: a type of incision that is made in the back wall of the vagina

intrauterine cannula: a hollow, rigid tube designed to place dyed fluid into the uterus to determine a perforation

laparoscopy: a surgical procedure in which a fiber-optic instrument is inserted through the abdominal wall to view the organs in the abdomen

sterilization: a permanent method of birth control

tenaculum: a surgical clamp with sharp hooks at the end, used to hold or pick up small pieces of tissue such as Fallopian tubes

INDICATIONS AND PROCEDURES

Tubal ligations are performed strictly for sterilization of a female patient. While there has been some success with reversing the procedure, it must be considered permanent. The woman must be well informed and certain that she does not want additional children under any circumstances.

The most common technique for tubal ligation is laparoscopy. As an outpatient, the woman receives local anesthetic and a light sedative. A small incision is made in the navel, and gas is used to inflate the abdomen, allowing easy visibility of the patient's Fallopian tubes. An instrument called an intrauterine cannula is inserted through the vagina, and a clamp called a tenaculum is positioned on the cervix. Both are used to manipulate the tubes into position. A laparoscope, a thin tube containing a camera and light, is inserted through the incision in order to view the tubes. An instrument to block the tubes is inserted through the laparoscope. The tubes may be blocked by burning, cutting, or applying rings or clips. The incision is sewn closed.

In a minilaparotomy, a small incision is made above the woman's pubic bone. The tubes are brought through the incision and are tied and cut. Tubal ligations can also be performed through a woman's vagina (culdoscopy or colpotomy).

Many tubal ligations are done immediately, or within a day, following the delivery of a baby. If a patient has a cesarean section, then tubal ligation is often done as part of the same surgical procedure. Following a vaginal delivery, a woman desiring a tubal ligation is usually brought to the operating room the next day. In cases in which there is a problem with the baby (including extreme prematurity, anomalies, or sepsis), the sterilization procedure is often delayed, pending a good outcome for the infant.

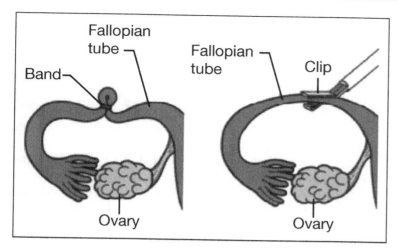

A common means of sterilization for women is tubal ligation, in which the Fallopian tubes through which eggs must pass to reach the uterus are severed or interrupted with clips or bands. © EBSCO

potential problems are those associated with any abdominal surgery, including unintentional damage to other internal organs, bleeding, and infection. One recent study indicated that there is no change in the level of hormones produced by women prior to or following tubal ligation.

It is essential that women are well informed by their medical professional before these procedures are done. Historically women of color and/or of low socioeconomic status have been encouraged or even pushed to undergo sterilization procedures. This should be a well-thought-out decision, without any pressure on the woman from others.

—*Karen E. Kalumuck, Ph.D.;*
Updated by Robin Kamienny Montvilo,
R.N., Ph.D.

USES AND COMPLICATIONS

The only purpose of tubal ligation is sterilization. It is highly effective (with a 0.2 percent failure rate) and largely irreversible. Depending on the type of blockage used, it is about 30 percent reversible; however, only 10 percent of women become pregnant after undergoing tubal reconstruction. Other forms of birth control are recommended for any patient who is not absolutely certain about the procedure.

Tubal ligations take only thirty minutes to perform, and there is only minor postsurgical pain. A rare complication may be an ectopic pregnancy within the Fallopian tube, which could rupture. Other

FOR FURTHER INFORMATION

Berek, Jonathan S., ed. *Berek and Novak's Gynecology.* 15th ed. Philadelphia: Lippincott Williams & Wilkins, 2012.

Gentile, Gwen P., et al. "Hormone Levels Before and After Tubal Sterilization." *Contraception* 73, no. 5 (May, 2006): 507–511.

Health Library. "Tubal Ligation—Laparoscopic Surgery." *Health Library,* April 22, 2013.

MedlinePlus. "Tubal Ligation." *MedlinePlus,* May 13, 2013.

Zollinger, Robert M., Jr., and Robert M. Zollinger, Sr. *Zollinger's Atlas of Surgical Operations.* 9th ed. New York: McGraw-Hill, 2011.

U

Ultrasonography

CATEGORY: Procedure

KEY TERMS:

Doppler effect: the relationship of the apparent frequency of waves, such as sound waves, to the relative motion of the source of the waves and the observer or instrument; the frequency increases as the two approach each other and decreases as they move apart; an effect also known as the Doppler shift

duplex scan: an ultrasound representation of echo images of tissues and blood vessels combined with a Doppler representation of blood flow patterns

frequency: the number of complete cycles, such as sound cycles, produced by an alternating energy source; sound is measured in cycles per second, and one cycle per second is equal to 1 hertz

oscilloscope: an instrument that displays a visual representation of electrical variations on the fluorescent screen of a cathode-ray tube

transducer (probe): a device designed to transfer ultrasound waves into the body noninvasively, receive the returning echoes, and transform those echoes into electrical voltages

ultrasonic: referring to any frequency of sound that is higher than the audible range-that is, higher than 20,000 cycles per second (20 kilohertz)

INDICATIONS AND PROCEDURES

Sound waves are mechanical pressure waves that can propagate through liquids, solids, and, to some extent, gases. A sound wave is composed of cyclic variations that occur over time; one cycle per second is called 1 hertz (Hz). Ultrasound waves have a frequency of oscillation that is higher than 20,000 hertz, placing ultrasound above the audible range for humans. The useful frequency range for medical diagnostic ultrasound is between 1 and 10 megahertz (10 million hertz), although surgical instruments often use carrier frequencies greater than 20 megahertz.

The basic ultrasound system has two principal components. The first, and perhaps more important, component is the transducer, or probe. The transducer converts electrical pulses into mechanical pressure (sound) waves that are transmitted into the tissues. It then detects the echoes that are reflected from the tissues and transforms those echoes into electrical voltages. The second component is the audiovisual electronic component, which processes and displays the reflected echoes in the form of an image of internal organs and structures or an image of the movement of red blood cells.

Ultrasound waves are created when the crystalline material within the transducer is excited by an electrical voltage produced by the instrument's oscillator. The application of an electrical charge causes the crystalline particles to expand and contract, producing mechanical waves and pulses. These pulses of sound pass from the face of the transducer into the body, where they strike the organs, bones, and blood vessels. The reflected echoes in turn strike the face of the transducer, again causing the crystalline particles to vibrate and produce an electrical charge. Such crystalline material is said to have piezoelectric (a combination of the Greek word *piesis*, meaning "pressure," and the word "electric") properties.

Ultrasound systems commonly employ sound in two modalities. The transducer uses sound waves to create an echo image of body structures. The audiovisual component uses the Doppler shift theory to analyze the range of velocities over which red blood cells are moving.

To create an echo image, millions of pulses of sound must be transmitted into the body each second. For each transmitted pulse, one line of echo information is received by the transducer crystal. To build up an image rapidly and depict the real-time motion of body structures, the pulses are sent into the body from many angles as the sound beam is moved over the body surface. The depth of the echoes is displayed as a function of time, and a two-dimensional image is created by relating the sound's direction of propagation to the direction of the echo-image trace that appears on the instrument's oscilloscope.

The time required for a sound pulse to travel from the transducer to its target within the body, reflect, and return to the transducer can be used to measure the distance to the target, as radar does. In body tissues, sound travels at a speed of 1,540 meters per second. It takes approximately thirteen microseconds for a sound pulse to travel 1 centimeter into the body and return to the transducer. The depth and orientation of echoes may be determined by using this information.

As a sound beam travels through tissues, it is attenuated, or reduced in amplitude and intensity. Attenuation occurs as the energy from the beam is absorbed by the tissues and transformed into heat. Additionally, a part of the beam may be reflected into the surrounding tissues at an angle away from the incident angle or backscattered as the long wavelength of the sound beam strikes the smaller red blood cells. Only a small fraction of the returning echoes reaches the face of the transducer.

Because the attenuation of the sound beam increases as the depth of penetration increases, the echoes that return from the deepest part of the image field will be reduced in intensity when compared to the echoes that return from the structures nearer the skin surface. The echo intensity is dependent on the degree of change and impedance of each tissue through which the echo passes, the strength of the incident sound beam, and the degree of attenuation of the beam. To equalize the intensity of the echoes from all depths of the image field, the echoes that travel farthest, and therefore take the longest time to reach the transducer, are amplified over time by using time-gain compensation methods.

For medical imaging applications, the returning echoes may be displayed in several ways. The amplitude mode (A-mode) depicts the returning echoes as deflections on the instrument's oscilloscope; the height of the deflection depends on the strength of the returned signal, and the distance between the deflections depends on the depth of the signal. The brightness mode (B-mode) depicts the strength of the echoes as shades of gray, with the strongest echoes appearing the brightest. The B-mode display makes it possible to differentiate tissue texture

characteristics. The time-motion mode depicts movement over time by moving the B-mode trace across the face of a high-persistence oscilloscope, showing the depth, orientation, and strength of echoes with respect to time.

The transducer crystal determines the shape and focus of the sound beam and the frequency of the sound waves, features that are important in resolving echo information into complex images. The beam may be divided into three parts: the near field, the focal zone, and the far field. The beam width, close to the face of the transducer, is equal to the width of the transducer. The beam converges as it travels away from the transducer and then diverges at its narrow focal zone. In order for tissue targets to be resolved into discrete image points, both the lateral and the axial planes of the beam must be narrow. The focusing of the beam is facilitated by placing convex acoustic lenses in front of the transducer crystal to shorten the near field to a narrow focal point, thereby increasing the lateral resolution.

Axial resolution is the ability to distinguish targets along the sound beam. If a single pulse is emitted from the transducer, echo sources lying close together in the axial path of the beam may not be separated. Multiple short bursts of sound are used to separate the echo sources; each echo is captured as a discrete burst. Because axial resolution is inversely proportional to the duration of the ultrasound pulse (and the resonant frequency of the crystal is inversely proportional to its diameter), small-diameter, high-frequency crystals are used to obtain maximum axial resolution.

Ultrasound may be used to determine the velocity of blood flow. This velocity is determined in relation to the frequency of the incident sound beam according to the Doppler theory. Several different techniques may be used to process and display the echoes from moving red blood cells. The ultrasound system's computers may be programmed to perform fast Fourier transform analysis, a complex mathematical method for ranking the speed of the echoes returning over time. The signals may be displayed either as spectral tracings of the range of Doppler frequency shifts, represented in the returned echoes recorded throughout the cardiac cycle, or as color-coded Doppler-shifted signals from within the blood vessels, superimposed on a gray-scale image of the surrounding tissues.

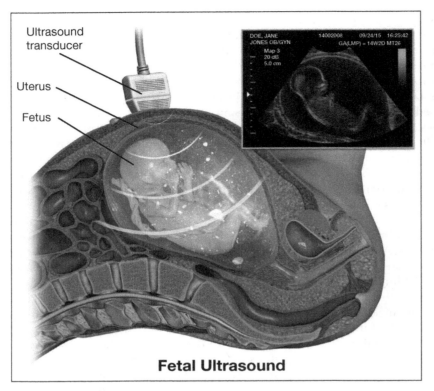

Fetal Ultrasound

Ultrasound transducer

Uterus

Fetus

(BruceBlaus via Wikimedia Commons)

USES AND COMPLICATIONS

High-resolution abdominal ultrasonography is a valuable technique for the visualization of intra-abdominal organs and disease processes. For example, liver conditions such as parenchymal abnormalities, abscesses, hematomas, cysts, and cancerous lesions can be identified easily by means of this technique. B-mode and Doppler color-flow imaging are particularly valuable technologies that can be used to evaluate the tissue characteristics and blood flow patterns of transplanted organs. An ultrasound examination of the gallbladder may reveal gallstones, obstruction of the common bile duct, or inflammatory disease. Ultrasound imaging of the pancreas is used to identify pancreatitis, pancreatic pseudocysts, and carcinoma of this organ. An ultrasound examination of the spleen may reveal spleno-megaly, or enlargement of the spleen in response to disease or trauma. Additionally, ultrasonography can be used to evaluate splenic volume and to identify hematomas, congenital cysts, infarctions, and tumors within the organ. The technology is particularly well suited for the study of tumors and abscesses within the abdomen. Ascites and other fluid collections may be recognized, and primary tumors and lymph node metastases within the abdominal cavity may be identified by means of pulse-echo imaging.

Ultrasound has certain characteristics that make it particularly valuable for examining the kidneys and the genitourinary tract. The ability to image both native and transplanted kidneys noninvasively from the longitudinal and transverse planes provides additional diagnostic information in uremic patients for whom the injection of contrast agents is undesirable or may fail to provide sufficient information. Urologic ultrasonography may be used to determine renal size and position or to identify cysts and masses, kidney or bladder stones, obstruction of the ureters, and bladder contour. Transabdominal scanning of the pelvic organs, which is used to determine the presence or absence of suspected lesions, makes possible the precise localization and quantitative mapping of pelvic abdominal masses, facilitating the determination of disease stages and the positioning of radiation ports. The technology is used to differentiate cysts from solid tumors and to determine if pelvic tumors are of uterine, ovarian, or tubal origin.

The sonographic resolution of deep abdominal structures is achieved by internal scanning; endorectal or endovaginal approaches are used to reduce the distance between the transducer and the target organ. During these procedures, the transducer probe either is in direct contact with the genital organs or prostate gland or is separated from them by the thin walls of the bladder or rectum. The information obtained with these techniques is thought to be submacroscopic, observed at approximately twenty to thirty times light magnification. Ultrasonography plays a major role in the evaluation of obstetrical cases. Ultrasonic imaging is used to study early pregnancy and high-risk cases, as well as to confirm ectopic pregnancy (development of the fetus outside the uterus).

In cases of spontaneous abortion, ultrasound procedures are used to indicate whether the fetus and placenta have been retained. Ultrasonography is often used to determine fetal growth rate and placental development and to confirm intrauterine fetal death, threatened abortion, and fetal abnormalities.

It is the best method for guiding amniocentesis (the sampling of placental fluids). A study published in the *Journal of the American Medical Association* in 2013 confirmed that ultrasound is the best detector of ectopic pregnancies. Echocardiography, the ultrasound evaluation of the heart, is a reliable and useful tool for the study of patients with congenital and acquired heart disease. The role of cardiac ultrasound in the investigation of cardiac dysfunction, tetralogy of Fallot, transposition of the great vessels, and atrial septal defect has been well defined. Echocardiology is used to detect pericardial effusion; is coupled with Doppler ultrasound to evaluate the pulmonic, mitral, tricuspid, and aortic valves; and is used to investigate primary myocardial disease and atrial tumors. Improved resolution of cardiac structures and patterns of blood flow can be achieved by using endoesophageal (transesophageal) imaging and Doppler color-flow technology.

The vascular system of the body can be studied by combining pulse-echo imaging of the blood vessels and Doppler ultrasound detection of red blood cell movement. This combined technology, known as duplex scanning, not only offers information that is relevant to the anatomy and morphology of blood vessels but also—and this is most important—provides the opportunity to evaluate the dynamics of blood flow and the pathophysiology of vascular disease. Duplex technology is used to demonstrate the presence and characteristics of atherosclerotic disease and to define the severity of vascular compromise resulting from the progression of disease or the presence of blood clots in vessels (thrombosis).

Applications of the technology have been extended to the evaluation of arteries and veins of the extremities, the abdomen, and the brain. Advances in computer technology have made it possible to color-code the Doppler-shifted signals returning from moving red blood cells within the vessels.

Ultrasonography has proven to be particularly useful in the fields of obstetrics and gynecology. Physicians involved in maternity care use ultrasonography to determine the position of a fetus, measure the amniotic fluid index, locate the placenta, and measure cardiac activity in a fetus. More advanced skills involve assessing gestational age, ascertaining accurate dating, and using ultrasonography to guide amniocentesis during the second and third trimesters of a pregnancy.

Ultrasonography has additional benefits for women. Three-D ultrasonography can be used to diagnose congenital anomalies. In one study, almost 17 percent of women prone to miscarriages had congenital uterine anomalies; 3-D ultrasound can diagnose these with anywhere from 88 to 100 percent accuracy. Further, the procedure can be used to locate fibroids and polyps, identify uterine adhesions (also known as uterine synechiae), and examine the placement of intrauterine devices (IUDs). In the case of IUD placement, ultrasound can improve detection of IUDs that have become embedded in the uterine tissue, usually causing pain and bleeding. Further, transvaginal ("through the vagina") ultrasonography is used by physicians to evaluate postmenopausal bleeding in women. This bleeding can be caused by endometrial cancer, which can be spotted by ultrasound as an alternative to sampling of endometrial tissue.

Doppler color-flow imaging has facilitated the investigation of vascular disorders that result in slow or reduced blood flow (venous thrombosis or preocclusive narrowing of vessels) or that affect the vascularity of organs and tissues (tumors or transplanted organs). Therefore, vascular ultrasonography plays a major role in the evaluation of patients with arterial occlusive disease and those suspected of having thrombosis of the deep or superficial venous systems.

Perspective and Prospects

Ultrasonic techniques have assumed a preferred role in the diagnosis of many diseases and have become an essential component of quality medical care. In contrast to the rapid development and use of x-ray technology in medical diagnosis, the application of diagnostic ultrasound has been relatively slow. Progress depended in large part on the development of high-resolution electronic devices and transducers. Early research into medical applications involved the adaptation of instruments that had been designed for industrial or military purposes.

The first attempts to locate objects with ultrasound probably occurred following the sinking of the

Titanic in 1912. Improvements in the technology led to the widespread industrial and military use of ultrasound for the detection of flaws in metals, for the determination of range and depth information, and for navigation. The first application of ultrasound to medical diagnosis occurred in 1937, when K. T. Dussik attempted to image the cerebral ventricles by measuring the attenuation of a sound beam transmitted through the head. In 1947, Douglas H. Howry pioneered the ultrasonic imaging of soft tissues and constructed a pulse-echo system that utilized a transducer submerged in water. The system utilized surplus Navy sonar equipment, a high-fidelity recorder power supply, and a metal cattle-watering trough in which the patient and the transducer were immersed.

In the 1960s, Howard Thompson and Kenneth Gottesfeld performed obstetric and gynecologic examinations using the first contact scanner, which had been produced in 1958 by Tom Brown, an engineer, and Ian Donald, a professor of midwifery, at Glasgow University in Scotland. The first commercial scanner marketed in the United States was designed by William L. Wright, an engineer at the University of Colorado. The two-dimensional scanning system was developed in 1953 by John Reid, an engineer, in cooperation with John Wild, a physician who demonstrated that ultrasound could detect differences between normal tissues, benign tumors, and cancers. The collaboration between medicine and engineering has propelled diagnostic ultrasonography forward at a phenomenal rate of development since that time.

The field of echocardiography was pioneered by Inge Edler, who discovered in the 1950s that echoes from the moving heart could be received and displayed by using a time motion ultrasonic flow detector. Using this technology, Edler diagnosed mitral stenosis, pericardial effusion, and thrombus in the left atrium.

The use of ultrasound to evaluate blood flow was first described by S. Satomura in 1959. This investigator observed that ultrasound could be transmitted through the skin to derive information about the velocity of blood flow by using the Doppler effect to analyze the reflected signals from the moving blood cells. The first transcutaneous continuous-wave Doppler system was developed at the University of Washington in the 1960s. The instrument was first used to detect fetal life by demonstrating the fetal heartbeat.

This application of Doppler ultrasound spurred research under the guidance of Eugene Strandness Jr. that ultimately led to the development of duplex scanners, instruments that combine pulse-echo imaging with analysis of blood flow patterns derived from the Doppler effect. As a result of the efforts of these early investigators and others, diagnostic medical ultrasonography has evolved into a highly useful tool with diverse clinical applications.

—*Marsha M. Neumyer*

FOR FURTHER INFORMATION

American College of Obstetricians and Gynecologists, "The Role of Transvaginal Ultrasonography in Evaluating the Endometrium of Women with Postmenopausal Bleeding," ACOG Committee Opinion, May 2018, http://bit.ly/2UkroKa.

Bates, Jane A. *Abdominal Ultrasound: How, Why, and When.* 3d ed. New York: Churchill Livingstone/Elsevier, 2011.

Griffith, H. Winter. *Complete Guide to Symptoms, Illness, and Surgery.* Revised and updated by Stephen Moore and Kenneth Yoder. 6th ed. [N. p.]: Perigee/Penguin Group, 2012.

Kremkau, Frederick W. *Diagnostic Ultrasound: Principles and Instruments.* 7th ed. St. Louis, Mo.: Saunders/Elsevier, 2006.

Voyatzis, Diane. "Doppler Ultrasound." *Health Library,* November 19, 2012.

Umbilical cord

CATEGORY: Anatomy

KEY TERMS:

allantois: a hollow sac-like structure filled with clear fluid that forms part of a developing embryo; helps the embryo exchange gasses and handle liquid wastes

amnion: the innermost membrane that encloses an embryo and eventually fills with amniotic fluid

chorion: the outermost membrane surrounding an embryo; contributes to the forming of the placenta

cryopreservation: the use of very low temperatures to preserve structurally intact living cells and tissues

extraembryonic membranes: the term for the collective layers enclosing the embryo inside the uterus

hemangioma: a birthmark that most commonly appears as a rubbery, bright red nodule of extra blood vessels in the skin

yolk sac: a membrane outside the human embryo that is connected by a tube (the yolk stalk) though the umbilical opening to the embryo's midgut; an early site for the formation of blood and is eventually enveloped by the embryo's primitive gut

STRUCTURE AND FUNCTIONS

The umbilical cord is composed of a thickened fibrous covering over a gelatinous material that protects three blood vessels, which connects the mother with her unborn child. Two umbilical arteries carry blood from the baby to the placenta and coil around the single umbilical vein. Blood containing oxygen and other essential nutrients returns from the placenta through the umbilical cord.

At term, the umbilical cord measures approximately 20 inches. The cord may be short if there is little amniotic fluid and if the baby has a muscular weakness, limiting movement inside the uterus. Umbilical cord lengths of less than 14 inches have a high incidence of traumatic separation and fetal blood loss at the time of a vaginal delivery.

DISORDERS AND DISEASES

Normally, the umbilical cord dries rapidly after birth, with most of its fluid content evaporating in two days. The base of the cord is then colonized by bacteria. An immune system response to the bacteria and chemicals released by white blood cells are required for the final shedding of the dried cord. The untreated umbilical cord is shed approximately seven to ten days after birth. Any treatment (such as alcohol) used to dry or delay cord bacterial colonization allows the cord to persist for nearly twice as long as in the untreated condition.

Persistence of an umbilical cord beyond three weeks after drying may be caused by a persistent blood supply and may require evaluation by a pediatric surgeon. Conditions that are associated with a persistent cord blood supply include a hemangioma, a connection from an artery in the skin to the vein of the umbilical cord, a small outpouching of the lining of the abdominal cavity, or retained elements of tissue connected to the bladder.

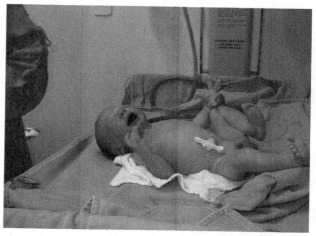

A newborn with umbilical cord clamp. (Eduardo Marquetti via Wikimedia Commons)

Once the cord has been fully shed, a reactive overgrowth of tissue may occur at the base of the cord. This is termed an umbilical granuloma and is readily managed by the application of silver nitrate, which cauterizes the tissue. There should be no further drainage from the base of the umbilicus beyond six weeks after birth.

During normal embryonic development, the umbilical cord is associated with a portion of two extraembryonic membranes, the yolk sac and the allantois. In late embryonic stages, the umbilical region normally herniates out of the embryo's body wall and is then fully retracted. If part of the herniated bowel is not returned to its normal position, then a connection between the base of the umbilical cord and the small intestine may occur. This is known as a Meckel's diverticulum of the ileum. Similarly, if the allantois does not completely degenerate, then it can leave a connection between the umbilical cord and the top of the bladder, known as a patent urachus. Both conditions are usually easily corrected by surgery.

PERSPECTIVE AND PROSPECTS

Within the last decades, the umbilical cord has taken on new significance as the source of embryonic stem cells. Blood from the umbilical cord taken immediately after the infant has been born can be isolated and cryopreserved for many years. Should the infant (or even individuals who are not perfectly matched immunologically) require new blood stem cells to repopulate the immune system after chemotherapy or radiation therapy, then the cord blood stem cells can be thawed and injected into the recipient. A host of diseases have been successfully treated using cord blood, including many genetic diseases, and thousands of parents have opted to bank their infant's cord blood. The cost of harvesting and maintaining cord blood, however, is a source of controversy. Harvesting and storing cord blood is expensive, and the chances of an individual spontaneously acquiring a childhood neoplasm or serious genetic disease that would require cord cell therapy is not high. In addition, alternative therapies, such as bone marrow transplants, are sometimes available. On the other hand, parents in which such diseases run in the family may seriously consider cord blood banking.

The hope of stem cell technology in the future lies in the possibility that specific differentiated cell lineages can be stimulated to cure disease and not simply to reconstitute the immune system. For example, diabetic patients might have stem cells in cord blood engineered to produce insulin-secreting cells under appropriate control of circulating glucose concentration. Using the patient's own cord blood to produce such differentiated stem cells would avoid the problem of host-graft rejection.

In July 2013, the *New York Times* reported on a study suggesting that doctors clamp umbilical cords too soon following birth. According to the study, waiting at least one minute before cutting the cord improves iron and hemoglobin levels in newborns. "Delayed cord clamping" is now medically indicated as to ensure the newborn babies get all the rich and healthy blood into their bodies. Since this is a relatively new change, the parents may still need to discuss this ahead of time or during delivery with their doctors to make sure they follow this process.

—*David A. Clark, M.D.;*
Updated by Alexander Sandra, M.D.

FOR FURTHER INFORMATION

Cunningham, F. Gary, et al., eds. *Williams Obstetrics.* 23d ed. New York: McGraw-Hill, 2010.

Kurtzberg, J., A. D. Lyerly, and J. Sugarman. "Untying the Gordian Knot: Policies, Practices, and Ethical Issues Related to Banking of Umbilical Cord Blood." *Journal of Clinical Investigation* 115 (October, 2005): 2592-2597.

Moore, Keith L., and T. V. N. Persaud. *The Developing Human.* 8th ed. Philadelphia: Saunders/Elsevier, 2008.

Preidt, Robert. "Later Clamping of Umbilical Cord May Benefit Newborns: Study." *MedlinePlus.* July 11, 2013.

Simkin, Penny, Janet Whalley, and Ann Keppler. *Pregnancy, Childbirth, and the Newborn: The Complete Guide.* 3d ed. Minnetonka, Minn.: Meadowbrook Press, 2008.

"Umbilical Cord Abnormalities." *March of Dimes.* February 2008.

"Umbilical Cord Care: Do's and Don'ts For Parents." *MayoClinic.* February 22, 2013.

Uremia

CATEGORY: Disease/Disorder

KEY TERMS:

amino acids: any of a number of nitrogen-rich compounds used by the body for the production of protein

antihypertensive drugs: medications designed to reduce and control elevated blood pressure

diuretics: medications used to increase urination and eliminate wastes from the bloodstream

edema: an abnormal accumulation of watery fluid in the connective tissues, resulting in swelling

hemolytic uremia: a type of uremia that afflicts mostly young children and infants

renal failure: the failure of the kidneys, making it impossible for the kidneys to function efficiently

urea: the waste product when proteins and other nitrogen-rich compounds are broken down

CAUSES AND SYMPTOMS

Uremia is a condition that results when waste products, notably urea and creatinine, accumulate in the bloodstream. Toxins are normally transported through the body by way of the bloodstream passed the liver, filtered in the kidneys and expelled in the urine. The kidneys purify the blood and are responsible for maintaining adequate levels of red blood cells, calcium, potassium, vitamin D and other micronutrients.

Individuals with end-stage renal disease often are those who present with uremia because their kidneys no longer work as a filter to rid the body of toxins. Other individuals may present with uremia due to acute injury to the kidneys (acute renal failure). The causes of acute renal failure may include heart failure, heavy hemorrhage, and severe dehydration. These conditions lead to kidney damage as a result of reduced blood supply.

Kidney damage may stem directly from other illnesses such as diabetes, lupus, glomerulonephritis and hemolytic uremic syndrome. In fact, the leading cause of end-stage renal disease in the US is diabetes. Additionally, anything that may prevent the urine from leaving the kidney (such as cancer compressing the ureters, a swollen prostate, kidney stones) will cause a backflow. Prolonged restrictions of this kind can lead to kidney damage.

Signs of patients suffering from uremia include fatigue, confusion and disorientation. Individuals may become nauseated and lose interest in eating. Some outward manifestations may include a rash, itching, excessive thirst, sores and/or edema in the mouth. They may present with anemia, high potassium levels in the blood, vitamin deficiencies, and unusual bone fracture from low calcium in the blood. Men can have low sexual performance, and childbearing age women may have infertility that is secondary to disrupted reproductive hormone regulation. High blood pressure, valvular heart disease, chronic heart failure, and angina may be seen. Uremia may cause platelets abnormalities resulting in gastrointestinal bleeding. If not treated promptly, uremia may lead to seizures, comas, cardiac arrest and ultimately, death.

TREATMENT AND THERAPY

Uremia is usually diagnosed in the presence of high urea levels in the blood and the aforementioned signs and symptoms. Once a patient presents with symptoms, the most effective way to manage the condition is hemodialysis to cleanse the blood of its impurities. Patients with end-stage kidney failure often have repeated episodes of uremia.

Currently, the only long-term solution for these individuals is a kidney transplant.

For years it's been debated whether diet changes can manage uremia syndrome. The topic continues to be debated and somewhat controversial.

PERSPECTIVE AND PROSPECTS

In most cases, uremia occurs in the presence of end-stage renal disease. These patients often present fatigue, confusion, and disorientation. Currently, the most effective management of uremia is hemodialysis.

—*R. Baird Shuman, Ph.D.*
Updated by Ashley Henry, MPH, RN

FOR FURTHER INFORMATION

Alper, A. (2019). Uremia: Background, Pathophysiology, Etiology. Retrieved from https://emedicine.medscape.com/article/245296-overview

———. (2019). Uremia Treatment & Management. Retrieved from https://emedicine.medscape.com/article/245296-treatmentBrenner, Barry M. *Brenner and Rector's The Kidney.* Philadelphia: Saunders/Elsevier, 2008.

Foris, L., & Bashir, K. (2019). Uremia. Retrieved from https://www.ncbi.nlm.nih.gov/books/NBK441859/

Gurland, Hans J., ed. *Uremia Therapy: Perspectives for the Next Quarter Century.* 1st ed. New York: Springer, 2012. Print.

Rosenberg, M. (2019). UpToDate. Retrieved from https://www.uptodate.com/contents/overview-of-the-management-of-chronic-kidney-disease-in-adults?search=uremic%20syndrome-&source=search_result&selectedTitle=1~150&usage_type=default&display_rank=1

Tamparo, Carol D. *Diseases of the Human Body.* Philadelphia: Davis, 2000.

Urinary disorders

CATEGORY: Disease/Disorder

KEY TERMS:

bacteriuria: the presence of bacteria in the urine

cystitis: inflammation of the urinary bladder, often characterized by pain and dysuria

dysuria: painful or difficult urination, often the result of urinary tract infection or obstruction

urethra: the tubular structure that drains the urine from the bladder

urethritis: inflammation of the urethra, often characterized by dysuria

urinary bladder: the muscular organ that stores urine to be discharged through the urethra *urinary tract infection:* infection involving any organs associated with the urinary system

CAUSES AND SYMPTOMS

Diseases of the urinary tract represent one of the most common forms of infection by microorganisms. In the United States, the prevalence of urinary tract infections is a reflection of both gender and age. By the age of five, bacteriuria is found in approximately 4 to 5 percent of girls, which is about ten times the rate among boys. Infections are far more common among female adolescents and young women than among men Between 50-80% of women will have a urinary tract infection (UTI) in their life. Data regarding prevalence of infection varies depending on what definition of infection is used. It has been suggested that more women experience urinary disorders because of the shorter length of the urethra and its closer relation to the anus. Insertive sex also contributes to the possibility of contracting a urinary disorder. The prevalence of infection among both men and women rises sharply among the elderly, often reflecting problems with aging, including enlargement of the prostate in men. Most infections are self-limiting, particularly among the young. If not treated properly, however, such infections have the potential to be more serious.

Normally, urine is free of microbial contamination. The much higher incidence of urinary tract infections in women reflects, to a large degree, the anatomical differences between males and females. In women, the close proximity of the urethra to the rectum permits relatively easy access of intestinal flora to the urinary tract. Not surprisingly, most urinary infections are caused by bacteria found in the body, particularly the gut. The most common infectious agent, *Escherichia coli.*

Urinary tract infections usually begin with the entry of the organisms into the opening of the urethra; the migration of microorganisms into the vagina may occur in a similar manner. Most bladder infections result from movement of the microbial agents along the urethra into the urinary bladder. Inflammation of the urethra (urethritis) or urinary bladder (cystitis) results from a combination of microbial colonization and the host's immune response to the infection. Often, such inflammation may be the first symptom of these infections.

Various factors appear to increase the likelihood certain individuals to urinary tract infections. Strains

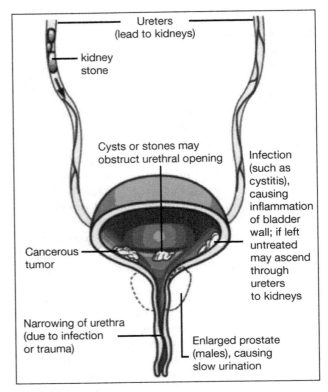

In addition to the variety of infections that may attack the urinary system, urinary disorders may be caused by cancerous tumors, cysts, stones that cause obstruction, reactions to trauma, and in males pressure from an enlarged prostate. © *EBSCO*

of *E. coli* that colonize the urethra appear to have a greater ability to adhere to the surface tissue. In particular, those strains that frequently ascend into the ureters or kidneys often possess unique types of fimbriae (filamentous structures), which promotes adherence to the epithelial cells that line the surface of the urinary tract; this bacterial structure may be of particular importance to the course of the infection, since the flushing action of urinary flow is a mechanism by which the body maintains the sterility of the urinary tract. Likewise, anything with the potential to interrupt micturition (urination), such as the presence of calculi or tumors, may predispose an individual to a urinary tract infection. Among children, congenital abnormalities at the site of ureter entry into the bladder may result in vesicoureteral reflux, or urine backflow, which may interfere with normal urine flow. Such abnormalities, which are not

Information on Urinary Disorders

Causes: May include bacterial infections, catheters, prostate gland enlargement, stones, tumors, STIs, cancer

Symptoms: Depends on the cause; may include abdominal pain, fever, vomiting, painful and frequent urination, abdominal heaviness, lower back pain

Duration: Typically acute

Treatments: Depends on cause; may include antibiotics, surgery, chemotherapy, radiation therapy

uncommon, are found in equal numbers among both young boys and girls; they frequently disappear naturally by the time of puberty. Nevertheless, such problems may contribute to infections among those in this age group.

Certain forms of birth control, in addition to the act of intercourse itself, may contribute to urinary infections. The colonization of *E. coli* may be associated with the use of diaphragms or spermicides. The reasons for this connection are unclear, but both appear to represent an alteration in the normal flora of the periurethral area and vagina. It is important for women to flush their urinary system after sexual intercourse, as there is a 60-fold increase in the oddd of developing cystitis in the first 48 hours after intercourse.

Clinical manifestations of urinary tract infections vary with age and are often nonspecific. The infiltration of leukocytes (white blood cells), resulting in inflammation, accounts for many of the symptoms. Among children, abdominal pain is often present, accompanied by fever and sometimes vomiting.

Among adults, cystitis and urethritis are often accompanied by difficulty in urination (dysuria), including painful urination and frequent urination, particularly in women. A sensation of abdominal heaviness or lower back pain, in addition to low-grade fever, is often observed. The urine may be bloody or turbid, reflecting a mixture of microbial agents and white blood cells.

Infection of the urinary tract may also result from a variety of sexually transmitted organisms. Chlamydial infections are common in both males and females, and they represent one of the most commonly observed forms of sexually transmitted disease (STI). *Chlamydia trachomatis* causes urethritis in both males and females; though many chlamydial infections are asymptomatic, they can lead to severe complications. Urethritis may also result from other microbial STIs, both viral and bacterial.

The use of catheters, particularly among hospitalized elderly persons, is a frequent cause of urinary infections. In most cases, these infections are inapparent, but such persons remain predisposed to cystitis or urethritis.

The urinary tract is also subject to other disorders, including cancer. The most common form of neoplasm of the urinary tract is bladder cancer. Such cancers tend to be highly aggressive, often occur as multiple growths, and are difficult to cure once metastasis has begun. Approximately two-thirds of cases of bladder cancer are diagnosed in men, perhaps in part a reflection of risk factors. Exposure to both cigarette smoke and carcinogens, particularly those used in the petrochemical industry, has been linked to an increased incidence of bladder cancers. The symptoms of bladder cancer resemble those of urinary tract infections: dysuria, cystitis, and the frequent need to urinate. If the tumor is diagnosed early enough, electrosurgery or resection may be sufficient to remove the lesion. If the tumor has begun to infiltrate the bladder tissue, complete removal of the bladder may be necessary. Radiation and chemotherapy are also commonly used in the treatment of certain forms of urinary tract cancers.

In May 2013, the journal *Science Translational Medicine* published a report suggesting that repeat urinary tract infections may be caused by a strain of *E. coli* bacteria present in the stomach or bladder. According to a study, an adaptable strain of *E. coli* that can survive repeated treatment efforts may be the cause of recurrent infections.

Urinary disorders in pregnant women can lead to more serious conditions. Two to ten percent of pregnancies are complicated by UTI's, and if left untreated, 25-30% of those women will develop pyelonephritis, a sever kidney infection that can be life threatening. This can cause premature birth and low birth weight. Pregnant women should be screened for bacteriuria 12 to 16 weeks after getting pregnant.

TREATMENT AND THERAPY

Standard treatment for urinary tract infections consists of a regimen of antimicrobial drugs. Ideally, the antibiotics of choice are secreted in the urine over a prolonged period, rather than achieving high concentrations in the blood serum. In this manner, the drug is directed at the infection itself, with minimal effect on the normal flora elsewhere in the body. Depending on whether the infection is limited to the lower urinary tract (urethra or bladder) or has spread to the upper tract (ureters or kidneys), the period of regimen may last for several days or up to two weeks. Generally, infections of the upper urinary tract require more prolonged treatment and may be subject to recurrence.

Standard therapy of conventional lower-tract infections routinely consists of a three-day regimen of trimethoprim-sulfamethoxazole (TMP-SMX) or TMP alone. Since most of the drug combination is excreted in the urine, there is a minimum of side effects and little danger to the normal flora within the body. The short duration of treatment also minimizes the chances of encouraging the growth of resistant populations of bacteria. Elderly patients or persons with diabetes mellitus may require longer treatment. If the person shows evidence of upper-tract infection, treatment is generally given over a two-week period.

If there is evidence of kidney involvement or inflammation (pyelonephritis), the patient is often hospitalized in order to monitor treatment, which usually involves a fourteen-day course of TMP-SMX. Severe illness or evidence of spreading may require more intensive therapy with other antibiotics. Since the flushing action of urine is itself a nonspecific means of removing bacteria from the bladder or urethra, patients are usually advised to drink as much water as possible. In this manner, weakly adherent or nonadherent bacteria may be flushed from the site of infection, reducing the number of bacteria and supplementing the course of antimicrobial therapy. In some cases, this action is sufficient to relieve symptoms or even cure the infection.

In situations in which the infection is asymptomatic, unless the situation warrants treatment (such as impending surgery), antimicrobial therapy may not be necessary, as the infection is self-limiting. Given the large proportion of persons, particularly women, who develop bacteriuria, forgoing therapy may minimize the chances for the artificial selection of resistant strains. In individuals with heart disease, renal failure, or diabetes, however, such therapy may be necessary as a preventive measure for later problems.

Bacteriuria during pregnancy represents a special situation. During early pregnancy, from 4 to 7 percent of women develop bacteriuria, which is probably related to such physiological changes as the dilation of the bladder and uterus, along with vesicoureteral (bladder and urethra) reflux. Even though the infection may be asymptomatic, urinary tract infection is associated with increased risk of both pyelonephritis and loss of the fetus; about one-third of women with untreated bacteriuria during pregnancy develop infections within the upper urinary tract by the third trimester.

For this reason, it is generally recommended that pregnant women be screened for such infections and undergo treatment if bacteriuria is present. Pregnant women generally undergo a three-day treatment regimen, though with alternative antibiotics considered safer in the presence of a developing fetus: ampicillin, nitrofurantoin, or cephalexin. Patients should be monitored at intervals during the pregnancy to prevent recurrence. If pyelonephritis should develop, the woman is routinely hospitalized to allow close monitoring of both the mother and the fetus during therapy.

Bacteriuria associated with catheterization is generally treated only when it is symptomatic since the recurrence of the infection is common; long-term treatment presents no advantage and may select for antibiotic-resistant strains. Since the catheter may harbor bacteria, it usually is removed at the start of therapy.

The treatment of sexually transmitted infections follows much the same pattern. Fortunately, most STIs can be treated or controlled. Both chlamydial infections and gonorrhea are generally treated with doxycycline, a derivative of tetracycline.

PERSPECTIVE AND PROSPECTS

Urinary tract infections are notoriously difficult to prevent. Because in most cases the associated etiological agents are the normal intestinal flora, vaccination or prophylactic use of antibiotics would be impractical. Proper hygiene appears to be the most effective means of prevention among young adults.

STIs can be a source of urinary tract disease. Either a decrease in sexual promiscuity or more effective use of physical barriers (such as condoms) is necessary to reduce the level of such forms of infection. While vaccines against some of the more prevalent forms of STI (gonorrhea, chlamydia) remain a possibility, antibiotic therapy continues to be the most reliable means to treat urinary infections within the individual. Catheters represent an important source of infection among the elderly, particularly those who are hospitalized. Since a single catheterization results in infection among less than 1 percent of patients, limiting catheterization, or avoiding it entirely, would appear to be the most effective preventive measure. The use of closed drainage systems has also reduced significantly the incidence of such infections.

Antiseptic solutions and ointments have had limited success in the prevention of urinary tract infections. The use of antibiotic therapy has been effective in the short term, but over time such therapy may simply select for resistant mutants among the microorganisms. Development of catheters that do not lend themselves to microbial colonization, or that actively inhibit microbial growth (such as silver-impregnated catheters), may reduce the chances of such types of urinary tract infections.

—*Richard Adler, Ph.D.*
Updated by Ashley Henry, MPH, RN

FOR FURTHER INFORMATION

Ammer, Christine. *The New A to Z of Women's Health: A Concise Encyclopedia.* 6th ed. New York: Checkmark Books, 2009.

Boston Women's Health Collective. *Our Bodies, Ourselves: A New Edition for a New Era.* 35th anniversary ed. New York: Simon & Schuster, 2005.

Gorbach, Sherwood L., John G. Bartlett, and Neil R. Blacklow, eds. *Infectious Diseases.* 3d ed. Philadelphia: W. B. Saunders, 2004.

Hooton, T.M. "Uncomplicated Urinary Tract Infection." *New England Journal of Medicine.* 366. (2012): 1028-1037.

Schrier, Robert W., ed. *Diseases of the Kidney and Urinary Tract.* 8th ed. Philadelphia: Wolters Kluwer Health/Lippincott Williams & Wilkins, 2007.

Stamm, W. E., and T. M. Hooton. "Current Concepts: Management of Urinary Tract Infections in Adults." *New England Journal of Medicine* 329. (1993): 1328-1334.

Urinary tract infections

CATEGORY: Disease/Disorder

KEY TERMS:

bladder: a membranous sac in which urine is collected for excretion

cystopathy: a chronic complication of diabetes characterized by a classic triad of symptoms that consist of decreased bladder sensation, increased bladder capacity, and impaired detrusor contractility

kidney stones: a hard mass formed in the kidneys, typically consisting of insoluble calcium compounds

oxalate: a salt or ester of oxalic acid, which is capable of forming an insoluble salt with calcium and interfering with its absorption by the body

urinary tract: the organs of the body that produce, store, and discharge urine; these organs include the kidneys, ureters, bladder, and urethra

voiding: the discharging of waste matter from the body

WHAT WE KNOW

A urinary tract infection (UTI) is an infection that occurs anywhere within the urinary tract system, which includes the kidneys, ureters, bladder, and urethra. The majority of UTIs are caused by the bacteria *Escherichia coli*, which lives in the bowel, and are most likely to occur in the bladder and the urethra. Although most UTIs are minor, infection can become serious if the kidneys are affected, particularly if the bacteria reach the bloodstream (i.e., septicemia).

Women are more susceptible to UTIs than men and are more prone to recurrent infection. In addition to making certain lifestyle changes (e.g., taking showers instead of baths, voiding after sexual intercourse), initiating dietary strategies can reduce the likelihood of UTI recurrence. Dietary strategies include maintaining adequate hydration, avoiding alcohol and caffeine, and regularly consuming cranberry juice.

Signs and symptoms of a UTI include the following:

- Dark, cloudy, or bloody urine that had a strong odor;
- Fever above 101 °F/38.3 °C may indicate kidney involvement (pyelonephritis)

- Pain or a burning sensation with urination;
- sensation of incomplete emptying of the bladder;
- urinary frequency and urgency;
- Lower abdominal, back, side, or groin pain and/or cramping;
- Nausea and vomiting.

RISK FACTORS

Risk factors for developing a UTI include the following:

- Women are more likely to develop UTIs due the anatomic feature of having a shorter urethra that is close to the bowel as a source of bacteria.
- Menopause increases the likelihood of developing a UTI.
- Diabetes increases the risk of developing a UTI due to the following:
- High glucose content in the urine.
- Diminished function of the immune system.
- Complications such as neuropathy, cystopathy, and renal papillary necrosis
- Urinary retention or blockage of urinary flow (e.g., narrowed urethra, enlarged prostate).
- Use of a urinary catheter because it increases urinary tract exposure to bacteria.
- Bowel incontinence.
- Kidney stones.
- Immobility.

RESEARCH FINDINGS

Researchers have repeatedly documented the benefits of cranberry intake for the prevention of UTIs in women, men, children, and patients who have neurogenic bladder due to spinal cord injury. Cranberries are rich in phytochemicals that inhibit bacterial growth. However, studies to date have not definitively shown the efficacy of cranberry intake in preventing recurrent, uncomplicated UTIs in women. For women with recurrent UTIs who are already using cranberry products or who are interested in trying cranberry products for UTI prevention, there is likely little harm in doing so aside from the increased caloric intake.

In response to an increase in antimicrobial resistance to treatment of UTIs caused by *E. coli*, researchers have been seeking alternative treatment options. Results of one study indicate that, although no direct antibacterial activity was exhibited, dandelion contains active constituents that help to protect against *E. coli* infection by decreasing bacterial colonization of bladder epithelial cells.

Individuals experiencing a UTI should become knowledgeable about dietary recommendations based on personal characteristics and health needs. Individuals should be aware of the importance of adequate hydration for maintaining urinary tract health, as proper hydration promotes flushing of bacteria out of the urinary tract and inhibits bacterial growth in the bladder. Healthy adults should consume six to eight 8 oz portions of water/day, while children require about 1.5 oz of water per pound of body weight/day. Individuals with a history of UTIs should avoid consuming alcohol and caffeine, as they can irritate the bladder. Individuals who can tolerate cranberry products can trial these products as there are generally few side effects. Individuals that have a history of kidney stones should be aware that cranberry consumption can increase risk for kidney stones because cranberry extract contains high amounts of oxalate, a primary component of kidney stones.

—*Cherie Marcel, BS*
Updated by Adrienne Jaeger, RN

FOR FURTHER INFORMATION

Bass-Ware, A., et al. "Evaluation of the effect of cranberry juice on symptoms associated with a urinary tract infection." *Urologic Nursing*, vol. 34, no. 3, 2014, 121-127.

Luthje, P., et al. "*Lactuca indica* extract interferes with uroepithelial infection by *Escherichia coli*." *Journal of Ethnopharmacology*, 135, no. 3, 2011, 672-677.

National Institutes of Health (NIH). "Urinary tract infections in adults." *National Institute of Diabetes and Digestive and Kidney Diseases (NIDDKD)*. U.S. Department of Health and Human Services. https://www.niddk.nih.gov/health-information/urologic-diseases/bladder-infection-uti-in-adults.

"Urinary Tract Infections." *MedlinePlus*, U.S. National Library of Medicine, 28 June 2018, medlineplus.gov/urinarytractinfections.html.

Uterus

CATEGORY: Anatomy

Also known as: Womb

KEY TERMS:

cervix: narrow passage forming the lower end of the uterus

corpus uteri: the main body of the uterus above the constriction behind the cervix and below the openings of the fallopian tubes

endometrium: the mucous membrane lining the uterus, which thickens during the menstrual cycle in preparation for possible implantation of an embryo

fallopian tubes: a pair of tubes along which eggs travel from the ovaries to the uterus

menstruation: the process of discharging blood and other materials from the lining of the uterus at intervals of about one lunar month from puberty until menopause, except during pregnancy; interruptions or abnormalities of the menstrual cycle can be symptoms of a larger condition

myometrium: the smooth muscle tissue of the uterus

ovulation: a time during the menstrual cycle when an ovary releases an egg or ovum

vagina: the muscular tube leading from the external genitals to the cervix of the uterus

STRUCTURE AND FUNCTIONS

The uterus provides a space for a fetus to grow. Situated in the pelvis, in front of the rectum and behind the bladder, the uterus is a bulb-shaped pouch about 3 inches (8 centimeters) in length that has heavily muscled walls and is held firmly in place by several ligaments. The uterus has two main parts: the body (corpus) includes the area above the opening to the two Fallopian tubes, while the fundus is the larger area below the Fallopian tubes to the cervix, all positioned at about a ninety-degree angle to the vagina; the cervix is a funnel that connects the body to the vagina. During a woman's reproductive years, the body is about double the size of the cervix, but that proportion reverses after menopause. The thick muscle (myometrium) of the uterus is lined with mucous membrane, the endometrium.

During ovulation, sperm can enter the body through the cervix on its way to fertilize an egg in a Fallopian tube. During menstruation, blood and excess endometrium exit the uterus through the cervix. During gestation, the uterus expands to accommodate the growth of the fetus, and during labor the walls contract to impel the fetus through the cervix and vagina.

DISORDERS AND DISEASES

Among common disorders specific to the uterus are various noncancerous growths. Fibroids are masses of muscle and fibrous tissue, of unknown cause, in the uterine wall that occur in about 20 percent of women more than thirty-five years old. If small, they are seldom noticed, but large fibroids can affect urination and menstruation and cause pain. Adenomyosis involves enlargement of the uterus after glandular tissue obtrudes into the myometrium; it can result in heavy, painful periods, sensations of pressure, and bleeding between periods. Endometriosis occurs when bits of the endometrium grow outside the uterus, which may produce pain in the lower abdomen or pelvis. The uterus is also subject to abnormal bleeding and vaginitis, inflammation caused by chemical irritants, bacteria, or yeast (candidiasis). Sometimes, because of pregnancy or birth, the uterus sags and protrudes into the vagina, a condition known as prolapsed uterus.

Two cancers in the uterus are among the most common to afflict women. Endometrial cancer grows in the membrane lining the body. It usually develops between the ages of fifty and sixty and has a high cure rate if detected early. Cervical cancer usually develops between the ages of thirty-five and fifty-five, following infection by the human papillomavirus, and is also curable if detected early. Untreated, both penetrate the uterine wall and spread to nearby organs.

—*Roger Smith, PhD*

FOR FURTHER INFORMATION

Beers, Mark H., ed. *The Merck Manual of Medical Information*. 2d ed. Whitehouse Station, N.J.: Merck Research Laboratories, 2003.

Fortner, Kimberley B., ed. *The Johns Hopkins Manual of Gynecology and Obstetrics*. Philadelphia: Lippincott Williams & Wilkins, 2007.

Thibodeau, Gary A., and Kevin T. Patton. *Structure and Function of the Body*. 14th ed. St. Louis: Mosby/Elsevier, 2012.

"Uterine Diseases." *MedlinePlus*, May 28, 2013.

V

Vaginal birth after cesarean (VBAC)

CATEGORY: Procedure

KEY TERMS:

cesarean section: a surgical operation for delivering a child by cutting through the wall of the mother's abdomen and uterus

eclampsia: a condition in which one or more convulsions occur in a pregnant woman suffering from high blood pressure, often followed by coma and posing a threat to the health of mother and baby

placenta previa: a condition in which the placenta partially or wholly blocks the neck of the uterus, thus interfering with normal delivery of a baby

prolapse: a slipping forward or down of one of the parts or organs of the body

vaginal birth: a birth in which the child is pushed out of the mother's uterus via the vagina, as opposed to being delivered surgically

INDICATIONS AND PROCEDURE

Women who have had a Cesarean section (C-section) may want to attempt a vaginal birth with their next child. A C-section is the delivery of a baby through an incision in the abdomen and uterus and is often used when pregnancy complications occur that prevent a vaginal birth. Historically, once a C-section was used to deliver a baby, future births required scheduled C-sections. In recent years, women and their physicians are considering a vaginal birth after a C-section. This procedure is called Vaginal Birth After Cesarean or VBAC. When all indications are positive for VBAC, approximately 75 percent of attempts at vaginal delivery are successful.

Cesarean sections account for 32 percent of all deliveries in the United States according to the National Center for Health Statistics, Centers for Disease Prevention and Control. Vaginal deliveries are considered safer for both the mother and baby. While vaginal births are considered the optimal way to deliver, C-sections may be necessary when labor slows, often due to a too small cervical opening or a large baby. The physician may be concerned that the baby is not receiving sufficient oxygen often indicated by a slowing heart rate. A problem with the umbilical cord such as prolapse (falling out through the cervix before the baby) may also be an indicator of need. If the baby is in an abnormal position such as feet first (breech) or positioned horizontally across the abdomen, a C-section may be the safest option. This is particularly true if the mother is carrying twins or multiple babies or if labor started too early in the pregnancy (premature).

Placenta Previa, where the placenta covers the cervix, often requires a C-section for the safe delivery of the baby. The health of the mother may also indicate a need for a C-section such as with gestational diabetes or eclampsia (high blood pressure with potential damage to other organs). Congenital defects in the baby such as hydrocephalus (an abnormal head size due to excessive spinal fluid in the brain) may require surgical delivery. Having a previous C-section may also require surgical delivery based on a variety of factors such as previous births and reason for C-sections.

The procedure to attempt VBAC begins with a decision between the physician and the pregnant woman and, once labor contractions begin, a trial labor is allowed. A Trial of Labor After Cesarean (TOLAC) is the term that defines the initial step in the procedure. The benefits of vaginal birth include a shorter recovery time, no abdominal surgery, less blood loss and a decreased chance of infection. Depending on the number of children the woman wants, VBAC may decrease the problems with multiple Cesarean deliveries. This Trial of Labor After Cesarean (TOLAC) procedure allows labor to progress normally until either the baby is safely delivered vaginally, or failure necessitates an immediate C-section. The procedure should follow a prescribed protocol to enhance patient safety. The American College of Obstetricians and Gynecologists provides a Patient Safety Checklist to determine the appropriateness of a TOL.

The decision to attempt VBAC and a Trial of Labor is determined by several factors. Steps in the VBAC procedure and Trial of Labor After C-section begin with a discussion of benefits, risks, potential for success and potential for failure and written information should be provided to the woman. The ability of the woman's chosen hospital to provide emergency care should be determined and a decision made to move to an alternate facility if necessary. A careful history and physical is taken to include health of the mother and baby, previous births, potential complications, and chance of success. If the woman wants more children, VBAC is an option as multiple C-sections often have substantial associated risks. Labor should begin naturally close to the actual due date of the mother. If labor must be induced, VABC is usually less successful.

USES AND COMPLICATIONS

When a woman becomes pregnant again after a C-section, she has two potential options. The first is scheduling another C-section and the second is attempting a vaginal birth after Cesarean. The decision to attempt a VBAC should be made between the physician and the woman after carefully considering the benefits and risks. Having a VBAC avoids another scar on the uterus, creates less pain after delivery when compared to a C-section, minimizes the chance of infection, results in a shorter hospital stay with better recovery and allows the mother's partner to participate more actively in the delivery.

The Agency for Healthcare Research and Quality, U.S. Department of Health and Human Services, has developed a Vaginal Birth After Cesarean (VBAC) Risk Calculator that predicts the probability of a successful vaginal delivery after a C-section. Factors included in the risk analysis include maternal age in years, height, weight, body mass index, race Hispanic or African-American, number of previous vaginal deliveries, any vaginal deliveries since last C-section, indications for last C-section.

Even when the decision to attempt VBAC is made, changes to the delivery plan due to happenings later in the pregnancy may prevent the procedure. If a woman chooses a C-section over VBAC, her physician may still advise VBAC if she goes into labor before the scheduled C-section procedure or if she comes into the hospital with labor well advanced and the baby is healthy.

The primary risk of a TOLAC is the possible rupture of the existing C-section scar or the rupture of the uterus itself. The incidence of ruptured uterus is 43.8 times per 100,000 live births according to the CDC. According to the American College of Obstetricians and Gynecologists, the risk of uterine rupture is less than two percent. A side to side incision, or low transverse incision, is least likely to rupture and women with one or two C-sections with this type of incision may be eligible to try TOLAC. Up and down incisions, or high vertical incisions, carry the highest risk of rupture and TOLAC should not be considered. Both ruptures may harm the baby and the mother, and if the physician deems the mother to be at high risk of uterine rupture, TOLAC should not be tried. While no set number of C-sections dictates the ability of a woman to try VBAC, doctors often feel that multiple C-sections increase the risks associated with the procedure.

A successful VBAC procedure is more likely when the woman has only one, or at the most two, previous low transverse uterine incision. This transverse incision is the most common approach. If the pregnancy is progressing normally and the reason for the previous C-section is not a current factor, the chance of success is improved. If a previous successful vaginal delivery occurred, chance of success is also enhanced. An unsuccessful VBAC procedure is more likely if labor does not start at or near the expected due date. Having a large baby, having two or more previous C-sections, a previous uterine rupture and/or a vertical incision in the uterus are all factors that may compromise a successful VBAC procedure.

A failed TOLAC requires a C-section which brings its own set of risks, including blood loss (hemorrhage), infection, the need to remove the uterus (hysterectomy), bladder or bowel complications, blood clots and maternal and/or fetal loss. An unplanned hysterectomy occurs 51.1 times per 100,000 live births. The need for anesthesia for an emergency C-section may be a risk factor for complication.

Vaginal birth after C-section can be a safe alternative for the pregnant woman if a careful assessment of all potential factors occurs. Prenatal care for both C-section and potential VBAC are the same. Once the labor trial begins, the woman is more carefully monitored than for that of a normal vaginal delivery. If any problems arise, an emergency C-section is done. There is no statistically significant difference in morbidity between vaginal and C-section deliveries so attempting a Trial of Labor for most women post C-section is a viable possibility according to the Center for Health Statistics.

Patricia Stanfill Edens, PhD, RN, LFACHE

FOR FURTHER INFORMATION

Cunningham, FG, and CE Wells. Patient education: Vaginal birth after cesarean delivery (VBAC) (Beyond the Basics) *UpToDate Wolters Kluwer*. Available from: http://www.uptodate.com/contents/vaginal-birth-after-cesarean-delivery-vbac-beyond-the-basics?source=search_result&search=vbac&selectedTitle=1%7E2

Practice Guideline: Planning for Labor and Vaginal Birth After Cesarean Delivery: Guidelines from the AAFP American Academy of Family Physicians. American Academy of Family Physicians. Available from: http://www.aafp.org/afp/2015/0201/p197.html.

Vaginal Birth after Cesarean Delivery-Deciding on a Trial of Labor After Cesarean Delivery. *American College of Obstetricians and Gynecologists*. Available from: https://www.acog.org/Patients/FAQs/Vaginal-Birth-After-Cesarean-Delivery-Deciding-on-a-Trial-of-Labor-After-Cesarean-Delivery.

Vaginal Birth after Cesarean Section Risk Calculator. *Agency for Healthcare Research and Quality, U.S. Department of Health and Human Services*. Available from: https://innovations.ahrq.gov/qualitytools/vaginal-birth-after-cesarean-vbac-risk-calculator

What is vaginal birth after cesarean (VBAC)? *Eunice Kennedy Shriver National Institute of Child Health and Human Development*. Available from: https://www.nichd.nih.gov/health/topics/labor-delivery/topicinfo/Pages/vbac.aspx.

Vertigo

CATEGORY: Disease/Disorder

KEY TERMS:

ataxia: coordinated movement difficulties

auditory nerve: the eighth cranial nerve, which conveys information from the ear to the brain

disequilibrium: off-balance sensation

dizziness: non-specific term that includes vertigo, fainting, and disequilibrium

electronystagmography: specialized eye movement measurements

endolymph: inner-ear fluid

labyrinth: mazelike system of canals in the inner ear

Ménière's disease: a disorder affecting endolymph

nystagmus: rhythmic involuntary movements of the eyes

oscillopsia: the sensation of bouncing vision

otoliths: granular bones of the inner ear

otorhinolaryngologist: the ear, nose, and throat (ENT) specialist

proprioception: the ability to locate the body in space

tinnitus: ringing in the ear

vestibular: the inner ear, vision, and nervous systems responsible for balance

CAUSES AND SYMPTOMS

Vertigo is a sensation of spinning or movement. Dizziness and disequilibrium are broader terms that include vertigo in some cases.

Vertigo results from disorders of the inner ear or central nervous system. Inner-ear causes include vestibular injury, labyrinthitis, vestibular neuritis, acute or recurrent vestibulopathy, benign positional vertigo, Ménière's disease, perilymphatic fistula, and vestibular toxicity from drugs. Labyrinthitis or vestibular nerve dysfunction can result from trauma, cancer (acoustic neuroma), benign tumor, infection, connective tissue disorders, autoimmune disorder, otosclerosis, or middle-ear infection. Central nervous system causes of vertigo include brain stem stroke, cervical vertigo, tumors adjacent to the brain stem, migraines, multiple sclerosis, cranial nerve injury or degeneration, seizure disorders, hereditary familial ataxia, and inflammatory paraneoplastic syndromes. Problems with peripheral nerves and vision can contribute to vertigo.

Three systems work together to provide balance. The first is the inner-ear labyrinth system of tiny canals filled with a fluid called endolymph and tiny bones called otoliths. These canals contain tiny hair cells that sense endolymph movement. Information from the inner ear is conveyed to the brain through the eighth cranial nerve (auditory nerve) as well as branches of the seventh cranial nerve (facial nerve). The second system, vision, provides information to the brain via the optic nerve. The third system is proprioception, the ability to orient the body in space using input from the musculoskeletal system and from peripheral nerves. Specialized areas of the brain process information from these three systems to provide balance and maintain the vestibular ocular reflex and the vestibular spinal reflex. Adaptation to variations in input from these systems allows for activities such as figure skaters being able to tolerate high-speed spins. Balance is also possible with just two of three balance systems, allowing normal individuals to stand with eyes closed and not lose balance. Disruption of one or more balance systems causes vertigo.

Additional symptoms may include tinnitus, disequilibrium, hearing loss, sensitivity to sound, nausea, blurred vision, oscillopsia, nystagmus, ataxia, clumsiness, or headaches. Symptoms of underlying disease may be present. Onset and additional symptoms; examination of the ear, nose, and throat; and a general neurological examination will help in diagnosis. Specialized techniques include the Hallpike maneuver (tilting the head over the edge of the examination table) and the fistula test, done by plugging one ear.

Women are more likely than men to experience vertigo and dizziness. For example, hormonal changes can result in dizziness during PMS or menopause. Dizziness many accompany anemia in both pregnant and non-pregnant women of diverse ages. Women who skip meals due to a busy lifestyle may have dizziness associated with low blood sugar or diabetes. Exercise activities such as yoga or Pilates often require the participant to lie down with the head held in an extended position which can produce dizziness.

Diagnosis of the underlying disorder is necessary for treatment. Testing may include complete eye examination, computed tomography (CT) scan, magnetic resonance imaging (MRI), electronystagmography, hearing test, and rotational chair testing

TREATMENT AND THERAPY

Treatment of vertigo depends on the cause. Ménière's disease and other inner-ear conditions such as vestibular neuronitis may be treated with a salt-restricted

Information on Vertigo

Causes: Inner ear or central nervous system disorders
Symptoms: Sensation of movement or spinning, sometimes accompanied by tinnitus, nausea, disequilibrium, clumsiness, ataxia
Duration: Varies depending on cause; may be episodic
Treatment: Depends on cause; may include otolith repositioning, inner ear surgery, low-salt diet, medications, vestibular rehabilitation therapy, treatment of underlying diseases

diet, diuretics, motion sickness medication, antinausea medication, steroid injections, lifestyle modification including stress reduction, or inner- ear surgery. Otolith repositioning involves specialized physical therapy maneuvers that may be helpful for benign positional vertigo. Perilymphatic fistula may respond to bed rest. Middle-ear infections are treated with antibiotics.

Vertigo requires treatment aimed at correcting the underlying disorder. For example, acoustic neuromas may be treated with surgery and radiation. Symptoms from multiple sclerosis may respond to oral or intravenous steroids. Diagnosis and treatment of vertigo will require a team of specialists, including a family physician, otorhinolaryngologist, neurologist, audiologist, internist, physical therapist, and occupational therapist.

Vestibular rehabilitation treats vertigo and other balance and dizziness problems through adaptation. Because vision is an important part of the balance system, significant vision impairment might limit rehabilitation effectiveness. Exercises prescribed by a physical or occupational therapist target activities that are problematic and may be done at home, in a rehabilitation center, or both. Exercises include targeted movements such as bending over, walking with one foot in front of the other, or walking with the head turned. Rehabilitation can take several weeks to several months.

PERSPECTIVE AND PROSPECTS

Vertigo and dizziness are common symptoms. Because of the variety of causes, some otolaryngologists and neurologists focus solely on the diagnosis and treatment of vertigo and dizziness.

Ménière's disease is the best-known cause of vertigo, first presented by Prospère Ménière to the French Academy of Medicine in 1861. Other inner-ear problems cause similar symptoms, but Ménière's disease specifically affects the endolymph fluid, causing vertigo and tinnitus. With modern diagnosis, Ménière's disease is now known to be less common than once thought.

Several famous people may have suffered from Ménière's disease or other forms of vertigo. Julius Caesar was said to have "falling disease" attributed to Ménière's disease or epilepsy. Other famous sufferers include artist Vincent Van Gogh, poet Emily Dickinson, and film star Marilyn Monroe.

Fortunately, vertigo does not usually indicate serious or life-threatening disease. However, it can take time and numerous tests to pinpoint the cause. With patience and persistence, most people can find a treatment or combination of treatments to reduce or eliminate their symptoms.

—*E. E. Anderson Penno, M.D., M.S., FRCSC*
Updated by Marylane Wade Koch, MSN, RN

FOR FURTHER INFORMATION

Alan, Rick, and Kari Kassir. "Meniere's Disease." *Health Library*, Sept. 10, 2012.

"Causes of Dizziness." *Vestibular Disorders Association*, 2012.

"Dizziness During Menopause." *Menopause Now, 2019.* https://www.menopausenow.com/dizziness

"Dizziness and Vertigo." *MedlinePlus*, May 17, 2013.

Brady, Krissy. 8 "Things You Need to Know About Vertigo." *Women's Health*, Apr 13, 2017. https://www.womenshealthmag.com/health/a19972073/vertigo-facts/

Fauci, Anthony, et al. *Harrison's Principles of Internal Medicine.* 18th ed. New York: McGraw-Hill. 2012.

Jasmin, Luc, et al. "Vertigo-Associated Disorders." *MedlinePlus*, Nov. 2, 2012.

Poe, Dennis. *The Consumer Handbook on Dizziness and Vertigo.* Sedona, Ariz.: Auricle Ink, 2005.

Schroeder, Karen, and Rimas Lukas. "Vertigo." *Health Library*, Apr. 25, 2013.

West, John. *Best and Taylor's Physiological Basis of Medical Practice.* 12th ed. Baltimore: Williams & Wilkins, 1991.

Vision disorders

CATEGORY: Disease/Disorder

KEY TERMS:

aqueous fluid: a clear, watery liquid that fills the region inside the front of the eyeball between the lens and cornea

cataract: a loss of transparency in the lens of the eye, commonly associated with aging

cornea: the transparent, curved front surface of the eyeball, providing protection and focusing light onto the retina; most of the focusing power of the eye occurs here

glaucoma: an increase in the eye's internal pressure that can damage the optic nerve and eventually lead to blindness

laser: a very intense beam of light; used in eye surgery for glaucoma, a detached retina, or hemorrhaging blood vessels

lens: the transparent part of the eye behind the cornea that is responsible for changing shape to allow the eye to accommodate and fine-tune focus

macular degeneration: a common disorder primarily affecting the elderly that causes deterioration of the macula. The macula is the visual center of the retina and is responsible for high acuity color vision. Patients with macular degeneration often complain of central vision loss

retina: a thin membrane, lining the inside back surface of the eyeball, where light is transformed into electrical signals that are transmitted to the brain

vitreous fluid: the clear, watery liquid in the center of the eyeball

CAUSES AND SYMPTOMS

Women are affected by blindness and visual impairment to a much greater degree than men. One systematic review of global population-based blindness surveys carried out between 1980 – 2000 showed that blindness is about 40 percent more common in women compared to men (in persons older than 50 years). Since 2000, further research has shown that several rapid assessments of avoidable blindness studies (RAABs) have confirmed the earlier findings. It appears that being a woman is a significant risk factor for some eye diseases, but it is also an important factor in the use of eye care services. Women account for about 64 per cent of the total number of blind persons globally (a summary value). Furthermore, in many areas, men are twice as likely as women to be able to access eye care.

The visual pathway in the eye consists of two main components: light focusing and light transformation. When light enters the eye, it first passes through the cornea and lens. The cornea and lens focus the light onto the retina similar to the way a camera lens focuses light on film. Focused light then passes through the vitreous humor and reaches the retina, where photoreceptor cells transform light information into electrical and chemical signals that are transmitted through the optic nerve to the brain. Disruptions at any point in this pathway may cause a variety of visual impairments.

The most common defects in the visual system affect the cornea, lens, and the muscles that control the lens. These include nearsightedness (myopia), farsightedness (hyperopia), and astigmatism. Together, these conditions are called refractive errors because the cornea-lens focusing system fails to appropriately bend light onto the retina. Fortunately, refractive errors are easily corrected by eyeglasses or contact lenses.

Myopia and hyperopia are caused by a mismatch between the focusing power of the cornea and lens and the length of the eye. For a nearsighted person, light comes to a focus in front of the retina; a diverging lens is needed to move the image farther back. For a farsighted person, light is focused at a point past the retina, so a converging lens is needed instead.

Astigmatism is caused by a deformity of the eye. Not all eyes are perfect spheres – as a result, the eye's horizontal curvature may require a different prescription than the vertical curvature. This can be visualized by imagining a ball being squeezed on two sides and forming an oval or football-like shape. Astigmatism can be corrected by prescribing glasses with different focal lengths in the horizontal and vertical planes. The prescription must specify the angle at which the deformation of the eyeball is maximized.

Cataracts are caused by clouding of the inside surface of the lens and are typically seen in older adults. While cataracts are a normal part of the aging process, they may also be seen at birth or after an injury. The cause of cataracts is not fully understood and has been tied to a long-term reaction between glucose and protein molecules that results in lens clouding. Onset of cataracts may be delayed by healthy lifestyle behaviors. Cataracts are progressive and may eventually require surgical removal of the lens and implantation of an artificial replacement. Women have a slightly higher incidence of cataract and tend to have longer life expectancy than men. Therefore, ideally, women should account for 60–65 percent of all cataract operations. However, many studies have shown that more men than women received cataract surgery.

Glaucoma typically affects individuals over the age of 40 and is caused by excess fluid pressure inside the eye. There are two forms of glaucoma – acute angle closure glaucoma and chronic open angle glaucoma. Acute angle closure glaucoma occurs spontaneously or is caused by eye disease, trauma, or medications and is characterized by sudden onset eye pain and loss of vision. Often, the pupil is unable to dilate or constrict. Acute angle closure glaucoma is a medical emergency that may result in permanent vision loss without urgent treatment. In contrast, chronic open angle glaucoma is characterized by long-term pressure buildup in the eye and is characterized by slow loss of peripheral vision that may not be noticed at first. Pressure caused by acute and chronic glaucoma can cause damage to the optic nerve and lead to blindness. Epidemiological studies in eastern Asia have shown that women have a higher incidence of primary angle-closure glaucoma (PACG) compared to men. However, there appears to be no sex-specific difference in incidence of primary open-angle glaucoma.

The retina is a thin membrane at the back of the eye that is fed by a network of tiny blood vessels. The retina is made of multiple layers of different types of cells that are responsible for transforming light into electrical and chemical information. Damage to the retina disrupts this process and results in vision loss and potential blindness.

There are two critical types of photoreceptor cells in the retina. Rod cells, which exist at the edges of the retina, are responsible for black and white, low-contrast vision that enables night-time and peripheral vision. Cone cells are in the center of the retina and are responsible for high acuity color vision. The center of the retina is called the macula, which has a high density of cone cells and is responsible for high-acuity visual tasks like reading.

Diabetic retinopathy is a disease associated with diabetes that is characterized by long-term damage to the vessels feeding the retina. Patients with diabetes are at a higher risk of vascular disease, and the vessels feeding the retina often become enlarged and bleed. This is an irreversible cause of blindness in diabetic patients, who are strongly encouraged to see an ophthalmologist on a yearly basis.

Macular degeneration (AMD) is a condition that commonly affects older adults. In the dry stages of macular degeneration, a yellow substance called drusen begins to deposit on the surface of the retina. While this may cause some visual disturbances, full vision loss may not occur until the wet stages of macular degeneration, during which long-term damage to the retina results in blood vessel growth and hemorrhage. Typically, patients with AMD complain of loss of central vision that cannot be corrected by glasses.

Finally, retinal detachments vision loss that requires urgent care. Trauma or leakage of fluid under the retina can result in the separation of the retina from the underlying epithelium. Depending on the size of the separation, this may be known as a retinal "tear" (if small) or "detachment" (if large). Detachment of the retina in the macular area can lead to sudden loss of vision. Retinal detachments require urgent surgical correction and may lead to permanent vision loss if left untreated. Patients are recommended to see an ophthalmologist immediately if they notice a cascade of black shapes known as "floaters," sensations that a curtain is falling over their vision, or new onset of flashing lights.

TREATMENT AND THERAPY

Optometrists are trained to detect deviations from normal vision and to measure patients' nearsightedness, farsightedness, and astigmatism. After measuring the degree of each of these abnormalities, they can prescribe corrective lenses. Ophthalmologists are able to take a closer look at the eye and treat cataracts, glaucoma, and retinal diseases.

The history of eyeglasses has been traced back to the thirteenth century, when Roger Bacon, a Catholic scholar, described the use of convex glass to enlarge writing. Some medieval paintings show elderly noblemen wearing eyeglasses. However, no significant medical innovations were made until

Benjamin Franklin invented bifocals in 1780. Plastic lenses were introduced in the late 1940s with the advantages of lighter weight and greater durability.

An alternative to eyeglasses came in the 1950s with the development of contact lenses. Contact lenses rest over the surface of the cornea. While hard contact lenses are convenient, many wearers experience eye dryness and irritation. Daily-wear soft contact lenses became available in the 1970s. Soft contact lenses have the advantage of being more comfortable and gas-permeable than hard contacts but are also more prone to infection and must be cleaned regularly. Most recently, soft contacts for extended wear (up to two weeks without removal), bifocal gas-permeable contacts, and inexpensive, disposable contacts (to be discarded after two or three weeks) have been introduced.

In the 1970s, eye specialists began to investigate the possibility of reshaping the eyeball to do away with eyeglasses completely. The first attempt involved pressing directly against the cornea with a hard lens to temporarily flatten it. A Soviet physician, Svyatoslav Fyodorov, later developed Radial Keratotomy (RK), a surgical procedure to flatten the cornea permanently. Here, a series of shallow incisions are made in the outer part of the cornea. As the incisions heal, the cornea bulges slightly near the edges and flattens near the middle. While thousands of patients underwent RK surgery between 1980 and 1993, the procedure remained controversial. The main problem was that the procedure could overcorrect or under-correct the patient's prescription. Some ophthalmologists were also concerned about possible long-term effects of scars on the cornea.

Another technique to alter the shape of the cornea is called keratomileusis. The outer half of the patient's cornea is removed and frozen, and then reshaped with a computer-controlled lathe to a predetermined curvature. After thawing, the cornea is sewn back into place, where it acts as a permanent contact lens. Keratomileusis can correct both myopia and hyperopia.

Laser-assisted in situ keratomileusis (LASIK) was popularized at the end of the twentieth century. In LASIK surgery, the cornea is reshaped to help patients overcome myopia, hyperopia, or astigmatism. The procedure is done with a cool beam laser that removes thin layers of tissue from selected sites on the cornea to change its curvature. Success rates are high: 90 to 95% of patients achieve 20/40 vision, and 65 to 75% of patients achieve 20/20 vision or better. Patients with 20/20 vision are able to see objects 20 feet away that others are able to see at 20 feet. Patients with 20/40 vision need to stand at 20 feet to see an object that others are able to see at 40 feet.

The standard treatment for cataracts is surgical removal of the defective lens followed by implantation of an artificial, plastic lens. Ophthalmologists routinely perform cataract surgery using only local anesthetic so that the patient can go home without an overnight hospital stay. Cataract surgery has been well-documented over the past several decades and has attained inspiring success rates.

First line treatment for chronic glaucoma includes eyedrops to reduce pressure in the eyeball. These eyedrops work by either improving the drainage of aqueous humor from the eye or by decreasing the production of aqueous humor in the eye. These eyedrops include a variety of medications, including prostaglandins, beta blockers, alpha-adrenergic agonists, and carbonic anhydrase inhibitors. Laser or ophthalmologic surgery can also achieve similar results by enlarging the drainage channel of the eye. By creating an opening at the edge of the iris, aqueous fluid is able to drain between the lens and cornea. While glaucoma damage to the optic nerve cannot be repaired, prompt treatment can prevent vision deterioration and full loss of vision if addressed early.

There are a variety of treatment approaches for AMD and diabetic retinopathy. The majority of these treatments are geared towards reducing the overgrowth of blood vessels in the retina. This may involve anti-vascular endothelial growth factor (anti-VEGF) injections or the use of laser therapy to burn new blood vessels.

Retinal detachment is a medical emergency that requires surgery. The most common surgical procedure for repairing a retinal detachment is vitrectomy, during which surgeons use small instruments and enter through the outside of the eye to flatten the retina against the back of the eye. Surgeons often insert a gas or fluid bubble into the eye to ensure that the retina remains flattened against the eye. Patients may also have a procedure known as a

---

Information on Vision Disorders

Causes: Infection, disease, allergies, injury, cataracts, glaucoma, refractive errors (nearsightedness, farsightedness, astigmatism)

Symptoms: Vary; may include eye redness, itchiness, or inflammation; blurred or disrupted vision; bleeding or hemorrhaging from eyes

Duration: Acute to chronic

Treatments: Depend on cause; may include medicated eye drops, corrective lenses, laser surgery, antibiotics, corneal transplantation

---

scleral buckle, where a buckle is stretched around the outside of the eye to help hold the retina in place. The FDA has recently approved the use of electrical stimulation to restore retinal function in certain diseases; however, further testing is needed before this technology is fully implemented in patients.

Perspective and Prospects

The eyes provide humans with a vast array of information about the outside world. Any defect or deterioration of normal vision can profoundly impact patients' quality of life and individuals' social, economic, and educational well-being. However, society is gradually becoming more sympathetic to handicapped individuals and is increasing access for patients who suffer from blindness. Braille printing, guide dogs, and books recorded on audiotape are helpful developments for the blind. The U.S. Congress in 1992 passed the Americans with Disabilities Act, which mandates improved access for the visually impaired in facilities that serve the general public. Nevertheless, retaining good vision and preventing further deterioration will continue to be a vital part of overall health care.

—*Hans G. Graetzer, Ph.D.*
Updated by Derrick Cheng, BSc, BA, and Carol Shi, BA

For Further Information

"Eye Health and Safety." *Prevent Blindness America*, 2011.
"Healthy Eyes." *National Eye Institute*, 2013.
Parker, James N., and Philip M. Parker, eds. *The Official Patient's Sourcebook on Myopia.* San Diego, Calif.: Icon Health, 2004.

"Refractive Errors." *MedlinePlus*, May 20, 2013.

Sutton, Amy L. *Ophthalmic Disorders Sourcebook*. 3d ed. Detroit, Mich.: Omnigraphics, 2008.

"Vision Impairment and Blindness." *MedlinePlus*, May 28, 2013.

"What Is Low Vision?" *EyeSmart*. American Academy of Ophthalmology, 2013.

Von Willebrand's disease

CATEGORY: Disease/Disorder

Also known as: Pseudohemophilia, angiohemophilia, vascular hemophilia

KEY TERMS:

autosomal dominant: one of many ways that a trait or disorder can be passed down through families; if an individual gets the abnormal gene from only one parent, they can get the disease

autosomal recessive: one of many ways that a trait or disorder can be passed down through families; both parents must pass down the abnormal gene

menorrhagia: abnormally heavy bleeding at menstruation

platelet: a small colorless disk-shaped cell fragment without a nucleus, found in large numbers in blood and involved in clotting

postpartum hemorrhage: the loss of more than 500 ml or 1,000 ml of blood within the first 24 hours following childbirth

CAUSES AND SYMPTOMS

Von Willebrand disease (vWD) is a genetic disorder affecting the normal clotting function of platelets in the blood. There are three types of vWD found within families, all due to inheriting mutations in the *VWF* gene. The VWF gene encodes the von Willebrand factor (vWF) protein, which is an integral member of the blood clotting machinery within the body. After an injury, blood clots seal off damaged blood vessels and staunch further blood loss. vWF works to glue blood clots together and prevent the breakdown of other blood clotting proteins. Failure of proper vWF function prevents normal blood clot formation, which can cause prolonged bleeding episodes.

The pattern of inheritance of vWD may be autosomal dominant or autosomal recessive, although

with either, both males and females are affected equally; some persons could be carriers of the defective gene without exhibiting any symptoms. There is another form of vWD called "acquired von Willebrand syndrome." This disease is not caused by inheriting mutations in *VWF*, and, therefore, does not run in families.

This disease is characterized by the qualitative or quantitative deficiency of von Willebrand factor (vWF). vWF is found in platelets and the endothelium (lining) of blood vessels and facilitates the adhesion of platelets to one another to form a stable clot when blood vessels have been injured. Therefore, patients with vWD exhibit the signs and symptoms of blood clotting abnormality that manifests as excessive bleeding. Three types of vWD are recognized: type I vWD, with decreased levels of the protein vWF; type II vWD, with normal levels but decreased activity of vWF; and type III vWD, the most severe form of the disease, with a nearly complete deficiency of vWF.

Patients with mild or moderate vWD (type I or type II) can become symptomatic at any age and usually exhibit one or more of the following symptoms: easy bruising, bleeding gums, frequent nosebleeds, bleeding points under the skin (subcutaneous hemorrhages), prolonged bleeding after injury or surgery of any kind, and, in women, menorrhagia, or excessive bleeding during menstrual periods. Since vWD is the most prevalent inherited bleeding disorder among American women, the presence of chronic menorrhagia should be addressed by a proper medical evaluation, performed by a healthcare professional.

If heavy menstrual bleeding intervenes with daily activities, the use of progestin-only contraceptives such as *Nexplanon*, DMPA or levonorgestrel-releasing intrauterine device may help. Timely vWD diagnosis becomes very important for pregnancy management to avoid serious complications in case of spontaneous abortion, performing epidural anesthesia, addressing a selection of delivery method and managing postpartum hemorrhage.

Patients with severe type III vWD become symptomatic at an early age and exhibit symptoms similar to hemophilia, with bleeding into and pain in the joints (hemarthrosis), spontaneous bleeding into the gastrointestinal tract and from the mucous membranes that is potentially life-threatening, and painful bleeding into the muscles (hematomas). Some patients with type III disease also have multiple episodes of acute gastrointestinal bleeding and are often misdiagnosed. Some patients also have decreased factor VIII, which is deficient in hemophilia. The symptoms of vWD appear to decrease with advancing age, and they are milder in pregnancy, when factor VIII levels are high. Typically, bleeding time is prolonged in all patients with vWD.

The disease is diagnosed in the laboratory using specialized blood tests, such as the von Willebrand factor antigen (which measures the amount of vWF in blood), Ristocetin cofactor (which measures the function of vWF in blood), vWF multimers, and factor VIII levels. A careful family history of the disease should help distinguish it from the rarer hemophilia. A correlation of family history, laboratory findings, and clinical findings may be needed in order to diagnose the condition in mild cases of vWD, in which diagnosis is difficult. A few cases of acquired vWD have been identified, with antibodies against vWF being present. Such persons may be otherwise healthy or may also exhibit other immune-mediated diseases.

TREATMENT AND THERAPY

The aim of therapy for vWD is to stop the bleeding and to prevent further episodes. Both goals can be met by increasing vWF and/or factor VIII levels in the blood. This result can be achieved by many methods, the most common being the administration of the drug DDAVP (desmopressin acetate) by a nasal or intravenous route. This drug does not seem to have a beneficial effect in type III disease, and these patients may need intravenous infusions of concentrates of factor VIII and vWF. For women with heavy menstrual bleeding, estrogen therapy in the form of oral contraceptive (birth control) pills is a good alternative, as it has been observed that estrogen increases the levels of vWF in the blood. Local antifibrinolytic drugs, which delay the dissolution of the clot, are useful in milder presentations of the disease (such as nosebleeds) or following dental procedures.

Preventive care should be taken by all persons suspected of having vWD. Adequate care and treatment taken prior to any dental procedure or surgical intervention should prevent the excessive loss of blood. Children with the disease are advised against engaging in rough and vigorous sports activities with a high

> ### Information on Von Willebrand's Disease
>
> **Causes:** Genetic disorder
> **Symptoms:** Depend on type; may include easy bruising, bleeding gums, frequent nosebleeds, subcutaneous hemorrhages, prolonged bleeding after injury or surgery, menorrhagia in women, spontaneous bleeding, hematomas
> **Duration:** Chronic
> **Treatments:** DDAVP (desmopressin acetate) nasally or intravenously, intravenous factor VIII and vWF, progestin-only contraceptives, antifibrinolytic drugs, care prior to dental or surgical procedures

potential for injury. Patients should also be cautioned against the excessive intake of aspirin and other nonsteroidal anti-inflammatory drugs (NSAIDs), as they worsen the symptoms of vWD.

PERSPECTIVE AND PROSPECTS

In 1925, Finnish physician Erik von Willebrand identified a bleeding disorder in the natives of the Aland Islands and named it after himself. Later, it was found that the disease was caused by a defect in one of the clotting factors, and the factor was also named after the brilliant physician. Today, vWD is recognized as the most common inherited bleeding disorder. It is estimated to affect 1-3 percent of the population, with an equal distribution between the two sexes. It is important to distinguish this condition from the better-known hemophilia. The diagnosis of vWD in women is significant, since it is a popular misconception that bleeding disorders occur only in men. The present drug therapy available to combat the disease is quite effective in reducing the bleeding that occurs. Modern day medicine has reduced the problems of blood infections associated with the administration of cryoprecipitates. Further research is being conducted to develop an effective recombinant vWF.

—*Rashmi Ramasubbaiah, M.D., and Venkat Raghavan Tirumala, M.D., M.H.A.*
Updated by Maria Haslip, PhD, RN

FOR FURTHER INFORMATION

Fauci, Anthony S., et al, eds. *Harrison's Principles of Internal Medicine.* 20th ed. New York: McGraw-Hill, 2018.

Greer, John, et al., eds. *Wintrobe's Clinical Hematology.* 12th ed. Philadelphia: Wolters Kluwer/Lippincott Williams & Wilkins Health, 2014.

Hoffmanm R et al, eds. *Hematology: basic principles and Practice*, 7th ed. Philadelphia: Elsevier, 2018

"Platelet Disorders." *MedlinePlus*, February 28, 2019.

Rosenblum, Laurie, and Michael Woods. "Von Willebrand Disease." *Health Library*, Nov. 26, 2012.

Ruggeri, Zaverio M., ed. *Von Willebrand Factor and the Mechanisms of Platelet Function.* New York: Springer, 1998.

"von Willebrand Disease" *National Heart, Lung, and Blood Institute*, February 28, 2019.

Von Willebrand disease in women. Committee Opinion No. 580. *American College of Obstetricians and Gynecologists*, 122: 2013.

W

Weaning

CATEGORY: Procedure

KEY TERMS:

engorgement: an uncomfortable, often painful condition in which the breasts are overly full of milk

overfeeding: the provision of more milk or formula for an infant than is necessary; may result in regurgitation

INDICATIONS AND PROCEDURES

For a woman who is well-informed about breast-feeding, the appropriate time to wean her infant will become clear if she is sensitive to the child's cues. Other factors affecting a mother's decision to wean her child include family or cultural pressures, pressure from the partner, and personal beliefs about when weaning should occur. Often, weaning takes place between periods of great developmental activity for the child: between eight to nine months, twelve to fourteen months, eighteen months, two years, or three years of age.

Most babies are weaned before nine months of age. Mothers who want to wean their children from breast milk to a bottle before nine months of age need to prepare the child for the process by introducing a bottle when the infant is about six to eight weeks old. They can do so without compromising the nutrition of breast milk by pumping and offering breast milk occasionally through a bottle. Infants who are not used to the bottle after that age are more reluctant to accept it later. If the mother decides to wean the baby before one year of age, a commercial formula should be used for supplementation. Cow's milk is not appropriate for infants under one year of age. Honey should never be used to sweeten the formula because of the danger of infant botulism.

When a mother decides to wean her child from breast milk, she should supplement one bottle (or cup) of formula for the least important breast-feeding session of the day. This should be done over a period of two days to a week. If weaning is conducted abruptly, the mother's breasts may become painfully engorged with milk. Breast-feeding sessions associated with meals can be easily forgone, as the child has less desire for milk during those times. Gradually, the mother can substitute more breast-feeding sessions with bottle-feeding. Many mothers continue to breast-feed their infants in the morning and/or in the evenings for many months before weaning is completed. This has many advantages, in that both the baby and the mother will have time to adjust to their new feeding schedule. Weaning mothers should continue to drink plenty of fluids, as restricting fluid intake will not prevent engorgement. Typically, this late form of engorgement passes in one or two days after the weaning process begins.

When bottle-feeding babies, mothers should assume the same position with their infants as they did when breast-feeding. Most women cradle their infants in the crook of their arm for comfort and intimacy. The bottle's nipple should have a hole big enough to allow milk to flow in drops when turned upside down. Too big a hole, however, can lead to overfeeding and regurgitation by the baby. Cleanliness is important when bottle-feeding; appropriate methods of formula preparation and the sterilization of bottles must be followed.

Related to weaning is getting an infant to discontinue the use of a pacifier. Just as in weaning a baby from breast milk, this process has to be gradual and gentle. The best time to wean a baby from a pacifier is when he or she becomes more mobile, in order to prevent the pacifier from becoming a habit. The parent can remove the pacifier after the baby is asleep. Gradually, pacifier use can be restricted to nap time and bedtime. Parents should encourage the baby to stop using the pacifier by offering praise and being patient.

Once a baby starts to use a cup, it is important to make sure that the cup is heavy enough to be stable on a flat surface such as a table or high chair tray. The cup needs to be small enough for the baby to hold properly. Special training cups with spill proof tops are widely available. Using a floor mat often saves the parent time in cleaning up after a spill.

USES AND COMPLICATIONS

If both the mother and the child are comfortable with the timing of the weaning, it can be accomplished with minimal difficulty. Nevertheless, weaning is a time of emotional separation for mother and child, and they may be unwilling to give up the closeness that nursing offers. Hence, it is important to plan comforting, consoling, and play activities to replace breast-feeding. Weaning is best conducted in a gradual manner.

One worry that mothers often express when switching from breast to bottle is uncertainty as to how much milk an infant needs. Parents should avoid overfeeding or feeding infants every time they cry. They should also avoid setting artificial goals such as "the baby must consume 8 ounces," feeding the infant until the goal is reached even though the baby may no longer be hungry. Overfeeding results in obesity.

PERSPECTIVE AND PROSPECTS

In recent years, the American Pediatrics Association has emphasized the importance of breast-feeding through a baby's first year. Physiologically, breast milk helps the infant fight infections by supplying antibodies and by coating the intestines with bacteria-fighting liquids. Developmentally, it has been found that breast-feeding mothers are more likely to engage in frequent interactive behavior with their infants, report that their infants have "easy temperaments," and engage in more flexible caregiving. It has been found that infants who are breast-fed retain an advantage in cognitive ability as measured by intelligence quotient (IQ) tests well into their third year of life.

For a majority of women who end breast-feeding prior to one year, inadequate milk supply and employment are the major reasons cited. Whether the result of choice or necessity, weaning is a natural process and a milestone for both mother and child.

—*Gowri Parameswaran*

FOR FURTHER INFORMATION

Arvedson, Joan. "Weaning Preparation for Children Fed by G-Tube." *The Oley Foundation*, June 26, 2013.

"Breastfeeding." *womenshealth.gov*, August 1, 2010.

Hillis, Anne, and Penelope Stone. *Breast, Bottle, Bowl: The Best Fed Baby Book*. Rev. ed. Pymble, N.S.W.: HarperCollins, 2008.

Meek, Joan Younger, and Sherill Tippins, eds. *American Academy of Pediatrics New Mother's Guide to Breastfeeding*. New York: Bantam Books, 2006.

"Solid foods: How to get your baby started." *Mayo Clinic*, June 6, 2013.

Weight loss and gain

CATEGORY: Biology

KEY TERMS:

basal metabolism: the energy used to fuel the involuntary activities necessary to sustain life (respiration, circulation, and hormonal activity)

energy balance: the state in which kilocalories from ingested food are equal to kilocalories expended

energy-yielding nutrient: nutrients that supply the body with energy (fat provides 9 kilocalories per gram, while carbohydrates and protein provide 4 kilocalories per gram)

kilocalorie: the amount of heat necessary to raise the temperature of a kilogram of water 1 degree Celsius; the unit of measure for the energy content of foods, also called a Calorie

nutrient density: the amount of nutrients provided per kilocalorie of food

wasting: severe weight loss characterized by the loss of muscle tissue and body fat deposits

PROCESS AND EFFECTS

Weight loss or gain is dependent on a variety of factors, a major one being the balance of energy expended versus energy ingested. Thus, weight is determined by how many kilocalories of energy are expended. Normal day-to-day fluctuations in weight are typically minor changes attributed to shifts in body fluid and are not related to energy balance (input versus output). Input kilocalories refer to those from fat, protein, carbohydrates, and alcohol. Although alcohol is not considered an energy yielding nutrient, it provides 7 kilocalories per gram. Output kilocalories are used to maintain the body's basal metabolism; to chew, digest, and process food; to fuel muscular activity for physical exercise; and to help the body adapt to environmental changes. Simply put, when energy intake exceeds output, a person gains weight. When energy output exceeds intake, a person loses weight. However, weight gain and loss are more complex than this simple algorithm implies. A person's food choices are affected by a lifetime of eating habits that may be informed by cultural and family values, past traumas, food insecurity, poverty, and not having access to healthy foods or a safe place to exercise.

Excluding all social context and thinking exclusively on the scientific aspect of weight, body weight is determined by the amounts of body fat, water, lean tissue (muscle), and bones. Ideally, what people want to lose when dieting is body fat, not lean tissue. It takes approximately 3,500 excess kilocalories to store a pound of body fat, whereas approximately 2,000 to 2,500 kilocalories are required to gain one pound of lean tissue. Any excess food kilocalories—whether from fat, carbohydrates, protein, or alcohol—can be converted into body fat. There is no limit to body fat stores.

During periods of caloric deficit (meaning that input is less than output), a person will lose weight. A deficit of 500 kilocalories per day translates into a loss of about one pound per week. Not all the body weight lost is fat. During a deficit or fasting, the body draws on stores to provide energy. During the first four to six hours without eating, either while sleeping during the night or while awake and active during the day, the body draws its energy primarily from liver carbohydrate stores called glycogen. If no food is consumed after these periods, the body begins to break down muscle (also called lean body tissue) as fuel. Although people lose weight under these circumstances, it is the result of muscle loss and fluid shifts, not fat loss. Body fat supplies fuel during fasting but cannot prevent muscle wasting unless a regular supply of carbohydrates is present. The fat used during fasting is not efficiently metabolized and can cause medical problems if the fast continues for more than a few days. Fat loss can be accomplished by eating balanced regular meals that contain fewer kilocalories than those typically eaten. If diet alone is insufficient to address weight concerns, Medical interventions for weight loss include medications and bariatric surgery.

Caution should be used before an individual undergoes either a weight loss or a weight gain plan.

Starvation diets or very low kilocalorie diets and meal skipping are not wise. These diets promote water and muscle loss, not a steady body fat loss. Depending on a person's initial weight, a reduction in kilocalories of about 500 per day will promote safe, effective fat loss without medical hazards. The central nervous system, i.e. the brain, cannot use stored body fat as fuel, making prolonged fasting a dangerous practice. If diet alone is insufficient to address weight concerns, Medical interventions for weight loss include medications and bariatric surgery.

By consuming a balanced diet that contains all five food groups in moderate portions, exercising, and modifying poor dietary behaviors (such as snacking while watching television), an individual can achieve lasting weight loss. Nutrient-dense foods—those that are low in kilocalories and fat yet still contain ample amounts of vitamins and minerals—should be chosen. Understanding the caloric content of foods is not always necessary if a person uses exchange lists (diabetic exchanges), which are portion-controlled groupings of foods with similar energy contents that can be used to form an adequate diet. Exercise is important because it not only tones the body but also promotes energy expenditure. Research has shown that regular exercise speeds up the basal metabolic rate, which also helps control weight.

Usually individuals seeking weight gain want to gain muscle, not body fat. Weight gain of this type can be accomplished by physical conditioning and a high kilocalorie diet. The amount of muscle gained is under hormonal control. In healthy individuals, an excess of 700 to 1,000 kilocalories per day is sufficient to add 1 to 2 pounds per week. This excess must be accompanied by exercise training, however, or only body fat deposits will increase.

Healthy individuals desiring weight gain need to exercise and to ingest more kilocalories in order to increase muscle size. Consuming more kilocalories can be problematic, especially for athletes. These individuals must take time to eat perhaps five to six times per day. These individuals should eat more calorically dense foods—the exact foods avoided during weight loss. Emphasis should still be placed on nutrient-wise choices, not simply empty kilocalories. If someone is underweight, increasing fat in the diet is not considered a major heart disease risk because the fat will prevent muscle wastage.

COMPLICATIONS AND DISORDERS

Not all weight gain or loss is voluntary. Weight changes can be warning signs or consequences of disease. Several diseases are frequently accompanied by severe weight loss and wasting, such as acquired immunodeficiency syndrome (AIDS), cancer, colitis, chronic obstructive pulmonary diseases (such as emphysema), cystic fibrosis, kidney diseases, anorexia, and bulimia. Wasting is characterized by decreased muscle mass and depleted fat stores. This is a result of inadequacies in both kilocalories and nutrient intake. Lack of appetite, could be a consequence of disease, drug therapy, or both, complicating a person's desire to eat. Severe weight loss is compounded by other nutrient losses caused by diarrhea, loss of blood, or drug interactions. Individuals with AIDS can experience extreme weight loss, perhaps losing up to 34% of ideal body weight.

Thus, with illness a vicious cycle occurs: A lack of adequate food energy promotes the risk of infection; infections require more food energy for healing, further depleting energy reserves; and patients lose more weight, placing them at greater risk for subsequent infections. Extreme weight loss makes AIDS patients prone to other infections, which subsequently compromise weight status because more kilocalories are needed to combat these infections. Similarly, patients with cancer, colitis, and chronic obstructive pulmonary disease who experience weight loss become nutritionally compromised, placing them at risk for infections and delayed wound healing. Extra kilocalories are required to support the labored breathing accompanying chronic obstructive pulmonary disease. People with emphysema, a type of this disease, are often too weak to ingest enough food to prevent weight loss. Diseases of the gastrointestinal tract magnify poor nutritional status because energy-yielding nutrients cannot be absorbed.

Weight loss is also a symptom of cystic fibrosis. Cystic fibrosis is a genetic disorder that affects the pancreas and lungs. Individuals with this disease become malnourished because the normal release of pancreatic digestive enzyme secretions is impaired and because of high nutritional needs to combat lung infections. In an effort to clear congested lungs, individuals with severe cystic fibrosis cough so forcefully that frequently they vomit any food substances that they were able to consume.

Treatment for illness-related weight loss is complex. Individuals do not always want to eat, for both physical and psychological reasons. More frequent meals, higher fat intakes, and even special nutritional supplements are required. In severe cases, intravenous solutions, tube feedings, and hyperalimentation (feeding higher-than-normal amounts of nutrients through tube feeding or veins) may be implemented. Some medications can be used to improve appetite.

Sudden, dramatic weight loss could be a sign of dehydration. Athletes exercising during hot weather must pay attention to weight loss after practice and replenish fluids immediately. Rapid weight loss in teenagers, especially girls, may be attributable to eating disorders such as anorexia nervosa (self-induced starvation) and bulimia (periods of binge eating followed by intentional vomiting, or purging). While both genders can suffer from anorexia and bulimia, they tend to affect women more. Our society places unrealistic beauty expectations on women, and those expectations can contribute to disordered eating. Anorexia can lead to severe cardiac complications and cause infertility in women. The complications of anorexia can be deadly; anorexia is the mental illness with the highest mortality rate. In childhood, patterns of weight gain or loss are important indicators of childhood health. Rapid changes may signal illnesses or psychological problems that have manifested themselves as overeating or undereating. Tracking weight gain during pregnancy is also important. Gaining weight too rapidly may be a sign of fluid imbalance forewarning pregnancy complications. Gaining too little weight during pregnancy can also be harmful to the fetus. Weight gain may be a factor in Type 2 Diabetes Mellitus. Although people with this type of diabetes are often characterized as overweight, they are hungry because the energy that they ingest cannot enter the body's cells; consequently, they continue to overeat, fostering further weight gain. The location of excess weight on the body is also important. Individuals who gain excess weight in the waist area are considered to be at risk for hypertension, type 2 diabetes, and other disorders.

PERSPECTIVE AND PROSPECTS

It is now well known that weight loss, the predominant goal of people with nonmedical weight-related concerns, cannot usually be achieved and sustained by dieting. It is estimated that one-fifth to one-third of the otherwise healthy adult population in the United States is "on a diet" at any given time.

Going on a diet is not the way to get control of weight. Diets can produce weight loss; they rarely produce weight control over the long term. Repeated cycles of weight loss through deprivation of favorite high-calorie foods and weight gain when the motivation to tolerate this deprivation wanes, so-called yo-yo dieting, are hazardous. The cycles usually reduce individual metabolic rates, reduce lean tissue, discourage the individual, and make subsequent weight loss extremely difficult.

Weight management is a long-term endeavor resulting from myriad short-term decisions. Success comes with setting and achieving realistic goals. Family or group support, positive and tolerant attitudes, regular meals representative of all food groups, and behavioral modification will sustain healthy weight. Twenty to thirty minutes of exercising the large muscle groups, every other day, can prove a modest, effective way to burn fat and increase one's metabolic rate. It also produces more lean muscle tissue, a goal for both dieters and gainers.

Whether weight gain or loss is the goal, healthful eating habits require one to make wise choices and understand that weight control is a lifestyle, not a quick fix. Individuals experiencing a weight gain or loss who are not voluntarily altering exercise or food intake should have a thorough physical examination to determine the root cause. In June 2013, the American Medical Association voted to classify obesity as a disease. The decision spurred a nationwide conversation about obesity treatment and prevention. In addition, it led some members of the United States Congress to consider expanding Medicare coverage to include weight-loss drugs and weight-reduction treatments.

—Wendy L. Stuhldreher, Ph.D., R.D., and Paul Moglia, Ph.D.;
Updated by LeAnna DeAngelo, Ph.D. and Julia Lockamy, RN

FOR FURTHER INFORMATION

Pollack, Andrew. "A.M.A. Recognizes Obesity as a Disease." *New York Times.* New York Times Co., Web. 18 June 2013.

Prescription Weight-Loss Drugs: Can They Help You?" *Mayo Clinic.* June 7, 2013.

Rolfes, Sharon Rady, Kathryn Pinna, and Eleanor Noss Whitney. *Understanding Normal and Clinical Nutrition.* 8th ed. Belmont, Calif.: Thomson/Wadsworth, 2009.

Wardlaw, Gordon M., and Anne M. Smith. *Contemporary Nutrition.* 7th ed. New York: McGraw-Hill, 2008.

"Weight Loss: Gain Control of Emotional Eating." *Mayo Clinic.* December 1, 2012.

"Weight Loss: Choosing a Diet That's Right For You." *Mayo Clinic.* June 22, 2012.

Weight loss medications

CATEGORY: Treatment

KEY TERMS:

body mass index: a value derived from the mass (weight) and height of an individual, calculated by dividing the body mass by the square of the body height and used to determine whether a person is underweight, or normal weight, overweight, or obese

ephedrine: causes constriction of the blood vessels and widening of the bronchial passages, and is typically used to relieve asthma and hay fever

obesity: a condition characterized by the excessive accumulation and storage of fat in the body

INDICATIONS AND PROCEDURES

By the mid-1990s, several drugs had come onto the market showing promise in helping people achieve weight loss. The most widely sought and prescribed of these were Fen-Phen (combining serotonergic fenfluramine and amphetamine-like phentermine) and Redux (dexfenfluramine, with similar properties and actions to fenfluramine). Fen-Phen inhibited the brain's utilization of the neurochemical serotonin, which acts on the brain's appetite control center in the hypothalamus, and suppressed appetite directly, much as traditional over-the-counter diet pills do. Other drugs, less widely used, included phentermine, mazindol, and fluoxetine.

The hope and early evidence were that these medications would produce improved cardiac function, cholesterol and triglyceride profiles, blood sugar concentrations, and blood pressure; assist in the treatment of bulimia; and reduce weight in the obese and prevent weight gain in those at high risk for it, such as individuals who recently have quit smoking. The drugs were intended to assist those with morbid obesity, obese persons with serious medical conditions, and obese persons who had failed to manage their weight using more conservative nutritional and behavioral methods. At no point did researchers intend the medications as quick fixes for those unwilling to exercise or unwilling to change their eating habits. Nevertheless, many physicians prescribed them to patients who were not significantly obese or who were merely overweight.

USES AND COMPLICATIONS

Multiple studies across many different populations have tended to show the same results: Measurable weight loss in those taking the drugs was between 5 and 15 percent, with weight regained one year after patients had stopped taking the drug. The medications had few initial side effects—dry mouth, constipation, and drowsiness being the most common—and were unlikely to become physically addicting.

Health providers across all disciplines were particularly concerned, however, that some patients were coming to rely on these medications as alternatives to the sustained, hard work of developing lifestyle habits of healthy, proportional eating and exercise. In addition, concerns grew over the drugs" potential to cause neurotoxicity and primary pulmonary hypertension. Fen-Phen, in particular, was responsible for numerous reports of valvular heart disease and pulmonary hypertension.

The issue of weight loss affects women and men differently. Men typically lose weight more quickly than women do because they usually have more muscle and women have more fat. Muscle burns more calories than fat, so men burn more calories at rest than women do. Further, because men on average are larger than women and have more muscle to support, they usually can consume more calories compared to women and still lose weight. Accordingly, portion control is particularly important for women.

Meanwhile, in the wake of the Fen-Phen issue, other drugs were developed to help with weight loss. The five that have been approved by the Food and Drug Administration for long-term use as of 2018 were bupropion-naltrexone (*Contrave*), liraglutide (*Saxenda*), lorcaserin (*Belviq*), orlistat (*Xenical*), and phentermine-topiramate (*Qsymia*). A doctor may recommend use of one of these medications for obese women—those with a body mass index of 30 or more—as well as for those who are overweight (BMI of 27 or more) and have health problems related to excess weight such as high blood pressure, high blood cholesterol, and diabetes; and for those who have been watching their diets and exercising for six or more months with weight loss of less than a pound per week. These medications, however, can cause birth defects, so they are not recommended for women who could become pregnant.

PERSPECTIVE AND PROSPECTS

In 1997, the Food and Drug Administration (FDA) withdrew approval of Fen-Phen and Redux for treating obesity, and their marketing and distribution were discontinued. Class-action lawsuits were filed—former Fen-Phen users alone have filed approximately fifty thousand lawsuits against the makers of the drug—and large settlements were reached for those who had used Fen-Phen and other such drugs. As of 2017, more than 570,000 claims were filed against Wyeth, with more than $21 billion in settlements paid out.

The government then set its sights on dietary products containing ephedra. Manufacturers claimed that ephedra, a botanical source of ephedrine, is a "fat-burning" supplement that could boost energy and enhance athletic performance, but reports began to surface about seizures, strokes, heart attacks, and even deaths in otherwise healthy users. In 2003, the FDA banned the use of ephedra.

—*Paul Moglia, Ph.D.;*
Updated by LeAnna DeAngelo, Ph.D.
and Michael J. O'Neal

FOR FURTHER INFORMATION

Finn, R. "Pharmacotherapy May Help Some Obese Teens." *Internal Medicine News* 38, no. 19 (June, 2005): 45.

Lawler, Moira. *These 5 Weight-Loss Drugs Really Work-but Here's What Else You Need to Know.* Women's Health, 22 June 2016, www.womenshealthmag.com/weight-loss/a19997110/fda-approved-weight-loss-prescriptions/.

Marcovitz, Hal. *Diet Drugs.* Farmington Hills, Mich.: Lucent Books, 2007.

Mayo Clinic Staff. "Pros and Cons of Weight-Loss Drugs." *Mayo Clinic,* Mayo Foundation for Medical Education and Research, 18 Sept. 2018, www.mayoclinic.org/healthy-lifestyle/weight-loss/in-depth/weight-loss-drugs/art-20044832.

Well-baby examinations

CATEGORY: Procedure

KEY TERMS:

alopecia: hair loss

dehydration: excessive loss of the body's water content; in infants, manifests as increased pulse, sunken fontanelle, decreased blood pressure, dry mucous membranes, and decreased skin turgor

periodic breathing: rapid breathing followed by several seconds of no breathing; more than ten-second pauses are abnormal

trichotillomania: excessive hair pulling

INDICATIONS AND PROCEDURES

A pediatrician or nurse practitioner usually performs the routine physical examination of an infant. Because the child may be frightened, some steps in the examination may be performed while the baby is being held in the parent's lap. If the baby or child is ill, the health care provider will look for signs of dehydration and possible lethargic mental status. Dehydration is always checked in cases where fever is present. A child's normal oral temperature is similar to an adult's (98.6 degrees Fahrenheit). A rectal temperature will typically be 1 degree higher. It is not uncommon for a young child to have a temperature of 105 degrees with even a minor infection. Respiration and pulse are measured. Young children and infants breathe with their diaphragm; therefore, the movements of the abdomen can be counted. Periodic breathing is common in infants. Respiratory rates for newborns are 30 to 50 respirations per minute. Toddlers average rates of 20 to 40 respirations per minute. The pulse of a newborn baby is detected best over the brachial artery. The rate is usually in the range of 120 to 160 beats per minute; this figure declines as the child grows older.

Blood pressure, length, weight, and head circumference are measured and checked against charts showing norms. Infants are weighed without clothing and are measured on a firm table. The head is measured at the maximum point of the occipital protuberance posteriorly and at the mid forehead anteriorly. The shape of the child's head, such as flatness or swelling, is observed. Hair is checked for quantity, color, texture, and infestations. The presence of a fungus can be indicated by alopecia (hair loss), but

this cause must be distinguished from trichotillomania. Hypothyroidism can be indicated by dry, coarse hair.

An eye examination can give information about systemic problems and about the eyes themselves. The eyes are observed working together; reaction to light, pupil size, cornea haziness, excess tearing, vision, visual fields, and the distance between the eyes are checked. Observations for nystagmus (involuntary movement of the eyes) and for the abnormal upward outward eye slant and epicanthal folds associated with Down syndrome are also made. Newborns have about 20/400 vision, which improves to 20/40 by six months of age. During an ear examination, the tympanic membrane is checked for perforations, color, lucency, and bulging (indicating pus and/or fluid) in the middle ear. A rough hearing acuity may be determined by eliciting from the child a startle reflex to sound.

The nose is checked interiorly, and the nasal mucus is checked for watery discharge (indicating allergy) and mucopurulent discharge (indicating infection). The nasal septum and passages are also checked, and any foreign bodies are removed.

The oral cavity examination consists of checking the lips for asymmetry, fissures, clefts, lesions, and color. The tongue is examined for color, size, coating, and dryness. The tonsils are observed for signs of infection and color, while the palate is observed for arch and possible lesions. The throat is examined for signs of inflammation and other problems. The neck is checked for tilt and range of motion. The thyroid gland is palpitated and evaluated for symmetry, consistency, and surface characteristics. Any other swellings are noted, and their causes determined.

The neurologic examination is extensive and begins with an assessment of a child's milestones. An infant's primitive reflexes—Moro, asymmetric tonic neck, Babinski, palmar grasp, rooting, and parachute reflexes—are checked. Cranial nerves that can be assessed at the child's stage of development may be assessed. General sensation and response to touch and muscle tone and movement are checked for unusual responses. The musculoskeletal system and extremities are checked for gross deformities and congenital anomalies. Gait and stance are observed, as well as muscle tone and range of motion. Posture in older children may be observed for spinal curvatures.

The lungs are checked to evaluate air movement, to identify breath sounds and chest sounds, and to inspect the shape of the chest. The physician will note any physical deformities and listen to rhythms that could indicate abnormal blood circulation. Indications of circulatory system problems in infants are cyanosis, clubbing of fingers or toes, tachycardia (rapid heart rate), peripheral edema, and tachypnea (rapid breathing). Examination of the abdominal contour and auscultation and palpation of the abdomen are done. In newborns, the genitals are checked for ambiguity, and the rectal area is checked for fissures or anal prolapse. Skin is checked for color, pigmentation, rashes, or burns.

Vaccinations—either oral or by injection—and boosters are a part of some well-baby visits. Occasionally, blood or urine samples are taken for analysis.

USES AND COMPLICATIONS

The challenge of keeping the child calm enough for the clinician to perform a valid exam is important in the diagnostic process. Although an older child can usually be examined easily in standard adult order, this does not work well for pediatric patients. The younger the patient, the more important it is that crucially affected areas be examined first, before the child becomes upset or cries. Clinicians and parents should work together to minimize a child's fears during the examination.

—*Patricia A. Ainsa, M.P.H., Ph.D.*

FOR FURTHER INFORMATION

Albright, Elizabeth K. *Pediatric History and Physical Examination.* Updated and revised ed. Laguna Hills, Calif.: Current Clinical Strategies, 2003.

Barness, Lewis A. *Manual of Pediatric Physical Diagnosis.* 6th ed. St. Louis, Mo.: Mosby Medical, 1991.

"Children's Health." *MedlinePlus,* June 26, 2013.

Hay, William W., Jr., et al., editors. *Current Diagnosis and Treatment in Pediatrics.* 19th ed. New York: Lange Medical Books/McGraw- Hill, 2009.

"Middle Childhood (9-11 years of age)." *cdc.gov,* August 15, 2012.

"Preschoolers (3-5 years of age)." *cdc.gov,* August 12, 2012.

Sanghavi, Darshak. *A Map of the Child: A Pediatrician's Tour of the Body.* New York: Henry Holt, 2003.

Schwartz, M. William, ed. *Schwartz's Clinical Handbook of Pediatrics.* 4th ed. Philadelphia: Wolters Kluwer/ Lippincott Williams & Wilkins, 2009.

Zitelli, Basil J., and Holly W. Davis, eds. *Atlas of Pediatric Physical Diagnosis.* 5th ed. St. Louis, Mo.: Mosby/Elsevier, 2007.

Y

Yoga

CATEGORY: Treatment

KEY TERMS:

asana: from Sanskrit, meaning "sitting down"; the physical aspects of yoga, including poses and stretches

pranayama: from Sanskrit, meaning "extension of the breath"; the regulation of the breath through certain techniques and exercises

samyana: from Sanskrit, meaning "holding together," "binding," "integration"; combined practice of concentration (Dh ra), meditation (Dhy na) and union (Sam dhi); a term to summarize the process of psychological absorption during meditation

INTRODUCTION

The word "yoga" comes from the Sanskrit word *Yuj*, meaning to "yoke," "join," or "unite." The word implies joining or integrating all aspects of the body with the mind to achieve a healthy and balanced life. The true purpose of the ancient practices of yoga is to bring a proper balance between the physical and mental aspects of a person and to awaken what yoga practitioners understand to be subtle energies of the body. Yoga cultivates muscular strength, endurance, and flexibility and enhances the practitioner's mental acuity. Meditative breathing calms a person's nerves and sharpens a person's focus. With regular yoga practice, individuals are known to gain physical health, mental relaxation, and inner tranquility.

Yoga has been practiced in India, in one form or another, for more than four thousand years. More than two thousand years ago, the Indian scholar Patanjali codified the various yoga practices into a written collection called the *Yoga Sutras*. According to Patanjali, there are three critical components of yoga: physical postures (*asanas*), breath control (*pranayama*), and meditation (*samyana*). The main purpose of *asanas* and *pranayam* is to cleanse the body, increase energy, and raise the level of consciousness.

Yoga styles have come to include a strong component of meditation to enhance the union of mind, body, and soul. Patanjali showed how, through the practice of yoga, one could gain mastery over mind and emotion. Advanced yoga practitioners are known to have incredible control over several autonomic functions such as respiration, heart rate, and blood flow.

While the ancient practice of yoga focused more on access to a higher level of consciousness and spirituality, modern yoga focuses more on the physical and mental health benefits of the practice. Yoga has enjoyed rising popularity in recent years in the U.S., particularly among younger, college-educated females.

HEALTH BENEFITS

Research, mostly performed in India, suggests a wide variety of positive health effects from the daily practice of yoga, including, but not limited to, pain reduction in arthritis and carpal tunnel syndrome, reduction of coronary artery disease, and relief from asthma and other respiratory ailments. Situated in Bangalore, India, the Swami Vivekananda Yoga Anusandhana Samsthana (SVYASA) University treats people with such ailments as asthma, arthritis, heart disease, high blood pressure, psychiatric ailments, and eating disorders. The center uses an integrated approach of yoga therapies that includes *asanas*, chanting, *kriya* (yoga cleansing techniques), meditation, *pranayam*, and lectures on yoga philosophy. The system, according to their research, has been shown to benefit people with asthma, intellectual disabilities, rheumatoid arthritis, and type 1 diabetes mellitus. It is believed to improve visual perception, manual dexterity, and spatial memory. However, the quality of the research in Indian institutes must be taken into consideration, since a Cochrane Airways Group review of literature found that "no reliable conclusions could be drawn concerning the use of breathing exercises for asthma in clinical practice. This was a result of methodological differences among the included studies and poor reporting of methodological aspects in most of the included studies."

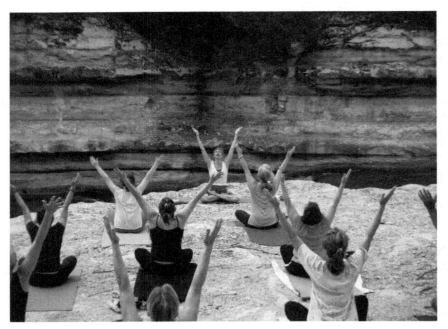

Women performing yoga. (Wikimedia Commons)

With support from other organizations, SVYASA has been engaged in a vast variety of research, including studies regarding the use of yoga to treat obsessive-compulsive disorder; the effects of yoga on people with multiple sclerosis; and the use of yoga for assessing alertness, ability to focus, flexibility, balance, quality of life, and fatigue in healthy elderly people. *Pranayam* has been shown to lower blood pressure in people with hypertension, to alleviate discomfort from gastritis, and to reduce stress and anxiety. One difficulty with the work in India, however, has been a lack of rigor in research design and protocol. For example, the yoga practices are traditionally combined with chanting, discourse, and other activities, and it is difficult to determine the effects of such extra variables when comparing the results of one study with another. Currently Yoga is being used in many mental health treatments centers, such as substance abuse treatment and in the healing of other emotional struggles.

Studies suggest that yoga can have benefits on several parameters including physical and mental health, quality of life, and pain relief, though no association has been shown with decreased mortality. Benefits in cardiovascular fitness have been shown primarily among older adults. Evidence suggests that yoga is associated with improved flexibility, balance and pain relief, particularly for patients with low back pain and rheumatologic conditions. There may also be benefits for pregnant patients, particularly with regards to decreased pelvic pain and improved perinatal outcomes. Evidence from randomized trials also indicate improvements in sleep quality and fatigue in cancer survivors.

PERSPECTIVE AND PROSPECTS

With growing interest in alternative therapies, several individuals and institutions have initiated extensive studies on the effects of yoga. For example, researchers at Ball State University found that fifteen weeks of yoga training brought a 10-percent improvement in lung capacity. Yoga has been found to help fight cardiovascular disease when used in conjunction with other lifestyle changes, such as a low-fat diet; however, the *European Journal of Preventative Cardiology* reviewed the literature on yoga and heart disease and concluded that only "weak recommendations can be made for the ancillary use of yoga for patients with coronary heart disease, heart failure, and cardiac dysrhythmia." The National Institutes of Health (NIH) is supporting research on yoga, including its use for treating insomnia and chronic lower back pain.

In a study at the University of Iowa, some patients with chronic fatigue syndrome were shown to benefit from yoga. Yoga prevailed among numerous conventional and alternative therapies as an effective fatigue fighter. At the end of the two-year study, yoga was the only therapy linked to a statistically significant positive outcome by linear regression analysis.

Marian Garfinkel, a yoga teacher turned researcher, has demonstrated that practicing certain yoga postures can relieve the symptoms of carpal tunnel syndrome, the common ailment resulting from repetitive hand activities such as typing. Patients practicing prescribed yoga postures showed significant improvement in grip strength and suffered less pain. There was also improvement on a nerve test used to measure the severity of carpal tunnel syndrome. Studies are in progress to observe the effect of yoga on osteoarthritis of the knee and on repetitive strain injuries. However, later work reviewing the effects of yoga on carpal tunnel syndrome has come to more modest conclusions.

Because each patient is unique in their different abilities and weaknesses, a yoga approach should be tailored to specific problems as well as specific potentials. It is also important to look at the studies in which yoga did not prove effective and to determine which variables led to these failures.

IMPACT ON WOMEN

Yoga in the United States is heavily dominated by women, the majority being educated upper middle class (due to the cost of joining a studio). It is estimated that yoga is a $27 billion-dollar industry in the US, with more than 20 million participants- of that 83% of them being female. Some believe that this has to do with the marketing of yoga with young beautiful thin peaceful women. If women desire to have these attributes in their lives, they may be more likely to sign up for yoga. Despite the marketing advantages the yoga industry may utilize, overall, practicing yoga is believed to serve as an emotionally and physically beneficial practice. The physical exercise and stretching of the practice will benefit the heart and physical body. The overall meditation practice and mindfulness approach is proven beneficial for emotional well-being. Therefore, yoga is considered to be a healthy addition to a woman's life. Although it is very costly to join a professional yoga studio, yoga itself can be practiced anywhere. Practicing the techniques at home or out in the community or utilizing online yoga practices are a great way for anyone to have access to this beneficial art.

—*Tulsi B. Saral, Ph.D*
Updated by Ananya Anand, M.Sc.
and Kimberly Ortiz-Hartman, Psy.D., LMFT

FOR FURTHER INFORMATION

Cramer, H., et al. "A Systematic Review of Yoga for Heart Disease." *European Journal of Preventative Cardiology* (2015); 22(3): 284-95. doi: 10.1177/204748-7314523132.

Freitas, Diana A, et al. "Breathing exercises for adults with asthma." *Cochrane Database of Systematic Reviews* (2013); 10: DOI: 10.1002/14651858.CD001277.pub3.

Mayo Clinic. "Yoga: Fight Stress and Find Serenity." *Mayo Foundation for Medical Education and Research,* January 15, 2013.

National Center for Complementary and Alternative Medicine. "Yoga for Health." *National Institutes of Health,* May 2012.

Wren, A. A., et al. "Yoga for Persistent Pain: New Findings and Directions for an Ancient Practice." *Pain* 152 (2011): 477–80.

Government Agencies

Centers for Disease Control and Prevention (CDC)
800-232-4636
https://www.cdc.gov/

Food and Drug Administration (FDA)
1-888-463-6332
https://www.fda.gov/

National Center for Homeless Education (NCHE)
1-800-308-2145
https://nche.ed.gov/

National Institutes of Health (NIH)
301-496-4000
https://www.nih.gov/

National Cancer Institute (NCI)
1-800-422-6237
https://www.cancer.gov/

National Eye Institute (NEI)
301-496-5248
https://nei.nih.gov/

National Heart, Lung, and Blood Institute (NHLBI)
301-592-8573
https://www.nhlbi.nih.gov/

National Institute on Aging (NIA)
Aging information
1-800-222-2225

Alzheimer's disease information
1-800-438-4380
https://www.nia.nih.gov/

National Institute on Alcohol Abuse and Alcoholism (NIAAA)
301-443-3860
https://www.niaaa.nih.gov/

The National Institute of Allergy and Infectious Diseases (NIAID)
1-866-284-4107
https://www.niaid.nih.gov/

National Institute of Arthritis and Musculoskeletal and Skin Diseases (NIAMS)
Arthritis, musculoskeletal, and skin diseases:
1-877-226-4267

Osteoporosis and other bone diseases:
1-800-624-2663
https://www.niams.nih.gov/

Eunice Kennedy Shriver National Institute of Child Health and Human Development (NICHD)
1-800-370-2943
https://www.nichd.nih.gov/

National Institute on Drug Abuse (NIDA)
1-877-643-2644
https://www.drugabuse.gov

National Institute of Diabetes and Digestive and Kidney Diseases (NIDDK)
1-800-860-8747
https://www.niddk.nih.gov/

The National Institute of Environmental Health Sciences (NIEHS)
919-541-3345
https://www.niehs.nih.gov

National Institute of General Medical Sciences (NIGMS)
301-496-7301
https://www.nigms.nih.gov/

National Institute of Mental Health (NIMH)
1-866-615-6464
https://www.nimh.nih.gov

NATIONAL INSTITUTE ON MINORITY HEALTH AND HEALTH DISPARITIES (NIMHD)
301-402-1366
https://www.nimhd.nih.gov/

NATIONAL INSTITUTE OF NEUROLOGICAL DISORDERS AND STROKE (NINDS)
1-800-352-9424
https://www.ninds.nih.gov/

NATIONAL INSTITUTE OF NURSING RESEARCH (NINR)
301-496-0207
https://www.ninr.nih.gov/

NATIONAL LIBRARY OF MEDICINE (NLM)
1-888-346-3656
https://www.nlm.nih.gov/

OFFICE ON WOMEN'S HEALTH (OWH)
1-800-994-9662
https://www.womenshealth.gov/

SUBSTANCE ABUSE AND MENTAL HEALTH SERVICES ADMINISTRATION (SAMHSA)
877-726-4727
https://www.samhsa.gov/

U.S. DEPARTMENT OF HEALTH AND HUMAN SERVICES (HHS)
1-877-696-6775
https://www.hhs.gov/

Crisis Organizations and Hotlines

ABORTION

All-Options

All-Options (formerly Backline) uses direct service and social change strategies to promote unconditional, judgment-free support for people in all of their decisions, feelings, and experiences with pregnancy, parenting, abortion, and adoption.
1-888-493-0092

Connect & Breathe

Connect & Breathe creates safe space to talk about abortion experiences by offering a talkline providing unbiased support and encouragement of self-care.
1-866-647-1764

National Abortion Federation Hotline

The largest national, toll-free, multi-lingual Hotline for abortion referrals and financial assistance in the U.S. and Canada.
1-800-772-9100

National Office of Post Abortion Reconciliation and Healing

Networks researchers and psychotherapeutic professionals working in the field within the U.S. and abroad, consults on the formation of post-abortion support services within secular and religious settings, provides training for care providers and maintains a national "800" referral line for those seeking assistance in reconciling an abortion experience.
1-800-593-2273

Project Rachel

An outreach of the Catholic church, this ministry is composed of a network of specially trained clergy, spiritual directors and therapists who provide compassionate one-on-one care to those who are struggling with the aftermath of abortion.
1-888-456-4673

ABUSE

Adult Protective Services and Elder Abuse Hotline

Assists vulnerable and elder adults to stop and prevent abuse, neglect, or exploitation.
1-800-222-8000

Childhelp - National Child Abuse Hotline

The largest organization dedicated to helping victims of child abuse and neglect as well as at-risk children. Provides a direct link to professional crisis counselors who have access to a database of 55,000 emergency, social service, and support resources.
1-800-4-A-CHILD (422-4453)

National Center for Missing and Exploited Children

Provides a wide range of support services for victims and their families including peer support, reunification assistance, and mental health referrals.
1-800-THE-LOST (843-5678)

Rape, Abuse, and Incest National Network (RAINN)

The nation's largest anti-sexual violence organization, RAINN created and operates the National Sexual Assault Hotline in partnership with more than 1,000 local sexual assault service providers across the country and operates the DoD Safe Helpline for the Department of Defense.

Phone Hotline:
1-800-656-HOPE (4673)
Online Hotline:
online.rainn.org

ADDICTION

Alcoholics Anonymous
212-870-3400

Families Anonymous
A twelve-step program for relatives and friends of addicts.
1-800-736-9805

Marijuana Anonymous
1-800-766-6779

Narcotics Anonymous
1-818-773-9999

National Association for Children of Alcoholics
The only national membership organization focusing on the children of parents struggling with alcohol or substance abuse.
1-888-554-2627

National Drug Hotline
Provides accessible resources and contact information to anyone who may be in need of substance abuse or mental disorder help.
1-888-633-3239

Substance Abuse and Mental Health Services Administration (SAMHSA)'s National Helpline
A free, confidential, 24/7, 365-day-a-year treatment referral and information service (in English and Spanish) for individuals and families facing mental and/or substance use disorders.
1-800-662-HELP (4357)

CANCER

American Cancer Society
Funds and conducts research, shares expert information, supports patients, and spreads the word about prevention.
1-800-227-2345

Cancer Support Helpline
Staffed by counselors and resource specialists who have over 170 years of combined experience helping people affected by cancer. They are available to provide emotional support as well as information and referral to local, regional and national resources to anyone impacted by a cancer diagnosis.
1-888-793-9355

CARE GIVERS

Elder Care Locator
A public service of the U.S. Administration on Aging connecting seniors to services for older adults and their families.
1-800-677-1116

Well Spouse Association
A nonprofit membership organization advocating for and addressing the needs of individuals caring for a chronically ill and/or disabled spouse/partner.
1-800-838-0879

CHRONIC ILLNESS/PAIN

U.S. Pain Foundation
A nonprofit organization dedicated to serving those who live with pain conditions and their care providers, U.S. Pain Foundation helps individuals find resources and inspiration.
1-800-910-2462

DOMESTIC VIOLENCE

Between Friends
A nonprofit agency dedicated to breaking the cycle of domestic violence and building a community free of abuse.
1-800-603-4357

Love Is Respect
Highly-trained advocates offer support, information and advocacy to young people who have questions or concerns about their dating relationships. Also provides information and support to concerned friends and family members, teachers, counselors, service providers and members of law enforcement.
1-866-331-9474
Text loveis to 22522

National Domestic Violence Hotline

Provides an immediate link to lifesaving help for victims. and information and assistance to adult and youth victims of family violence, domestic violence, or dating violence.
1-800-799-SAFE (7233)

Safe Horizons

The largest non-profit victim services agency in the United States. Partners with governmental and other community agencies and also advocates for policies on a local, state, and national level on behalf of those affected by violence and abuse.

Crime Victims Hotline:

1-800-621-4673

Rape and Sexual Assault & Incest Hotline:

212-227-3000

EATING DISORDERS

National Eating Disorders Association

The largest nonprofit organization dedicated to supporting individuals and families affected by eating disorders. NEDA supports individuals and families affected by eating disorders, and serves as a catalyst for prevention, cures and access to quality care.
1-800-931-2237

National Association of Anorexia Nervosa and Associated Disorders

The oldest organization aimed at fighting eating disorders in the United States. ANAD assists people struggling with eating disorders and also provides resources for families, schools and the eating disorder community.
630-577-1330

The Meadows Ranch

The Meadows Ranch helps women and girls recover from eating disorders. Treatment is led by a well-qualified multidisciplinary team that is dedicated to providing assistance and support 24 hours a day to help patients achieve medical stabilization and support them in the following stages of recovery.
866-330-1456

HOMELESSNESS

American Family Housing

AFH provides a continuum of housing and an array of services to support homeless and low income families and adults to secure a stable home, to be an active part of their community, and to achieve a self-sustaining way of life.
714-897-3221

Covenant House

Offer housing and support services to young people in need – reaching 80,000 boys and girls every year.
1-800-999-9999

Directory of Covenant Houses:

https://www.covenanthouse.org/homeless-shelters

National Coalition for the Homeless

A national network of people who are currently experiencing or who have experienced homelessness, activists and advocates, and community-based and faith-based service providers.
202-462-4822

Homeless Shelter Directory:

https://www.homelessshelterdirectory.org/

LGBTQIA+

LGBT National Help Center

A non-profit, tax-exempt organization that provides vital peer-support, community connections and resource information to people with questions regarding sexual orientation and/or gender identity.
1-888-843-4564

Youth Talkline:

1-800-246-7743

Senior Hotline:

1-888-234-7243

Pride Institute

Pride Institute is committed to providing LGBTQ+ people a safe place for recovery through evidence-based treatment for substance abuse, sexual health and mental health.
1-800-547-7433

Trans Lifeline
A national trans-led organization dedicated to improving the quality of trans lives by responding to the critical needs of our community with direct service, material support, advocacy, and education.
877-565-8860

Trevor Hotline (Suicide)
The Trevor Project is the leading national organization providing crisis intervention and suicide prevention services to lesbian, gay, bisexual, transgender, queer & questioning (LGBTQ) young people under 25.
1-866-488-7386
Text START to 678678

True Colors United
The True Colors Fund is working to end homelessness among lesbian, gay, bisexual, transgender, queer, and questioning youth, creating a world in which all young people can be their true selves.
212-461-4401

MENTAL HEALTH

Anxiety and Depression Association of America
An international nonprofit membership organization dedicated to the prevention, treatment, and cure of anxiety, depression, OCD, PTSD, and co-occurring disorders through education, practice, and research.
Find a Therapist:
https://members.adaa.org/page/FATMain

Children and Adults with Attention-Deficit/Hyperactivity Disorder
The organization is composed of dedicated volunteers from around the country who play an integral part in the association's success by providing support, education and encouragement to parents, educators and professionals
1-800-233-4050

Depression and Bipolar Support Alliance
DBSA offers peer-based, wellness-oriented support and empowering services and resources available when people need them, where they need them, and how they need to receive them.

Find a Support Group:
https://www.dbsalliance.org/support/chapters-and-support-groups/find-a-support-group/

Postpartum Support International
Dedicated PSI members, leaders, and friends work tirelessly across all levels to meet goals of the shared PSI mission of support, education, advocacy, and research for people living with mental illness through various activities
1-800-944-4773

PREGNANCY

American Pregnancy Association
A national health organization committed to promoting reproductive and pregnancy wellness through education, support, advocacy, and community awareness.
1-800-672-2296

Birthright International
Birthright is committed to providing confidential, non-judgmental support to any woman who is pregnant or thinks she might be pregnant, no matter her age, race, circumstances, religion, marital status or financial situation.
1-800-550-4900

National Life Center
Offers support and services to any girl or woman who suspects she may be pregnant. All services are free and confidential.
1-800-848-5683

RUNAWAYS

Boys Town National Hotline
One of the largest nonprofit child care agencies in the country, providing compassionate treatment for the behavioral, emotional and physical problems of children and families.
1-800-448-3000

National Runaway Safeline
The National Runaway Safeline is the federally designated national runaway and homeless youth crisis hotline and online service in the United States.
1-800-786-2929
Text 66008

SEXUAL ADDICTION

COSA
A Twelve Step recovery program for men and women whose lives have been affected by another person's compulsive sexual behavior.
866-899-2672

Project Know
ProjectKnow.com aims to inform parents and family members of those struggling with addiction, as well as addicts and alcoholics themselves, about the options available for treating addiction.
1-877-429-2572

Sex Addicts Anonymous
A twelve-step program for people who want to stop their addictive sexual behavior.
1-800-477-8191

SUICIDE & SELF-HARM

American Foundation for Suicide Prevention
AFSP raises awareness, funds scientific research and provides resources and aid to those affected by suicide.
1-888-333-2377

National Suicide Prevention Lifeline
The Lifeline provides 24/7, free and confidential support for people in distress, prevention and crisis resources for you or your loved ones, and best practices for professionals.
1-800-273-8255
Deaf Hotline:
1-800-799-4889

S.A.F.E. (Self Abuse Finally Ends)
A nationally recognized treatment approach, professional network, and educational resource base, which is committed to helping you and others achieve an end to self-injurious behavior.
1-800-366-8288

YOUTH CRISIS

Crisis Text Line
Crisis Text Line is free, 24/7 support for those in crisis.
Text RISE to 741741

Stop it Now!
Prevents the sexual abuse of children by mobilizing adults, families and communities to take actions that protect children before they are harmed, along with support, information and resources to keep children safe and create healthier communities.
1-888-PREVENT

Teen Line
A nonprofit, community-based organization helping troubled teenagers address their problems.
310-855-4673
Text TEEN to 839863

Glossary

abdomen: the area of the body between the diaphragm and the pelvis; it contains the visceral organs.

abortion: the medical term for intended and unintended pregnancy loss.

abortive treatment: treatment focusing on reducing the duration or intensity of symptoms after they have already occurred.

abscess: a collection of infected fluid, which may be treated with antibiotics and drainage.

absence seizures: very brief seizures that usually last under 15 seconds and frequently go undetected by the person experiencing it.

abstinence: complete refrainment from the use of a substance of abuse.

acetaminophen: analgesic used to treat headaches and other minor pains and to reduce fever; proprietary names include Tylenol.

acne rosacea: a skin eruption that usually appears between the ages of thirty and fifty; unlike acne vulgaris, it is not characterized by comedones.

acne vulgaris: a skin eruption that usually occurs in puberty and is characterized by the development of comedones, which may be inflamed.

acquaintance rape: a forced sexual act perpetrated by someone known to the victim.

acquired immunodeficiency syndrome (AIDS): a severe and usually fatal disease caused by infection with the human immunodeficiency virus (HIV); infection results in progressive impairment of the immune system.

acromion: the outward end of the spine of the scapula or shoulder blade.

acute confusion syndrome: a transient condition caused by the action of various biological stressors on vulnerable older persons, who may experience inattention, disorganized thinking, other cognitive impairments, and emotional problems.

acute: referring to exposure to hazardous environmental agents or conditions that occur once or over a short period of time (typically fourteen days or less); environmental disease symptoms that appear rapidly.

adenohypophysis: another name for the anterior lobe of the pituitary gland.

adenomyosis: a noncancerous disorder in which cells resembling the lining of the uterus are found within the muscle layer of the uterus, leading to abnormal vaginal bleeding and pain.

adenopathy: the enlargement of any gland (often the lymph gland).

adequate intake (AI): recommended average nutrient intake level based on experimentally derived intake levels or the average intake levels observed in healthy populations.

adipocytes: cells specialized for the storage of fat, found in connective tissue.

adipose tissue: the tissue that stores fat.

adolescent scoliosis: curvature of the spine that is diagnosed in the early stages of puberty.

adrenal gland: an endocrine gland situated immediately above the upper pole of each kidney; it consists of an inner part or medulla, which produces epinephrine and norepinephrine, and an outer part or cortex, which produces steroid hormones.

AF: amniotic fluid.

AFI: amniotic fluid index; a quantitative estimate of the amount of amniotic fluid surrounding the fetus as ascertained by ultrasound.

afterbirth: the placenta and fetal membranes discharged from the uterus after birth.

AFV: amniotic fluid volume.

ageism: a negative or prejudiced view of aging endorsed by an individual or society.

alarmone: a type of intracellular hormone which alerts the cell to various chemical imbalances in the cellular environment.

allantois: a hollow sac-like structure filled with clear fluid that forms part of a developing embryo; helps the embryo exchange gasses and handle liquid wastes.

Alleles; one or more variations of a gene that reflects the genes passed from your parents; usually referred to as dominant and recessive genes; while other genes have more than two more alleles.

allergens: foreign substances in the surrounding environment thatmay cause an allergic response, such as a skin reaction.

allograft: a transplanted tissue or organ from a genetically different member of the same species as the recipient.

alopecia areata: loss of hair in patches.

alopecia: hair loss, especially if noticeable or significant.

alveolar cell: also known as an acinar cell; the fundamental secretory unit of the mammary glandular tissue.

alveoli: the many tiny air sacs at the ends of the terminal bronchioles, where oxygen and carbon dioxide are exchanged.

Alzheimer's beta peptide (Aβ): the principal proteinaceous component of certain brain lesions in Alzheimer's disease.

amaurosis fugax: temporary blindness in one eye.

ambulatory care: health care provided outside the hospital, usually in a clinic or office and sometimes in the patient's home.

amenorrhea: an abnormal absence of menstruation.

amino acids: any of a number of nitrogen-rich compounds used by the body for the production of protein.

amniocentesis: the drawing of amniotic fluid through the abdominal wall of a pregnant woman in the fifteenth or sixteenth week of pregnancy to test for fetal abnormalities, particularly Down syndrome.

amnion: the innermost membrane that encloses an embryo and eventually fills with amniotic fluid.

amniotic fluid: fluid within the amniotic cavity produced by the amnion during the early embryonic period (two to eight weeks) and later by the lungs and kidneys.

amniotic sac: a thin, tough, membranous sac that contains amniotic fluid and that encloses the embryo or fetus.

amyloid: extracellular proteinaceous deposits having distinctive tinctorial properties.

anagen: active growth phase of hair follicles.

anal intraepithelial neoplasia (AIN): precursor lesions to the development of anal cancer.

androgen: a hormone producing or stimulating the development of male characteristics.

anemia: a condition characterized by abnormally low concentrations of circulating red blood cells.

aneurysm: a bulge in a blood vessel that can leak or burst open causing a stroke.

angiogenesis: the development of new blood vessels.

angiography: radiological modality to visualize the arteries in the body; involves the placement of a catheter in an artery and the injection of dye.

annular bulge: protrusion of a disk beyond its normal circumference, usually due to compression from gravity, strain on the spine, or aging.

Anomaly: abnormality or deviation from the norm.

anorexia nervosa: a psychiatric disease characterized by a distorted body image in which the individual severely limits food intake because of fear of weight gain.

anoscopy: examination of the anal canal via a small tubal instrument inserted a few inches into the anus.

anovulation: a condition in which a woman does not ovulate normal or at all.

antenatal steroids: medications given to pregnant women expecting preterm delivery; they have been shown to reduce the morbidity and mortality of hyaline membrane disease.

anterior: forward, in the customary direction of motion; equivalent to ventral in humans, but the same as cranial in other animals.

antianxiety medication: a medication that acts in the brain to decrease negative reactions to stress and anxiety and to decrease avoidance behavior.

antibodies: proteins manufactured by the body to attack and neutralize foreign substances, such as bacteria.

antibody: a protein found in the blood and produced by the immune system in response to contact of the body with a foreign substance.

anticonvulsants: drugs typically used to manage conditions involving brain seizures and sometimes used to treat bipolar disorders.

antidepressant: a medication that acts in the brain to decrease a sad or depressed mood and other behaviors associated with depression.

antifungal agents: drugs that can result in the inhibition of growth or killing of fungi; these drugs may be topical or systemic in application.

antigen: a protein or related molecule that is seen as foreign and therefore induces antibody formation in an individual.

antihypertensive drugs: medications designed to reduce and control elevated blood pressure.

anti-inflammatory drugs: drugs to counter the effects of inflammation locally or throughout the body; these drugs can be applied locally or introduced by electric currents (in a process called iontophoresis), by injections into the joint or into the muscles, or by mouth; the three classes of these drugs are steroidal, immunosuppressant, and nonsteroidal.

antinuclear antibody (ANA): an unusual antibody that is directed against structures within the nucleus of cells.

antiphospholipid syndrome: also known as Hughes syndrome, a disorder of the immune system that causes an increased risk of blood clots.

antiretroviral treatment: treatment with drugs that inhibit the ability of the human immunodeficiency virus or other types of retroviruses to multiply in the body.

antiviral agent: a drug that acts against a virus, usually by preventing it from reproducing itself; may be used at the first evidence of symptoms to reduce the severity and length of an episode or continually to prevent episodes from occurring.

anxiety: a condition characterized by nervousness or agitation; in older people, it is often caused by the existence of a psychiatric disorder such as depression, a general medical condition such as hypothyroidism, or a side effect of medication.

apnea: lack of airflow for more than ten seconds.

apnea-hypopnea index (AHI): the average number of apneic and hypopneic episodes in one hour.

aqueous fluid: a clear, watery liquid that fills the region inside the front of the eyeball between the lens and cornea.

architectural distortion: when a mammogram shows a region where the breasts normal appearance looks like an abnormal arrangement of tissue strands, but without any associated mass as the apparent cause of this distortion.

areola: the pigmented tissue immediately surrounding the nipple.

arteriovenous malformation (AVM): a genetic disorder in which the capillary beds that connect the arteries and the veins are abnormal or defective, resulting in malnourishment of tissues, especially in the brain and spinal cord.

arthritis: a condition that causes the joints to be inflamed from degeneration of cartilage.

arthroscopy: minimally invasive surgical procedure on a joint in which an examination and sometimes treatment of damage is performed using an arthroscope, an endoscope that is inserted into the joint through a small incision.

articular cartilage: cartilage found in joints in the body.

asana: from Sanskrit, meaning "sitting down"; the physical aspects of yoga, including poses and stretches.

asexual: an individual who identifies on a spectrum of non-sexuality, not having sexual attraction and/ or not having romantic attraction.

aspirate: to remove a substance using suction; a cyst can be aspirated using a needle and syringe to withdraw its .

aspiration: to draw in or out using a sucking motion; either breathing in a foreign object, or, as in the case of culdocentesis, removal of fluid and cells via suction.

assessment: the systematic process of collecting, validating, and communicating patient data; these data will include information gathered from the patient's history and from physical examination and laboratory test results.

assisted reproductive technology: any treatment or procedure involving the manipulation of sperm or eggs outside the body in order to achieve pregnancy.

asthma: a condition in which spasms of the bronchial smooth muscle cause narrowing and constriction of the airways.

asymptomatic: not causing any symptoms.

ataxia: coordinated movement difficulties.

atherosclerosis: narrowing of the internal passageways of essential arteries caused by the buildup of fatty deposits.

atopic: a form of allergy in which the hypersensitivity reaction may occur in a part of the body not in contact with the allergen.

atopy: the genetic tendency to develop allergic diseases such as atopic dermatitis, rhinitis, or asthma.

atresia: the programmed process of cell death.

atria: the chambers in the right and left top portions of the heart that receive blood from the veins and pump it to the ventricles.

atrial fibrillation: a quivering or irregular heartbeat (arrhythmia) that can lead to blood clots, stroke, heart failure and other heart-related complications.

attachment: the development of a nurturing relationship between an infant and its caretaker(s).

auditory nerve: the eighth cranial nerve, which conveys information from the ear to the brain.

augmentation: an increase in the volume or size of the breast.

aura: symptoms (often visual) that precede a migraine.

autoantibodies: antibodies that attack the body's own cells and tissues.

autoantibody: an antibody which binds to a protein that is a normal part of the human body from which it originates, as opposed to part of a bacteria, virus, or another human being;.

autograft: tissue transplanted from one site to another in the same patient.

autoimmune: a term describing a disease in which the body produces antibodies against its own cells.

autoimmunity: a condition in which the immune system fails to recognize its own tissues as "self" and mounts an immune response against its own cells.

autonomic symptoms: runny nose, congestion, watery eyes, sweating, pupil constriction, and other symptoms that commonly accompany a cluster headache.

autosomal dominant: one of many ways that a trait or disorder can be passed down through families; if an individual gets the abnormal gene from only one parent, they can get the disease.

autosomal recessive: one of many ways that a trait or disorder can be passed down through families; both parents must pass down the abnormal gene.

avoidance: a conscious or unconscious defense mechanism by which a person tries to escape from unpleasant situations or feelings, such as anxiety and pain.

axillary dissection: removal of lymph nodes found in the armpit (also known as axilla) to determine the spread of breast cancer; this procedure helps in planning therapy and in preventing spread of the cancer.

Ayre spatula: a wooden spatula with U shaped openings on one side and a flat surface on another.

B cells: also known as B lymphocytes; the antibody-producing cells of the immune system.

B lymphocytes: also referred to as B cells; white cells of the immune system that produce antibodies; produced within the bone marrow.

baby blues: depression affecting a woman after giving birth; symptoms usually lessen without medical intervention.

Bacillus Calmette-Guérin (BCG): an inactive strain of *Mycobacterium bovis* that stimulates the immune system in nonspecific ways.

bacteria: microscopic single-celled organisms that multiply by means of simple division; bacteria are found everywhere, and most are beneficial - only a few species cause disease.

bacteriuria: the presence of bacteria in the urine.

barrier method: a contraceptive that physically prevents sperm from meeting an egg.

Bartholin's glands: small glands located on each side of the vaginal opening; produce fluid that keeps the vagina tract moist.

basal cells: cells at the base of the epidermis that migrate upward and become the principal source of epidermal tissue.

basal metabolism: the energy used to fuel the involuntary activities necessary to sustain life (respiration, circulation, and hormonal activity).

benign tumors: tumors that grow relatively slowly, do not interfere with normal body functions, and do not metastasize.

benign: refers to a non-malignant tumor made up of a mass of cells that do not metastasize (leave the site where they develop).

benzodiazepines: minor tranquilizers used to treat anxiety.

bifidus factors: factors in colostrum and breast milk that favor the growth of helpful bacteria in the infant's intestinal tract.

bifidus factors: factors in colostrum and breast milk that favor the growth of helpful bacteria in the infant's intestinal tract.

biguanide: a type of medication to lower blood glucose by increasing sensitivity to insulin and possibly lowering the liver's glucose production.

bimanual examination: an internal exam of the pelvis conducted by a medical professional, often with a supervising "chaperone" in the room.

binge eating: frequent periods of rapid food consumption in a short time period, often followed by overwhelming feelings of guilt and shame.

biofeedback: the technique of making unconscious or involuntary bodily processes perceptible to the senses in order to manipulate them by conscious mental control.

biomedical model: a way of viewing and understanding psychiatric disorders which emphasizes customary medical practice in identifying and treating a particular disorder from which a person suffers.

biopsy: the removal of sample tissue for microscopic inspection and analysis by a pathologist.

biopsychosocial model: a model that examines the effects of illness on all spheres in which the patient functions-the biological sphere, the psychological sphere, and the social sphere.

bipolar disorders: mood disorders characterized by significant swings in mood from depression to persistent feelings of elation; also known as manic-depressive illness.

bipolar I: less formally known as manic-depressive disorder; a condition that involves both severe symptoms of mania and depression and includes at least one episode of mania.

bipolar II: a condition that involves both hypomania (milder symptoms of mania) and severe symptoms of depression and includes at least one episode of hypomania.

birth canal: the passageway from the uterus to the outside of the mother's body formed by the fully opened cervix in continuity with the vagina.

birth defect: a genetic or developmental abnormality which occurs in utero that leads to anatomic or functional problems after birth; the defect can be serious, with potentially significant consequences for the fetus or mother, or the defect can be minor.

bisexual: an individual who is sexually, and/or romantically, attracted to both men and women, or to more than one gender of people.

bisexuality: the capacity to be sexually attracted to and aroused by both genders; the term also implies a significant and consistent capacity for such arousal and does not refer to occasional attraction to or activity with both genders.

bladder: the pouch in the abdominal cavity that collects urine until it can be eliminated from the body; while not a part of the reproductive system, it is located adjacent to the reproductive organs and is an important landmark.

blastocyst: A five to six-day-old human embryo that consists of a hollow sphere of cells with flat, placenta-making trophoblast cells outside and round, embryo-making inner cell mass cells inside.

blighted ovum: a condition in which the gestational sac and placenta grow without a developing child inside.

body dysmorphic disorder: a distinct mental disorder in which a person is preoccupied with an imagined physical defect or a minor defect that others often cannot see.

body mass index (BMI): a weight-to-height ratio, calculated by dividing one's weight in kilograms by the square of one's height in meters and used as an indicator of obesity and underweight.

bonding: a process in which a mother forms an affectionate attachment to her infant immediately after birth.

bone mineral density (BMD): a measure of bone density, reflecting the strength of bones as represented by calcium content.

boosting: the combination of an anti-HIV drug (usually a protease inhibitor) with another agent (e.g., ritonavir) that inhibits the liver enzymes that metabolizes that anti-HIV drug, which increases the serum concentration of the anti-HIV drug and its efficacy.

bottom surgery: broad spectrum of surgeries some trans people undergo to construct genitalia consistent with their internal sense of sex/gender and/or to alleviate dysphoria (intense discomfort or sense of body not aligning with identity).

Bouchard's nodes: osteophytes or bony spurs that develop as a result of destruction of joint cartilage in proximal interphalangeal joints.

brachial plexus: complex of nerves that carry motor and sensory function to the arm.

bradycardia: slowness of the heartbeat.

brain imaging: any of several techniques used to visualize anatomic regions of the brain, including X rays, magnetic resonance imaging, and positron emission tomography.

brain imaging: any of several techniques used to visualize anatomic regions of the brain, including X rays, magnetic resonance imaging, and positron emission tomography.

BRCA1: an abbreviation for breast cancer 1; the mutant chromosomal factor, when found in chromosome 17, which indicates that a woman is vulnerable to developing breast cancer.

breech presentation: fetus presents to birth canal buttock or feet first.

breech: a commonly encountered abnormal fetal presentation in which any part other than the head presents first.

bronchi: the branching airways from the single large trachea to the multiple terminal bronchioles.

bronchoscopy: a procedure that uses a flexible or rigid fiberoptic telescope to visualize the bronchial tree directly; it also permits samples of tissue to be removed for analysis.

bulimia nervosa: an eating disorder in which a large quantity of food is consumed in a short period of time, often followed by feelings of guilt or shame and purging or vomiting.

bursa: a fluid-filled sac or sac-like cavity, especially one countering friction at a joint.

caffeine: stimulant of the nervous system, often added to NSAIDs; given with acetaminophen or ibuprofen, it can improve the drugs' pain-relieving properties.

calisthenics: exercises (as push-ups and jumping jacks) to develop strength and flexibility that are done without special equipment.

calories: units used to measure the energy value of food.

cancer: a tumor (or growth) of abnormal, genetically transformed cells that invade and destroy normal tissue; also referred to as a malignancy.

cancer: diseases in which abnormal cells divide uncontrollably and may enter nearby tissues or migrate to other parts of the body; malignant growth or tumor.

cannula: a narrow tube used in surgery to drain fluid or to deliver cell suspensions for a transplant.

cannula: a tube used to drain body fluids or to administer medications.

capsule: the wall that encloses a cyst.

carcinogen: a cancer-causing substance; usually a chemical that causes mutations.

carcinogen: a natural or artificial substance inducing the transformation of cells toward the malignant state.

carcinoma: a solid tumor malignancy occurring in cells of the epithelium or tissues surrounding the major organ systems of the body.

cardiac arrhythmia: a disturbance in the heartbeat.

cardio: a common shortening of cardiovascular exercise; any activity that increases heart rate and respiration while using large muscle groups repetitively and rhythmically.

cardiomyopathy: disease of the heart muscle.

carpal tunnel: a narrow tunnel formed by a U-shaped cluster of eight bones called carpals, that lie at the base of the palm and the inelastic transverse carpal ligament that lies across the arch.

carrier: a person infected by an organism who can transmit that organism to other people but who is asymptomatic.

cartilage: a firm, but soft and flexible connective tissue that is found in areas throughout the body including primarily joint surfaces, but as well in the respiratory tract.

case management: an interdisciplinary approach to medical care characterized by the inclusion of physical, psychological, social, emotional, familial, financial, and historical data in patient treatment.

catagen: transition between growth and resting phases of hair follicles.

cataract: a loss of transparency in the lens of the eye, commonly associated with aging.

catheter: a thin tube that is inserted into the groin area and pushed through arteries during embolization procedure.

caudal: toward the tail.

causation: a relationship between two events where one event is affected by the other.

cauterization: burning the skin or flesh of a wound with a heated instrument or caustic substance, typically to stop bleeding or prevent the wound from becoming infected.

CD4 lymphocytes (T cells): help coordinate the immune response by stimulating other immune cells, such as macrophages, B lymphocytes (B cells), and CD8 T lymphocytes (CD8 cells), to fight infection; HIV weakens the immune system by destroying CD4 cells.

CD4: a type of white blood cell (specifically a type of T-cell) that is affected by the human immunodeficiency virus (HIV).

CDC: Centers for Disease Control and Prevention; serves as the national focus for developing and applying disease prevention and control, environmental health, and health promotion and health education activities designed to improve the health of the people of the United States.

celibacy: originally meaning "unmarried," it also refers to the willful or circumstantial refraining from sexual intercourse and, by implication, erotic behavior; though sometimes misconstrued as asexual, celibates are no less sexual than noncelibates.

cell cycle: a step-by-step process whereby one cell duplicates itself to form two cells; it is the way in which most growth occurs, and the cycle leads to cancer if it becomes defective.

cell: the basic functional unit of the body, each of which contains a set of genes and all the other materials necessary for carrying out the processes of life.

cell-mediated immune response: an immune response that involves cells rather than antibodies, particularly T lymphocytes rather than B lymphocytes.

cell-mediated immunity: protection mediated by thymus derived lymphocytes; this type of immunity is particularly important for certain types of pathogenic organisms such as *Candida*.

cellular transformation: carcinogenesis; the biochemical conversion of a cell from a normal state to a cancerous one of uncontrollable proliferation.

cephalopelvic disproportion: baby's head or body is too large to fit through pelvic opening of the mother.

cerebral venous thrombosis: an obstruction in a blood vessel formed by a blood clot.

cerebral: pertaining to the brain.

cervical cancer: cancer of the cervix, the lower end of the uterus that projects into the vagina.

cervical cerclage: the process of encircling a cervix with sutures or synthetic tape that is abnormally liable to dilate (an incompetent cervix) with a ring or loop to prevent a miscarriage.

cervical ectopy: when the soft cells (glandular cells) that line the inside of the cervical canal spread to the outer surface of the cervix.

cervical spine: the highest of three parts of the spine, consisting of seven vertebrae, named C1 (top of the neck) to C7, in a natural lordosis.

cervicitis: inflammation of the cervix, most often contracted through sexual activity; may cause bleeding between menstrual cycles, pain during intercourse, and abnormal vaginal discharge.

cervix: a ring of tissue at the lowest and narrowest part of the uterus forming a canal that opens into the vagina.

cesarean section: a surgical operation for delivering a child by cutting through the wall of the mother's abdomen and uterus.

chancre: a painless ulcer, particularly one developing on the genitals as a result of venereal disease such as syphilis.

chaos: a disorderly shift from predictable, linear behavior to nonlinear randomness, a situation which often occurs in stress and homeostatic breakdown.

cheilosis: painful, dry, cracking, inflamed skin around the corners of the mouth.

chemical peeling: a skin-resurfacing procedure in which a chemical solution is applied to the skin to remove the top layers; the skin that grows back after a chemical peel is smoother and younger looking.

chemotherapy: the use of chemicals to kill or inhibit the growth of cancer cells.

Chlamydia pneumoniae: a type of bacteria that can cause respiratory tract infections, such as pneumonia.

chlamydia: a sexually transmitted infection caused by the bacterium Chlamydia trachomatis; often asymptomatic.

chlamydial conjunctivitis: an infection of the conjunctiva of the eye that is caused by chlamydia.

chlamydoconidia (chlamydospores): budding organisms that form directly from vegetative mycelia (molds); they differ from true spores, which are the result of sexual reproduction.

cholecystectomy: the surgical removal of the gallbladder.

cholestasis: any condition in which substances normally excreted into bile are retained; bile flow is decreased due to impaired secretion by hepatocytes or by obstruction of bile flow though intra- or extrahepatic bile ducts.

chondrocytes: the cells found within cartilage that are dispersed throughout the cartilage and that maintain and support the cartilage.

chorion: the outermost membrane surrounding an embryo; contributes to the forming of the placenta.

chorionic villi: the fingerlike projections of the placenta that function in oxygen, nutrient, and waste transportation between a fetus and its mother.

chromosomal defect: an abnormality in the chromosomes, the threadlike, darkly staining bodies found in all cells that carry genetic information in the form of deoxyribonucleic acid (DNA).

chromosome: a structure found in the cell nucleus that is composed of deoxyribonucleic acid (DNA) and associated proteins; chromosomes are responsible for carrying genetic information and can be observed under a microscope.

chronic: referring to exposure to environmental risk factor or agent occurring over a long period of time, typically more than one year; symptoms of environmental diseases that take a long time to appear after first contact with the causative agent.

chyme: the semiliquid state of foods that have gone through the first stage of digestion in the stomach.

cilia: minute, hair-like, extensions of the apical surface of the cell membrane that decorate the surfaces of certain cells and beat in rhythmic waves to move fluids along the surfaces of cell layers.

cirrhosis: chronic liver disease characterized by the loss of normal liver cells and the replacement of normal liver tissue with fibrous tissue.

cisgender: someone who is not trans. Someone who identifies with a sex and gender consistent with the sex they were assigned when they were born. For example, a baby boy who grows up to identify as a man is a cisgender man.

classic migraine: Migraine with an aura. An aura is a sensation prior to a seizure or a migraine that manifests as flashes of light, shimmering shapes, strange visual sensations, odd smells, or tingling in the hands and feet.

cleavage: the process by which the fertilized egg undergoes a series of rapid cell divisions, which results in the formation of a blastocyst.

climacteric: that phase in the aging process of women marking the transition from the reproductive stage of life to the nonreproductive stage.

clitoridectomy: the removal of the entire clitoris, the prepuce, and adjacent labia.

clomiphene: a synthetic estrogenic substance used to induce ovulation in women who do not ovulate regularly; it is taken orally as a medication.

cluster headache: headaches characterized by excruciating, unilateral, stabbing pain with autonomic symptoms; attacks occur in clusters over weeks to months.

cluster period: a time period, from two weeks to four months, during which cluster headaches occur; they usually disappear, or "enter remission," after the cluster period ends.

Cobb angle: the commonly used measure of spinal curvature; the angle created by perpendicular lines to the tops of the first and bottom of the last vertebrae in a curve.

cognitive behavior psychotherapy: talk therapy consisting of cognitive interaction between a patient and a mental health professional.

cognitive behavioral therapy: a type of psychotherapy in which people learn to recognize and change negative and self-defeating patterns of thinking and behavior.

cognitive functioning: a general term describing mental processes such as awareness, knowing, reasoning, problem solving, judging, and imagining.

cold sore: also known as a fever blister; a sore, frequently on the lips but sometimes on the chin, cheeks, nostrils, and occasionally the gums or palate, that causes itching, burning, or tenderness, followed by crusting over.

collagen: a fibrous protein substance in connective tissue, bone, tendons, and cartilage.

collecting duct: a tubular canal that transports milk from the milk duct to the nipple.

colon: the large intestine.

colonoscopy: the use of a small-diameter, flexible tube of optical fibers with an external light source to visually examine the interior of the body, specifically the colon.

colostrum: thin, yellow milky secretions of the mammary gland just a few days before and after childbirth; it contains more proteins and less fat and carbohydrates than does milk.

colposcopy: a procedure to closely examine the cervix, vagina and vulva for signs of disease.

colpotomy: a type of incision that is made in the back wall of the vagina.

comedo (pl. comedos, comedones): the major lesion in acne vulgaris; it occurs when a hair follicle fills with keratin, sebum, and other matter, and may become infected.

common migraine: Migraine without an aura. Classically described as a throbbing, pounding headache associated with nausea, vomiting, or photophobia.

complex migraine: Migraine with other, non-aura neurological complications. An example is migraine plus complete loss of strength in one arm.

compulsion: a persistent, irresistible urge to perform a stereotyped behavior or irrational act, often accompanied by repetitious thoughts (obsessions) about the behavior.

computed tomography (CT) scan: a technique that generates detailed pictures from a series of X rays.

concordance: the condition among twins of having the same physical or psychological trait.

cone biopsy: a biopsy to remove abnormal tissues high in the cervical canal; called a cope biopsy because a cone-shaped wedge of tissue is removed for examination.

congenital disorders: abnormalities present at birth that occurred during fetal development as a result of genetic errors, exposure to toxins and microorganisms, or maternal illness.

congenital malformation: any anatomical defect present at birth.

congenital: existing at birth; often used in reference to certain mental or physical malformations and diseases, which may be hereditary or caused by some influence during gestation.

congenital: inborn, inherited.

conjunctivitis: inflammation of the conjunctiva, which lines the back of the eyelid, extends into the space between the lid and the globe of the eye, and goes over the globe to the transparent tissue covering the pupil.

connective tissue: the supporting framework of the body, particularly tendons and ligaments.

contact tracing: also known as partner referral; a process that consists of identifying sexual partners of infected patients, informing the partners of their exposure to disease, and offering resources for counseling and treatment.

contraception: the prevention of pregnancy.

contraction: a squeezing action of the uterus that results in birth.

contractures: permanent shorting of muscles or joints.

contrasexual pubertal development: development of male characteristics in pubescent girls.

contrast: a substance used to increase the contrast of structures or fluids within the body in medical imaging.

Cooper's ligament: projections of breast parenchyma covered by fibrous connective tissue that extend from the skin to the deep layer of superficial fascia.

cornea: the transparent, curved front surface of the eyeball, providing protection and focusing light onto the retina; most of the focusing power of the eye occurs here.

coronary arteries: blood vessels surrounding the heart that provide nourishment and oxygen to heart tissue.

coronary artery disease: heart disease caused by obstruction of the main coronary arteries.

corpus luteum: a yellow cell mass produced from a Graafian follicle after the release of an egg.

corpus luteum: the structure that develops from an emptied ovarian follicle after ovulation.

corpus uteri: the main body of the uterus above the constriction behind the cervix and below the openings of the fallopian tubes.

correlation: statistical measure that indicates the extent to which two or more variables fluctuate together; does one variable causes the fluctuation in the other.

cortisol: also called hydrocortisone, a steroid hormone produced by the adrenal cortex present in a mother's breast milk; could potentially reduce stress and symptoms of postpartum depression.

cosmetic surgery: the application of plastic surgical techniques to alter one's appearance for purely aesthetic reasons.

CPAP: Continuous Positive Airway Pressure; a constant flow of air pressure to ensure that the airway stays open during sleep.

CRAFFT: short clinical assessment tool designed to screen for substance-related risks and problems in adolescents; stands for the key words of the 6 items in the second section of the assessment: Car, Relax, Alone, Forget, Friends, Trouble.

cranial: toward the head; the same as superior in humans.

crepitus: the scraping or grinding sound heard or felt when bone rubs over bone in joint spaces.

cretinism: a severe hypothyroidism in which infants are born with insufficiently developed thyroid tissue.

Crohn's disease: a disease characterized by inflammation of all layers (full thickness) of the intestines or any part of the digestive tract; early symptoms may resemble those of irritable bowel syndrome.

crusting: the appearance of slightly elevated skin lesions made up of dried serum, blood, or pus; they can be brown, red, black, tan, or yellowish.

cryogenic agent: a substance (such as liquid nitrogen) that produces low temperatures.

cryopreservation: the use of very low temperatures to preserve structurally intact living cells and tissues.

cryoprobe: a liquid nitrogen-cooled, probelike tool used in cryosurgery.

cryosurgery: surgery using the local application of intense cold to destroy unwanted tissue.

cul-de-sac of Douglas: also called a recto-uterine pouch, the extension of the peritoneal cavity between the rectum and the posterior wall of the uterus.

culdoscopy: an endoscopic procedure performed to examine the rectouterine pouch and pelvic viscera by the introduction of a culdoscope through the posterior vaginal wall.

culture: the propagation of organisms, such as fungi, on artificial media; *Candida* organisms grow in many kinds of media in both the yeast and mold forms.

cuticle: cutaneous or skin tissue that surrounds the nail plate on its proximal sides and provides a protective barrier to the nail bed; it is attached to the proximal nail fold and to the nail plate.

cyanosis: a bluish discoloration of the skin resulting from poor circulation or inadequate oxygenation of the blood.

cyclothymia: a mood disorder characterized by fewer and less intense symptoms of elevated mood and depressed mood than bipolar disorders.

cyst: a closed sac having a distinct border that develops abnormally within a body space or structure.

cystitis: inflammation of the urinary bladder, often characterized by pain and dysuria.

cystopathy: a chronic complication of diabetes characterized by a classic triad of symptoms that consist of decreased bladder sensation, increased bladder capacity, and impaired detrusor contractility.

cystoscope: a thin, tube-like instrument used to look inside the bladder and urethra; has a light and a lens for viewing and usually equipped with a tool to remove tissue.

cystoscopy: examination of the bladder and urethra using a cystoscope inserted through the urethra and into the bladder.

cytobrush: a long cotton swab with a conical head used to collect cervical cell samples.

cytochrome P450s: enzymes found predominantly in liver cells, but also gastrointestinal cells, associated with the endoplasmic reticulum that chemically transform foreign chemicals called xenobiotics into more water-soluble derivatives that are more easily eliminated from the body by means of oxidation, reduction, hydrolysis, and hydroxylation reactions.

cytokines: proteins secreted by immune cells which contribute to immune responses and inflammation.

cytoscopy: a minor operation performed so that the urologist can examine the bladder.

cytotoxic: having a damaging effect on cells.

cytotoxicity: toxic to human cells.

cytotrophoblast: The inner layer of the trophoblast (the outermost layer of the embryo) that helps implant the embryo into the endometrial layer of the uterus. Together with the syncytiotrophoblast, the cytotrophoblast, and other cells form the placenta.

danger assessment tool: An instrument that helps determine the level of danger an abused woman has of being killed by her intimate partner.

date rape: a forced sexual act that occurs between people involved in a romantic relationship.

debridement: the excision of contused and devitalized tissue from a wound surface.

degenerative: marked by progression to a state below what is considered normal or desirable.

dehydration: excessive loss of the body's water content; in infants, manifests as increased pulse, sunken fontanelle, decreased blood pressure, dry mucous membranes, and decreased skin turgor.

deinfibulation: an anterior episiotomy.

deletion: the loss of a portion of a chromosome as a result of induced or accidental breakage.

delirium tremens: severe alcohol withdrawal syndrome, with symptoms including confusion, delirium, visual hallucinations, severe tremors, and clinically unstable involuntary body functions.

deltoid muscle: the muscle forming the rounded contour of the human shoulder.

dementia: a diseased state in which intellectual ability is ever decreasing; personality changes, decreased interest or ability to care for one's self, and long-term and short-term memory loss can indicate dementia.

demyelination: the destruction of myelin.

dendritic cell: an antigen-presenting cell that acts as a key regulator of the adaptive immune response that is capable of activating naïve T cells and stimulating the growth and differentiation of B cells.

deoxyribonucleic acid (DNA): genetic material contained in cells, which can definitively identify an individual.

depression: a condition characterized by a persistent mood of sadness, weight loss, greatly decreased interest in life, and sometimes psychotic episodes; biological factors, family history of depression, underlying medical problems, and medication side effects all can contribute to these symptoms.

dermabrasion: the removal of superficial layers of skin with a rapidly revolving abrasive tool, as a technique in cosmetic surgery.

dermatitis perpetiformis: a blistering, itching rash on the skin often resulting from celiac disease.

dermatitis: a general term for nonspecific skin irritations that may be caused by bacteria, viruses, or fungi.

dermatologist: a physician who treats the skin and its structures, functions, and diseases.

dermatoses: disorders of the skin.

dermis: the layer of skin directly beneath the epidermis, consisting of dense connective tissue and numerous blood vessels.

desquamation: shedding of the outer layer of skin.

Diagnostic and Statistical Manual of Mental *D*isorders: the handbook the American Psychiatric Society uses to categorize and diagnose mental disorders.

diagnostic codes: the method used in the *Diagnostic and Statistical.*

diaphragmatic hernia: a protrusion of the stomach into the diaphragm.

differentiation: The process by which immature cells become mature cells capable of executing specialized functions.

differentiation: the process of gradual remodeling of tissues in the embryo or fetus; in this context, the process of formation of the male or female reproductive organs.

dihydrotestosterone: male hormone, a derivative of testosterone that plays a key role in androgenic alopecia.

dilation and curettage (D&C): a procedure in which the cervix is stretched, and the lining of the uterus is scraped.

dilation: the opening of the cervix to allow passage of the fetus through the birth canal.

dimorphism: the ability of a fungus to exist in two forms, yeasts and molds; yeasts are unicellular round, oval, or cylindrical cells, and molds are branching tubular structures called hyphae.

discoid rash: raised red patches.

disequilibrium: off-balance sensation.

dishidrosis: also known as dyshidrotic eczema or pompholyx; a skin condition characterized by the formation of small blisters that appear on the palms of the hands and sides of the fingers and sometimes, the soles of the feet.

disimpaction: removal of feces, usually manually, in fecal impaction.

disseminated sclerosis: another name for multiple sclerosis (MS).

distal interphalangeal joints: the distal joints of the fingers.

distal: away from the point of origin.

distillation: the use of heat to separate or purify mixtures of liquid chemicals that boil at different temperatures by vaporization and cooling back into the liquid state.

diuretic: an agent that promotes the secretion of urine.

diverticulitis: inflammation of a diverticulum, especially in the colon, causing pain and disturbance of bowel function.

diverticulosis: a condition in which diverticula are present in the intestine without signs of inflammation.

dizygotes: fraternal twins; born from two ova separately fertilized by two sperm.

dizziness: non-specific term that includes vertigo, fainting, and disequilibrium.

dopamine: Neurotransmitter that inhibits the release of prolactin.

Doppler effect: the relationship of the apparent frequency of waves, such as sound waves, to the relative motion of the source of the waves and the observer or instrument; the frequency increases as the two approach each other and decreases as they move apart; an effect also known as the Doppler shift.

dorsal: toward the back.

dose-response: the relationship between the dose (a quantitative measurement of exposure usually expressed in terms of concentration and duration) and the quantitative expression of change to the status of human health and well-being resulting in disease.

Down syndrome: a common genetic disorder characterized by mental retardation and other abnormalities, including heart malformations.

dual diagnosis: a broad term used among professionals to indicate that an individual has two disorders needing integrated care and often used in psychiatry to indicate that an individual has received the diagnosis of a substance use disorder and another major clinical syndrome, such as a bipolar disorder.

duplex scan: an ultrasound representation of echo images of tissues and blood vessels combined with a Doppler representation of blood flow patterns.

dysmenorrhea: painful menstruation.

dysmorphic: abnormal in shape or appearance.

dyspareunia: painful sexual intercourse.

dysplasia: the presence of cells of an abnormal type within a tissue, which may signify a stage preceding the development of cancer.

dysthymia: a mood disorder characterized by symptoms similar to depression that are fewer in number but last for a much longer period of time.

dysuria: painful or difficult urination, often the result of urinary tract infection or obstruction.

dysuria: painful urination, usually as a result of infection or an obstruction; the patient complains of a burning sensation when voiding.

eating disorder: weight gain or loss resulting from compulsive overeating, anorexia nervosa, or bulimia.

eclampsia: a condition in which one or more convulsions occur in a pregnant woman suffering from high blood pressure, often followed by coma and posing a threat to the health of mother and baby.

ectopic pregnancy: a pregnancy in which the implantation of the fertilized egg occurs anywhere outside the uterus, usually in the Fallopian tube.

ectopic: occurring in an abnormal location (e.g. ectopic pregnancy, ectopic focus in the heart); in the case of pregnancy, referring to extrauterine sites of implantation.

edema: an abnormal accumulation of watery fluid in the connective tissues, resulting in swelling.

ejaculation: the reflex activated by sexual stimulation that results in sperm mixed with fluid being expelled from the male's body.

elastin: the major connective tissue protein of elastic structures.

electroconvulsive therapy (ECT): the use of electric shocks to induce seizure in depressed patients as a form of treatment.

electronystagmography: specialized eye movement measurements.

elementary body: a resting form of *Chlamydia trachomitis* that infects host cells.

emaciation: the state of being abnormally thin or weak.

emboli: substances that are released into the blood vessel for the purpose of their occlusion.

embolus: a clot or other piece of matter that may travel through the circulatory system to tiny blood vessels (as in the brain) and block the path that normally allows blood flow.

Embryo: from the 3rd through approximately the end of the 10th week of gestation.

emotional dysregulation: the inability of a person to control or regulate their emotional responses to provocative stimuli.

emphysema: progressive destruction of the alveolar walls, leading to highly inflated and stiffened lungs.

encephalitis: inflammation of the brain.

endarterectomy: a surgical technique in which an atherosclerotic plaque is excised.

endocrine pancreas: specialized secretory tissue dispersed within the pancreas called islets of Langerhans, which are responsible for the secretion of glucagon and insulin.

endocrine system: a series of ductless glands that deliver hormones to target cells directly through the bloodstream.

endocrine: the secretion of hormones directly into the bloodstream, rather than by way of a duct.

endolymph: inner-ear fluid.

endometrial curettage: a surgical procedure in which the endometrial lining of the uterus is scraped to remove tissue or growths.

endometriosis: a condition whereby cells of the uterine lining are found in abnormal locations, such as the pelvic cavity or ovary; endometriosis can lead to pelvic pain and the development of scars that can block the Fallopian tubes.

endometrium: Innermost layer of the uterus that responds to hormones and cycles through periods of proliferation and differentiation, followed by programmed cell death and sloughing of dead tissue.

endoplasmic reticulum: a network of membranes found throughout the cell and connected to the nucleus.

endorphins: hormones, found mainly in the brain, that bind to opiate receptors, reducing the sensation of pain and affecting emotions.

endoscopy: procedure with a flexible tube that allows direct viewing inside the body.

endotracheal tube: a tube placed in the trachea to assist with breathing or facilitate the delivery of oxygen and other medications directly into the lungs.

energy balance: the state in which kilocalories from ingested food are equal to kilocalories expended.

energy-yielding nutrient: nutrients that supply the body with energy (fat provides 9 kilocalories per gram, while carbohydrates and protein provide 4 kilocalories per gram).

engorgement: an uncomfortable, often painful condition in which the breasts are overly full of milk.

enterostomy: a surgical operation in which the intestine is diverted to an artificial opening in the abdominal wall or in another part of the intestine.

environmental epidemiology: the systematic study of the distribution and determinants of environmental diseases in a population.

environmental infection: human exposure to infectious agents of diseases (including bacteria, fungi, parasites, and viruses) through contact with environmental media such as contaminated water, air, food, and soil.

environmental radiation: human exposure to electromagnetic radiation at doses and durations that can produce adverse impacts on human health.

environmental toxicity: human exposure to chemical or biochemical substances at doses that produce harmful modification to the body's physiological mechanisms, leading to diseases.

ephedrine: causes constriction of the blood vessels and widening of the bronchial passages, and is typically used to relieve asthma and hay fever.

epidermis: the outermost part of the skin, composed of four or five different layers called strata.

epilepsy: a neurological disorder marked by sudden recurrent episodes of sensory disturbance, loss of consciousness, or convulsions, associated with abnormal electrical activity in the brain.

episiotomy: the incision of the labia.

Erb's palsy: stereotyped clinical presentation of neonatal brachial plexus palsy resulting from injury to the C5, C6, and sometimes C7 spinal nerve roots.

erogenous zones: bodily areas that are especially sensitive to touch, leading to sexual arousal; although a dozen or so such zones are common (for example, the clitoral glans and labia, penile glans and shaft, breasts, buttocks, inner thighs), these zones can differ from person to person.

erotic: referring to sensory perceptions that are sensual (gratifying or pleasurable) and sexual; the context in which they occur will determine whether the perceptions become erotic (for example, breast and testicle examinations are typically not erotic, while caressing these same body parts in romantic settings typically is).

erythematosus: characterized by redness of the skin.

erythematous: related to or marked by reddening.

erythrocytes: red blood cells of the circulatory system that contain hemoglobin and are responsible for delivering oxygen to the tissues.

erythropoietin: the hormone protein that is produced in the kidneys and acts on the bone marrow helping in red blood cell synthesis.

Escherichia coli: bacteria found in the intestines that may cause disease elsewhere.

estimated average requirement (EAR): intake level of a nutrient at which the needs of half the population will be met.

estradiol: the primary human female hormone before menopause.

estriol: female hormone produced primarily during pregnancy.

estrogen: a group of steroid hormones synthesized from cholesterol that promote the development and maintenance of female characteristics.

estrone: hormone produced by ovaries, placenta, and, in men and postmenopausal women, adipose tissue.

etiology: the science of causes or origins, especially of diseases.

excisional biopsy: a biopsy in which an entire lesion is removed.

exocrine gland: a gland that releases its secretions via ducts to external surfaces.

exocrine gland: a gland that secretes fluid into a duct.

exogenous: originating outside an organ or part.

exposure assessment: a systematic process of discovering the pathway through which humans are exposed to specific environmental agents and risk factors, and of ascertaining the quantity and duration of that exposure.

external genitalia: in the male, the penis and scrotum; in the female, the clitoris, the vaginal opening, and the folds (labia) around it.

extraembryonic membranes: the term for the collective layers enclosing the embryo inside the uterus.

eye movement desensitization and reprocessing (EMDR): a structured therapy that encourages the patient to briefly focus on the trauma memory while simultaneously experiencing bilateral stimulation (typically eye movements), which is associated with a reduction in the vividness and emotion associated with the trauma memories.

failure to thrive: a lack of healthy growth that may result from the absence of a nurturing presence and support, both emotionally and physically.

Fallopian tube: one of a pair of open-ended ducts branching from the top of the uterus, which collects eggs released from the ovary and in which fertilization usually occurs.

Fallopian tube: one of two structures that conduct the egg, as it is released from the ovary, into the uterus.

Fallopian tubes or oviducts: tubular structures attached at their lower ends to the uterus; the passageways for ova following ovulation.

false negative: a test result which incorrectly indicates that the individual is not pregnant.

false positive: a test result which incorrectly indicates that the individual is pregnant.

fast: to abstain from food.

feedback: the mechanism whereby a hormone inhibits its own production; often involves the inhibition of the hypothalamus and tropic hormones.

female sexual dysfunction: persistent, recurrent problems with sexual response, desire, orgasm **or painhormone replacement therapy:** treatment with hormones to replace natural hormones when the body does not make enough.

feminizing genitoplasty: male-to-female surgical procedures including penectomy, orchiectomy, and vaginoplasty.

ferritin: the primary intracellular storage form of iron.

fertilization: The fusion of male and female gametes, sperm and eggs, to form a new living organism.

fetal alcohol syndrome: a congenital syndrome of infants born to mothers who excessively consumed alcohol during pregnancy that is characterized by retardation of mental development of the infant, and impedance of normal physical growth, particularly of the skull and face.

fetal fibronectin: a protein produced by fetal cells; found at the interface of the the fetal sac and the uterine lining; it can be thought of as an adhesive or "biological glue" that binds the fetal sac to the uterine lining; when it starts "leaking" into the vagina it indicates a possible preterm delivery.

fetal macrosomia: a newborn who's significantly larger than average.

fetal: in humans, a term normally referring to the developmental period following eight weeks of gestation; in fetal tissue transplantation, refers to tissue from earlier developmental stages as well.

fetoscopy: an endoscopic procedure during pregnancy to allow surgical access to the fetus.

fetus: an unborn baby more than eight weeks after conception.

fibrillation: wild beating of the heart, which may occur when the regular rate of the heartbeat is interrupted.

fibrocartilage: tough, very strong tissue found predominantly in the intervertebral disks and at the insertions of ligaments and tendons.

fibrocystic breasts: the lumpy breasts that some women routinely develop, particularly in the seven or eight days before menstruation.

fibroid: a noncancerous tumor of the uterus, also known as leiomyoma; when large, these tumors can cause heavy menstrual bleeding leading to anemia or cause pressure symptoms in the pelvis.

fibromyalgia: a condition of generalized chronic pain that shares many symptoms with chronic fatigue syndrome.

fibrositis: an earlier, less common term for fibromyalgia.

fight-or-flight response: a stressful biochemical reaction in animals, usually involving the adrenal hormone epinephrine, that prepares the animal for confrontation with predators or competitors.

fine needle aspiration: a surgical procedure in which a thin, hollow needle is used to withdraw tissue from the body.

Fitz-Hugh-Curtis syndrome: a condition associated with pelvic inflammatory disease that includes inflammation of the Glisson's capsule that surrounds the liver.

flare-up: an episode of heightened pain and debilitation in fibromyalgia; sometimes flare-ups do not have an immediate, precipitating cause that is identifiable, while other times they are associated with humidity, cold, physical exertion, or psychological stress.

flatulence: the presence of excessive gas in the stomach and intestines, which is expelled from the body.

follicle: a small, spherical, secretory structure in the ovary that releases the ovum or "egg".

follicle-stimulating hormone: a peptide hormone secreted by the anterior lobe of the pituitary gland, also called follitropin, that stimulates the growth of the ovum-containing follicles in the ovaries.

forceps: curved metal blades that are carefully placed around the fetal head through the vagina to facilitate delivery.

foremilk: the milk released early in a nursing session, which is low in fat and rich in nutrients.

free radical: an uncharged molecule (typically highly reactive and short-lived) having an unpaired valence electron.

frequency: the number of complete cycles, such as sound cycles, produced by an alternating energy source; sound is measured in cycles per second, and one cycle per second is equal to 1 hertz.

full-term: referring to a gestation period of a full nine months.

functional somatic syndromes: a continuum or spectrum of disorders (such as chronic fatigue syndrome, Epstein-Barr virus, and primary headaches) characterized by complex interactions between symptoms and patients' personal stress.

fused labia: a condition where the two flaps of skin on either side of the opening to the vagina (the labia minora) are joined together.

GABA/benzodiazepine receptor: an area on a nerve cell to which gamma aminobutyric acid (GABA) attaches and that causes inhibition (quieting) of the nerve; benzodiazepine drugs enhance the attachment of GABA to the receptor.

galactorrhea: a physiologic condition in which the body produces a milk-like discharge outside of pregnancy and breastfeeding. While it usually occurs in women, it can occur in males and even in children.

galactosemia: a rare genetic metabolic disorder that affects an individual's ability to metabolize the sugar galactose properly.

gametes: the egg (ovum) and sperm cells that unite to form the fertilized egg (zygote) in reproduction.

ganglia: clusters of nerves.

gastroenterology: study of the function and diseases associated with the stomach, intestines, and other organs of the digestive tract such as the liver and pancreas.

gastrointestinal: referring to the small and large intestines.

gastrulation: A complex process during animal development in which the single-cell-thick embryo is rearranged into a multi-layered structure.

gay: may refer to same-sex attraction (i.e. male-male or female-female) generally. Self-identified men who are attracted to other men may consider themselves gay.

gender dysphoria: a distressed state arising from conflict between a person's self-identified gender and the sex the person has or was identified as having at birth.

gender expression: characteristics in personality, appearance, and behavior that in a given culture and historical period are designated as masculine or feminine. While most individuals present socially in clearly masculine or feminine gender roles, some people present in an alternative gender role such as genderqueer or specifically transgender.

gender fluid: identity label that may be used by individuals whose gender identity may fluctuate between masculine and feminine or an alternative gender.

gender identity: a person's inner sense and feeling of maleness/ masculinity or femaleness/femininity, or both; it implies that one clearly identifies with one gender more than the other, although some people identify with both genders equally or near equally.

gender nonconforming/gender diverse: adjective to describe individuals whose gender identity, role, or expression differs from what is normative for their assigned sex in a given culture and historical period.

gender presentation: how a person outwardly expresses their identity, may or may not conform to what is typically expected of men or women, or align with characteristics typically associated with the sex someone is assigned at birth.

gender role: behaviors and self-presentations that are associated with being a boy/man or a girl/woman and that one uses to identify or recognize others as a boy/man or a girl/ woman; the term also implies the sociocultural expectations of boys/men and girls/women.

gender: generally classified by societal expectations of feminine or masculine roles in social, psychological, or emotional expression.

gender-affirming hormone therapy (GAH): hormonal medication that helps patients develop secondary sex characteristics to achieve masculinizing or feminizing effects, relieve gender dysphoria, and overall support gender affirmation.

gender-affirming surgery: surgery to change primary and/or secondary sex characteristics to affirm a person's gender identity, often an important part of medically necessary treatment to alleviate gender dysphoria.

gender-confirming surgery or gender-affirming surgery: also known as sex reassignment surgery; surgery aimed to alter a person's primary and/or secondary sex characteristics to resemble that of their expressed gender (e.g., vaginoplasty or phalloplasty).

gender-nonconforming: person whose behavior or appearance does not conform to prevailing cultural and social expectations about what is appropriate to their gender.

genderqueer: identity label that may be used by individuals whose gender identity and/or role does not conform to a binary understanding of gender as limited to the categories of man or woman, male or female.

gene: a master molecule that encodes the information needed for the body to carry out one specific function; many thousands of genes working together are needed to sustain normal human life.

general anesthesia: anesthesia that induces unconsciousness.

general anesthesia: anesthesia that induces unconsciousness.

general practice: a primary care field with care provided by physicians who usually have completed less than three years of residency training; the organization from which family medicine evolved.

generalism: a medical and political movement concerned with primary care, often associated with the medical specialties of family medicine, general internal medicine, general pediatrics, and sometimes obstetrics and gynecology.

genetic: inherited.

genital herpes: a disease characterized by blisters in the genital area, caused by a variety of the herpes simplex virus.

genital warts: warts occurring in the genital and anal areas acquired by sexual contact and caused by HPV infection.

genitalia: the internal and external reproductive organs.

geriatrics: a medical specialty focused on the care of elderly patients.

germ tube test: an initial laboratory test used to identify unknown yeasts and performed by microscopi-

cally examining a colony of yeast inoculated into rabbit or human plasma.

gerontology: the formal study of the phenomena of aging from maturity to old age.

gestation: the period from conception to birth, in which the fetus reaches full development in order to survive outside the mother's body.

gestational age: the age of a fetus, as determined from the first day of the last menstrual period, which is approximately two weeks before the date of conception; when the date of the last menstrual period is not known, the gestational age can be estimated via ultrasound.

gestational hypertension: blood pressure of at least 140/90 mm Hg at or after 20 weeks' gestation.

gingivostomatitis: inflammation of the gums and mouth.

glandular cells: cells found in the cervix and the lining of the uterus that are involved in the menstrual cycle and in the production of cervical mucus; glandular cells found on a Pap test may be normal, abnormal, or cancerous.

glaucoma: an increase in the eye's internal pressure that can damage the optic nerve and eventually lead to blindness.

gliadin: a major component in gluten, gliadin is a class of proteins present in wheat and several other cereals within the grass genus Triticum.

glucose: a simple sugar which is an important energy source in living organisms and is a component of many carbohydrates.

gluten: substance present in cereal grains, especially wheat, that is responsible for the elastic texture of dough.

glycosaminoglycan: any of a group of compounds occurring chiefly as components of connective tissue. They are useful to the body as a lubricant or as a shock absorber.

goiter: a swelling of the neck resulting from enlargement of the thyroid gland.

gonad: the internal organ in either sex that produces the reproductive cells (ova and sperm): the ovary in the female and the testis in the male.

gonadal intersex: an individual with both ovarian and testicular tissue; this may be in the same gonad (an ovotestis), or the person might have one ovary and one testis; the individual may have XX chromosomes, XY chromosomes, or both; the external genitals may be ambiguous or may appear to be female or male.

gonadotropin releasing hormone: a peptide hormone synthesized in and secreted by the hypothalamus that stimulates the anterior lobe of the pituitary gland to secrete gonadotropins, which include follicle-stimulating hormone and luteinizing hormone.

gonadotropin: hormone secreted by the pituitary gland; the primary gonadotropic hormones are luteinizing hormone (LH) and follicle-stimulating hormone (FSH).

gonads: the reproductive organs; the ovaries in females and the testes (testicles) in males.

gonorrhea: a venereal disease involving inflammatory discharge from the urethra or vagina.

Graafian follicle: any of the ovarian follicles that produce eggs.

granuloma: a nodular, inflammatory lesion that is usually small, firm, and persistent and usually contains proliferated macrophages.

Graves' disease: a common type of hyperthyroidism in which the thyroid gland produces an oversupply of hormone.

gumma: a soft, non-cancerous growth that results from the tertiary stage of syphilis.

gynecomastia: Breast development in men.

Hashimoto's disease: the autoimmune system produces antibodies that attack the thyroid gland leading to underproduction of thyroid hormone.

head: the part of the body containing the major sense organs (such as the eyes and ears) and the brain.

healing: the restoration to a normal physical, mental, or spiritual condition.

health maintenance: the practice of anticipating, finding, preventing, and/or dealing with potential or established medical problems at the earliest possible stage to minimize adverse effects on the patient.

health: a condition in which all functions of the body, mind, and spirit are normally active.

helper T cells: a type of lymphocyte that recognizes foreign antigens and secretes signaling molecules called cytokines to regulate the immune response; there are two different subtypes of helper T cells, one of which (Th1) activates cell-mediated immune responses for defending against intracellular viral and bacterial pathogens, and the other (Th2) of which drives B cells to produce antibodies against antigens in the humoral response.

hemangioma: a birthmark that most commonly appears as a rubbery, bright red nodule of extra blood vessels in the skin.

hematopoiesis: the process by which blood cells are made in the bone marrow from hematopoietic stem cells.

hematuria: the abnormal presence of blood in the urine.

hemoglobin: the pigmented protein that imparts red color to the blood and carries oxygen from the lungs to the rest of the body.

hemolysis: the rupture of red blood cells and release of hemoglobin into the blood, which can cause anemia.

hemolytic anemia: anemia attributable to increased destruction of red blood cells.

hemolytic uremia: a type of uremia that afflicts mostly young children and infants.

hemorrhage: uncontrolled bleeding.

hemorrhagic stroke: caused by a weakened blood vessel that has burst or is leaking blood into the brain causing intracranial pressure to rise and to kill brain cells.

hemorrhagic stroke: stroke caused by the rupture of a blood vessel in or on the surface of the brain with bleeding into the surrounding tissue.

hemorrhagic: weakened blood vessel ruptures, as a result of aneurysm or arteriovenous malformation.

Herberden's nodes: osteophytes or bony spurs that develop as a result of destruction of joint cartilage in distal interphalangeal joints.

herniated disk: prolapse of the nucleus through a rupture or weakness in the annulus.

heterosexual: being principally attracted to and aroused by a person of the opposite gender; a synonymous term, "straight," refers to persons of either gender who are primarily Heterosexual.

hiatal hernia: a protrusion of the stomach into the opening normally occupied in the diaphragm by the esophagus.

highly active antiretroviral therapy (HAART): the use of a combination of three or four anti-HIV drugs in an HIV positive individual to suppress replication of new HIV particles and slow the progression to full-blown AIDS.

hind milk: the milk obtained in the latter part of one session of breastfeeding.

hirsutism: excess facial hair.

histopathology: the study of the appearance and structure of abnormal or diseased tissue under the microscope.

holistic: the philosophy that individuals function as complete units or integrated systems and are not understood merely through their parts.

homeostasis: the maintenance of constant, linear conditions within a system, such as the maintenance of human body temperature, pH, and hormonal levels at stable states.

homologous chromosomes: chromosome pairs of the same size and centromere position that possess genes for the same traits; one homologous chromosome is inherited from the father and the other from the mother.

homophobia: obsessive fear of and anxiety about homosexuals and their social and sexual activities; while several causes of homophobia are known, the most common is a homophobe's private, often unconscious fear and doubt about his or her own sexuality and sense of sexual adequacy.

homosexual: being principally attracted to and aroused by persons of one's own gender; two synonymous terms are "gay," which can refer to all homosexuals or to homosexual boys/men exclusively, and "lesbian," which refers only to homosexual girls/women.

hormone receptor: a molecule contained in or on a cell that allows it to respond to a hormone; if receptors are not present, the hormone will have no effect.

hormone: a chemical carried in the blood that acts as a messenger between two or more body parts.

Horner's syndrome: ptosis (eyelid drooping), miosis (abnormal constriction of the pupil of the eye), and anhydrosis (decreased sweating on the face).

HRT estrogens: estrone, estradiol, and estriol.

HRT: hormone-replacement therapy.

human chorionic gonadotropin (hCG): a glycoprotein hormone similar in structure to luteinizing hormone that is secreted by the placenta during early pregnancy to maintain corpus luteum function and is commonly tested for as an indicator of pregnancy.

human papilloma virus (HPV): a virus with subtypes that cause diseases in humans ranging from common warts to cervical cancer.

humeral: relating to the humerus bone, the bone of the upper arm or forelimb, forming joints at the shoulder and the elbow.

hyaline cartilage: translucent, bluish-white type of cartilage present in the joints, the respiratory tract, and the immature skeleton.

hydronephrosis: swelling (distension) of the kidney.

hyperandrogenism: higher-than-normal levels of androgens in the blood.

hypercortisolemia: refers to high amounts of circulating cortisol and may be a pathological or non-pathological condition.

hyperkeratosis: excessive proliferation of skin cells accompanied by accelerated sloughing.

hyperlipidemia: an excess of lipids (for example, cholesterol and triglycerides) in the blood.

hyperthermia: environmentally influenced elevated body temperature.

hyperthyroidism: the thyroid gland produces too much hormone.

hypnosis: the induction of a state of consciousness in which a person apparently loses the power of voluntary action and is highly responsive to suggestion or direction.

hypochondriasis: a condition in which the patients believe strongly that they are suffering from one or more serious illnesses, even when this belief is unsupported by medical evidence.

hypogonadism: Underdevelopment of the gonads.

hyponychium: cutaneous tissue underlying the free nail at its point of separation from the nail bed; structurally similar to the cuticle.

hypopnea: a decrease in airflow greater than 50 percent.

hypospadias: a congenital condition in males in which the opening of the urethra is on the underside of the penis.

hypothalamic hamartomas: tumors in the hypothalamic region of the brain, which are usually benign.

hypothalamohypophysial: relating to the hypothalamus and the hypophysis (pituitary gland).

hypothalamus: a region of the forebrain below the thalamus which coordinates both the autonomic nervous system and the activity of the pituitary, controlling body temperature, thirst, hunger, and other homeostatic systems, and involved in sleep and emotional activity.

hypothermia: environmentally influenced lower-than-normal body temperature.

hypothyroidism: a condition in which the thyroid gland produces an insufficient supply of hormone.

hypotonic: the presence of a low osmotic pressure.

hypoxemia: subnormal oxygenation of arterial blood.

hysterectomy: a surgery that removes part or all of the uterus.

hysteroscopy: a procedure that uses a thin, lighted scope to look inside the uterus and diagnose uterine conditions.

hysteroscopy: a procedure using a thin, lighted tube with a camera and tool to examine visually and remove part of the endometrium.

ibuprofen: synthetic compound used as an analgesic and anti-inflammatory drug; proprietary names include Advil.

idiopathic: referring to a medical condition with no known cause.

ileum: distal part of the small intestine, closest to the starting part of the colon; can be involved in ulcerative colitis.

illness: the condition of being sick or diseased.

immortalized: the state of a cancer cell that allows it to divide an unlimited number of times.

immunity: the capacity to resist a disease caused by an infectious agent.

immunocompromised: the state of having a weakened immune system.

immunoglobulin E (IgE): ordinarily, a relatively rare antibody; in patients with atopic dermatitis, levels can be significantly higher than in the general population.

impaction: the condition of being or process of becoming impacted, especially of feces in the intestine.

implant: a section of endometrial tissue found outside the uterus.

implantation: an early stage during pregnancy in which the fertilized embryo attaches within the wall of the uterus, or "womb".

in utero: the Latin term for "inside or within the womb".

in vitro fertilization (IVF): the fertilization of eggs outside the body with subsequent implantation of embryos in the uterus.

in vitro: a Latin term used to indicate a process that has taken place outside an organism, such as in a laboratory test tube or petri dish.

incest: a sexual act between close relatives such as father-daughter or brother-sister.

incidence: probability or risk of contracting a disease within a population.

incision: a cut made with a scalpel during a surgical procedure.

incisional biopsy: a biopsy in which a piece of tissue is removed from a lesion or mass; the tissue is then tested to find out what it is.

incontinence: inability to control the bladder or bowel.

incubator: in the nursery, a Plexiglas unit that encloses the premature or sick infant to allow strict temperature regulation.

infant: a young child from birth to twelve months of age.

infectious mononucleosis: acute self-limiting infection of lymphocytes by the Epstein-Barr virus.

inferior: downward; toward the ground or the feet.

infertility: the inability to produce offspring by a person in the childbearing years who has been having sex without contraception for twelve months.

infibulation: a clitoridectomy followed by the sewing up of the vulva.

inflammation: a response of the body to tissue damage caused by injury or infection and characterized by redness, pain, heat, and swelling.

inflammatory: irritation that causes swelling, heat, and discomfort.

inherited disorder: a disorder caused by an alteration of a gene and passed through families.

initiation: the first abnormal change that starts a cell along the pathway to cancer.

insomnia: disturbed sleep, which occurs in older people more often than in any other age group; insomnia in older people can be caused by many factors, such as dysfunctional sleep cycles, breathing problems, leg jerking, underlying medical and psychiatric disorders, and the side effects of medication.

insulin: a hormone produced in the pancreas by the islets of Langerhans, which regulates the amount of glucose in the blood.

integrase: an enzyme associated with the HIV virion that can insert the retroviral dsDNA and insert it into the genome (i.e. the chromosomes) of the host cell.

interleukin-2: a protein messenger that regulates T cell activity and differentiation during the immune response.

internship: a synonym for the first year of residency training.

intersex: also called "difference in sexual development"; any of a number of chromosomal or anatomical differences that someone is born with that vary from what is biologically associated with "male" or "female". Some intersex conditions will yield what medical providers may call "ambiguous genitalia". Many cultures worldwide recognize intersex conditions as normal variance.

interstitial pulmonary fibrosis (IPF): the scarring and thickening (fibrosis) of the lung tissue, which causes breathing difficulty, chest pain, coughing, and shortness of breath; the lungs become increasingly stiffer until heart failure ensues.

interventional radiology: the specialty of radiology in which techniques such as X-ray imaging, computed tomography (CT) scans, ultrasounds, or magnetic resonance imaging (MRI) are used for guidance to navigate and introduce catheters or electrodes for various purposes.

intervertebral disk: the flexible, cylindrical pad between each two vertebrae, consisting of the nucleus pulposus (gelatinous center) and the annulus fibrosis (concentric rings of cartilage); the flexibility, moistness, and thickness of the disk decreases naturally with age.

intrauterine cannula: a hollow, rigid tube designed to place dyed fluid into the uterus to determine a perforation.

intrauterine growth retardation: the condition of infants who are born significantly smaller than the standard for the number of weeks that they have spent in the uterus.

irritability: a state of general overreaction to external stimuli.

ischemia: a local anemia or area of diminished or insufficient blood supply as a result of mechanical obstruction of the blood supply (commonly narrowing of an artery).

ischemic colitis: inadequate blood supply to the colon.

ischemic stroke: stroke caused by a blood clot that blocks or plugs a blood vessel in the brain.

isograft: a transplanted tissue or organ from a genetically identical individual (identical twin).

isoimmunization: the development of antibodies against antigens from the same species.

isthmus: a narrow organ, passage, or piece of tissue connecting two larger parts.

joints: the junctions at the ends of bones that allow for movement.

Kaposi's sarcoma: a form of blood vessel tumor that produces pink to purple splotches or plaques on the skin in about 25 percent of persons with AIDS and may also affect internal organs; caused by sexual transmission of human herpes virus 8 (HHV8).

karyotype: the chromosomal makeup of an individual; also refers to the arrangement of chromosomes in standard paired fashion on a photomicrograph, which can facilitate analysis of the chromosomes.

keratin: a family of fibrous structural proteins that compose skin, nails, and hair.

keratinocytes: matrix basal epithelial cells that differentiate, fill with keratin, and form the dead horny substance making up the nail plate.

ketone: an organic compound containing a carbonyl group bonded to two hydrocarbon groups, made by oxidizing secondary alcohols; the simplest such compound is acetone.

ketosis: a metabolic state characterized by raised levels of ketone bodies in the body tissues, which is typically pathological in conditions such as diabetes, or may be the consequence of a diet that is very low in carbohydrates.

kidney stones: a hard mass formed in the kidneys, typically consisting of insoluble calcium compounds.

kilocalorie: the amount of heat necessary to raise the temperature of a kilogram of water 1 degree Celsius; the unit of measure for the energy content of foods, also called a Calorie.

Korsakoff's psychosis: mental illness named after Sergei Korsakoff that involves severe confusion and inability to remember recent memories, usually caused by alcoholism.

Kupffer cells: specialized cells in the liver that perform the function of removing bacterial debris from the blood that has circulated throughout the body.

kyphosis: backward curvature of the spine or a section of the spine.

labia majora: relatively large, fleshy folds of tissue that enclose and protect the other external genital organs.

labia minora: a pair of thin cutaneous folds that form part of the vulva, or external female genitalia.

labioscrotal: relating to or being a swelling or ridge on each side of the embryonic rudiment of the penis or clitoris which develops into one of the scrotal sacs in the male and one of the labia majora in the female.

labor: the period in the birth process in which forceful and rhythmic uterine contractions are present.

labyrinth: mazelike system of canals in the inner ear.

lactation: the production and secretion of milk by the mammary glands.

lactiferous duct: a single excretory duct from each lobe of mammary glandular tissue that converges yet opens separately at the tip of the nipple; the mammary gland has fifteen to twenty lactiferous ducts.

lactoferrin: a breast milk factor that binds iron, preventing it from supporting the growth of harmful intestinal bacteria; it may also promote the ability to absorb dietary iron.

lactose: a sugar found in milk and milk products; some people cannot digest lactose, causing lactose intolerance, which can produce symptoms that resemble those of irritable bowel syndrome.

laparoscope: a small surgical tube which can be inserted through a small incision into the abdominal cavity to view and perform surgery on abdominal organs.

laparoscopy: a minimally invasive surgery technique that utilizes small incisions through the skin to pass a camera and other surgical instruments into the abdomen or pelvis; typically results in decreased postoperative pain and length of recovery compared to traditional open procedures.

laparotomy: a surgical procedure, often exploratory in nature, carried out through the abdominal wall; it may be used to correct endometriosis.

larynx: the hollow muscular organ forming an air passage to the lungs and holding the vocal cords in humans and other mammals; the voice box.

laser: a concentrated, high-energy light beam often used to destroy abnormal tissue.

latent: lying hidden or undeveloped within a person; unrevealed.

lateral: away from the midline.

laxative: an agent that promotes evacuation of the bowel.

leiomyomas: also known as fibroids, benign smooth muscle tumor occurring frequently in the uterus.

lens: the transparent part of the eye behind the cornea that is responsible for changing shape to allow the eye to accommodate and fine-tune focus.

lentivirus: a classification of retroviruses characterized by a very long incubation period (ten to twenty years) before symptoms of a disease appear.

lesbian: a self-identified woman who is sexually, or romantically, attracted to other women.

lesion: any pathologic change in tissue.

let-down reflex: the reflex that forces milk to the front of the breast.

lipid: any of a class of organic compounds that are fatty acids or their derivatives and are insoluble in water but soluble in organic solvents.

lithium: a drug composed of lithium carbonate used in the treatment of bipolar disorders.

lobule: a small gland that, when sent appropriate hormonal cues, produces milk.

local anesthesia: anesthesia that numbs the feeling in a body part, administered by injection or direct application to the skin.

lordosis: forward curvature of the spine or a section of the spine.

lower extremities: the thigh, lower leg, and foot.

lumbar puncture: also known as a spinal tap; a procedure that involves insertion of a needle into the lumbar spinal column.

lumbar spine: the lowest of three parts of the spine, consisting of five vertebrae, named L1 to L5 (just above the sacrum), in a natural lordosis.

lumpectomy: a surgical operation in which a lump is removed from the breast, typically when cancer is present but has not spread.

lunula: a white, crescent-shaped area at the end of the proximal nail fold that marks the end of the nail matrix and is the site of nail growth.

luteal phase: the second half of the menstrual cycle after ovulation; during this phase, the corpus luteum secretes progesterone.

luteinizing hormone: a peptide hormone secreted by the anterior lobe of the pituitary gland that stimulates: ovulation of ova from Graafian follicles and the development of the corpora lutea after ovulation in the.

lymphocytes: a form of small leukocyte (white blood cell) with a single round nucleus, occurring especially in the lymphatic system.

lymphoma: one of a number of cancers of the lymphatic system.

lysine: a basic amino acid which is a constituent of most proteins; an essential nutrient in the diet of vertebrates.

macrocytic anemia: anemia with red blood cells of increased size.

macrophages: professional phagocytic cells that detect, phagocytose, and destroy bacteria and other harmful invading organisms, and regulate the immune response by presenting antigens to T cells and initiating inflammation by releasing signaling molecules known as cytokines that activate other cells.

macular degeneration: a common disorder primarily affecting the elderly that causes deterioration of the macula. The macula is the visual center of the retina and is responsible for high acuity color vision. Patients with macular degeneration often complain of central vision loss.

magnetic resonance imaging (MRI): a radiologic technique that uses radio signals and magnets and a computer to produce highly detailed images of tissues.

major depressive disorder: a pattern of major depressive episodes that form an identified psychiatric disorder.

major depressive episode: a syndrome of symptoms characterized by depressed mood; required for the diagnosis of some mood disorders.

malaise: a general feeling of discomfort, of being "out of sorts".

malar rash: a redness or rash on the face covering the cheeks and the bridge of the nose; also called butterfly rash.

malignant: cancerous; able to spread into and destroy nearby tissues and to spread to distant areas.

malnutrition: a physical state characterized by an imbalance of dietary proteins, carbohydrates, fats, vitamins, and minerals, given an individual's physical activity and health needs.

mammary gland: a group of milk-producing cells consisting of lobules and ducts.

mammography: a technique using X-rays to diagnose and locate tumors of the breasts.

mandatory reporting requirements: laws designating groups of professionals that are required to report specific types of violence, abuse, and neglect. In the U.S. these laws vary by state.

manic episode: a syndrome of symptoms characterized by elevated, expansive, or irritable mood; required for the diagnosis of some mood disorders.

Manual of Mental Disorders (DSM): to record psychiatric diagnoses for statistical and administrative purposes.

masculinizing vaginoplasty: female-to-male surgical procedures including metoidioplasty and phalloplasty.

mastectomy: surgical removal of the breast.

mastitis: inflammation of the glands in the breast.

masturbation: self-stimulation of the genitals for sexual pleasure.

medial: toward the midline.

median nerve: a nerve running through the carpal tunnel that carries sensory impulses from the thumb, index and middle fingers, and half of the ring finger to the central nervous system; it has a motor branch that supplies the thenar muscles on the thumb side of the hand.

megaloblastic anemia: a type of anemia that results from inhibition of DNA synthesis during red blood cell production, which results in abnormally large red blood cells.

meiosis: the type of cell division that produces the ova and sperm, which contain one-half of the chromosome number found in the original cell before division.

melanin: a polymer made up of several compounds (including the amino acid tyrosine) that causes pigmentation in the skin, hair, and eyes.

melanocytes: cells in the upper layer of skin which produce the pigment melanin.

memory loss syndrome: a condition in which a person gradually but progressively loses capacity in many cognitive areas, but especially in the ability to remember; Alzheimer's disease is considered the most common factor causing serious memory loss in older people.

menarche: the first occurrence of menstruation.

menarche: the onset of menstrual cycles in a woman.

Ménière's disease: a disorder affecting endolymph.

menopause: the last menstrual period a woman experiences.

menopause: the permanent cessation of menstrual cycles, signifying the conclusion of a woman's reproductive life.

menorrhagia: abnormally heavy bleeding at menstruation.

menorrhagia: excessive uttering bleeding that lasts more than 7 days or loss of more than 80 mL of blood per cycle.

menses: the monthly flow of blood and cellular debris from the uterus that begins at puberty in women.

menstrual cycle: the cycle of hormone production, ovulation, menstruation, and other changes that occurs on an approximately monthly schedule in women.

menstruation: a cyclical discharging of blood, secretions, and tissue debris from the uterus that recurs in non-pregnant breeding-age women.

mental status exam: a comprehensive evaluation assessing general health, appearance, mood, speech, sociability, cooperativeness, motor activity, orientation to time and reality, memory, general intelligence, and other cognitive functioning.

mesenchyme: loosely organized tissue that may form connective tissues, bone, or several other types of tissues.

messenger ribonucleic acid (mRNA): a single-stranded RNA that arises from and is complementary to double-stranded DNA; it passes from the nucleus to the cytoplasm, where its information is translated into proteins.

messenger RNA: The messenger ribonucleic acid molecule is encoded from DNA in a process called transcription; this molecule is then translated into protein.

metabolism: the full complement of biochemical reactions that occur within an organism that consist of the degradation of energy-rich molecules from food to generate energy (catabolism), and the use of that energy to build cellular structures from simpler precursors for growth, reproduction, healing and maintenance of organismal homeostasis (anabolism).

metastasis: the process by which malignant tumors invade other tissues either locally or distally.

methemoglobin: a stable oxidized form of hemoglobin which is unable to release oxygen to the tissues.

methotrexate: a powerful drug, originally developed to treat cancer, that is used to treat patients with severe cases of psoriasis.

microbicidal: any biocidal compound or substance whose purpose is to reduce the infectivity of microbes, such as viruses or bacteria.

microcalcifications: calcium deposits within breast tissue; they appear as white spots or flecks on a mammogram.

microcytic anemia: anemia with red blood cells of decreased size.

microvascular angina: angina cause by the failure of very small heart arteries to supply blood and oxygen to the heart because of spasms or cellular disorders.

migraine headache: headaches characterized by throbbing, unilateral pain, often accompanied by nausea, vomiting, and photophobia, and occasionally accompanied by a visual or sensory aura.

migraine: a recurrent throbbing headache that typically affects one side of the head and is often accompanied by nausea and disturbed vision.

milk duct: a tubular canal that transports milk from the lobule to the collecting duct.

milk line: a line that originates as a primitive milk streak on each front side of the fetus; it extends from axilla to vulva, where rudimentary breast tissues or nipples could be located.

mitosis: the type of cell division that occurs in nonsex cells, which conserves chromosome number by equal allocation to each of the newly formed cells.

molar pregnancy: abnormal, cyst-like placental tissue that grows either in place of the developing child (complete mole) or in addition to the developing child (partial mole).

monoamine oxidase inhibitors (MAOIs): a class of drugs that relieve the symptoms of depression by inhibiting the enzyme monoamine oxidase (an enzyme that degrades monoamine neurotransmitters), and increasing levels of these neurotransmitters (dopamine, serotonin, and norepinephrine) in the brain.

monocytes: a type of large white blood cell that can differentiate into macrophages, or dendritic cells.

monosaccharides: any of the class of sugars (e.g., glucose) that cannot be hydrolyzed to give a simpler sugar.

monozygotes: identical twins; born of a single ovum that divides after a single sperm fertilizes it.

mood disorders: a group of disorders characterized by disturbance of mood and including symptoms of depression and/or mania that are not caused by any other physical or mental disorder.

mood stabilizers: drugs that decrease the frequency and intensity of mood fluctuation, including drugs such as lithium and anticonvulsants.

morula: Early stage embryo that consists of a solid ball of cells.

Müllerian ducts: the pair of tubes in the early embryo that will develop into the internal female organs (uterus, oviducts, and upper vagina).

multiaxial classification: the classification system used in the DSM to account for several factors when making psychiatric diagnoses, including present condition, developmental/ personality disorders, physical disorders, life stresses, and overall functioning.

multifactorial inheritance: the interaction of genetic and environmental factors, which leads to certain congenital malformations.

multigenetic: referring to a trait or characteristic that requires the product of more than one gene in order to be activated;.

multistep progression: the typical pathway of induction of cancer, beginning with an initial alteration to a gene and progressing to the fully malignant state.

mutation: a change in gene structure that disrupts the normal functions of the encoded protein.

myelin: a fatty substance wrapping nerves as a sheath that accelerates electric impulse propagation.

myocardium: the muscle tissue that forms the walls of the heart, varying in thickness in the upper and lower regions.

myoepithelial cell: a cell that is anatomically located next to the alveolar cells and contractile in nature to aid in the movement of milk from the alveoli into the ducts.

myometrium: the smooth muscle tissue of the uterus.

nail bed: The soft tissue directly beneath the nail unit that acts as a barrier between the nail plate and underlying soft tissue and osseous structures.

nail plate: The keratinized structure that serves as the visible nail unit extending from the skin outwards.

naproxen: synthetic compound used as an analgesic and anti-inflammatory drug; proprietary names include Aleve.

necrosis: cell death, usually involving the rupture of the cell membrane and the release of cell into the surrounding tissue.

necrotizing enterocolitis: the death of tissue in the intestine; occurs most often in premature or sick babies.

negative feedback: a common physiological process by which the product of a process feeds back to inhibit further stimulation (or reverse) the process.

neobladder: a urinary pouch made from 50 -60 cm of the intestine.

neonatal intensive care unit: a hospital nursery with advanced equipment and specially trained staff to maintain the vital functions of sick newborns and to monitor their progress closely.

neonatal period: the first month of life; derived from the Greek *neo* (meaning "new") and the Latin *natum* (meaning "birth").

neonatal: the period of time succeeding birth and continuing through the first twenty-eight days of life.

neonate: a newborn infant, typically aged between 0 and 28 days.

neonatologist: a physician who specializes in treating newborn infants.

neoplasia: the formation or presence of a new, abnormal growth of tissue.

nervous system: the system in the body, including the brain, that receives and interprets stimuli and transmits impulses to other organs; the brain is the center of thinking and behavior.

neural tube: the embryonic structure that gives rise to the central nervous system.

neurocognitive disorder (formerly known as organic brain syndromes: clusters of condition that frequently lead to behavioral and psychological symptoms involving impaired brain function, where etiology is unknown; includes delirium, delusions, amnesia, intoxication, and dementias.

neurodevelopmental outcomes: a broad term referring to measures of neurologic development among cognitive, language, and motor domains.

neuroendocrine: both neural (relating to the nervous system) and endocrine (relating to hormones) in structure or function.

neurofibrillary tangles: a hallmark lesion of Alzheimer's disease and several other disorders consisting of intracellular aggregates of the structural protein tau.

neurogenesis: the growth and development of nervous tissue.

neurohypophysis: another name for the posterior lobe of the pituitary gland.

neuropathy: malfunction of the nerves.

neuroscience: the scientific specialization that seeks to understand mental processes, occurrences, and disturbances in terms of underlying mechanisms in the brain and the nervous system.

neurotransmitter: a chemical in the brain that sends a signal from one brain cell to another.

nevus: a pigmented site on the skin which is composed of melanocytes.

nitrates: a salt or ester of nitric acid, often used in food preservation and fertilizer.

nodes: areas of electrochemical transmission within the heart that regulate the heartbeat.

nondisjunction: the failure of chromosomes to separate during cell division, resulting in new cells that either lack a chromosome or have an extra chromosome.

nonlinear system: a process which is unstable and unpredictable in nature; such a process often results from a disturbance to a linear, predictable system.

non-normative aging: significant factors that affect aging that are person-specific.

"no suicide" contract: an agreement, verbally or in writing, that a suicidal person will not act on his or her urges to commit suicide and instead will take other more adaptive action.

non-steroidal anti-inflammatory drug (NSAID): a class of analgesic medication that reduces pain, fever and inflammation.

normative age-graded: biological and environmental factors affecting aging that are correlated with chronological age.

normative history-graded: events affecting aging that are widely experienced within a particular culture at a given time.

normocytic anemia: anemia with red blood cells of normal size.

nuchal rigidity: stiffening of the back of the neck.

nulliparity: having never given birth.

nummular dermatitis: also known as discoid dermatitis; a skin condition characterized by coin-shaped or oval sores on the skin that often appear after skin injury.

nurture: the act or process of raising or promoting development and well-being.

nutraceutical: a food or part of a food allegedly containing health-giving additives and having medicinal benefit.

nutrient density: the amount of nutrients provided per kilocalorie of food.

nystagmus: rhythmic involuntary movements of the eyes.

obesity: a condition characterized by the excessive accumulation and storage of fat in the body which can be measured in many ways, including BMI, abdominal circumference, and body fat percentage.

obsession: a recurrent, unwelcome, and intrusive thought.

obsessive-compulsive disorder: a psychiatric disorder that causes a person to ruminate on a particular thought and then act out a ritualistic behavior.

obsessive-compulsive: having a preoccupation with a specific idea (such as body image) and showing uncontrollable related behavior (such as dieting).

Oligohydramnios: abnormally decreased amniotic fluid volume.

oncogene: a gene directly or indirectly inducing the transformation of cells from the normal to the malignant state; most oncogenes have normal counterparts in body cells.

onychomycosis: common nail disorder in which fungal organisms invade the nail bed causing progressive changes in the color, texture, and structure of the nail.

oocyte: a female germ cell that differentiates to become a mature ova.

oophorectomy (or ovariectomy): removal of the ovaries, which is often necessary in cases of severe endometriosis.

oophoritis: inflammation of the ovary.

opioid: pain-relievers that include both legal (Vicodin) and illegal (heroin) drugs; proprietary names include Oxycontin and Demerol.

opportunistic infection: an infection caused by any type of pathogen in individuals who have an impaired immune system.

orchitis: inflammation of the testis.

organic disease: a disease caused or accompanied by an alteration in the structure of the tissues or organs.

organic mental disorders: mental and emotional disturbances from transient or permanent brain dysfunction, with known organic etiology; includes drug or alcohol ingestion, infection, trauma, and cardiovascular disease.

organic: arising from an organ.

organogenetic period: the period of embryonic development, from approximately fifteen to sixty days after fertilization, during which most body organs form.

oscillopsia: the sensation of bouncing vision.

oscilloscope: an instrument that displays a visual representation of electrical variations on the fluorescent screen of a cathode-ray tube.

osmotic pressure: the pressure between two solutions separated by a membrane.

osteoarthritis: degeneration of joint cartilage and the underlying bone, most common from middle age onward.

osteopenia: reduced bone mass.

osteoporosis: a condition characterized by a loss of bone density and an increased susceptibility to fractures.

otoliths: granular bones of the inner ear.

otorhinolaryngologist: the ear, nose, and throat (ENT) specialist.

ovarian follicle: a fluid-filled sac that contains an immature egg, or oocyte.

ovariectomy: the removal of the ovaries.

ovaries: the female reproductive organs, which contain the ova (eggs); the ovaries are almond-shaped and are found in the lower pelvic area.

ovary: the female gonad located in the pelvic cavity, where egg production occurs; the principal organ that produces the hormones estrogen and progesterone.

overfeeding: the provision of more milk or formula for an infant than is necessary; may result in regurgitation.

oviduct: the thin tube that leads from near the ovary to the upper part of the uterus; also called the Fallopian tube.

ovulation: the process by which an ovum is released from its follicle in the ovary; occurs in the middle of each menstrual cycle ovum (*pl. ova*): the egg or reproductive cell produced by the female, which when fertilized by a sperm from the male will develop into an embryo.

ovum (pl. ova): an egg cell.

oxalate: a salt or ester of oxalic acid, which is capable of forming an insoluble salt with calcium and interfering with its absorption by the body.

oxidation: an imbalance in antioxidants and free radicals in the body.

oximeter: noninvasive device worn over a finger that measures the oxygen level in the bloodstream.

oxygenation: the addition of oxygen to any system, including the human body.

oxygenation: the process of getting oxygen into the bloodstream.

oxytocin: a hormone secreted by the pituitary gland that causes increased contraction of the uterus during labor and stimulates the ejection of milk into the ducts of the breasts.

palliative treatments: therapies that reduce symptoms without completely eradicating a disorder.

palpation: a digital examination of affected parts of the body.

pancreas: the gland located under the stomach that produces insulin and glucagon, the hormones responsible for control of the body's blood sugar level; it also produces enzyme- containing digestive juices.

panic: a sudden episode of intense fearfulness.

pan-plexopathy: a form of neonatal brachial plexus palsy comprising of injury to all of the spinal nerve roots manifesting as a flaccid arm.

Pap smear: a test carried out on a sample of cells from the cervix to check for abnormalities that may be indicative of cervical cancer.

Pap test: a screening test for precancer and cancer of the cervix; it is performed by placing a sample of cervical cells on a microscope slide along with a preservative solution or by placing the cells into a small container filled with preservative solution.

Pap testing: a screening test to detect precancerous and cancerous cells of the cervix.

parafollicular cells: neuroendocrine cells in the thyroid for which the primary function is to secrete calcitonin; also called C cells.

paralysis: a loss of muscle function for one or more muscles.

paraphilias: the experience of intense sexual arousal to atypical objects, situations, fantasies, behaviors, or individuals.

parathyroid gland: one of four small endocrine glands situated underneath the thyroid gland, whose main product is parathyroid hormone, which regulate serum calcium levels.

parathyroid: a gland next to the thyroid which secretes a hormone (parathyroid hormone) that regulates calcium levels in a person's body.

parenteral nutrition: intravenous feeding or a way of getting nutrition into the body through the veins.

Parkinson's disease: a disease in which the dopamine-secreting cells of the midbrain degenerate, resulting in reduced levels of the neurotransmitter dopamine, tremors, uncontrolled and slow movement, and rigidity.

pathogen: a bacterium, virus, or other microorganism that can cause disease.

pathology: the study of the nature and consequences of disease.

patient advocacy: the representation of the patient's interest in medical diagnosis and treatment decisions, in which the physician acts as an information source and counselor for the patient.

pelvic inflammatory disease (PID): an extensive bacterial infection of the pelvic organs, such as the uterus, cervix, Fallopian tubes, and ovaries.

periareolar: around the areola (dark part of the breast just around the nipples).

periductal: around the duct (drainage system of the mammary glands).

perimenopause: a period of years around the menopause, during which changes occur in the balance among the reproductive hormones, leading to the cessation of menses and the end of fertility; this time of transition from reproductive to post-reproductive life is also known as the climacteric.

perinatal mortality: number of stillbirths and deaths in the first week of life per 1,000 total births.

perinatal period: the period immediately before and after birth, commencing at 20 weeks of gestation and ending at 28 weeks after birth (140 days total).

perineum: the short bridge of flesh between the anus and vagina in women and the anus and base of the penis in men.

periodic breathing: rapid breathing followed by several seconds of no breathing; more than ten-second pauses are abnormal.

peristalsis: a series of muscular contractions that move food through the intestines during the process of digestion.

peritoneal cavity: the abdominal cavity that contains the visceral organs.

peritoneum: a membrane enclosing most of the organs in the abdomen.

perpetrator: an individual who commits **a crime sexual harassment:** physical behavior of a sexual nature that is aimed at a particular person or group of people, especially in the workplace or school.

personal trauma narrative: the story of a traumatic experience will be told repeatedly through verbal, written, or artistic means; sharing and expanding upon a trauma narrative allows the individual to organize their memories, making them more manageable, and diminishing the painful emotions they carry.

petechiae: tiny, round, purple spots on the skin that result from bleeding underneath the skin.

phagocytes: white cells of the immune system that destroy invading foreign bodies by engulfing and digesting them in a nonspecific immune response; include macrophages and neutrophils.

phagocytosis: the progress of ingestion and digestion by cells that are part of the immune system; this process is one of the ways that mammals use to defend themselves against infectious invaders, including *Candida* organisms.

pharaonic circumcision: another term for infibulation.

pharmacodynamics: changes in tissue sensitivity or physiologic systems in response to pharmacological substances.

pharmacokinetics: the action of pharmacological substances within a biological system; pharmacologic substance absorption, distribution, metabolism, and elimination by an organism.

pharmacotherapy: the treatment of disease with medication.

pheromones: excreted or secreted chemicals that trigger a social response in members of the same species.

phobia: an extreme or irrational fear or aversion to something.

phocomelia: a rare congenital deformity in which the hands or feet are attached close to the trunk, the limbs being grossly underdeveloped or absent.

photonutrient: a substance found in certain plants which is believed to be beneficial to human health and help prevent various diseases.

photophobia: dread or avoidance of light.

photosensitivity: a sensitivity to light or sunlight.

physical deconditioning: a condition that results when a person who has previously been exercising (has become conditioned) stops exercising.

physical modalities: the physical means of addressing a disease, which include heat, cold, electricity, exercises, braces, assistive devices, and biofeedback.

physiological dependence: a state of tissue adaptation to a substance of abuse marked by tolerance and/or withdrawal.

phytochemicals: chemical compounds produced by plants, generally to help them thrive or thwart competitors, predators, or pathogens.

pilosebaceous: referring to hair follicles and the sebaceous glands.

pituitary gland: the body's master gland that produces various hormones which in turn stimulate other glands in the body to produce their own hormones; in women, the pituitary produces follicle-stimulating hormone and luteinizing hormone, which stimulate the ovary to produce estrogens and progesterone.

pituitary: the endocrine gland responsible for the functioning of the thyroid, along with many other central control activities.

placenta abruptio: placenta prematurely separates from uterus before childbirth.

placenta previa: a condition in which the placenta partially or wholly blocks the neck of the uterus.

placenta: a fetomaternal organ that joins mother and offspring; it secretes endocrine hormones and selectively exchanges soluble, blood-borne substances through its interior structures.

plaque: an accumulation of matter within artery walls that can impede blood flow.

plastic surgery: the branch of operative surgery concerning the repair of defects, the replacement of lost tissue, and the treatment of extensive scarring; it accomplishes these ends by direct union of body parts, grafting, or the transfer of tissue from one part of the body to another.

platelet: a small colorless disk-shaped cell fragment without a nucleus, found in large numbers in blood and involved in clotting.

pleurisy: the inflammation and swelling of the pleurae, the membranes that enclose the lungs and line the chest cavity; a complication of several pulmonary diseases.

Pneumocystis pneumonia: a form of pneumonia caused by the fungus *Pneumocystis carinii* and commonly seen in persons with AIDS.

pneumonia: an inflammation of the lung tissue in which the alveolar sacs fill with fluid.

polycystic ovary: an ovary containing multiple cysts, may occur as part of a hormonal condition known as polycystic ovary syndrome (PCOS).

Polyhydramnios/Hydramnios: abnormally increased amniotic fluid volume.

polymerase chain reaction: a laboratory method used to increase the amount of DNA found in small quantities.

polymicrobial infection: an infection caused by multiple microorganisms such as bacteria and viruses.

polypeptide chains: chains of amino acids and essential portions of proteins in cells.

polysaccharides: a carbohydrate (e.g. starch, cellulose, or glycogen) whose molecules consist of a number of sugar molecules bonded together.

polysomnography: a sleep study used to diagnose a variety of sleep disorders.

positive feedback: a physiological process in which a product feeds back to stimulate the process, resulting in additional production or the continuation of that process.

posterior: toward the rear, opposite to the customary direction of motion; equivalent to dorsal in humans, but the same as caudal in other animals.

postpartum hemorrhage: the loss of more than 500 ml or 1,000 ml of blood within the first 24 hours following childbirth.

postpartum: following childbirth or the birth of young.

posttraumatic stress disorder: A maladaptive condition resulting from exposure to events beyond the realm of normal human experience and characterized by persistent difficulties involving emotional numbing, intense fear, helplessness, horror, reexperiencing of trauma, avoidance, and arousal.

pranayama: from Sanskrit, meaning "extension of the breath"; the regulation of the breath through certain techniques and exercises.

preeclampsia: a complication of pregnancy that can be characterized by high blood pressure and signs of possible damage to another organ such as the liver or kidney.

premature adrenarch: the appearance of public hair without any other signs of puberty.

premature menarch: the onset of periods without other signs of puberty.

premature ovarian failure: cessation of menses prior to the age of forty because of the early loss of ovarian follicles.

premature thelarche: development of breasts without any other sign of puberty.

premature: referring to a birth that is less than full term.

prematurity: strictly defined, birth before a full-term pregnancy (thirty-eight weeks); more commonly associated with birth before thirty-five weeks.

premenstrual dysphoric disorder (PMDD): a severe form of premenstrual syndrome characterized by affective symptoms causing significant disturbances in relationships or social adaptation.

PrEP: pre-exposure prophylaxis; taking of a prescription drug as a means of preventing HIV infection in an HIV-negative person.

prepuce: the covering of the clitoris.

presenilins: proteins linked to several forms of inherited Alzheimer's disease, which are believed to play a role in the production of Aβ.

prevalence: the proportion of infectious cases in a population at a given time.

primary aging: aging intrinsic to a person as determined by inherent or hereditary influences.

primary care: first-line or entry-level care; the health care that most people receive for most illnesses.

primary progressive MS: the most aggressive form of MS, characterized by the absence of remissions and continual decline.

probability judgments: a technique used for the purposes of evaluating the probability of a human error occurring throughout the completion of a specific task.

procollagen: the precursor of collagen; it is formed in fibroblasts and converted to collagen by a peptidase.

prodrome: a forewarning symptom of a disease.

progesterone/progestin: a hormone produced in the ovaries that sustains pregnancy; birth control pills are composed primarily of progesterone, which works by suppressing ovulation.

progesterone: a hormone produced in the ovary that prepares and maintains the uterus for pregnancy.

prohormone: a hormone that must be cut or modified in a specific way in order to achieve full activity.

prolactin: a hormone released by the anterior lobe of the pituitary gland that stimulates milk production by the mammary glands.

prolapse: a slipping forward or down of one of the parts or organs of the body.

prolapsed cord: umbilical cord of the baby comes out of mother's uterus ahead of baby.

proline: an amino acid which is a constituent of most proteins, especially collagen.

promotion: the second step in tumor development, which causes initiated cells to begin growing into tumors.

pronation: rotation of the medial bones in the midtarsal region of the foot inward and downward so that in walking the foot tends to come down on its inner margin.

prone: lying face-downward.

proof: a designation of beverage alcohol content that is defined as twice the percentage of alcohol by volume.

prophylactic treatment: a treatment focusing on preventing or reducing the number of headaches.

prophylaxis: a method of preventing a disease.

proprioception: the ability to locate the body in space.

prostaglandins: chemical messengers that are not carried in the blood and that function only locally.

prostaglandins: cyclic fatty acids with varying hormone-like effects, notably the promotion of uterine contractions.

prostaglandins: one of a number of hormone-like substances that participate in a wide range of body functions such as the contraction and relaxation of smooth muscle, the dilation and constriction of blood vessels, control of blood pressure, and modulation of inflammation.

protease inhibitors: any drug that inhibits the assembly of HIV.

proteinuria: the presence of protein (typically albumin) in the urine.

proteoglycan: a core protein containing oligosaccharide chains covalently bound to glycosaminoglycans.

protozoan: a single-celled organism that is more closely related to animals than are bacteria; only a few drugs are available that will kill protozoa without harming their animal hosts.

protozoan: a unicellular organism with an organized nucleus.

proximal interphalangeal joints: the proximal joints in the fingers.

proximal: toward the point of origin.

psoralens: chemicals found in plants that make the skin more sensitive to light.

psychodynamic model: a way of viewing and understanding psychiatric disorders which emphasizes the recognition and treatment of underlying psychological and developmental traumas.

psychogenic fatigue: fatigue caused by mental factors, such as anxiety, and not attributable to any physical cause.

psychogenic: psychologic in origin.

psychological dependence: need for a substance provided by its reinforcing properties, causing

persistent desire to cut down or control use, use across varied situations to the exclusion of other behavior, use despite other worsening physical or psychological conditions, and/or great amounts of time spent finding, using, or recovering from substance effects.

psychopharmacology: the use of drugs to study effects on brain chemistry; drugs are used to treat mental disorders, study brain chemistry, and promote new disease classifications.

psychosis: a severe mental state characterized by loss of normal social function and being either withdrawn from or unable to accurately perceive reality.

psychosocial interventions: treatments that enhance individual psychological and social functioning by assisting with the development of the skills, attitudes, or behaviors necessary to function as independently as possible.

psychosocial treatment: a significant specialization in treating people with psychiatric disorders through employing principles of psychology, human behavior, family and group dynamics, and social and occupational learning.

psychosomatic: referring to physical symptoms interacting with psychological problems.

Psychostimulant medication: a medication used for the treating ADHD that acts on the central nervous system to reduce hyperactivity, improve concentration, focus attention, and for many induce a calming effect.

psychosurgery: the surgical removal or destruction of part of the brain of depressed patients as a form of treatment.

psychotherapy: the "talk" therapies that target the emotional, social, and other contributors to and consequences of depression.

psychotherapy: treatment using the mind to remedy problems related to disordered behavior or thinking, emotional problems, or disease.

puberty: the physiological sequence of events by which a child acquires the reproductive capacities of an adult; the growth of secondary sexual characteristics occurs, reproductive functions begin, and the differences between males and females are accentuated.

pulmonary: the Latin word for lung, used to describe both the lung tissue and the bronchial tree.

punch biopsy: a biopsy that is performed by using a punch, an instrument for cutting and removing a disk of tissue.

purging: regularly compensating for binge eating with self-induced vomiting, laxative abuse, diuretics, or enemas.

PUVA: a treatment for psoriasis in which the patient is exposed to ultraviolet A (UVA) light after receiving one of the psoralens.

quadrantectomy: a form of lumpectomy that removes more tissue than the usual lumpectomy, leaving little visible scarring but slightly diminishing the size of the affected breast.

queer: sexual or gender identity that is categorized outside of established gender roles or sexuality. Usually a self-identification. May be considered offensive term by some in LGBT community but has been increasingly reclaimed by community members.

quickening: the point at which a fetus first begins to move in the uterus.

radial: on the medial side (or thumb side) of the arm, forearm, and hand.

radiculopathy: also called nerve root entrapment or pinched nerve; irritation or compression of the root of a spinal nerve between vertebrae, caused by annular bulge, herniated disk, or spinal injury.

range of motion: movement of a joint from full flexion to full extension.

rational suicide: suicide to avoid suffering when there is no underlying cognitive or psychiatric disorder.

Raynaud's phenomenon: discoloration and pain in the fingertips induced by cold.

receptor: a molecular structure at the cell surface or inside the cell that is capable of combining with hormones and causing a change in cell metabolism or function.

recommended dietary allowance (RDA): the estimated amount of nutrient, nutrients or calories per day considered necessary for the maintenance of good health as established by the Food and Nutrition Board.

reconstructive surgery: the application of plastic surgical techniques to repair damaged tissues.

recurrent miscarriage: a condition in which a woman experiences three consecutive miscarriages.

recurrent: repeated.

reduction: a decrease in the total volume or mass of breast tissue.

refeeding: the reintroduction of nutritional substances into the diet of a patient suffering from malnutrition.

referred pain: any pain whose origin is elsewhere in the body from where it is felt; with radiculopathy in the lumbar spine, the pain is typically in the leg.

rehabilitation: a physician-led program to evaluate, treat, and educate patients and their families about the sequelae of birth defects, trauma, disease, and degenerative conditions, with the goals of alleviating pain, preventing complications, correcting deformities, improving function, and re-integrating individuals into the family and society.

reinforcement: a process that increases the frequency or probability of a response.

relapsing-remitting MS: the most common form of MS, characterized by unpredictable attacks (relapses) followed by periods free of symptoms (remission).

remyelination: the repair of myelin.

renal failure: the failure of the kidneys, making it impossible for the kidneys to function efficiently.

renal: pertaining to the kidney.

residency training: medical training provided in a specialty after graduation from medical school; similar to an apprenticeship and designed to mimic real-life practice as closely as possible.

respiration: a process that includes both air conduction (the act of breathing) and gas exchange (oxygen and carbon dioxide transfer between the air and blood).

respirator: a machine that inflates and deflates the lungs, imitating normal breathing; connected to the patient through a tube placed into the windpipe (endotracheal tube).

respiratory distress syndrome: a disease of lung immaturity that can be fatal and is found in children who are born prematurely.

reticulate body: the metabolically active form of *Chlamydia trachomitis* that the elementary body transforms into after penetrating a host cell that appropriates the host cell resources to divide and form elementary bodies, which culminates in host cell lysis and liberation of elementary bodies for future infective cycles.

retina: a thin membrane, lining the inside back surface of the eyeball, where light is transformed into electrical signals that are transmitted to the brain.

retrovirus: a virus with ribonucleic acid (RNA) as its genetic material that produces a deoxyribonucleic acid (DNA) copy of the RNA to be integrated into a chromosome of the host cell from which it will make new infectious copies of the RNA during the viral life cycle.

reuptake: the absorption by a presynaptic nerve ending of a neurotransmitter that it has secreted.

revascularization: procedures to reestablish the circulation to a diseased portion of the body.

reverse transcriptase: an enzyme associated with the HIV virion that copies or replicates the viral single-stranded RNA molecule into a double-stranded DNA copy of it.

Rh isoimmunization: a condition in which a woman who is lacking a substance on red blood cells called Rh factor carries a fetus with the Rh factor on its red blood cells; in these cases, the woman may produce antibodies that attack the red blood cells of the fetus, leading to fetal anemia.

Rh: a human blood factor, originally identified in rhesus monkeys, that can be either positive (present) or negative (absent).

Rh0(D) immune globulin: also known as RhoGAM; a type of gamma globulin protein injected into Rh-negative mothers who may have an Rh-positive fetus to protect the fetus from an immune reaction called isoimmunization.

rhinitis: inflammation of the nasal mucous membrane.

ritual suicide: a formal, ceremonial, and proscribed form of suicide performed for social reasons in Japanese history.

rotator cuff: a capsule with fused tendons that supports the arm at the shoulder joint and is often subject to athletic injury.

saline infusion sonography: an ultrasound scan of the uterus while the it is being filled with sterile saline (salt water). This helps outline the uterine wall and cavity.

salivary glands: the glands that produce saliva.

samyana: from Sanskrit, meaning "holding together," "binding," "integration"; combined practice of concentration (Dh ra), meditation (Dhy na) and union (Sam dhi); a term to summarize the process of psychological absorption during meditation.

satiety: the state of feeling full or fed and free from hunger.

scaling: a buildup of hard, horny skin cells.

sciatica: intense pain in one buttock and down the back of that leg, caused by inflammation of the sciatic nerve, the largest nerve in the body; in some cases this inflammation is due to sciatic nerve radiculopathy (originates between L4 and the sacrum).

sclerosis: a process of hardening of tissues.

scoliosis: sideways curvature of the spine or a section of the spine.

screening procedures: tests that are carried out in populations which are usually asymptomatic and at high risk for a disease in order to identify those in need of treatment.

screening procedures: tests that are carried out in populations, which are usually asymptomatic and at high risk for a disease, in order to identify those in need of treatment.

seasonal affective disorder (SAD): a mood disorder associated with the winter season, when the amount of daylight hours is reduced.

sebaceous glands: glands in the skin that usually open into the hair follicles.

sebaceous: pertaining to glands in the skin that secrete an oily substance called sebum.

seborrheic: characterized by overactivity of the sebaceous glands that results in oily coating, crusts or scales on the skin.

sebum: a semifluid, fatty substance secreted by the sebaceous glands into the hair follicles.

secondary aging: changes in a person caused by hostile factors in the environment, which could include trauma, pollution, and acquired disease.

secondary infection: a bacterial, viral, or other infection that results from or follows another disease.

secondary progressive MS: a form that occurs in patients who initially had relapsing-remitting MS and transition to a more aggressive MS.

secondary sexual characteristics: in females, the development of breast tissue and pubic hair.

seizure: a misfiring of cortical neurons that alters the patient's level of consciousness; the seizure may or may not involve muscular convulsions.

selection: the process by which developing immune system cells are either allowed to continue to maturation or destroyed before they can enter the circulation;.

selective norepinephrine reuptake inhibitors (SNRIs): a class of antidepressants that inhibits the reuptake of the neurotransmitters norepinephrine and serotonin, thus making more of them available to the brain, potentially improving the mood of the patient.

selective serotonin reuptake inhibitors (SSRIs): a class of antidepressant drugs that inhibit the reuptake of the neurotransmitter serotonin, thus making more of it available to brain cells.

semen analysis: analysis of a recently ejaculated semen specimen, which includes a sperm count and an estimate of the percentage of motile sperm.

senile plaques: a hallmark lesion of Alzheimer's disease, composed of Aβ amyloid.

seroconversion: the detection of anti-HIV antibodies in the blood of an HIV-infected person, who is then said to be HIV-positive.

serositis: inflammation of the lining of the lung or heart.

serotonin: the neurotransmitter associated with pain perception, sleep, impulsivity, and aggression; implicated in disorders associated with anxiety, depression, and migraines.

service: work done or duty performed for another or others.

sex: sex is assigned at birth as male or female, usually based on the appearance of the external genitalia. For most people, gender identity and expression are consistent with their sex assigned at birth; for transgender and gender-diverse individuals, gender identity or expression differ from their sex assigned at birth.

sexual harassment: physical behavior of a sexual nature that is aimed at a particular person or group of people, especially in the workplace or school.

sexuality: an individual's sexual preference or orientation, also refers to feelings about sexual intercourse, arousal, and one's relationship to sexual activity.

sexually transmitted disease (STD): a disease that is usually transmitted from person to person through contact between the vaginal or urethral discharges from an infected person and the genital mucous membranes of a person susceptible to infection.

sexually transmitted infection: an infection caused by organisms transferred through sexual contact (genital-genital, orogenital, or anogenital); transmission of infection occurs through exposure to lesions or secretions which contain the organisms.

shoulder dystocia: diagnosed when the delivery of the fetal head is not followed by the emergence of the shoulder due to impaction of the fetus' shoulder in the birth canal.

shoulder impingement: common cause of shoulder pain, often caused by repeated activity of the shoulder; also called "swimmer's shoulder".

sigmoid: the distal part of the large colon, just before the rectum.

sigmoidoscopy: similar to colonoscopy, with the tubular instrument with light instead inspecting only the anus, rectum, and sigmoid colon.

signal-to-noise: a measure used in science and engineering that compares the level of a desired signal to the level of background noise.

sinoatrial node: the section of the right atrium that determines the appropriate rate of the heartbeat.

Skene glands, or Skene's glands: also known as the lesser vestibular glands, paraurethral glands, or homologous female prostate; located on the anterior wall of the vagina, near the lower end of the urethra; fluid that lubricates the urethral opening.

sleep apnea: cessation of breathing during sleep, which may result from either an inhibition of the respiratory center (central apnea) or an obstruction to the flow of air (obstructive apnea).

sleep disorders: conditions resulting in sleep interruption, interfering with the restorative functions of sleep.

somatic treatment: the treatment of people with psychiatric disorders using specialized drugs and electroconvulsive therapy; some major drug groups used are antidepressants, antipsychotics, mood stabilizers, anxiolytics, and psychostimulants.

somatoform disorder: a mental disorder whose symptoms focus on the physical body.

sonogram: an image of body organs produced through focusing sound waves on the part to be examined.

spasm: an involuntary muscle contraction; a painful spasm is called a cramp.

specialist: any physician who practices in a specialty other than the generalist areas of family medicine, general internal medicine, general pediatrics, and obstetrics and gynecology.

speculum: a metal or plastic instrument that is used to dilate an orifice or canal in the body to allow inspection.

sperm: the motile cells produced within the male that carry his genetic material.

spermicide: a chemical that kills sperm after it is ejaculated.

spina bifida: a birth defect involving malformation of vertebrae in the lower back, often resulting in paralysis and lower-body organ impairment.

statin: any of a group of drugs that act to reduce levels of fats, including triglycerides and cholesterol, in the blood.

statutory rape: a sexual act with a child below the legal age of consent, even if the act is consensual.

stem cells: multipotential precursor cells within the bone marrow that develop into white cell populations, including lymphocytes and phagocytic cells.

stereotaxic computed tomography (CT): a method of imaging using a series of X rays that are compiled by a computer to give a three-dimensional image of internal structures.

sterilization: a permanent method of birth control.

stoma: an artificial opening made into a hollow organ, especially one on the surface of the body leading to the gut or trachea.

stratum corneum: the outermost layer of the epidermis; its cells are normally dead, hard, and removed by normal bathing.

stress: physical, environmental, or psychological strain experienced by an individual that requires adjustment.

stroke: a complete loss of blood flow to a region of the brain that is of sudden onset and causes abrupt muscular weakness, usually to one side of the body.

stroma: the deeper layer of breast tissue.

subcutaneous: under the skin.

substance abuse: the continued use of a psychoactive substance despite repeated impairment, within a twelvemonth period, of social, occupational, or legal functioning or continued exposure to physical hazards.

suicide cluster: the occurrence of several suicides immediately following a much-publicized suicide.

suicide gesture: a superficial suicidal action in which the intention is not to die but to solicit help.

sunna circumcision: the removal of the tip of the clitoris and/ or the prepuce.

superior: upward; toward the top of the head.

supine: lying face-upward.

suppressor T cell: a type of T lymphocyte that is believed to modulate the immune response.

suspiciousness: a range of symptoms from increasing distrust of others to paranoid delusions of conspiracies; changes related to aging are thought to be major factors causing increased suspiciousness in older people.

synaptogenesis: the formation of synapses between neurons in the nervous system.

syncytiotrophoblast: The multinucleate, outermost layer of the trophoblast of the embryo that aggressively invades the endometrial layer of the uterus to implant the embryo into it and find uterine blood vessels of nourish it. Together with the syncytiotrophoblast, the cytotrophoblast, and other cells form the placenta.

syndrome: a collection of complaints (symptoms) and signs (abnormal findings on clinical examination) that do not match any specific disease.

synovial fluid: fluid contained in the synovium of joint margins that reduces friction during movement of the joints.

synovium: the cellular lining of a joint, having a blood supply and a nerve supply; the synovium secretes fluid for lubrication and protects against injury and injurious agents.

systemic shock: a shock to any system that perturbs a system enough to drive it out of equilibrium.

T cells: also known as T lymphocytes; the immune system cells involved in cellular immunity and regulation of the immune response;.

T lymphocyte: a type of immune cell that kills host cells infected by bacteria or viruses and secretes chemicals (interleukins) that regulate the immune response.

T4 cells: also called CD4 cells or T-helper cells; a specific type of white blood cell (lymphocyte) which regulates the entire immune system and is the preferred target for HIV infection, resulting in immunodeficiency.

tachycardia: rapid beating of the heart.

tamoxifen: is the oldest and most-prescribed selective estrogen receptor modulator that is used to treat estrogen receptor-positive breast cancers.

target cell or organ: a cell or organ possessing the specific hormone receptors needed to respond to a given hormone.

telogen effluvium: a form of temporary hair loss that usually happens after stress, a shock, or a traumatic event.

telogen: the resting phase of hair follicles.

telomerase: the enzyme that synthesizes the repeated sequences called telomeres at the ends of chromosomes.

telomere: the repeated sequences at the end of chromosomes.

tenaculum: a surgical clamp with sharp hooks at the end, used to hold or pick up small pieces of tissue such as Fallopian tubes.

tend-and-befriend response: a neuroendocrine-linked stress response observed in females characterized by a tendency to respond to stressful situations by protecting self and young through nurturing behaviors and forming alliances with a larger social group.

tender points: specific, precise, and localized areas of moderately to severely intense pain.

tendonitis: inflammation of a tendon, often caused from overuse.

tension headache: a type of headache characterized by bandlike or cap-like pain over the head.

teratogen: an agent or factor which causes malformation of an embryo.

teratogen: an agent or factor which causes malformation of an embryo.

teratogen: an environmental factor that can induce the formation of congenital malformations.

teratogens: substances that induce congenital malformations when embryonic tissues and organs are exposed to them.

teratology: the study of congenital malformations.

teratoma: a tumor composed of tissue not normally found at that site.

terminal hair: thick, pigmented hairs found on the scalp and other parts of the body.

testes: the male reproductive organs and the site of sperm production; also known as the testicles.

testosterone: the male sex hormone produced by the testes and responsible for the male sexual traits; a small amount is also produced by the adrenal glands in females and is responsible for the growth of hair during adolescence in both sexes.

thermolabile: unstable when heated.

thoracic spine: the middle of three parts of the spine, consisting of twelve vertebrae, named T1 (top of the chest) to T12, in a natural kyphosis.

thorax: the bone and cartilage cage attached to the sternum; generally referred to as the rib cage.

threatened abortion: when the symptoms of a miscarriage first occur.

thrombophilias: an abnormality of blood coagulation that increases the risk of blood clots in blood vessels.

thrombosis: the aggregation of platelets and other blood cells to form a clot.

thrombus: a blood clot that is attached to the interior wall of a blood vessel.

thyroid gland: a 20-gram endocrine gland that sits in front of the trachea and consists of two lateral lobes connected in the middle by an isthmus.

thyroiditis: Inflammation of the thyroid gland.

thyroxine: the main hormone produced by the thyroid gland, acting to increase metabolic rate and so regulating growth and development.

tinnitus: ringing in the ear.

Tocolytic agents: drugs that prevent preterm labor by suppressing uterine contractions.

tolerable upper intake level (UL): highest level of nutrient intake that is likely to cause no risk of adverse health effects for most people within a population.

tolerance: a condition in which the same dose achieves a lesser effect, or in which successively greater doses of a substance are required to achieve the same desired effect.

tonic-clonic seizures: also known as grand mal seizures. These produce bilateral, convulsive muscle contractions.

top surgery: refers to breast augmentation ("implants") to create/shape breasts or chest surgery to remove breast tissue and shape chest to pectoral muscles.

torsion: "twisting", as in the case of an ovary twisting around itself and cutting off the blood supply.

total iron-binding capacity (TIBC): a measure of the iron-binding capacity in blood (via transferrin).

tourniquet: a device for stopping the flow of blood through a vein or artery, typically by compressing a limb with a cord or tight bandage.

toxic shock syndrome: an infection normally caused by staphylococci that can develop rapidly into severe untreatable shock, which can be fatal.

toxin: a poisonous substance that is a specific product of the metabolic activities of a living organism and is usually very unstable, notably toxic when introduced into the tissues, and typically capable of inducing antibody formation; counter intuitively, toxins can be used to treat a variety of diseases.

trans fat: also known as trans-unsaturated fatty acids, are a type of unsaturated fat whose carbon-carbon double bonds have hydrogens on opposite faces of the molecule rather than on the same side of the molecule.

trans man: a person born female who has transitioned to male.

trans or transgender: an umbrella term often used to describe those who do not ascribe to a binary means of gender, as it relates to their gender assigned at birth or their cultural norms. Transgender is a self-identified term and some gender nonbinary (i.e. not identifying as "men" or "women") individuals do not use this term.

trans woman: a person born male who has transitioned to female.

transdermal: through the skin; transdermal medications are those which are applied as creams, gels, or patches and are then absorbed through the skin.

transducer (probe): a device designed to transfer ultrasound waves into the body noninvasively, receive the returning echoes, and transform those echoes into electrical voltages.

transfection: a technique used to introduce genes into cells by exposing the cells to fragmented deoxyribonucleic acid (DNA) under conditions that promote the uptake and incorporation of DNA.

transferrin: the primary transport form of iron; transferrin exhibits an inverse relationship to ferritin.

transformation: genetic change in cancer cells which results in loss of growth control and often immortalization.

transgender: adjective to describe a diverse group of individuals who cross or transcend culturally defined categories of gender. The gender identity of transgender people differs to varying degrees from the sex they were assigned at birth.

transgender: an umbrella term for anyone whose sense of gender identity does not correspond to the designation given at birth (gender-variant people); includes transsexual people.

transient ischemic attacks (TIAs): commonly known as mini strokes; associated neurological deficits last less than twenty-four hours and usually only minutes.

transition: the experience of changing genders. Can be social (i.e. asking friends to refer to you with a new pronoun (i.e. he/she/they) or name), medical (taking estrogen or testosterone), and/or surgical (having surgery to change your body to align with how you feel or see yourself).

translocation: an aberration in chromosome structure resulting from the attachment of chromosomal material to a nonhomologous chromosome.

transman; refers to a person assigned female at birth who identifies as a masculine gender identity, male, or a man. People may alternatively use "FTM" (female-to-male) or "man of trans experience" to refer to themselves.

transsexual: one who wishes to assume a sexual identity different from that assigned at birth, or someone who has undergone surgery to change the sexual organs; pertains to sexual characteristics but not necessarily to sexual activities.

transvaginal ultrasound (TVUS): a test used to look at a woman's uterus, ovaries, tubes, cervix and pelvic area; the ultrasound probe is placed inside the vagina.

transvaginal ultrasound: an ultrasound scan obtained via a probe inserted into the vagina; it is used to examine female reproductive organs.

transwoman: a person assigned male at birth who identifies as a feminine gender identity, female or a woman. People may alternatively use "MTF" (male-to-female) or "woman of trans experience" to refer to themselves.

treatment: any specific procedure used for the cure or improvement of a disease or pathological condition.

Treponema pallidum: spirochete bacterium visible only by using dark field illumination.

trichotillomania: excessive hair pulling.

tricyclic antidepressants: antidepressant drugs that interfere with the recycling of several neurotransmitters, particularly norepinephrine and serotonin, making more of them available to the brain, and improving the patient's mood.

trigeminal nerve: the nerve that is responsible for sensation in the face, including light touch, temperature, and pain. When cluster headaches involve this nerve, it creates the sensation of an extremely sharp, "icepick-like", stabbing pain in the eye.

trigeminal pathway: originating from the base of the brain that is activated **during cluster attacks unilateral:** occurring only on one side (for example, on one side of the head or behind one eye).

trimester: any of the three consecutive three-month periods during pregnancy; the first trimester generally refers to weeks zero to twelve of gestation, the second trimester refers to weeks thirteen to twenty-four of gestation, and the third trimester refers to weeks twenty-five to forty-two of gestation.

trisomy 18: a condition caused by an extra chromosome 18 in the cells of the fetus; characterized by mental retardation and other abnormalities, often including severe heart malformations.

trophoblasts: cells forming the outer layer of a blastocyst, which provide nutrients to the embryo and develop into a large part of the placenta.

tropic: hormones that feed a particular physiological state.

tropin: hormones that cause a "turning toward" a particular physiological state.

tropocollagen: a subunit of collagen fibrils consisting of three polypeptide strands arranged in a helix.

trunk: the central part of the body, to which the extremities are attached.

tubal ligation: a permanent form of birth control in which a woman's fallopian tubes are surgically severed or blocked off to prevent pregnancy.

tubal ligation: a surgical procedure to prevent the possibility of pregnancy permanently by blocking the Fallopian tubes, thus preventing eggs from passing into the uterus.

tumor suppressor gene: a gene that, in its normal form, inhibits cell division.

tumor suppressor genes: genes that normally keep cell division in check, orderly, and properly timed; when mutated, they can cause cancer.

tumor: a mass of cells characterized by uncontrolled growth; can be either benign or malignant.

turgor: fullness and firmness; the quality of normal skin in a healthy young person.

turgor: the state of turgidity and resulting rigidity of cells or tissues, typically due to the absorption of fluid.

type A behavior: a psychological behavior classification for individuals who exhibit stressful, time-conscious lifestyles.

type B behavior: a psychological behavior classification for individuals who exhibit unstressed, relaxed lifestyles.

ulcerative colitis: an inflammatory disease that causes superficial ulcers in the colon and rectum.

ulnar: on the lateral side (or little finger side) of the arm, forearm, and hand; the same side that contains the ulna.

ultrasonic: referring to any frequency of sound that is higher than the audible range-that is, higher than 20,000 cycles per second (20 kilohertz).

ultrasonography (ultrasound): the use of sound waves, directed at the body, to create visual images of the tissues being examined.

ultrasonography: an imaging modality in which sound waves penetrate bodily tissues in order to generate an image; in obstetrics, this technique is commonly used to assess the fetus, amniotic fluid, and uterus and ovaries.

ultrasound: a non-invasive, diagnostic imaging modality that uses high-frequency sound waves to produce images that are interpreted by a physician; does not result in radiation exposure as in the case of X-ray or computed tomography (CT).

ultraviolet light: invisible light composed of waves that are shorter than the ordinary light waves able to be seen by humans.

umbilicus: the cord that contains the blood vessels connecting the fetus to the placenta.

undifferentiated patient population: patients seen by family physicians regardless of age, sex, or type of problem.

unipolar depression: a term used by professionals to indicate that a person has the condition of depression with no evidence of having experienced a manic or hypomanic episode.

unipolar mania: a very rare condition in which a person experiences periods of mania but has no experience of depression; is not caused by another disorder or condition.

upper extremities: the arm, forearm, and hand.

urea: the major waste product produced in the kidneys that, when gathered in sufficient quantity and liquefied, flows into the bladder for elimination as urine.

ureters: the two tubes that carry urine from the kidneys to the bladder.

urethra: the tube that drains the bladder; the urethra opens in front of the vagina but does not have a reproductive function.

urethritis: inflammation and infection of the urinary tract.

urinary bladder: the muscular organ that stores urine to be discharged through the urethra.

urinary tract infection: infection involving any organs associated with the urinary system.

urinary tract: the organs of the body that produce, store, and discharge urine; these organs include the kidneys, ureters, bladder, and urethra.

urogenital development: early development of the urinary system and genitals.

uropathy: any disease of the urinary tract.

urothelial: pertaining to a layer of cells that line the bladder and some other organs of the urinary system.

uterine fibroid embolization (UFE): embolization procedure to stop blood supply for uterine fibroids (benign tumors in the uterus).

uterine fibroid: benign smooth muscle tumors of the uterus.

Uterine rupture: tearing of the uterus, typically during labor.

uterus: a hollow, muscular organ located in the pelvic cavity of females, in which a fertilized egg develops.

uvulopalatopharyngoplasty: surgical removal of excess soft tissue including the tonsils in the back of the mouth.

uvulopalatoplasty: procedure in which a laser is used to remove parts or all of the uvula.

vacuum: a device with a suction cup that is applied to the fetal head through the vagina to assist in delivery of the infant.

vagina: the muscular tube leading from the external genitals to the cervix of the uterus.

vaginal birth: a birth in which the child is pushed out of the mother's uterus via the vagina, as opposed to being delivered surgically.

vaginitis: inflammation and infection of the vagina.

vaginoplasty: the surgical construction of a vagina & vulva (clitoris, labia minora, majora, female urethral location).

varicocele: the condition in which the varicose vein of the scrotum enlarges and causes extreme pain; this condition is also associated with infertility.

vas deferens: the tubes in the male reproductive system that carry sperm.

vasectomy: a surgical procedure for preventing sperm from being released during ejaculation; involves the removal of a portion of the vas deferens.

vasoconstrictive: the narrowing of the blood vessels resulting from contraction of the muscular wall of the vessels.

vellus: short, fine, unpigmented hair that covers most of the person's body from childhood.

ventral: toward the belly surface.

ventricles: the chambers in the right and left bottom portions of the heart that receive blood from the atria and pump it to the arteries.

vertebra (pl. vertebrae): the individual bones that are stacked upon one another to form the vertebral column, or spine.

vesicle: also called a blister; a collection of fluid under the epidermis, or topmost layer of the skin.

vestibular: the inner ear, vision, and nervous systems responsible for balance.

viability: the point at which a fetus is able to survive outside the uterus.

viral load: a measurement of the amount of HIV present in the blood; often used to monitor the effectiveness of anti-HIV therapy.

virus: a noncellular particle of protein and nucleic acid; viruses, which can reproduce only inside cells, usually cause damage to their hosts by killing the cells they enter.

vitamins: a group of organic compounds essential for normal growth and nutrition that cannot be synthesized by the body, and are required in small quantities in the diet.

vitreous fluid: the clear, watery liquid in the center of the eyeball.

voiding: the discharging of waste matter from the body.

wasting: severe weight loss characterized by the loss of muscle tissue and body fat deposits.

Wernicke-Korsakoff syndrome: a brain disorder caused by thiamine deficiencies, but since alcohol use disorder causes malabsorption of thiamine, this condition is a long-term consequence of it. Symptoms include confusion, loss of muscular coordination (ataxia), leg tremors, vision changes, memory loss, hallucinations and psychosis.

wheal: a small swelling in the skin.

WHI: Women's Health Initiative, a large, double-blind, placebo-controlled trial involving 27,000 healthy postmenopausal women.

whitlow: a herpes infection on the finger; it is found commonly in health care workers who must put their fingers into others' mouths and can occur even with the use of protective gloves.

withdrawal: a physical and mental condition following decreased intake of an abusable substance, with symptoms ranging from anxiety to convulsions and seizures.

Wolffian ducts: the pair of tubes in the early embryo that will develop into the internal male organs (the epididymis, vas deferens, and seminal vesicles).

WPATH: World Professional Association for Transgender Health.

X and Y chromosomes: the chromosomes that determine genetic sex; females carry an XX pair, and males carry an XY pair.

xenograft: a transplanted tissue or organ obtained from a member of a species different from that of the recipient.

yolk sac: a membrane outside the human embryo that is connected by a tube (the yolk stalk) though the umbilical opening to the embryo's midgut; an early site for the formation of blood and is eventually enveloped by the embryo's primitive gut.

zygote: the single cell formed after fertilization that is the result of the fusion of egg and sperm; it can develop into a new individual organism.

INDEXES

Category Index

Subject Index